Breaking the Adolescent Parent Cycle

Valuing Fatherhood and Motherhood

Jack C. Westman

UNIVERSITY PRESS OF AMERICA,® INC.

Lanham • Boulder • New York • Toronto • Plymouth, UK

University Press of America,® Inc.
4501 Forbes Boulevard
Suite 200
Lanham, Maryland 20706
UPA Acquisitions Department (301) 459-3366

Estover Road
Plymouth PL6 7PY
United Kingdom

Library of Congress Control Number: 2009924130
ISBN: 978-0-7618-4536-2 (paperback : alk. paper)
eISBN: 978-0-7618-4537-9

Dedicated to our grandchildren
and to their generation:

Matthew, Laura, Carly,
Peter, Megan, Eric,
Luke, Clay and Alexander

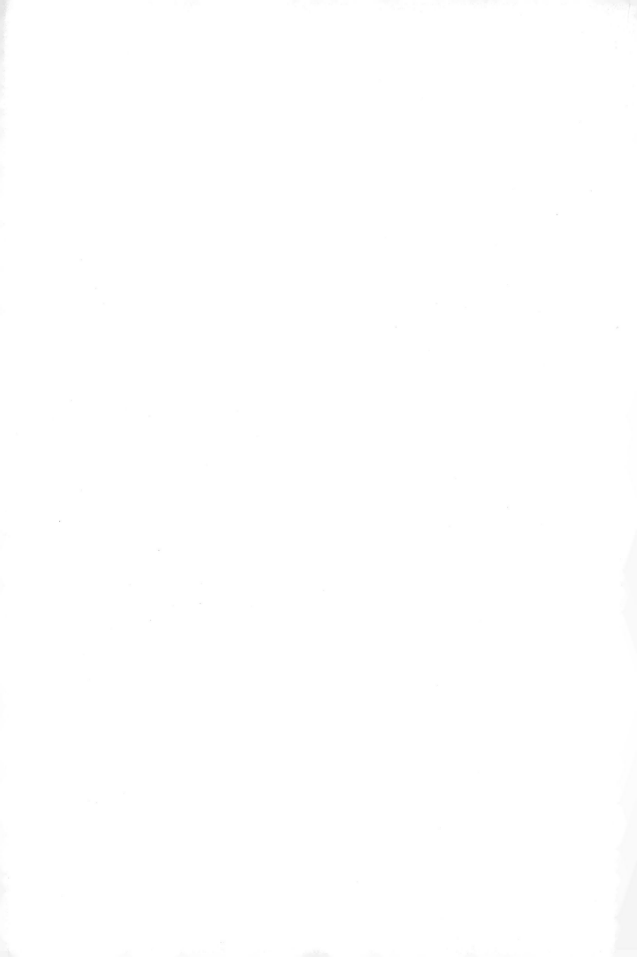

Contents

Preface

Our personal experiences as adolescents are relevant for readers of this book. Each one of us had a unique experience during this formative stage of life. For me, reading Sigmund Freud's *Introductory Lectures to Psychoanalysis* as an adolescent revealed that human motives are not always what they seem to be. Discovering hidden motives behind the façades of adult behavior appealed to me. This curiosity led me to become a psychiatrist.

In order to understand the behavior of individuals, I need information ranging from molecules to environments. In order to understand the behavior of individuals in groups, I need information about families, societies and cultures. The living system and chaos/complexity theories help me make sense out of all of this information.

Over forty-five years of clinical practice and research, I participated in the lives of many poor and affluent young people and their families. My interest is in connecting systems that influence them and their families—childcare, schools, neighborhoods, communities, health and mental health care, social services, law enforcement, courts and corrections. I was inspired to write this book by the growing strain on these systems created by the intractable cycle of adolescent parents—the most preventable cause of crime and welfare dependency.

My book *Child Advocacy* played a role in the child advocacy movement in the 1980s. I developed the child advocacy team that brought an interdisciplinary focus on the family into courts. Similarly formed coordinated service and wraparound teams now integrate public and private services for families in many communities across the nation.

I learned that "child advocacy" actually diverted attention from the more important need for "family advocacy." I began to refer to myself as a family psychiatrist and joined the parent licensing movement in 1990s. That brought both positive and negative attention. I found that the word "family" is controversial and needs clarification. I decided to focus on public policies to strengthen "childrearing families."

All too often the words we use derail thoughtful dialog. Difficulty in finding the most appropriate language contributes to the lack of objective thinking about adolescent pregnancy and parenthood. It reflects the inherent ambiguity of adolescence as the "child-adult" stage of life. Referring to adolescent girls and boys as "women" and "men" ignores adolescence as a vital developmental stage in life. Any words used to refer to minority groups can evoke positive and negative stereotypes.

The words used in this book inevitably will evoke negative associations, especially "adolescence" and "adoption." Adolescents may prefer to be referred to as "teenagers," "teens," "kids" or "youth" because "adolescence" connotes immaturity when they are trying to be mature. "Adoption" can evoke images of taking babies away from their mothers.

Legal adulthood also complicates thinking about adolescence. Two-thirds of all adolescent mothers are eighteen and nineteen. They are at a different stage of adolescent development than those under eighteen. Although still adolescents, they are considered legal adults in most respects in our society. To further complicate matters, the term "woman" often is used to refer to a pregnant minor. Even "adolescent pregnancy" takes the focus off the male contributor. In a broader sense, "sexually active" has replaced "promiscuous"; "affair" has replaced "adultery"; and "hooking up" has replaced "dating."

This book approaches cultural differences by referring to minorities, particularly those who live in poverty, as Asians, American Indians, Blacks, Hmong, Latinos and Muslims. Referring to the nation's second largest minority group as colored, African-American, Negro, black or Black is an especially sensitive issue, although each of these terms have been used by Black luminaries.[1]

The term "white" is even more confusing because it covers a wide variety of backgrounds and is gradually being overshadowed by the "browning" of America. Lower case "black" and "white" often is used to de-emphasize racial backgrounds consistent with an effort to minimize racial differences between people. As did Beverly Tatum in her book *Why Are All the Black Kids Sitting Together in the Cafeteria*, I capitalize "Black" and "White" to follow the capitalization of "African-American" and the names of other ethnic groups and to acknowledge the fact that ethnic background is important.[2]

"Latino" is preferred over "Hispanic" by Latin America activists.[3] For them, Latino describes their cultures better than the language they speak.

The term "American Indian" is ambiguous. It and "Native American" encompass all indigenous Indians on the American Continent but refer to Indians in the United States and Alaska, where the latter also may be referred to as Native Alaskans.

Ethnicity does matter. For the sake of consistency, I capitalize ethnicity in the United States as American Indian, Asian, Black, Hmong, Latino, Muslim and White. There may come a time when ethnicity no longer matters, but we are not there yet.

It is easy to overlook the importance of brain development in adolescents who appear to be young adults. Consequently, I refer to "teenagers," "teens" and "youth" as "adolescents" and as "girls" and "boys." I also refer to "infants" as "babies" to acknowledge the nurturing feelings they evoke. Referring to "babies" as "infants" makes it possible to deal with them as objects rather than as human beings.

All of these words used to describe people still can be misinterpreted because of the sensitive nature of the topics addressed in this book. For this, I ask the reader's indulgence.

I cite research in the social sciences recognizing that their methodologies cannot achieve the validity and reliability of research in the physical sciences. At the same time, I know that all physical and social science research is subject to bias. I acknowledge my bias in favor of the interests of babies, girls, boys and parents committed to the career of parenthood.

I hope that sharing my perspective will highlight the vital role of parenthood in our society and help to bring adolescent parenthood into public awareness as a public health crisis that can be resolved.

Jack Westman
Madison, Wisconsin

Acknowledgments

Without the encouragement and editorial assistance of my wife and life companion, Nancy Baehre Westman, I could not have written this book. Without the experience of raising three sons, growing to love three daughters-in-law and participating in the growth of nine grandchildren, I would not know the rewards and vicissitudes of family life firsthand.

My work with child and family related systems over the years introduced me to professionals from a variety of disciplines who retired when I did. I am deeply indebted to Norma Berkowitz, Paul Brandl, Glen Cain, Jack DeWitt, Tom Corbett, Ethel Dunn, Marty Fliegel, Vern Haubrich, Jim Hickman, Margo Melli, Frank Newgent, David Nordstrom, Florian Smoczynski, Bob Sundby and Sherwood Zink. Through the nonprofit organization Wisconsin Cares, Inc., we are devoted to stimulating awareness of how struggling families affect their members, their communities and society and to strengthening those families, many of which began with adolescent parents.

I want to thank the following persons for their comments and cooperation on aspects of this book: Jacqueline Allen, Francene Ambrose, Teresa Arnold, Laila Al-Narayati, James Bates, Eli Berger, Jerry Bread, Valin Brown, Kenneth Bryson, Paula Callahan, Shannon Carstens, Ronald Chance, Meda Chesney-Lind, Terry Cross, Paul Devantier, Denis Donovan, Van Dougherty, Sydney Duncan, James Dwyer, Lisa Edwards, Julie Felhoelter, Denise Gordon, Kirk Greenway, Martin Guggenheim, John Hagedorn, Beth Hall, Hilari Hauptman, Anne Hardenbergh, Steven Hartley, Saul Hoffman, Andrea Kane, Barbara Kates, Jacqueline Williams Kaye, Tammy Gillespie, Kirk Greenway, Ann Kirwan, Julie Keown-Bomar, Dale Langer, Tamarah LeMay, Gordon Limb, Michael Males, Janice Matthews, Rebecca May, Rebecca Maynard, Sara McLanahan, Jody Miller, Joan Moore, Kirstin Moore, Paul Nadasdy, Larry Nesper, Carolyn Newberger, Jeannine Nielsen, Rigel Oliveri, Sandra Opdycke, Patricia Owens, Patricia Paluzzi, Peter Pai, Adam Pertman, James Pierce, Timothy Potter, Karen Pridham, Sally Pope, Patricia Quinn, Leslie Raneri, Mary Roach, Azara Santiago-Rivera, Roccco Scalzi, Mary Shanley, Helena Silverstein, Stephen Small, Vincent Smeriglio, Donald Malcolm Smith, Lee SmithBattle, Jennifer Souders, Scott Spear, Catherine Stevens-Simon, Michele Stockwell, Mary Beth Styles, Bret Vlach, Beth

Wachter, Michael Wallace, Catherine Webb, Dianne Weber, Kathy Webster, Daniel Westman, Eric Westman, John Westman, Barbara Woodhouse, Claire Wyneken, Phelan Wyrick, Michael Yellow Bird and Franklin Zimring.

As one accustomed to decades of hands-on library research of books and journals, I am in awe of the accessibility the internet provides to the literature. The extensive bibliography in this book would not have been possible without it.

I am most grateful to all of the persons who have permitted me to share their lives in clinical settings. Where I specifically refer to an individual or family, I have altered names and identifying circumstances to protect their privacy. When information about persons is in the public domain, I have used actual names, situations and places.

Introduction

Question*: What would our nation be like if parenthood was valued as much as paid work and if every child had a competent parent?*

Answer*: We would see dramatic reductions in our social problems and dramatic improvements in personal well-being.*

Question*: Can we really do this?*

Answer*: Yes.*

WHY SHOULD YOU READ THIS BOOK?

Every four minutes a minor gives birth to a baby. Each year over 6,000 are 14 and younger. These births create dilemmas for the adolescents, their babies, their families and our society. I will describe the issues, identify the causes and outline possible solutions for this preventable source of our social problems.

If you believe all babies should have a chance to become productive citizens, you will see how ensuring that all babies have competent parents will achieve this goal. If a baby grows up to be a productive citizen, we all benefit. If a baby grows up to be a criminal or welfare dependent, we all pay for the consequences.

If you believe little can be done to solve our social problems, you will find that solutions are within our reach if we recognize that parenthood entails more than simply being a parent. If you are concerned about the increasing costs of government, you will see how valuing parenthood as a life-long career will reduce our taxes.

We all have a stake in ensuring that children have competent parents. Each child they raise contributes $1.2 million to our economy. Regardless of social class, each child neglected and abused by an incompetent parent costs our economy $2.4 million. If every child had a competent parent, we would reduce our total state expenditures by at least a quarter and our county expenditures by almost one half. We would reap the profound humanitarian benefits of people living productive lives.

The focus of this book is on adolescent parenthood because it is the most obvious and common rebuttal of the belief that genetic parents are inherently capable of assuming the custodial guardianship of another human being – of being competent parents.

Babies born to adolescent parents have one, two or three strikes against them. The first strike is having immature parents and no legal custodial guardian. The second strike is being born handicapped by prematurity or prenatal drug or alcohol abuse. The third strike is being neglected or abused, or both.

Even though adolescent childbirth was declining in the United States because of contraception and pregnancy termination, concern about adolescent childbearing began in 1976 with the publication of *Eleven Million Teenagers: What Can Be Done about the Epidemic of Adolescent Pregnancy in the United States* by the Alan Guttmacher Institute. Later President Clinton "declared war" on adolescent pregnancy in 1995.

My work with neglected and abused children and their families convinces me that we can dramatically reduce crime and welfare dependency by ensuring that every baby has a competent parent. We use science and technology to improve our personal comfort and abilities. We can use child development science and technology to improve the quality of our lives and of our society as well.

Over the last century, we *already have* applied our knowledge about child development. Child labor, education, abuse and neglect and immunization laws protect older children. We are focusing on early childhood to prepare children for school. Now we can apply our knowledge about competent parents *before birth* to ensure that every child has a healthy start in life.

Compelling scientific evidence now permits defining competent parents as:

• capable of assuming responsibility for their own lives;
• capable of providing food, shelter and clothing for their children;
• capable of arranging for health care and education for their children;
• willing to sacrifice some of their own interests for their children;
• able to provide limits for their children's behavior; and
• able to offer their children hope for their futures.

Competent parents need financial, educational and community resources in order to do these things.

How can we ensure that every child has a competent parent when the capacity to procreate precedes parental competence and when many parents do not have the financial and educational resources they need to raise their children? These questions make ensuring that every child has a competent parent seem like an overwhelming task. But it really is not if we would place a high priority on fulfilling the basic civil right of children to have competent parents.

An idealistic vision? Yes, if we really are not serious about improving our society. No, if we align our existing resources to make this vision come true. That it can be done is demonstrated by other societies in which child neglect and abuse and their most preventable cause—adolescent parents—are far below the levels in the United States. And we are reducing child neglect and abuse now in many of our communities.

The sense of helplessness created by adolescent parents calls for thoughtful consideration of all of the causes of adolescent parenthood and the barriers to constructive action. As the following pages reveal, we have the knowledge and resources to resolve the problem but lack the vision and the will to apply them.

Part 1 analyzes the consequences of the growing discrepancy between the family wealth that has created two sets of young people—those with educated, affluent parents living in safe neighborhoods and those with less educated, poor parents living in dangerous neighborhoods. It also outlines the demographics of adolescent pregnancy and childbirth.

Our failure to recognize and value parenthood as essential for the prosperity of our society is reflected in the variety of parenting styles that result from the materialistic values of the marketplace. The fragmentation, discontinuity and resulting ineffectiveness of our social service, educational and correctional systems impede effective and efficient responses to our social problems.

Part 2 sets the stage for understanding and dealing with incompetent parents by using chaos/complexity theory to organize the evolving "big picture" essential for understanding how to ensure that children have competent parents. It places the moral and legal rights of adolescents and parents in perspective.

The traditional legal view of babies as the property of their genetic parents presumes that parents are competent until they are found unfit by a court. This presumption ignores the fact that millions of parents are not competent when their babies are born. It has resulted in overwhelmed child protection services that are unable to intervene until children have been damaged by neglect or abuse.

Part 3 examines the developmental needs of young people and the influences that amplify or dampen the natural drift of their lives toward chaos. Human beings are complicated self-organizing systems in which nature and nurture interact through the anchoring process of attachment bonding. Both childhood and parenthood are developmental stages in life.

One of the most obvious reasons for the adolescent parenthood dilemma is the nature of adolescence itself. Adolescents are children becoming adults and vary widely in maturity. Adolescence has three phases reflecting development of the brain that continues into emerging adulthood:

- early from puberty through 13;
- middle from 14 through 17;
- late from 18 through 21; and
- emerging adulthood from 21 through 24.

Part 4 describes the initial conditions that set the stage for adolescent childbirth and the swirl of events and patterns that ultimately directly and indirectly affect our entire society. The short-term and long-term effects are most keenly felt by the adolescents themselves and by their children.

Powerful forces support adolescent parenthood, both as a life style to be sought and as a life style to be supported. Adolescents hear they are not mature enough to be mothers and fathers, but, when they become parents, they are presumed to be capable of entering parenthood with support. The status accorded by this support contributes to continuing the cycle of adolescent childbirth and its consequences.

Part 5 deals with the initial family circumstances that directly influence adolescent childbirth and with the later impact of those births on relatives. The families of adolescent parents play crucial roles in decisions their daughters and sons make to become parents. They also play active roles in second and even third generation childrearing.

There is a tendency to avoid dealing with adolescent problems because of the belief they will be outgrown, even though adolescence extends for years. When girls are pregnant, professionals often are reluctant to become involved in counseling them and their families because they lack professional and public support for doing so.

Part 6 illustrates the roles peers, neighborhoods, gangs and communities play in adolescents becoming parents and in amplifying and dampening the problems that emerge in the lives of all of those affected.

The causes of adolescent parenthood are disputed. Are they genetic, personality, morality, fertility, societal, cultural or economic? Social class is the most important correlate of adolescent parenthood and of child neglect and abuse. Some advocates highlight childbirth as a rational choice for adolescents living in poverty. They believe that delaying parenthood would not improve their already disadvantaged lives.

Part 7 reviews the cultural factors that dampen or amplify the degree of adversity in adolescent parents' lives. The goals of adolescence are the same in all cultures—to prepare young people for responsible roles in their society. However, some subcultural pressures in the United States encourage rather than discourage adolescent parenthood.

Our Black, Latino, American Indian, Hmong and Muslim subcultures have traditions and values that are relevant in research and in counseling related to adolescent parents. The possibility of privileged classes exercising a eugenic bias against disadvantaged classes is considered.

Part 8 reveals that parenthood no longer is a strictly private matter. Our society both absorbs the consequences of incompetent parents and plays a role in amplifying or dampening the problems they create.

Programs intended to promote the aspirations and maturity of adolescent parents have disappointing results because adolescent parents often are multiply disadvantaged. In addition, the varieties of resources they need are not effectively coordinated, are of low quality or have requirements that adolescents do not meet. Still, there are positive trends that can be amplified to the benefit of all concerned.

Part 9 suggests that if our society appropriately valued parenthood and responded to adolescent childbirth as a public health crisis, we would do everything we could to insure that every baby has a competent parent and that every adolescent has an opportunity to become a productive citizen.

Parenthood Planning Teams composed of existing family planning, prenatal care, child protective service, home visitation and legal professionals could be organized in the same way crisis intervention teams are formed in other health and child welfare matters. When adolescents and dependent adults choose parenthood, a legal procedure is needed to ensure that their babies have competent custodial guardians. This can be done by expanding the birth certificate to become a parenthood certificate.

When an adolescent's or dependent adult's baby is born, three feasible outcomes are proposed after all parties have carefully considered the options and their long-range consequences:

- relatives continue guardianship of the minor parent or legally dependent adult, assume temporary guardianship of the baby and assist the minor or dependent parent in childrearing;
- a voluntary adoption plan is made for the baby; and
- an involuntary termination of parental rights and adoption of the baby occurs when relatives cannot function as custodial guardians of the minor or dependent adult parent and baby.

Part 10 concludes that if all young people had competent parents who were able to provide the nurturance, housing, education and health care they need to grow up with skills and hope for the future, adolescent parents would no longer be a public issue.

Reducing adolescent parenthood has immediate and long-term effects on poverty. It removes the public costs of caring for and educating adolescent parents and raising additional disadvantaged children now. It enables adolescents to concentrate on their careers and become self-sufficient. It reduces poverty in the future by breaking the adolescent parent cycle.

We need to recognize parenthood as a life-long career and as the foundation of our society for which minimum standards are required. My hope is that the holistic perspective of this book will inspire interest in doing so.

Prolog

GOOD INTENTIONS[1]

Lillie, 14 and pregnant, needed a mom. Amy, 37 and already raising a big family, gave her a home. Neither was ready for what happened next.

It was just before midnight on Saturday, Jan. 14. Amy Chandler, a sonogram tech at Tampa General, had been sent to the emergency room to examine a young patient. The girl was six months pregnant and suffering from complications. She was biting her lip, trying not to cry.

Amy stroked the girl's forehead.

"Maybe it would help if I got your mom."

The girl looked up at Amy.

"I don't have a mom," she said. "Do you want to adopt me? Me and my baby?"

She said her name was Lillie. She was 14.

Amy and her husband, Mike, had five kids, ages 1 to 11. They had always wanted a big family and had decided early on they wouldn't put their kids in day care. So Amy worked nights at the hospital, and Mike worked days at a cement plant. It was a hectic schedule, but for years they had made it work.

Waking up that night, Mike noticed Amy's eyes were swollen. He saw something in her face, a mixture of sorrow and hope. Mike had seen that look before.

"I met this girl today . . . ," Amy began.

On the computer, she called up the Heart Gallery, a Web site filled with photos of foster children who want to be adopted. Lillie had told her to look for her picture there.

"I want you to see something," Amy told her husband.

Mike saw Lillie's freckled face, her forced smile. The Web site had an audio link. Amy turned it up.

"Hi, my name is Lillie." The voice was high-pitched, with a twang. "I'm sweet, smart. I'm a nice person in general. I love to sing, I love to dance to country music. . . . And I'm pregnant. I'm having a little boy. I'm kind of nervous. . . . I just want someone to be by me, and to believe in me."

In the glow of the computer, Amy saw Mike's cheeks shining. She wrapped her arms around him.

"You feel it too," she said.

Mike stroked his wife's hair.

"Let's see what we can do," he said.

That was all Amy needed to hear.

Lillie's case manager had warned her not to be too hopeful. It was hard enough to find a home for a 14-year-old girl, much less one with a baby. But if Lillie stayed in foster care, she knew the state would take her baby away. He'd end up lost in the system's maze, without a mother. Just like her.

For most of her life, Lillie had been raised in a tangle of bureaucracy, with an army of caseworkers and therapists and court-appointed lawyers looking after her. Lillie didn't want that life for her son. She wanted the two of them to have a real home, together. So that night at Tampa General, when she met Amy during the sonogram, Lillie asked for help. She didn't know anything about the woman or her house or kids. Amy had seemed kind. She had held Lillie's hand. It was enough.

Amy and Mike were gambling, too. They didn't know anything about Lillie, her background, the realities of the foster care system. All they saw was a girl who had grown up without a mother and was about to become a mother herself.

The Chandlers' friends told them they were crazy. With five kids of their own, why would they want to take on two more?

Because they need us, Amy kept saying.

Good intentions were all they had.

That Monday, after checking with adoption counselors, Amy learned she and Mike could be approved as foster parents quickly, without the usual classes and training, because this was considered an emergency case. Lillie was sleeping in a shelter with pregnant women and new moms. She needed a more permanent home.

Foster workers couldn't believe Lillie had found one. To them, the Chandlers seemed a godsend. As in other emergency placements, the workers waived the waiting period, expedited the court date and broke down the barriers.

Amy and Mike didn't worry about how a teenage daughter and her infant son would change their family. They told their kids they were lucky to be able to help. They didn't think about the money they would spend, the adjustments they'd all have to make.

The next day, three days after Amy met Lillie, the phone rang. Lillie was calling from the hospital. She'd had her baby almost three months prematurely. Thomas weighed 3 pounds, 9 ounces.

A few weeks later, Lillie sat at the shelter, waiting for Brenda Young, her caseworker from Camelot Community Care, to drive her to the Tampa courthouse. If the judge agreed, Lillie could go home with her new family that day.

"I can't wait to go home," Lillie said. "I don't want to stay here no more."

She still hadn't met Mike, or the couple's five kids.

Thomas, a month old now, was still in the hospital, tethered to a breathing monitor. He had sleep apnea and needed constant doses of iron. The hospital was ready to discharge him, but only when all the details were finalized with the Chandlers.

Sometimes during those first few weeks, when Lillie could beg a ride from the shelter to the hospital, she would hold Thomas, practice being a mom. Diapers and bottles were hard enough. She also had to learn to check his monitor, remember to give him medicine. Some of the nurses told Lillie she should give Thomas up for adoption.

"I'm keeping him," she remembered telling them. "My new mama's gonna help me."

At the courthouse, Amy rode the elevator to the second floor. When the doors opened, she saw Lillie sprinting toward her, arms outstretched.

"Mama! Mama!"

Amy hugged Lillie, kissed her cheek. "Did you pack everything? Are you nervous?"

Lillie nodded yes, then no. The two of them walked arm-in-arm. Amy explained that if the judge granted her and Mike temporary custody of Thomas, they could take him home from the hospital that day.

On a bench outside the courtroom, sitting with her caseworker and Amy, Lillie volunteered the scattered details of her life.

"We lived in a nasty trailer. Daddy was always drunk or passed out. Mama, she can't read or cook or nothing. We'd go to the neighbors and beg food."

Her dad's friend molested her when she was 5, she said. That same year, her dad went to prison—"for something with a gun."

Lillie said she had three older sisters and a big brother, and they'd all been raised in foster care. Lillie had lost track of them. In nine years, she had moved 10 times. The last place she had been was a group home. She had hated it, she told Amy, so she ran away. She had lived on the streets, on and off, for more than a year.

"I was 12 years old, doing crack, prostituting to pay for it."

Amy listened, trying not to look shocked. Lillie's caseworker winced and shook her head.

Lillie wasn't proud of her past. But she wasn't ashamed. She had made a lot of money, she said, sometimes having sex with 10 men in a day.

"The court's trying to find my baby's daddy right now," she told Amy. "But I don't even know who he is. I was so high all the time, I didn't even know I was pregnant till I got arrested."

That was two months ago, she said. Her friend had stolen a car, they had gone joy-riding and crashed into a fence. At the jail, she had found out she was five months pregnant.

"I'm glad now, though," Lillie said, beaming. "If I didn't have a baby, I wouldn't never have been adopted."

Amy didn't answer. What was she getting herself into?

"I'm so happy he actually did it," the caseworker told Amy, coming out of court. Then she handed Lillie's paperwork to Amy and said, "She's all yours." The caseworker explained that Lillie did not have to give up her parental rights to Thomas. If she wanted to keep her son, she would have to finish a parenting class and a drug education class, go back to school and promise not to contact friends from her former life. She was still on probation for a stolen car.

For now, the judge had ruled, Lillie couldn't be left alone with her baby. But he was allowing Lillie and Thomas to go home that day with the Chandlers.

"I'm a happy little kid today!" Lillie bubbled.

Her court-appointed attorney scowled at her.

"You just remember how you feel right now," said Norman Palumbo, Jr. "When you get mad, when you want to run again, just remember this chance you got. You won't get another one like this."

Lillie's new life started in Amy's van. From the courthouse to the shelter to pick up Lillie's bags. From the shelter to the hospital to gather Thomas and his breathing monitor and his medicine and diapers. From the hospital to the drive-through at Taco Bell for a chicken quesadilla, so Lillie's stomach would stop growling. Then, finally, home.

That evening, while everyone else ate dinner, Lillie unpacked. She'd never had her own room. She couldn't wait to settle in.

"Time for bed!" Amy called at 9:30.

Lillie looked surprised. It had been years since anyone had told her to go to bed.

That night, Thomas' breathing monitor went off seven times. Lillie slept through it. Amy got up every hour.

The first few days were a blur. Amy and Mike would get up at dawn, change three diapers. Then they'd fix breakfast, pack lunches, get all seven kids dressed and load the van. Their boys kept getting tardy slips at school.

While Mike was at work, Amy's days were spent driving Thomas to the pediatrician, signing Lillie up for her drug education and parenting classes, meeting with Lillie's probation officer. Everywhere Amy went, she had to haul four kids under age 6.

Amy was getting only four hours of sleep after her night shifts at the hospital. And Thomas' monitor kept going off. Amy would have to get up, make sure Lillie's baby was still breathing. Lillie never wanted to go to bed. Long after midnight, she would lie awake, watching TV. She was trying to get used to being part of a family, but she didn't know how. She felt that all these other people were constantly hassling her with chores, expectations, rules. She wasn't allowed to eat whenever she was hungry; Amy made her eat when everyone else ate, at the table instead of in her room. And she made her have a meal, not just Doritos. It was strange to be back in school, too. Amy had enrolled Lillie in a school for girls with special needs. Lillie should have been in ninth grade. But she had missed so many semesters, she had to start over in sixth.

"I want to go to college," Lillie told Amy. "I want to go to Harvard to be a social worker—either that or I want to do nails or something."

Lillie wanted so many things. She had never had anything before, so she figured she had nothing to lose by asking. Everywhere Amy took her, Lillie begged for clothes, DVDs, stuffed animals. She never said thank you. She wanted to get her nose pierced, wear short skirts and high heels, go on dates. Amy wouldn't let her. Lillie kept saying she was bored.

One night, a week after Lillie moved in, she crept into the hall and got the cordless phone. The other kids were asleep. Amy was at work. Mike was changing Thomas in his room. Lillie dialed a number she knew by heart. After Mike had gone to bed, headlights appeared in the driveway. Lillie tiptoed to the front door, crossed the yard, opened the gate. She threw her arms around the man in the truck. His name was Julio. He was 23. Lillie had stayed with him on the street.

Hours later, Lillie called Amy at work.

"Mommy," she said. "I did something bad."

Amy hadn't even known Lillie had a boyfriend. She certainly didn't want some 23-year-old who had lived on the streets coming over to her house in the middle of the night. But she and Mike weren't sure how to punish Lillie. Yes, she had violated their rules and her probation. But she had apologized. They didn't want to be too strict. What if she got upset and ran away?

The foster care system wasn't much help. Because this had been an emergency placement, Mike and Amy had taken no classes, received no training. The Chandlers were relying on experience. But nothing in their experience had prepared them to take care of a child with Lillie's sad history. In the end, Amy talked to Lillie about trust and made her promise she'd never call that man again. Amy disconnected the kids' phone line, just in case.

One morning, Lillie climbed into bed with Amy. "I want to show you my diary," she said. She leaned against Amy's shoulder so they could read together.

Dear Diary, the neat print began. Every day now is hard for me. She loved Thomas, she wrote. But with a job and school, she couldn't focus on him. I decided to give him up for adoption to my parents, the Chandlers. She was ready to give up her parental rights, just as her mother had done. Only this was different, Lillie said. Her mom had given her up to the foster care system. Lillie was giving Thomas to a good family. And she'd still be with him. Of course we'll raise Thomas, Amy told Lillie. But she urged her to think it over. Lillie said her mind was made up.

It was a Saturday night, April 1, and Lillie had been with the Chandlers for almost two months. Amy was at work and the little kids were asleep. Mike had gone into his room to change Thomas. Their ten-year-old son Coletin and Lillie were in the living room, watching TV. When Mike returned, Coletin and Lillie were gone. Lillie's door was locked. Mike pounded on it.

"Just a minute," Lillie said. When she finally opened the door, Coletin tumbled out and dashed into his room. Lillie said she had been showing Coletin her secret stash of candy. Coletin told his dad Lillie had wanted to show him something in a movie. In Lillie's room, Mike found a DVD: *Unfaithful*.

When Amy got home at 2 a.m. and heard what had happened, she started shaking. Lillie had asked her to buy *Unfaithful* a few days earlier. Amy had refused. Lillie must have bought it when she was working at the grocery. Before confronting Lillie, Amy skimmed through a few scenes. The R-rated movie was about a married woman having an affair. Watching a man and a woman slapping each other and having sex in a toilet stall, Amy felt sick. Her 10-year-old had seen that?

"What were you thinking?" Amy shouted, entering Lillie's room. "What gives you the right to introduce that world to my son?"

Amy told her she would have to move out.

Lillie, in bed, pulled the comforter over her head.

At 3 a.m., Amy called Brenda Young, Lillie's primary caseworker, and left a frantic message. Then she called the caseworker's boss. She left a third message with the adoptions supervisor for Hillsborough Kids Inc., the agency the state contracts with to manage its foster children. For the rest of the night, Amy paced in the dark, trying to figure out how to get this girl out of their house. She was still up at 8 the next morning, still wearing her hospital scrubs, when Lillie walked into the kitchen in a short dress and platform sandals.

"Aren't we going to church?" Lillie asked, as if nothing had happened.

Amy sat her down. She needed to understand. Why? As Amy would later recall, Lillie told her she missed her freedom, her old life, her boyfriend. The movie had made her feel better.

"But why drag Coletin into it?"

Lillie didn't answer.

The caseworker finally called back—32 hours after the crisis.

"You're telling me it'll take three weeks to get her out of my house?" Amy asked. The system is slow, the caseworker told her. Besides, Amy remembers her saying, you knew Lillie had problems when you took her in. Amy was incredulous. She knew about Lillie's past only because Lillie told her. The caseworker had never talked about Lillie's background, never warned Amy that she was taking a former child prostitute into her house.

"I feel like you all set us up to fail," Amy told the foster worker. "And now, when we need help, you're abandoning us."

Mike called Hillsborough Kids Inc. "We're bringing Lillie back. If you all won't come get her, we'll drop her on your doorstep."

As Amy describes it, the next day went like this: She packed Lillie's belongings while Lillie was at school. When Amy picked her up and Lillie saw the suitcases inside the van, her face crumbled.

"You don't have to do this," Lillie said.

She was sobbing. So was Amy. The other kids were in the van, watching.

When Amy turned into the office of Hillsborough Kids Inc., Lillie told Amy to pick up her paycheck from Winn-Dixie that Friday.

"You have to send me my money," Lillie told her. She narrowed her eyes. "And I'm not going to let you adopt Thomas now."

Amy parked the van. "Don't do that to your baby," she told Lillie. "He'll end up bouncing around in foster care all his life, just like you did. You can come see him with us," Amy said. "You know we love him and will take care of him."

Lillie wasn't listening. She unbuckled Thomas and carried him across the parking lot. She stood outside the office door, kissing and kissing her son. Amy finished unloading the suitcases and reached for Thomas. Lillie cradled him. She glared at Amy, turned her head and finally handed over her baby. She ran into the office building, crying.

A week after Lillie went back to foster care, a caseworker called. They were coming to take Thomas.

"What?" Amy cried. "Why?"

Lillie didn't want her child in Amy's home, the foster worker said. Amy had been allowed to have Thomas only because she had agreed to take Lillie. Now the deal was off. Someone would be there to get Thomas in a half-hour.

"This is the only home that baby's known," Amy told Mike. "What's going to happen to him?"

The caseworkers arrived and took Thomas. On paper, Amy still had custody of the baby. The state had to take that away before foster workers could place him somewhere else. That meant there was still a chance the Chandlers could get Thomas back. Amy started looking for a lawyer. The emergency hearing was the next day.

Lillie was doing well, the assistant attorney general argued. She had gone back to school, gotten a job, enrolled in drug education and parenting classes.

Amy looked at Mike, her eyes wide. All those things they were praising Lillie for, Amy had done for her. Lillie just wanted to sit in her room and watch TV. For the state, Lillie and Thomas had been a package deal. The state's lawyer said the government wasn't sure the Chandlers could care for a child like Lillie, who had a history of abuse and neglect. The Chandlers already have five children of their own in the home, she said. Mike was so angry that he walked out of court. Their attorney noted that the state didn't have a problem with the Chandlers when they had placed Lillie and Thomas with them just two months before.

The judge wanted to know where Lillie and Thomas were staying now. The caseworkers explained that they had been unable to find another family to take them both. They couldn't even find a home for Lillie, they said. She was still in the shelter. Thomas was with a new foster family. In the end, the judge decided it was best to keep Thomas where he was, rather than move him again. After the hearing, Amy and Mike met the new foster dad and gave him the crib, the swing, the baby clothes—everything they'd bought for Thomas.

A month after Thomas was taken from the Chandlers, he is still living with his new foster family. His new foster dad says the breathing monitor isn't going off as much. Thomas is gaining weight, starting to smile. Lillie has vanished. She stayed at the shelter for three weeks, waiting for another family to take her. On April 23, she ran away.

Jeff Rainey, CEO of Hillsborough Kids Inc., said that by law he cannot discuss any child's specific case. Speaking generally, he said it is always hard to find appropriate homes for foster teenagers, many of whom have troubled pasts.

"This is a no eject, no reject situation," he said. "We have to take all of these kids, and we have to do our best with them. Does everything work out the way it should or the way we would like it to? No, not always.'"

Part 1

THE PROBLEM

*Each of our children represents either a potential addition to the productive capac-
ity and the enlightened citizenship of our nation, or, if allowed to suffer from neglect, a potential addition to the destructive forces of the community.*

Theodore Roosevelt
Special Message to Congress, 1909[1]

This section explains why I wrote this book. Although most are doing well, too many
of our young people are not. The growing discrepancy between the wealth of families
has created two sets of young people—those with educated, affluent parents living in
safe neighborhoods and those with less educated, poor parents living in dangerous
neighborhoods. The consequences of this discrepancy affect us all.

Disruptive behavior has increased in schools necessitating the presence of police.
Academic performance levels have deteriorated. Many students are unprepared for
college and drop out. A growing number of adolescents are uncontrollable and unreachable because they never learned how to empathize with other persons.

We are beginning to improve the quality of our *physically toxic environments*, but
we lag far behind in recognizing, understanding and reversing our *socially toxic
environments*.

Most importantly, anyone past puberty can be a parent in our nation. But being a
parent says nothing about childrearing competence. Having competent parents means
everything to babies, children and adolescents.

This book focuses on adolescent parents because they are the most common examples of dependent parents who require legal custodial guardians themselves. The principles and conclusions in this book about them also apply to dependent adult parents,
such as those who are developmentally retarded, adjudicated as unfit or incarcerated,
violent criminals.

Although decreasing, the adolescent birthrate in the United States is the highest of
any developed nation. Almost one in three sexually active adolescent girls has been
pregnant.

Family life is changing rapidly. We are on a trajectory in which more than one-half of all our children will spend some time in a one-parent home or homeless.

The crisis–recoil nature of our political system leads to overreaction to social crises followed by recoiling from their causes. It underlies our fragmented, discontinuous services that can adversely affect families and that result in enormous financial and humanitarian costs to our society.

We cannot afford to continue to ignore our young peoples' cries for help.

Chapter 1

The Neglect of Children and Adolescents in the United States

Never before have we subjected our children to the tyranny of drugs and guns and things or taught them to look for meaning outside rather than inside themselves, teaching them in Dr. King's words "to judge success by the value of our salaries or the size of our automobiles, rather than by the quality of our service and relationship to humanity."

Marian Wright Edelman, 1995
Children's Defense Fund[1]

The prevalent image of American parents centering their lives around their offspring suggests that our young people are doing very well. These parents provide unprecedented levels of lessons, sports, tutoring and camps for their children. But this image obscures the fact that almost 14 million children and adolescents do not live this way and over 11 million have been neglected or abused. A growing gap in family wealth has created two sets of young people—those with educated, affluent parents and those with less educated, poor parents. As a result, most middle and upper class adolescents are thriving and most lower class adolescents are not.[2]

This chapter outlines the actual status of children and adolescents in the United States where most adults live in homes without children. There are dire consequences for all of us when those of us without children do not see the connection between struggling families and the social problems that affect us all.

CONTEMPORARY URBAN AND SUBURBAN LIFE STYLES

Before reviewing the data on the well-being of children and adolescents, the overall urban and suburban context of their lives merits consideration. Both our affluent and poor young people are increasingly disconnected from the natural world.[3] Richard Louv, a futurist and journalist, notes that computers, television, video games and homework in addition to parents' fears of traffic, violence, strangers and diseases keep the young indoors. Louv argues for a return to an appreciation for Nature as a way of nurturing the creativity of young people. Nature also needs the young—as its future stewards. One parent summarized the consequences of contemporary urbanization:

> For my son to adapt to the demands of this high-performance culture, I have to medicate him with stimulants and stand beside him day in and day out, making sure he reads his books . . . If we lived in a village in which dozens of kids ran freely through the streets and there were nearby forests for building forts and creeks for trapping minnows, my son would be busy and satisfied.

The social, psychological and emotional implications of diminishing connections to nature are increasingly apparent, especially for those living near and in poverty. Activities in Nature can help such maladies as depression, obesity and attention deficit disorder.[4] Environmentally based education improves academic performance and develops skills in problem-solving, critical thinking and decision-making.

INDICATORS OF SOCIETAL WELL-BEING

The well-being of our nation is usually measured in economic terms, such as by the Gross Domestic Product (GDP)—the total value of goods and services produced. However, economic indicators do not accurately measure the well-being of people. In fact, the costs of crimes, disasters and illnesses actually increase the GDP.[5]

We need a better way to measure the well-being of our nation. The Human Development Index (HDI) has been used since 1993 by the United Nations to assess achievements in a country on three basic dimensions of human development: at birth, adult literacy rate, level of education and GDP per capita. The United States ranks eighth among developed nations on the HDI.[6] A general well-being (GWB) index has been proposed in Great Britain.

Index of Social Health

The Index of Social Health compiled by the Institute for Innovation in Social Policy at Vassar College measures the actual well-being of people.[7]

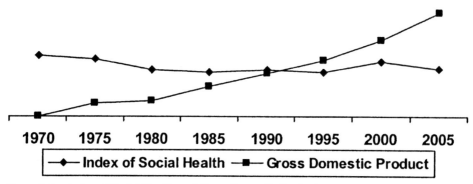

Figure 1.1.   Index of Social Health and Gross Domestic Product.

It focuses attention on preventing rather than on servicing social and health problems. It is the only current measure that examines sixteen social indicators for persons of all ages. Intriguingly, the Index of Social Health has been going down as our GDP has been going up.

Since 1970, ten indicators in the Index of Social Health have worsened as our Gross Domestic Product has risen:

- Child poverty
- Child abuse
- Teenage suicide
- Unemployment
- Average wages
- Health insurance coverage
- Out-of-pocket health care costs for 65 or over
- Food stamp coverage
- Access to affordable housing
- Income inequality

Six indicators have improved:

- Infant mortality
- High school dropouts
- Teenage drug abuse
- Poverty of those 65 and older
- Homicides
- Alcohol-related traffic deaths

Education Week

According to *Education Week*, 57% of our children do not have at least one parent with more than a high school diploma; 29% of our children do not have at least one parent working full time year-around; 16% of our children do not have parents who are fluent English speakers; and 11% of our children are not covered by health insurance.[8]

Kids Count

In the Annie E. Casey Foundation's *KIDS COUNT Data Book 2007* four of ten child well-being indicators worsened between 2000 and 2005:[9] children living below 100% of poverty increased by 1 million; the percentage of low-birth-weight babies increased; the number of children living in families where no parent has full-time, year-round employment increased; and the number of children living in single-parent families increased.

All of these indicators directly or indirectly affect the lives of adolescents.

Child and Youth Well-Being Index

According to the Foundation for Child Development Child and Youth Well-Being Index, after eight years of steady improvement from 1994 through 2002, the quality of life of our children and youth appears to be at a standstill.[10] The stall is reflected in reduced rates of improvement, flat-lines or actual declines across the majority of domains that comprise the Index. The overall stall in children's quality of life—underscored by a dramatic decline in children's health as well as persistent ethnic and racial disparities in education and poverty—sends a strong signal that America should be doing more to improve children's lives.

GROWING CHAOS IN THE LIVES OF ADOLESCENTS

Urie Bronfenbrenner, founder of the field of human ecology, identified the growing chaos in the lives of our children and adolescents.[11] The rising disarray in the lives of adolescents is emerging from changes in the social institutions that have the greatest impact on the development of competence and character:

- More children are growing up in disadvantaged one-parent homes.
- Growing conflict between the demands of employment and family life.
- The lack of positive adult models.
- The erosion of neighborhood ties between families.
- Increasing divorce and step-family formation.
- A widening gap between the rich and the poor.
- An increasing number of anti-social gangs.

Cross-cultural comparisons are intriguing. English-speaking countries lead other developed nations in adolescent births, one-parent homes, and divorce.[12] Alexis de Tocqueville observed in his 1830s classic *Democracy in America* that individualism had its roots in England. Hence, the "de Tocqueville hypothesis" for our times—Economically developed societies with the highest levels of social and developmental disarray will be English-speaking countries.

The "Syndrome of Alienation"

Both affluent and disadvantaged young people show evidence of the "syndrome of alienation" described by Bronfenbrenner.[13] The key elements of this syndrome are inattentiveness and misbehavior in school; academic underachievement; smoking and drinking; sexual activity; alcohol and substance abuse; dropping out of school; and ultimately violence, crime, homicide, suicide and welfare dependency.

Although genetic predisposition, pregnancy and birth complications, malnutrition, disabilities, poverty and racism all contribute to the vulnerability of children, whether or not children show the "syndrome of alienation" largely depends upon how they were parented. When parents are consumed by alcoholism, drug addiction or mental disorders or are preoccupied with their personal interests or vocations and neglect or abuse their children, boys are prone to become criminals and girls are prone to become welfare dependent.

In recent decades, the education, health, safety and economic status of our children has been insidiously eroded through both eras of economic prosperity and recession. The inescapable fact is that too many children are growing up in the United States under circumstances that prevent them from becoming responsible, productive citizens because they lack the abilities and the opportunities to learn essential social and work-related skills. A critical number of them swell the ranks of the criminal and the welfare dependent segments of the population. They become burdens for our society.

Developmental Assets & Mental Health

The Search Institute's Developmental Assets framework has two groups of twenty assets.[14] The twenty *external assets* are the positive experiences (social capital) young people receive from the world around them. These assets identify roles that families, schools, congregations, neighborhoods and youth organizations play in promoting healthy development. The twenty *internal assets* identify those characteristics and behaviors that reflect values, identities and social competencies that promote a commitment to learning. Having 31 of the 40 assets is the desirable level. Only 9% of our adolescents have 31 or more assets. The average young person has only 19.3. Boys have fewer assets than girls.

According to a Gallup survey developed by Child Trends and the Search Institute, only 31% of America's children have all or most of the five basic supports they need for healthy development: 1) caring adults; 2) safe places and constructive use of time; 3) healthy start in life and healthy development; 4) effective education for marketable skill and lifelong learning; and 5) opportunities to make a difference by helping others.[15]

Poverty

Harry J. Holzer, professor of public policy at Georgetown University estimates that the costs to our economy associated with childhood poverty total about $500 billion a year.[16]

In 2006, there were 73.5 million people in the United States under the age of eighteen (25% of the population): 58% were White, 19% Latino, 15% Black, 4% Asian and 4% other. Sixty-eight percent lived in two-parent homes, 23% lived with their mothers only, 5% lived with their fathers only and 4% lived in homes without either parent.[17]

In 2005, 18% of all persons under the age of eighteen lived in poverty (four times the rate in Scandinavia): Blacks—36%, American Indians—31%, Latinos—29%, Asians—14% and Whites—11%.[18] The percentages of children living in families where no parent has full-time employment were: American Indians—51%, Blacks—50%, Latinos—39%, Asians—32% and Whites—27%. The percentages of children living in one-parent homes were: Blacks—64%, American Indians—47%, Latinos—35%, Whites—23% and Asians—15%.

Crime

Adolescents and young adults experience the highest rates of violent crime victimization. Almost 25% of violent crimes are committed by juveniles.[19] The Uniform Crime Reporting Program reveals that from 1994 to 2003, the number of juvenile arrests increased by 23%. Between 1960 and 2004, juvenile court delinquency caseloads increased nearly 300%.

Homicide rates for males 15 through 24 in the United States are more than four times those in other developed countries.[20] Juvenile crime is rising especially in the form of increasing violence by girls in gangs. A decade ago, the ratio between boys and girls in arrests for assaults was ten boys for every girl. Now the ratio is four to one.

Overall crime remains near a 30-year low. However, violent crime at all ages increased by 3.8% from 2004 to 2006.[21] According to surveys conducted by the U.S. Department of Justice, the odds of being a violent-crime victim dropped nearly 60% since 1994, and those odds have not increased in recent years. At the same time, juvenile arrests showed a 20% increase from 2004 to 2005 for murder, an 11% increase for forcible rape, and an 11% increase for robbery. While violent crime has been at historic lows in cities like New York, Miami and Los Angeles, it is rising sharply in Milwaukee and in other cities across the nation. It is expected to increase as an increasing number of violent felons complete their sentences over the next five to ten years.

In the 1990s, homicides were in gang battles over drug turfs. Now they are over petty disputes.[22] One woman killed a friend in an argument over a silk dress. A man killed a neighbor whose 10-year-old son had mistakenly used his soap. Two men argued over a cell phone, pulled out their guns, and killed a 13-year-old girl in the crossfire. More weapons are on the streets making arguments potentially lethal. Milwaukee Police Chief Nannette H. Hegerty called it "the rage thing. We're seeing a very angry population, and they don't go to fists anymore, they go right to guns." In Chicago, two school-age children were killed in street fights every week during the first half of 2007.[23]

Disruptive Behavior in Schools

In 2003, there were 119,000 thefts from teachers and 65,000 violent offenses against teachers in school; 21% of students said street gangs were present in their schools; and 29% reported that someone had offered, sold or given them illegal drugs on school property.[24]

The number of student threats to teachers decreased from 342,100 in 1993–1994 to 253,100 in 2003–2004 because of increased security in schools. However, a 2006 AP-AOL Learning Services Poll found that two-thirds of the teachers surveyed said that student discipline and lack of interest in learning are major problems.[25] School bus drivers must deal with disrespectful and unruly young people.

Thirty years ago disciplinary problems in schools were chewing gum, stepping out of line, tardiness and occasional fist fights. Today they are attacks on teachers, rapes in hallways, murders and suicides. From 1992 to 2006, over 400 murders occurred at lower class, urban schools; 33 shootings occurred in middle-class schools. Many more deaths have been averted by early responses to warning signals.[26] Still children continue to shoot children, but these shootings no longer merit national media attention:

- When a 7-year-old-boy shot a 5-year-old three times, it was reported in the second section of the St. Petersburg Times.[27]
- 17-, 16-, and 13-year-olds talked about how a fight would be fun and stabbed a 34-year-old man to death.[28]
- An 18-year-old Cape Cod Regional Technical High School student made a pipe bomb and threatened to blow up the school.[29]
- A fifteen-year-old boy in Clearwater, Florida, said that he would do something like Columbine and was found to have a small arsenal in his room together with video files of Columbine, executions and images of the President and Vice President as targets.[30]
- Two seventeen-year-old boys had weapons and bombs in their homes with the intent of repeating the Columbine shooting in Green Bay, Wisconsin.[31]

Although there apparently is no typical profile of school shooters, they consistently report that they had no adults with whom they felt they could talk, including their own parents.[32]

The extent to which school safety is a significant issue is revealed by the No Child Left Behind Act's requirement that students attending a dangerous public elementary or secondary school, or students who become victims of a violent criminal offense while at a public school, be allowed to transfer to a safer public school.[33]

Education

The 1983 National Commission on Excellence in Education report *A Nation at Risk* called attention to our mediocre educational system. Its call to action has been repeated ever since with little evident progress.[34] In 2001, the United States ranked 13th of 15 developed countries in high school graduation rates. According to the National Assessment of Educational Progress, the average 17-year-old today is no more proficient at reading or mathematics than in 1970. The Program for International Student Assessment found that 15-year-old American students ranked 27th of 39 developed countries in mathematical literacy and problem-solving skills. Over 1 million adolescents ages 16–19 are neither in school nor working. Some progress has been made by 9- and 13-year-olds, but the gains evaporate by the end of high school. On the positive side, 15% of students in the class of 2007 had a grade predictive of college success or higher on an Advanced Placement Examination. This was up from 10% for the class of 2000.

In 2005, with the exception of students performing at the 90th percentile level, reading scores declined compared to 1992.[35] The percentage of students performing at or above the basic reading level decreased from 80% in 1992 to 73% in 2005. Sixty-one percent of high school seniors performed at or above the *Basic* mathematics level with 23% at or above *Proficient*.

In the United States, 29% of adults ages 25–29 have a bachelor degree.[36] Twenty percent of college students completing 4-year degrees and 30% of students earning 2-year degrees have only basic literacy skills. This means they are unable to estimate if their car has enough gasoline to get to the next gas station or calculate the total cost of ordering office supplies. These findings confirm low literacy levels among adults.

The percentage of high school graduates who go on to college are: Asian—66%; Whites—47%; Blacks—40% and Latinos—32%.[37] However, the percentage of students who graduate from urban public college campuses within six years ranges from 17% to 58%. Non-traditional students often take extra time to complete course work. Many are ill-prepared for college, have children and work full-time.

A national survey of more than 3,500 kindergarten teachers in the late 1990s revealed that 46% of teachers said that at least half of the children in their classrooms were having problems following directions, some because of poor academic skills and others because of difficulties working in a group.[38]

The earning power of dropouts has declined over the past three decades. In 1971, male dropouts earned $35,087 in 2002 dollars. This fell 35% to $23,903 in 2002. Earnings for female dropouts fell from $19,888 to $17,114.[39] Compared to a high school graduate, a single 18-year-old dropout earns $260,000 less over a lifetime and contributes $60,000 less in federal and state income taxes. Dropouts cost our nation more than $260 billion in lost wages, lost taxes and lost productivity over their lifetimes.

Dropping out of school is an epidemic in low-income communities.[40] Close to 60% of dropouts eventually do earn a General Equivalency Diploma (GED). Forty-four percent of those later enroll in two- or four-year colleges, but less than 10% earn a postsecondary degree. National Longitudinal Survey of Youth data reveal that young women possessing a GED do not generally do as well as high school graduates.[41]

A 2005 survey of school dropouts by Peter D. Hart Research Associates found that only 35% had failing grades; 47% thought classes were not interesting; 42% spent time with people who were not interested in school; and 38% said they had too much freedom and not enough rules.[42] However, focusing only on inadequate teachers and resources in schools diverts attention from the more important factors—a student's home, neighborhood and community.

Health

On the positive side, 82% of children and adolescents have very good or excellent physical health; 5% have severely disabling emotional and behavior disorders.[43] Suicidal ideation and suicide attempts among students in grades 9–12 decreased from 29% in 1991 to 17% in 2003. Still, suicide is the third leading cause of death for adolescents and young adults. Girls are more likely to attempt suicide than boys, who are more likely to actually commit suicide. American Indian/Alaskan Native boys have the highest suicide rate.

In 1979, I reviewed the available evidence and found that 16% of our children had significant physical, developmental, mental, educational and social handicaps.[44] Even more striking was the fact that at that time 37% of our children were thought to be at risk for maladjustment in later life. The intervening years have borne out that forecast. Now by the age of 18, 20% of young people have a diagnosed psychiatric disorder. A study of the mental health of young people found that of 15–18 year olds only 40% are flourishing; 54% are moderately mentally healthy; and 6% are languishing.

This generation of adolescents is more likely than their parents were to be from divorced or unstable families. It also is characterized by:[45]

- Increasing chronic mental and physical conditions related to the increasing numbers of premature babies.[46]
- Substance abuse and eating disorders occur at younger ages.
- Asthma and obesity have dramatically increased.
- Many of the Attention Deficit Disorder diagnoses in school-age boys would not occur if male rowdiness was seen as masked emotional pain.[47]
- Increased joint injuries among young athletes.
- One in five college students report self-injurious behavior correlated with a history of abuse and adverse health conditions in their lifetimes.[48]

Child Maltreatment

In one survey, one in three adolescents across all social classes reported having had direct or indirect exposure to violence or neglect.[49] In another survey, being left home alone as a child was reported by 42% of respondents followed by physical assault—28%; physical neglect—12%; and sexual abuse—5%. Over eleven million persons under 18 have been neglected or abused.

Although the number had been decreasing over the previous three years, in 2006 an estimated 3.3 million children were investigated by child welfare agencies. 905,000 were substantiated as victims of maltreatment:[50] 1,530 died; 63% were neglected; 17% were physically abused; 9% were sexually abused; and 7% were emotionally maltreated. The overall rates per 1,000 for ethnic groups were: Black—20, Pacific Islander—18, American Indian—16; White—11; and Latino—10. The perpetrators were: parents—79%, other relatives—7%, unmarried partners of parents—4% and "other"—10%. Fifty-eight percent of the perpetrators were female. Most perpetrators were in their 20s or 30s. Child maltreatment costs us $104 billion a year.

According to one study, 64% of children from 2 to 14 who came to the attention of the child welfare system did so because of alleged neglect; 36% of them also had allegations of physical abuse, 13% of sexual abuse and 12% of emotional abuse.[51] Nearly half had clinical emotional or behavioral problems at the time, but only 24% received mental health care.

The worldwide prevalence of childhood sexual abuse is 20% for females and 5–10% for males.[52] In California, childhood sexual abuse was reported by 25% of females and 16% of males in a study of over 17,000 adults.

Young children who have been abused may have severe emotional problems in later life.[53] Some boys may be genetically prone to be abused if they have a specific polymorphism on the X chromosome that predisposes them to overreact to events.

Compared to those reporting no sexual abuse, men and women who experienced childhood sexual abuse have twice the number of suicide attempts, a 40% increased risk of marrying an alcoholic and a 45% increased risk of having marital problems.[54] Two common sequelae of sexual abuse are substance abuse and running away from home. Brain changes from the trauma of abuse make it more likely that sexually abused adolescents using mood-altering substances will become chemically dependent. They may become prostitutes to buy drugs.

The tendency of victims to remain silent about rape and incest protects abusers who hold them in their thrall.[55] Sexual abuse may involve varying degrees of pleasure and guilt that complicate victim's responses. At the same time, some adolescents falsely allege abuse by their parents when their wishes are frustrated. Still, such an allegation is a cry for intervention to help the family.

Conscienceless Children

There is a growing cohort of children who are uncontrollable and unreachable because they never formed attachment bonds with people.[56] They do not have effective consciences. They become drug addicts, thieves, rapists and murderers. Many were disadvantaged at birth by suffering from cocaine withdrawal or prematurity and had frightening, insecure infancies. Their neglectful, often drug-using parents were unable to provide for their needs.

ALCOHOL AND DRUG ABUSE

The adolescent brain is affected more than the adult brain by alcohol, nicotine and other drugs because important neural circuits are being formed.[57] The same amount of alcohol produces more memory and learning impairment more rapidly, more severely and with less warning.

Some adolescents are vulnerable to addiction because of biological, psychological, social, cultural and environmental factors.[58] They use addicting drugs, like cocaine, for thrills and for self-treatment of emotional and personality disorders. Dopamine buildup in the nucleus accumbens in the limbic system appears to be responsible for the cocaine high.

The National Longitudinal Study of Adolescent Health found that suburban high school students drink, smoke, use illegal drugs and engage in delinquent behavior as often or more than urban high school students:[59]

- 37% of suburban 12th graders have smoked at least once a day compared to 30% of urban 12th graders;
- 63% of suburban and 57% of urban 12th graders drink away from family members;
- 40% of 12th graders in both urban and suburban schools have used illegal drugs;
- Urban and suburban students are equally likely to engage in fighting and stealing.

Half of adolescents have attended parties where drugs and alcohol were available.[60] One-third have attended a party at which alcohol, marijuana, cocaine, ecstasy or prescription drugs were available while a parent was present.

Girls metabolize drugs differently than boys, making them more sensitive to their effects and more likely to have harsher consequences. Paralyzed by shame, embarrassment and denial, many who struggle with substance abuse do not seek help. Six million girls and women meet clinical criteria for alcohol abuse or dependence, 15 million abuse illicit and prescription drugs, and nearly 32 million smoke cigarettes.[61] Of these, almost 70% report a history of sexual abuse. Forty-six percent of 9th to 12th grade girls drink, and more than half of 18 to 25-year-old women have used an illicit drug at least once in their lifetimes.

Alcohol Abuse

More adolescents in the United States drink alcohol than smoke tobacco or marijuana. Underage drinking accounted for at least 16% of alcohol sales in 2001. It led to 3,170 deaths and 2.6 million other harmful events.[62] The estimated $62 billion in costs of underage drinking included $5.4 billion in medical costs, $15 billion in work loss and other costs, and $41.6 billion in lost quality of life. Alcohol-attributable violence and traffic accidents dominate the costs.

Every day, three adolescents die from drinking and driving.[63] Every year, 5,000 young people under the age of twenty-one die as a result of drinking, including 1,900 deaths from motor vehicle crashes, 1,600 from homicides, 300 from suicide, and 1200 from other injuries, such as falls, burns and drownings.

Although adolescent drinking has declined since the 1970s, it remains a significant problem.[64] According to a study carried out by the National Center on Addiction and Substance Abuse, 47% of adolescents from 12 to 20 were frequent drinkers in 2005. 26% met clinical criteria for alcohol abuse and addiction, more than two and one-half times the percentage for adult drinkers. In 2003, 13% of 12-year-olds reported having had their first drink, according to a study by the National Institute on Alcoholism and Alcohol Abuse. In 2004, more than 7 million 12 to 20-year-olds reported binge drinking. In 2005, 11% of 8th, 21% of 10th, and 28% of 12th graders reported having five or more alcoholic beverages in a row in the last two weeks. Binge drinking by girls is increasing more rapidly than for boys.

The younger the age at which drinking starts, the greater the likelihood of alcohol addiction. Nearly half of a sample who became addicted to alcohol were first diagnosable by the age of twenty-one and two thirds by twenty-five.[65] Maternal alcohol use during pregnancy may increase the risk of adolescent alcohol abuse.

Illicit Drug Abuse

Illicit drug abuse peaked at 65% by the end of high school in 1980, reached a low of 40% in 1992 and returned to 52% in 2006; 16% of 8th graders, 32% of 10th graders and 42% of 12th graders had used marijuana.[66] In 2006, 9%, 17% and 23% of students in grades 8, 10 and 12 used illicit drugs during the previous 30 days. The estimated abuse rates for illegal drugs are: cocaine/crack (10%), ecstasy (8%), methamphetamine (8%) and heroin (5%). The weekly use at age 15 of marijuana increases the risk of dropping out of school.

In 2005, 62% of high school and 28% of middle school students attended schools in which drugs were readily available, up from 44% and 19% in 2002.[67]

In 2006, the Philadelphia School District acknowledged that the drug problem involving students from kindergarten through sixth grade was growing. Thirty-three students were found possessing drugs in first three months of 2006 compared with 26 for all of 2004–05.[68]

> Four bags of marijuana tumbled out when a 10-year-old took off his hat, and two more fell as he entered his classroom. Three fifth graders took turns holding a bag of marijuana, and the student who brought the drug to school had $920 in his pocket. When a 10-year-old was searched for a knife after he threatened to stab another student, school officials found cocaine.

From 1999 to 2003, the number of juvenile arrests for synthetic narcotic violations increased 81%, non-narcotics increased 55% and marijuana increased by 4%.[69] Arrests involving opium or cocaine decreased 28% during this period. Seventy percent of juvenile arrests were for marijuana.

Five percent of pregnant women of all ages in methamphetamine-prevalent areas used methamphetamine.[70] One quarter smoked tobacco, 23% drank alcohol, 6% used marijuana, and 1% used barbiturates prenatally.

Over the Counter and Prescription Drug Abuse

Adolescents are showing a trend toward using prescription drugs obtained from parents and from friends. They use illicit drugs for recreation and prescription drugs for specific effects: stimulants for studying, sedatives for sleep and tranquilizers to relieve stress.[71] In 2006, nearly 20% of all adolescents reported abusing prescription medications; 10% reported using cough medicine to get high. Nearly one-third believed there is nothing wrong with using prescription medicines once in a while and that prescription pain relievers are not addictive. They were influenced by advertising that suggests using pills to relieve discomforts. Twelve to seventeen-year-old girls were more likely to abuse these drugs than boys. They were more likely than boys to use addictive substances to control their weight, to alter their moods or to reduce inhibitions.

SMOKING

About 90% of smokers begin before the age of 21. Each day, 6,000 adolescents under 18 start smoking.[72] Of these, 2,000 will become addicted. According to a 2001 national survey, 28% of high school students smoked cigarettes. In 2005, 4% of 8th, 8% of 10th and 14% of 12th graders reported smoking daily. Most say they would like to quit, but are unable to do so.

Adolescents are particularly vulnerable to smoking addiction because their brains are more sensitive than adults to acetaldehyde and nicotine in tobacco smoke.[73] There also is evidence that genetic predisposition and depression influence adolescent smoking. Cigarette smoking during childhood and adolescence produces significant health problems among young people, including respiratory illnesses, diminished physical fitness and retarded lung growth.

SEXUALLY TRANSMITTED DISEASES

One in four sexually active adolescent girls and boys (4 million) contracts a sexually transmitted disease, accounting for 25% of all cases.[74] One in four of all girls (48% of Black and 20% of White) between 14 and 19 contracts a sexually transmitted disease. Of the some 900,000 adolescent runaways each year, over 6% test positive for the AIDS virus. They often engage in unsafe sex, prostitution and drug abuse. Each year up to 64,000 adolescents are spreading AIDS.

Of females of all ages, Blacks accounted for 67% of the estimated AIDS cases in 2004 while comprising only 13% of the female population.[75] Latinas accounted for 15% of the AIDS cases and 14% of the female population. In 2004, the AIDS rate for Black was 23 times, for Latina 5 times and for American Indian 3 times higher than the rate for White females.

Adolescent sexually transmitted disease rates are much higher in the United States than in most other developed countries: ten times higher for syphilis and gonorrhea and two to five times higher for chlamydia.[76] The age of sexual debut varies little across countries, yet American adolescents are the most likely to have multiple partners. The younger the sexual debut the more likely there will be health hazards.

OUR CHEMICALLY TOXIC ENVIRONMENT

Each one of us carries at least 250 toxic chemicals in our bodies. The *Handbook of Pediatric Environmental Health* highlights lead, mercury, PCB and pesticide poisoning as known hazards to children's health.[77] Numerous studies confirm that even slightly elevated blood lead levels can cause learning and behavioral disorders, decreased IQ and hearing impairments. Many environmental chemicals mimic hormones that can disrupt developing immune, nervous and endocrine systems. The greatest vulnerability to toxic chemicals is during the pre-natal phase of the life cycle. All of these chemical hazards are the greatest in the environments of disadvantaged, pregnant adolescents.

OUR SOCIALLY TOXIC ENVIRONMENT

James Garbarino, professor of psychology at Loyola University-Chicago, indicts our *socially toxic environment* as the reason for the larger number of our children with serious problems than in the 1950s and 1960s.[78] Social toxicity includes exposure to violence; economic pressures; disrupted family relationships; and behavior reflecting depression, paranoia, rudeness and alienation. All of these "social contaminants" demoralize families and communities.

Our violence-prone society appears to need delinquents and criminals who act out our own hidden impulses that we gratify through violent, sexually stimulating media. We then subject them to indignant censure.[79] In this sense, the "badness" of delinquents and criminals is a projection of our own impulses to be "bad" on to others. By punishing others who are "bad," we avoid facing our own "badness." We are fascinated by antisocial behavior and then demand "getting tough on crime" as we avoid facing our own contributions to it. This attitude obscures awareness of the need to strengthen struggling families as the antidote to antisocial behavior. Instead, we expect schools and governmental agencies to correct our social problems, as if parents had nothing to do with the outcomes of their children's lives.

Research on early brain development reveals that the elements of social toxicity most dangerous to the fetus and baby are parental neglect and abuse. Adolescents "home alone" are more vulnerable to social toxicity than those supervised by adults. The proliferation of handguns among adolescents means that conflicts and confrontations that once were settled with fists now result in shootings. More generally, children and adolescents must contend with frightening messages that undermine their sense of security. Some parents obtain DNA samples and fingerprints of their children in case they are kidnapped, run away or have accidents.[80] Fears of school violence, parental divorce and a future with dim employment opportunities are not uncommon for our young people.

We cannot expect our children to prosper when our society does not model, and actually undermines, the development of character. The good life is portrayed as gaining power, pleasure and possessions by any means. There is little emphasis on the strength of character needed to control our impulses, to tolerate frustration and to postpone gratification—essential qualities for life in a civilized society. Our children are not born with these qualities. They learn them from adults who model them. They learn them most indelibly from parents supported by a social environment that sets limits on behavior.

ELEVATED THRESHOLD OF DEVIANCY

Daniel Patrick Moynihan pointed out that societies under stress, much like individuals, turn to painkillers to cover up distressing social problems.[81] He noted that the tolerance of deviant behavior in our society increases over time. We redefine deviancy to exempt conduct we previously deplored. A prime example is homelessness that was not tolerated thirty years ago.

This numbing tendency reflects the human ability to adapt to stressful circumstances over which we perceive ourselves as having no control. A common metaphor is the failure of a frog to jump from water that is gradually heated to the point of extinguishing the frog's life.

JUVENILE AGEISM

The developmental needs of children will not be accorded appropriate attention until our society's inability to deal with incompetent parents is addressed. Unrecognized prejudice and discrimination against the young reflecting *juvenile ageism* stands in the way. As our nation's largest permanent minority, our young have no direct representation in the political process. The result is neglect of schools and resources for children, adolescents and their families.

The prejudice of juvenile ageism is as virulent as racism and as pervasive as sexism.[82] It is the greatest barrier to recognizing the true interests of adolescents and their babies. It is expressed through disregard of the developmental need of young persons for competent parents. Its most extreme form is seen in the belief that parents own their children as property. That belief is supported by the presumption that government can intervene only in extreme situations when parents damage their children by neglect or abuse. Juvenile ageism also is expressed when we treat adolescents as adults and ignore their developmental needs.

Our lack of awareness of juvenile ageism is understandable. First, it is eclipsed by our concern about racism and sexism. Second, we associate prejudice and discrimination based on age only with the elderly. Third, we all are juvenile ageists to some degree. Fourth, we all have difficulty recognizing our own prejudices, even when they are pointed out to us. As much as we might like to believe otherwise, all of our judgments are biased, or prejudiced, by our past experiences and by our current emotional states.

In some ways, to speak of juvenile ageism now resembles speaking of racism in the South in the 1850s. Then the economic interests and the latent guilt of plantation owners precluded recognizing the racism involved in slavery. Today, the economic interests and the latent guilt of many adults preclude recognizing juvenile ageism.

When children are oppressed, abused and neglected, it is easier to recognize juvenile ageism than when we believe we are helping them. Yet prejudice and discrimination can be expressed in benevolent and idealizing ways. Before racism was generally accepted as a social problem, many people believed that slaves were content and needed direction. Before sexism was openly revealed, many people believed that women were naturally dependent and were satisfied with subservient occupations. The idealization of motherhood still makes it possible for men to avoid their responsibilities in childrearing.

Now many of us under the influence of benevolent juvenile ageism believe that the wishes of adolescents should be gratified and that the interests of babies can be protected by supporting adolescent parenthood. In each of these instances, we do not recognize that indulgent or overly protective attitudes can harm adolescents by preventing them from learning how to handle life's challenges and to take advantage of life's opportunities in ways other than parenthood. We do not recognize that babies need competent parents.

CONCLUSION

The growing discrepancy in family wealth has created two sets of young people—those with educated affluent parents and those with less educated poor parents.

Only 31% of our children have all or most of the five basic supports they need for healthy development. Since 1970, ten indicators in the Index of Social Health have worsened as our Gross Domestic Product has risen. Disruptive behavior in schools has increased necessitating the presence of police. Academic performance levels have deteriorated, and many students are unprepared for college.

A enlarging cohort of children are growing up to be uncontrollable and unreachable because they did not form attachment bonds with people. They do not have functioning consciences.

Adolescents are oversensitive to damage and undersensitive to warning signs from alcohol abuse and smoking addiction. Underage drinking is estimated to cost our economy $62 billion. Half of adolescents have tried an illicit drug before they finish high school. Many use prescription drugs for specific effects: stimulants for studying, hypnotics for sleep and tranquilizers to relieve stress.

One in four sexually active adolescents contracts a sexually transmitted disease, accounting for 25% of all cases.

As the social environment becomes more socially toxic, our young—particularly the most vulnerable—show the effects first and the most. Social toxicity includes violence, poverty, family disruptions and economic pressures on parents and their children.

We have elevated the bar of tolerable deviant behavior to avoid facing the effort needed to heal our toxic society. Recognizing and overcoming juvenile ageism will help to restore our perspective on the plight of our disadvantaged young people.

For the prosperity of our nation, we can and must remove the barriers to developing a responsible, productive citizenry by helping the families of over 13 million young persons find pathways out of poverty and by addressing the needs of over 11 million who have been neglected or abused.

Chapter 2

Adolescent Pregnancy and Childbirth Trends

Causing the existence of a human being is one of the most responsible actions in the range of human life. To undertake this responsibility—to bestow a life which may be either a curse or a blessing—unless the being on whom it is to be bestowed will have at least the ordinary chances of a desirable existence is a crime against that being.

John Stuart Mill, 1859[1]

Statistical trends play a vital role in attracting public attention to social problems. When they rise, we become concerned. When they go down, as is the case with adolescent pregnancy and childbirth, we move on to another problem that is rising. In so doing, social problems seldom are effectively addressed. A more realistic approach is to attend to all of our social problems, especially those that affect family relationships, and use rates to assess progress.

ADOLESCENT PREGNANCY RATES

From 1990 to 2002, the pregnancy rate for 15 through 19-year-olds decreased 28%, from 111 to 76/1,000, a record low.[2] The pregnancy termination rate decreased 38% from 35 to 22/1,000. Of an estimated 757,000 pregnancies among 15 through 19 year-olds in 2002, 57% ended in childbirth, 29% in termination, and 14% in miscarriage. The pregnancy rate for 15 through 17-year-olds fell from 77 in 1990 to 44/1,000 in 2002, a 42% drop. This trend suggests increased motivation to avoid pregnancies and sexually transmitted diseases.[3]

Almost one third of all sexually experienced adolescent girls have been pregnant.[4] Over half of sexually active Latino girls have been pregnant compared to 40% of Black girls and 23% of White girls. Almost half of girls who first have sex before 15 have been pregnant. For all ages, the overall pregnancy rate for Latinas and Blacks is 60% more than for Whites.[5] Unintended pregnancies are 180% more for Latinas and 120% more for Blacks than for Whites. Girls with three or more partners are more likely to have been pregnant than girls with less.

In one survey, 22% of Black, 19% of Latino and 10% of White boys reported impregnating a girl.[6] These figures are believed to be low since males may not be informed about partners' miscarriages or terminations.

ADOLESCENT CHILDBIRTH

Two-thirds of all adolescent mothers are eighteen or nineteen and are adults by most legal standards.[7] In 2006, 145,325 births were to adolescents under the age of 18. 38% were to Latino, 32% were to White, 27% to Black and 3% to American Indian adolescents.[8] At this rate, 2.5 million children and adolescents were born to mothers under 18. An estimated 8% of all girls under eighteen are mothers (2.8 million). The birth rate for ages 15 through 19 declined from a peak in 1991 of 62 to 42/1000 in 2006 although it increased by 3% from 2005 to 2006.[9] The birth rate for ages 15 through 17 decreased by 43%.[10] For 10 through 14, it was 0.6/1000 in 2006 (6,405 births).

Birth rates vary greatly by race, ethnicity and economic status. Between 1991 and 2006, the birth rate for Black adolescents dropped almost by one-half, whereas rates for White adolescents dropped 38% and for Latina adolescents 21%.[11] The decline for Black 15 through 17-year-olds from 1991 to 2005 was 59%, the steepest reduction

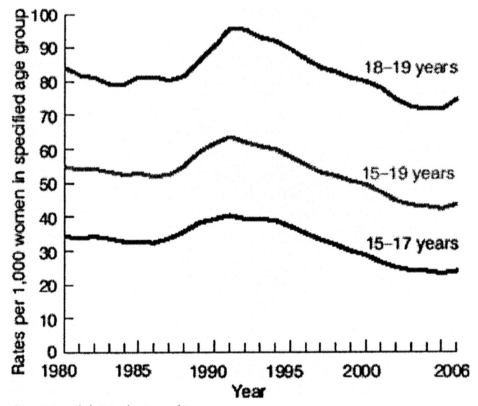

Figure 2.1.   Birth Rates by Age and Year.

overall by race or age group. Two-thirds of families begun by young, unwed mothers live in poverty.[12]

Surveys reveal that between 20% and 33% of births to 15 through 19-year-olds are planned before pregnancy.[13] Thirty-five percent had a repeat pregnancy within 18 months after the first birth. The second pregnancy often was associated with failure to return to school and an inability to become financially independent.[14]

The decline in adolescent birth rates was well under way before the 1996 welfare reform law was enacted. Increases in abstinence and contraception appear to be the most important reasons for the decline, although messages about the propriety of early childbearing may have been factors as well.[15]

Reliable and valid local prevalence data for adolescent mothers are not available. An estimate of the numbers in Madison and Milwaukee, Wisconsin, in 2003 revealed that 4% of all 15 through 17-year-old girls in Madison and 10% in Milwaukee were mothers. 24% in Madison and 20% in Milwaukee of all poor 15 through 17-year-old girls were mothers:[16]

Unwed Adolescent Births

In 2005, 37% of all births were to unwed girls and women.[17] 15 through 19-year-olds account for 12% of all births and for one-third of all unwed mothers.[18] Nearly half of all unwed first births occur to 15 through 19-year-olds, the largest single age group.[19]

Although the total adolescent birthrate has declined substantially since mid-century, the percentage of unwed adolescent births ages 15 through 19 soared from 15% in 1960 to 81% in 2003.[20] In 1960, adolescent childbearing occurred mostly in marriage with an employed husband. Now it occurs with unwed adolescents with limited prospects of marriage and economic security.

Fathers of Girls' Babies

According to the National Center for Health Statistics, the conception rate for boys ages 15 through 19 declined from a peak of 24/1000 in 1990 to 17/1,000 in 2002.[21] The conception rate for boys is much lower than the birth rate for girls because 39% of the fathers of children born to 15-year-olds and 47% of the fathers of children born to 16-year-olds are older than 20.

Geographic Variations

Although most poor adolescents live in rural areas, those growing up in large cities are more likely to give birth. In 2000, 15 through 19 birth rates ranged from a high of 174/1,000 in Miami, Florida, to a low of 17/1,000 in Glendale, California.[22] Thirteen percent of girls from all social class were pregnant in 2004 at Timken High School in Canton, Ohio.[23]

In 2003, New Hampshire had the lowest adolescent birth rate of 18/1,000. The highest were in Texas, New Mexico and Mississippi with rates over 62/1,000. Only 12% of adolescent births in New Hampshire were repeat births compared to 24% in Texas.

City	% of All Girls Who Are Mothers	% of All Poor Girls Who Are Mothers	% of All Black Girls Who Are Mothers	% of All Latina Poor Girls Who Are Mothers	% of White Poor Girls Who Are Mothers	% of Other Poor Girls Who Are Mothers	% of Black Girls Who Are Mothers	% of Latina Girls Who Are Mothers	% of White Girls Who Are Mothers
Madison	4%	24%	41%	28%	22%	9%	11%	15%	1%
Milwaukee	10%	20%	70%	22%	5%	3%	24%	24%	1%

Figure 2.2. Maternal Status of Girls Ages 15–17 in Madison and Milwaukee, Wisconsin.

However, fewer adolescent births were within marriage (11%) in New Hampshire than in Texas (27%). From 1993 to 2004, births to Wisconsin 15 through 19-year-olds decreased 27% from 41 to 30/1,000 as the rate for Latinos increased 15% from 84 to 96/1,000.[24]

International Comparisons

The adolescent birthrate in the United States is the highest of any developed nation, more than twice that of Canada; four times that of France, Italy and other Western European nations; and more than seven times that of Japan.

American adolescent sexual activity patterns are similar to those of peers in other developed countries, but Americans use contraception less effectively. Easily available contraception and education for adolescents through the schools and the media contribute to lower pregnancy and termination rates in Europe than in the United States.[25]

A lower proportion of adolescent pregnancies are terminated in the United States than in other developed countries; however, because of their high pregnancy rate, U.S. adolescents have the highest termination rate.

In the Union of South Africa, more than 30% of 19-year-old girls have had at least one birth.[26] Most find a way for their extended families to care for their children, and many continue their educations. The percentages of 15–19 year olds who have begun childbearing elsewhere are: Indonesia 10%, Turkey 10%, Pakistan 16%, Mexico 18%, Haiti 18% and Kenya 23%.

In Bangladesh, more than half of women marry before the age of 15.[27] Nevertheless, fertility in Bangladesh is on the decline. Women averaged 6.3 children in 1975 and 3 in 2004.

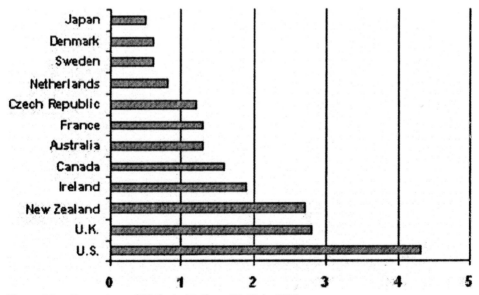

Figure 2.3.   Percentage of Births to Mothers 15–19 in 2002.

CONCLUSION

Eight percent of all girls under eighteen in the United States are mothers. Adolescent birth rates declined by one-third from 1991 to 2006 because of abstinence and contraception.

Black and Latino girls are more than twice as likely as White to become pregnant at least once before 20. Adolescents from low-income, single-parent families are far more likely to become pregnant and give birth than adolescents from affluent two-parent families.

Adolescents ages 15 through 19 account for 12% of all births and one-third of all unwed mothers. The percentage of unwed adolescent births ages 15 through 19 soared from 15% in 1960 to 81% in 2003. Up to one-third of births to 15–19 year olds are planned before pregnancy. Over one-third of these mothers have another pregnancy within 18 months.

The birth rate for boys is lower than for girls because 39% of the fathers of children born to 15-year-olds and younger and 47% of the fathers of children born to 16-year-olds are over 20.

Adolescent birth rates in the United States are the highest of any developed nation in part because of the higher level of multiple sexual partners among American adolescents.

Although most adolescents in poverty live in rural areas, those growing up in large cities are more likely to give birth.

One-third of sexually experienced adolescent girls have been pregnant. From 1990 to 2000, the pregnancy rate for ages 15 through 17 decreased by 33%. This trend suggests increased motivation to avoid pregnancies and sexually transmitted diseases.

Chapter 3

The Denigration of Parenthood

The proper officers will take the offspring of the good parents to the pen or fold, and there will deposit them with certain nurses who dwell in a separate quarter; but the offspring of the inferior, or of the better when they chance to be deformed, will be put away in some mysterious, unknown place, as they should be.

They (the nurses) will provide for their nurture, and will bring the mothers to the fold when they are full of milk, taking the greatest possible care that no mother recognizes her own child. . . Care will also be taken that the process of suckling shall not be protracted too long; and the mothers will have no getting up at night or other trouble, but will hand all this sort of thing to the nurses and attendants.

Plato

The Republic V[1]

Parenthood rather than *parenting* was deliberately chosen as the theme of this book. Parenting functions can be delegated to others. Parenting can be pieced together around children in foster homes, institutions and dysfunctional families without children actually having competent parents.

Even the word *parent* deserves attention. It derives from Latin for simply giving birth. Being a parent says nothing about childrearing. It means nothing in itself to babies, children and adolescents. Anyone past puberty can be a parent. Plato's Republic had parents but no parenthood.

To enter *parenthood* is to have a career—to make a lifelong commitment to a son or a daughter. It is a way for human beings to express their deepest values.[2] Parenthood means everything to babies, children and adolescents. The quality of their lives depends on having competent parents who can handle the responsibilities of parenthood. Unfortunately, our society does not distinguish between being a parent and parenthood and consequently fails to ensure that all of our children have competent parents. Advances in reproductive technology have even complicated determining who is a genetic parent.[3] All of this denigrates parenthood.

Our society does not recognize *parenthood* as a career. It does not formally acknowledge the fact that childrearing is skilled "hands on" work in which parents and children bond with each other and grow together. It awards any genetic parent regardless of age or ability full parental rights until the child is damaged by neglect or abuse.

Like any career, parenthood has its frustrations and rewards. Unlike any other career, it is based on affectionate attachment bonds between persons. It is a more important role in life than a paid career for most parents. This becomes especially evident during the later years of life. Louis Terman's Stanford study of eminent women and men found that, as they looked back on their lives, they valued their family relationships above their professional careers.[4]

We need to face the implications of parenthood as a lifelong career because family life is changing rapidly in the face of increasing maternal employment, father absence and cultural diversity. At the same time, children are being treated as commodities to be cared for by reimbursed systems. Many parents must have more than one income in order to make ends meet. In some families, parent-child roles are reversed. All of this is taking place in the context of increasing general ambivalence about committed relationships and questions about who is "the parent" of a child conceived through artificial fertilization.

Our society does not have formally articulated standards for parenthood except in agency requirements for adoption. Although unexpressed in our society, our culture does hold expectations for persons who enter parenthood through the birth of a child, as will be elaborated upon throughout this book. The vast majority of children are raised by parents who fulfill these cultural expectations of parenthood by living in committed relationships with their children, but an increasing number are not. T. Berry Brazelton, professor of pediatrics at Harvard University, and Stanley Greenspan, professor of child psychiatry at George Washington University, suggest that this fact underlies the general fragility of relationships in our society.[5] An increasing number of adults have difficulty sustaining committed relationships. They typically did not have parents who modeled caring, intimate relationships in their families.

There is an important caveat. Although parenthood contributes to fulfillment in life, life certainly can be fulfilling without directly participating in the reproductive cycle. Many persons choose not to enter the career of parenthood. Unfortunately, too many persons who are not able to assume its responsibilities choose to enter parenthood.

THE EVOLUTION OF PARENTHOOD IN WESTERN CIVILIZATION

The cohesion of human groups depends upon bonding based on love and commitment between members and on fear and hatred of enemies. Families evolved as our *species survival* instincts to bond and cooperate in groups dominated our *individual survival* instincts to compete with others and fight enemies. As resources became more abundant and families merged into tribes, competition for those resources led to fighting between tribes. Since then family ties have been disrupted during wars and strengthened during peaceful eras.

Against this background, the evolution of parenthood in Western civilization reveals an original pattern of nuclear families embedded in extended families and communities. Subsequently, nuclear and extended family ties were broken through migration from the countryside to cities. Then there was a gradual return of nuclear families in cities followed by a recent shift to a variety of family structures.

In the long-range, societies are held together by parenthood-transmitted integrative cultural values that promote accountability to others and that restrain unacceptable behavior. When individuals feel accountable to each other, the materialism of capitalism and the idealism of the American creed of equality and justice are reconciled in favor of the common good. But as the influence of parenthood-transmitted cultural values has diminished, moral constraints have been replaced by legal restraints. As a result, we have come to a time in our society in which individuals can successfully avoid accountability to others until they are convicted of crimes.

CONTEMPORARY PARENTHOOD IN THE UNITED STATES

Every generation in the United States has been concerned about the deterioration of families as they continually adapt to new social conditions.[6] In recent decades, the dominance of materialism and the shift away from the American creed has particularly affected family life. Following World War II, parents felt a strong commitment to give their children more material things than they had during their childhoods in the Great Depression. Overindulged children subsequently lost respect for their parents and for authority. Later decades were dominated by the Cold War and fear of nuclear attacks. The Vietnam War without an obvious national purpose intensified disillusionment of the young in their elders.

An anti-authority, "postmodern" philosophy now permeates our society with an emphasis on self-assertive individualism. There is an ethos of avoiding discomfort and frustration. Increasing options for both young and older persons permit choosing the options that are "best for me." The pursuit of perfection intensifies this ethos.

In ancient Greece, Plato's conception of the perfect republic was one in which children would be raised more efficiently by the state than by parents, who then would be free to pursue their own interests. Since then royalty and the wealthy have hired others to care for their children. This motif of delegating parenting functions to others permeates contemporary parenting styles in the United States where the self-assertive marketplace values only paid work.

Now motherhood brings one of the most difficult decisions in a woman's life. Stay at home or pursue a career or both? The dilemma produces internal conflicts and divides mothers into factions in the "mommy wars."[7] Mothers at home with their children have different viewpoints than those who hold full- or part-time jobs.

Parenthood is commonly seen as interfering with paid careers. Linda Hirshman, an emeritus professor of philosophy and women's studies at Brandeis University, believes that childrearing is not a fulfilling career for educated women.[8] She is concerned about the current trend in which women are leaving the work force to become full-time mothers. She believes that paid careers allow women to use their talents more fully and affect society in addition to providing income. The family with its repetitious, socially invisible tasks is a necessary social institution, but it does not give women opportunities to flourish as do careers in business or government where money and professional advancement

are the markers of success. Hirshman suggests that women devote the first few years after college to prepare for paid work. She wrote:

> Expensively educated mothers who stay at home are leading lesser lives. They bear the
> burden of work associated with lower social classes—housekeeping and childcare.

According to Leslie Bennetts, journalist and author, employed mothers are the best
kind for children because they teach resourcefulness and independence by example
and demonstrate the virtue of engaging in work one loves. She suggests that women
lose their humanity if they do not become all they can be through paid careers.[9]

In addition, contemporary philosophies about childrearing place intense demands
on busy parents and emphasize developing independent children. Annette Lareau, a
professor of sociology at the University of Maryland, notes that upper-middle-class
parents are involved in all aspects of their children's lives.[10] They make concerted efforts to provide learning experiences in what can be an exhausting pace. In contrast,
Lareau found that working-class parents seem to believe that adulthood will come
soon enough and that children should be left alone in their own playtime. Their children seem more relaxed and vibrant and have more intimate contact with their extended families. Lareau commented:

> Whining, which was pervasive in middle-class homes, was rare in working-class homes.
> Middle-class adolescents feel entitled to individual treatment and know how to navigate
> the world of organized institutions. Working-class adolescents feel constrained and are
> not as well prepared for the world of organizations and adulthood.

The rewards of parenthood are easily obscured for contemporary parents who have not
found the personal satisfactions and pleasures of parenthood and who pursue the goal of
trying to "have it all now" in a material sense for themselves and for their children.

Plato's idea of raising children away from their parents was not realized in ancient
Greece. It failed in all subsequent social experiments from those in the Israeli kibbutzim to the People's Republic of China.[11] Even the wealthy who delegate childrearing
often do not have rewarding intimate family relationships.

Because committed relationships are vital to the integrity and prosperity of our society, we need to articulate our cultural expectations of parenthood—the source of
committed relationships. Implicit cultural expectations of parents and children in the
United States include the moral right of children to have competent parents and the
obligations of children to respect and cooperate with their parents. These cultural expectations have evolved into societal expectations that become evident when parents
are brought into courts where they are codified in child abuse and neglect statutes. Because parenthood has been insufficiently valued by our society, courts are increasingly
involved in defining our cultural expectations of parenthood.

THE INCREASING ROLE OF COURTS IN DEFINING PARENTHOOD

Courts no longer recognize the tradition that the natural rights to conceive and to give
birth to a child also accord ownership of that child. When family matters are adjudi-

cated in courts, a variety of case and common law precedents set societal expectations of parenthood based on our cultural values.[12] These expectations are articulated in child abuse and neglect and divorce custody laws.

Expectations of Parenthood in Family Courts

In family courts, the positive expectations of parenthood are:

- Providing a home that legitimizes a child's identity in a community.
- Providing sufficient income for a child's clothing, shelter, education, health care, social and recreational activities.
- Providing the love, security and emotional support necessary for the healthy development of a child.
- Fostering the intellectual, social and moral development of a child.
- Socializing the child by setting limits and encouraging civil behavior.
- Protecting the child from physical, emotional and social harm.
- Maintaining stable family interactions through communication, problem solving and responding to individual needs.

When we look at these expectations of parenthood, we see that we rely on parents to instill our cultural values in our children so that they will become responsible citizens. The need to explicitly recognize the essential role of parenthood in our society and to support parents in their childrearing efforts becomes obvious. At the same time, neglect of the needs of young people at any point in their development can have long-range, unintended consequences. Still, instability and disadvantage in the lives of adolescents can offer opportunities for character growth, if we can identify and agree upon our expectations of adolescents.

Expectations of Adolescents in Juvenile Courts

Because adolescents are capable of being parents, it is important to consider the way in which our society expects them to relate to their own parents—their custodial guardians. In juvenile courts, adolescents are expected to learn how to respond to benign authority in order to interact comfortably and effectively with others. Without this ability, they remain self-centered and insensitive to others. Adolescents are expected:

- To learn and act in accordance with the values of our culture and society.
- To accept parental authority.
- To cooperate with their parents in protecting themselves from danger and in meeting their own physical, emotional and educational needs.
- To be loyal to their families.
- To perform appropriate family tasks and care for their material possessions.

All of these expectations of adolescents presume that their own parents are competently fulfilling the responsibilities of parenthood.

DEFINING COMPETENT PARENTS

Because we all fall short of our ideal images, most parents harbor doubts about their own competence. Our initial reaction to even the mention of competent parents might be to define ourselves as incompetent. This reaction creates a reluctance to deal objectively with parental incompetence, since to do so might adversely judge most parents. This reaction is unjustified because the vast majority of parents are competent.

Competent parents simply are people committed to parenthood. Their behavior shows they care about what happens to their children. They can restrain themselves from harming them. They do not neglect or abuse their children in a legal sense.

The definition of competent parents flows from our cultural expectations of parents. Competent parents are capable of assuming responsibility for their own lives, sacrificing some of their own interests for their children, providing limits for their children's behavior, and giving their children hope for the future. They have access to essential economic and educational childrearing resources.

Just as there are essential dietary elements for physical growth—vitamins, minerals, and proteins—there are essential experiences for healthy personality growth. Competent parents provide these experiences so their children can learn to delay gratifying their immediate urges, tolerate frustration, work and avoid harming others.

Children acquire these skills and values essential for success in our society through the influence of parents who possess these qualities. This does not mean that competent parents are socially conforming persons who raise conforming children who become conforming adults. Our democratic republic depends upon parents who initiate changes as well. Our way of life depends upon diversity in opinions and life styles.

Wealth does not ensure being a competent parent nor does poverty ensure being an incompetent parent. The empirical fact is that children raised by competent parents—including the handicapped and poor—seldom become criminals and or welfare dependent.

DEFINING INCOMPETENT PARENTS

A child's congenital handicaps and the lack of socioeconomic resources make parenthood a stressful experience for anyone. But incompetent parents are unable to handle responsibility for their own lives, much less for their children's lives. They have difficulty restraining themselves from harming their children. Their incompetence as parents can be due to immaturity or to personality, developmental or mental disorders. Most minimize or deny their incompetence. Even with support and treatment, many are unable to change in time to become competent parents for their own children. They are "unfit" parents in legal terms.

Because incompetent parents have difficulty controlling their own impulses, they are vulnerable to substance abuse and alcoholism. They are insensitive to the needs of others and are unreliable. They do not form dependable attachment bonds with their children. They mishandle the routine behaviors of children. They alternately neglect or overreact to their children's behavior with unpredictable and inconsistent sequences of indifference, idle threats and severe punishment. Their children are confused when what happens to them seems to bear little relationship to what they do. Their children's erratic behaviors aggravate their inconsistent childrearing practices. As a result their children lack sensitivity to the needs of other people and behave unpredictably as do their parents. Their children often become adults who do not control their impulses and who do not care about the effects of their behavior on other people.

The signs of incompetent parents are a lack of affectionate bonding between parents and their children; unpredictable and inconsistent reactions to their children's behavior; and a lack of involvement in the lives of their children in their communities.[13] These signs of incompetent parenting do not require subtle techniques or tests to detect. No unbiased person who has access to full information about a particular situation would have difficulty concluding that a particular parent is incompetent.

At any one time, about 4% of all parents are incompetent as conservatively inferred from reported child neglect and abuse cases.[14] This breaks down to 8% of one-parent and 3% of two-parent homes. Although small in percentage, the number is significant — almost 3 million. At least twice as many have not been identified as incompetent. Most people do not appreciate the enormous impact this comparatively small number of parents has on our society.

Neglect by incompetent parents is more harmful to children than physical abuse because it deprives children of the opportunity to develop the social skills they need to become responsible human beings. When children have prenatal or natal brain damage, the development of affectionate attachment bonds between those children and marginally incompetent parents is unlikely. In contrast, children who are abused but not neglected must cope with frightening experiences, but they may be able to relate to other people effectively and thereby acquire the social skills necessary for productive citizenship.

An example of the damage caused by parental neglect is evident in developmentally delayed babies who show "failure to thrive" because of the lack of affectionate attachment bonds with their parents. These babies do not feed properly and suffer from delays in their physical, social and cognitive development.

Parents also can be regarded as incompetent by default when they have not assumed the role of parenthood and are uninvolved in their children's lives.

The lack of preventive capabilities and the inability of child welfare services to therapeutically intervene with their families before children are damaged by neglect or abuse too often results in situations like the following:

Mary

Mary was born to a sixteen-year-old alcoholic mother, who subsisted on Aid to the Families of Dependent Children and divorced twice before Mary was first brought to the attention of child welfare services at the age of 3 because of repeated allegations of parental neglect.

At the age of 9, Mary began to be sexually abused by an older brother. When she was 10, she was placed in a special class for the emotionally disturbed. When 13, she was brought to juvenile court because of alcohol and substance abuse and a year later placed in a county juvenile home. Her destructive behavior led to subsequent placement in two adolescent treatment centers.

When 15, Mary was sent to a state correctional facility and thereafter to a state mental hospital. After her release at 18, her first child was born. She subsequently was married and divorced three times. Her second child was born when she was 20. When her children were 2- and 4-years-old, child welfare services intervened and placed the children in foster homes. Mary entered two alcohol and substance abuse treatment centers and did not complete treatment. She was arrested several times for drinking while driving, once in a near-fatal accident, and later for the sale of illegal drugs. She sought and obtained the return of her children after serving three months in jail. Within two months Mary resumed drinking. Her children were placed again in foster care at the ages of 4 and 6. By that time their behavior problems necessitated psychiatric treatment. When 25, Mary was sentenced to prison because of drug dealing. Her parental rights to her children were finally terminated, and they were placed in adoptive homes where they continued in psychiatric treatment and special education.

BethAnne

BethAnne was a 16-year-old bipolar child sexual abuse victim and crack-addicted prostitute with a pattern of threatening to kill her mental health worker. Child welfare services did not intervene until months after she left her baby with an ex-boyfriend's sister and an attempted murder charge was made against her.

These examples highlight the following facts. The capacity to procreate precedes the capacity to be responsible for one's own life. Too many parents do not make sacrifices for their children. Too many parents do not help their children learn self-discipline. Too many parents do not have hope for their own futures. Too many parents do not have the resources they need to rear their children.

We must recognize that not all persons who conceive and give birth to children are capable of being competent parents. When they are overwhelmed by the responsibilities of parenthood, help should be available for them. Identifying incompetent parents before they damage their children needs to be a high priority for our society. Those who cannot be competent parents need relief from the responsibilities of parenthood by expeditiously terminating their parental rights and adoption. Our society has a vital interest in ensuring that children have competent parents.

Adolescent parents need double protection from the incompetence of their own parents and from being incompetent parents themselves.

Society's most appropriate and cost-effective role is to support motherhood and fatherhood, rather than expect schools and childcare to take over parenting functions.

MOTHERHOOD

Women's labor force patterns have changed dramatically over the last twenty years. Many more mothers work both full-time and part-time. The wage gap between men and women has narrowed over the last few decades, but one study showed that it persists.[15] Mothers earn about $1.50 an hour less than childless women. If they continue to be largely responsible for childrearing, mothers will not be able to catch up to the wages of childless women or their male counterparts. Since the majority of women have children, this penalty continues to contribute to inequality in the workplace.

According to Syliva Ann Hewlett of the Centre for Work-Life Policy, 37% of all professional women leave employment at some point.[16] Even more have flexible schedules. Only 40% of those who return to employment find full-time jobs, usually with loss of earnings.

FATHERHOOD

Fatherhood varies more widely than motherhood. Fathers range from being the only parents to being totally absent from children's lives.[17] The division of labor by gender in domestic and breadwinning responsibilities is giving way to sharing them.

Fathers are involved with their children in three ways:[18]

- Living with their children.
- Responsible for their children's care regardless of physical proximity.
- Visitation with their children.

Of the estimated 5.5 million at-home parents in the United States, some 100,000 are fathers.[19] At-home fathers tend to be older than at-home mothers and are likely to perform paid work at home.

A University of Michigan Institute of Social Research study revealed that about half of all children do not live with their biological fathers at some point before adulthood.[20] Of the men who lived with their children's mothers at the time their children were born, 28% moved away at some point during a 30-year period. Men who cohabited with their children's mother were more than twice as likely as men who were married to live apart from their children. Forty-one percent of Black fathers do not live with their children compared to 24% of White fathers.

ESTABLISHING PATERNITY

The current prominence of establishing paternity symbolizes the vulnerability of parenthood in our society in which over one-third of all babies are born to unmarried parents.[21] To ensure that these babies obtain the support of both parents, federal policies encourage establishing paternity as soon as possible to increase the likelihood that the baby will have a lasting relationship with the father and that child support will be paid.

There are three ways to establish paternity: 1) marriage, 2) voluntary paternity acknowledgment and 3) either parent can file a law suit to establish the baby's paternity. According to one study, males who claim their paternity are right 96% of the time. Those who insist they are not fathers are wrong 70% of the time.[22]

Traditional paternity law relates support obligations solely to genetic connections.[23] Men with no intent to enter parenthood can be held for child support. In 1993, Congress required states to offer programs to establish children's paternity at birth. In 1996, Congress strengthened the contested paternity process. More recently, efforts have been made to encourage unmarried parents to consider marrying.

Almost 150,000 babies are born each year to unwed parents at least one of whom is a minor. As minors, they are not free to marry or bring a paternity suit without the permission of their parents.[24] In many states, boys must obtain their parent's permission to voluntarily acknowledge paternity. Adolescent mothers must provide information to locate the other parent in order to obtain Temporary Assistance to Needy Families and child support. Adolescent parents may be forced to choose between entitlement benefits or risk their safety, or their children's safety, by giving information that could reveal the current location of abusive partners.

As of 2005, six states enacted the Uniform Parentage Act. Other states vary in procedures for establishing parentage by presumption, genetic testing and voluntary acknowledgement.[25] Some fathers want to acknowledge paternity and exercise decision-making privileges. Others want to evade child support payments. Jurisdictions vary widely in paternity establishment rates and in child support awards.

Instead of setting unrealistic child support obligations, we should invest more effort in trying to find the father before childbirth, require him to participate in the paternity proceedings, set reasonable child support levels and encourage him to establish a relationship with his child.[26]

UNWANTED CHILDREN

Ideally, parenthood should be voluntarily assumed. Unwanted children pose burdens for their parents but also are at risk for physical, emotional and developmental damage. Swedish and Czechoslovakian studies revealed that children born to mothers who were denied pregnancy terminations showed long-term adverse psychological, emotional and social effects.[27] Much of the drop in crime in the 1990s was due to *Rowe v. Wade* in 1973. Millions of unwanted children simply were not born.[28] This does not imply support for pregnancy termination as a method of birth control. It does highlight the importance of preventing pregnancies or arranging for the adoption of unwanted children because of the hazards to the children and to their mothers who are not motivated or able to raise them.

CONCLUSION

Our society's presumption that all genetic parents are competent until they damage children by neglect or abuse denigrates parenthood. It implies that there are no proactive expectations of parents as we generally have for actions that affect other persons.

Anyone past puberty can be a parent in our society. But being a parent says nothing about the quality of childrearing. To enter parenthood is to make a lifelong commitment to a son or a daughter. Only competent parents are able to handle the responsibilities of parenthood.

Parenthood is the career that benefits everyone. Without progeny who become law-abiding citizens, our society cannot survive. Without productive consumers, our economy cannot prosper. In the long run parenthood is more important to our society than paid vocations.

We need to recognize that "work" is defined in our capitalistic economy as a paid activity. Unpaid activity like childrearing is not regarded as work. This obscures the fact that childrearing is work and has immense financial value for our economy.

From society's point of view, parents have an obligation to raise competent citizens or at least to not produce people who are dangerous to, or burdens for, others. This means that parents need help to be competent whenever possible. Society's most appropriate and cost-effective role is to define and support our cultural expectations of parenthood, rather than to have childcare and schools take over parenting functions.

Children prick our consciences. They painfully remind us that we are their flawed models, but they also evoke our highest ideals. Although inevitable conflicts exist between the interests of older and younger generations, it seems clear that the American cultural will is to promote competent parenthood. We need to recognize parenthood as a life-long career.

Chapter 4

Divergent Parenthood Styles

A woman is not married before eighteen, nor a man before twenty-two. If a man (or woman) is convicted of an illicit affair before marriage, he is severely punished and marriage is denied him for his whole life, unless a prince remits the punishment. The master and the mistress of the household in which the offense has occurred are in disgrace for having been remiss in their duty. The reason for punishing this offense so severely is the fear that few would unite in married love, to spend their whole lives with one person and put up with the annoyances of marriage, unless they were rigorously restrained from promiscuity.

Thomas More *Utopia*, 1551.[1]

Adolescents' motives to become parents are strongly influenced by the way society views parenthood. When parenthood generally referred to one of two married adults, single parenthood resulted from the death or divorce of a parent. Adolescent parenthood was not formally recognized then. In recent decades, parenthood has been increasingly defined by choice without regard to age. Personal choice has replaced cultural traditions in defining parenthood styles.

Although it may not seem so at first, words used to describe contemporary families are important. There are two-parent homes with and without marriage. When there is a nonresident parent, a family can be located in two homes. When a mother and father live separately, "single parent family" does not accurately define either home, which actually is a "one parent" home. Each of these styles can be with or without genetic parents. No wonder the word parenthood is confusing for children, parents and researchers.

This chapter reviews the literature on the various styles of parenthood. It illustrates why simply being a parent does not mean that one is living the life style of parenthood. Many parents are not actively involved in their offsprings' lives and have not entered the career of parenthood.

Marriage is the traditional arrangement for parenthood.

MARRIAGE

Marriage has been the most important marker of adulthood and respectability as well as a route to benefits, such as social security, health and unemployment insurance. Stephanie Coontz, professor of history and family studies at Evergreen State College, points out that married people are generally happier, healthier and better protected against economic setbacks and emotional problems than people in other living arrangements.[2] Some of these attributes may be because people already socially skilled, economically self-sufficient, healthy and emotionally stable are more likely to get and stay married than those with fewer of these qualities.

Marriage as a Social Institution

Marriage is not universal in human societies. The Na society in southeastern China has no husbands. Sexual affairs are casual and usually private. The partners owe each other nothing. Households are sibling-based with strong incest taboos.[3]

Still marriage is a vitally important human invention. Coontz's study of marriage reveals that for most of human history marriage was not a relationship based on mutual love. It was used to acquire wealth, power and property. One of its crucial functions was to forge cooperative networks beyond the immediate family or local tribe.[4]

Our ancestors understood that marriage was an economic and political institution with rigid rules.[5] For most of recorded history, it required women to suffer in silence when their hopes for love inside marriage were thwarted. Men sought sex outside of marriage. A man who fathered a child out of wedlock was seldom responsible for support of that child. An unwed woman who bore a child often could survive only by becoming a concubine or prostitute.[6]

As people began to expect romance and intimacy in their marriages, their unions became more fragile. No sooner did the idea of marrying for love take hold than the right to divorce if love died emerged. As the quality of a marital relationship became more important than the reproductive function of marriage, the committed love of two unmarried persons, including those of the same sex, ultimately came to be seen as deserving the same status as traditional marriage.[7]

Divergent parenthood styles have always existed in the Western world, but the traditional sequence has been marriage, mortgage and children in that order.[8] As families were expected to nurture children rather than exploit them as laborers, the social and legal consequences of "illegitimacy" for children were seen as inhumane. Marriage came to be seen as supporting middle-class values of foresight and self-sufficiency. It organized fathers and mothers around nurturing their children's development.

Decisions about marriage and parenthood style now are made by the individuals involved, not by extended families or tradition.[9] People tend to marry with the intent of finding a spouse who will make them happy. If that does not happen, they believe they chose the wrong partner. In a no-fault ethos, courts no longer need to find justification for a divorce. Individuals can divorce without a spouse's consent. Marriage has become a wager two people enter because of sexual attraction and personal friendship.

The wager is that if things do not work out, the bet is lost, and each party is free to end the relationship. The message seems to be that there is no reason to prefer one life style over another for childrearing, as revealed in the sentiment expressed by Nobel Laureate Toni Morrison in a Time magazine interview:[10]

> The little nuclear family is a paradigm that just doesn't work. It doesn't work for white or black people. Why we are hanging on to it, I don't know.

Paula Ettelbrick, Executive Director of the International Gay and Lesbian Human Rights Commission, put it this way:[11]

> Marriage of all institutions is to the liberationists a form of imprisonment; it reeks of a discourse that has bought and sold property, that has denigrated and subjected women, that has constructed human relationships into a crude and suffocating form.

The Supreme Judicial Court of Massachusetts in 2002 explicitly considered and then rejected the view that marriage is centrally concerned with bearing and raising children:[12] "the Commonwealth affirmatively facilitates bringing children into a family regardless of whether the intended parent is married or unmarried, whether the child is adopted or born into a family, whether assisted technology was used to conceive the child, and whether the parent or her partner is heterosexual, homosexual, or bisexual." This view separates marriage and procreation.

Others see modern families as regressing to the informal norms of tribal societies.[13] They hope to revitalize marriage as a way to regulate sexuality, legitimize children, organize the division of labor between men and women and redistribute resources to dependents.

For college-educated Americans, the motivation to marry appears to have grown stronger in recent years. For others, marriage continues to be unappealing. David Popenoe, founder of the National Marriage Project, believes that the "marriage gap" is generating a society of greater inequality.[14] America is becoming a nation divided not only by unequal education and income levels but by unequal family structures. Kay Hymowitz, Manhattan Institute fellow, posits that the separation of marriage from childrearing threatens to turn what the founders imagined as an opportunity-rich republic of equal citizens into a hereditary caste society with a married affluent class and an unmarried poor class.[15]

The current debate about marriage boils down to whether or not marriage is the optimal context for childrearing. Despite the advantages of a single life, the desire for children and adult companionship is a strong human force.

Marriage Statistics

One in five adults do not marry. Many who marry do not have an interest in parenthood. Fortunately, neither the survival of the species nor the fulfillment of individuals depends upon every person becoming a parent.

In 2003, 68% of homes with children were headed by married couples; 26% by mothers, and 6% by fathers.[16] In 2005, 51% of all households contained married couples with and without children.[17] 46% of all households included children; 29% consisted of married couples with children and 17% consisted of one-parent or unmarried couples, comprising 40% of all households with children.

Individuals are marrying later, divorcing more frequently and cohabiting more often. The median age at first marriage in the United States in 2003 was 27 and 25 for men and women respectively.[18] The marriage age for men and women was higher than the national averages in the Northeast. The divorce rate has been falling continuously over the past quarter-century. It peaked at 23/1,000 married couples in 1979 and fell to 17 by 2005. While marriage rates are also declining, those marriages that do occur are increasingly more stable. Fifty-three percent of couples who married from 1975 to 1979 reached their silver anniversary. In the United States, Russia and Scandinavia most divorces are likely to happen between five and 10 years into a marriage. Couples who marry young and those living in urban areas are more likely to divorce.[19]

Fewer families fit the traditional image of two married parents living with their own genetic children. Twenty-one percent of married couples and 59% of unmarried couples have children from more than one relationship.[20] Eight percent of births each year are to adolescent mothers with Southern states having higher and Northeastern states lower percentages.

In 2000–2003, 23% of all mothers with a birth in the previous year were below the poverty level as were 12% of all married mothers and 50% of all unmarried mothers. In 2005, 50% of all married mothers were employed full time and 17% part time.[21] 69% of single mothers were employed full time and 19% part time.

In 2005, 37% of all births were to unmarried girls and women (18% one-parent and 19% cohabiting) and 63% to married couples.[22] The U.S. Marriage Index that measures the integrity of marriage as a social institution dropped from 78 in 1970 to 63 in 2000.[23]

Attitudes toward Marriage

A 2007 Pew survey found that Americans of all ages believe that the link between marriage and parenthood has weakened.[24] Just 41% of Americans said that children are "very important" to a successful marriage, down from 65% in 1990. Children have fallen to eighth of nine on a list of items people associate with successful marriages — well behind "sharing household chores, good housing, adequate income, happy sexual relationship and faithfulness."

On the other hand, the Michigan Study of Adolescent Life Transitions revealed that despite greater acceptance since the 1960s of divorce, premarital sex and nonmarital cohabitation, positive attitudes toward marriage and parenthood remain strong among high school seniors.[25] Eighty-eight percent of males and 83% of females said it was quite or extremely important to have a good marriage and family life. Seventy-five percent of college freshmen in 2003 named raising a family as an important life goal, compared to 59% in 1977. However, only 1 in 1,000 chose "full-time homemaker" as their probable career.[26] Almost 70% of adolescent boys and 54% of girls agreed that: It is better for a person to get married than to go through life being single and that divorce is not the best solution to marital problems.[27]

In a National Marriage Project survey men expressed a desire to marry but were in no hurry to do so.[28] They:

- can get sex without marriage more easily than in the past;
- can have a companion by cohabiting rather than marrying;
- want to avoid divorce and its financial risks;
- are waiting for the perfect "soul mate;"
- face few social pressures to marry;
- are reluctant to marry a woman who already has children; and
- want to own a house before marrying.

More than half of the young men surveyed reported changing jobs and having a variety of living arrangements, including returning to their parents' homes. Friends were their stable attachments.

The Relative Value of Marriage

The idea of *relative value* explains how people can value marriage and yet act to the contrary. Our values compete with each other. Lawrence Bumpass, professor of sociology at the University of Wisconsin, attributes changes in family to a combination of *individualism* and the *market economy*.[29] Individualism creates a climate in which the attractiveness of childrearing is diminished. Our market economy encourages people to produce and consume—values that compete with parenthood. As one 28-year-old mother put it:

> I have to put my baby in day care now so I can work and afford to buy a home so that, when he is ready to enter school, we will be in the best school district.

A consequence of these competing values is a diminished willingness to make long-term commitments. As a result, children from unstable families tend to form unstable families.

In recent decades, public policies in the United States have avoided showing a preference for family structures. There has been little emphasis on the benefits of marriage or on the social and economic contributions of parents devoted to childrearing. As low-income men and women grow older, the chances they will have children with more than one partner increase substantially. A woman or man with children may not be a good marital prospect.

Adolescent Parenthood and Marriage

Despite a nearly one-third decline over the past decade in adolescent pregnancy and birth rates in the United States:[30]

- 60% of all girls ages 15–17 and 73% of ages 18–19 approve of unwed childbearing.
- Half of all first unwed births are to adolescents.

- Within one year of childbirth, 8% of adolescent mothers marry the genetic fathers.
- Only 30% of adolescent mothers who marry are still in that marriage at 40.

Public Welfare Marriage Policies

Until the late 1990s, public welfare policies tended to discourage marriage. Whether or not government should promote marriage is controversial now.

The Personal Responsibility and Work Opportunity Reconciliation Act of 1996 strove to end discrimination against married parents. However, Irwin Garfinkel, professor of urban problems at Columbia University, points out that single-parent families continue to get preference indirectly through the priority given to Temporary Assistance for Needy Families (TANF) and ex-TANF recipients for childcare subsidy programs.[31] One analysis found that over half of unmarried parents would lose their poverty-based benefits if they married.[32] Restrictions against ex-offenders in public housing also favor one-parent homes.

Emphasis on the employment of mothers can create disincentives for parents to care for their own children.[33] It is less expensive for mothers to raise their own babies during the first 6–12 months of life than to pay for childcare. Yet mothers may be required to work when their babies reach 6 weeks of age, threatening the breastfeeding and attachment bonding of poor children.

Wendy Sigle-Rushton, an associate at the London School of Economics and Political Science, and Sara McLanahan, professor of sociology and public affairs at Princeton University, assert that public policies should not penalize marriage.[34] Neither should they provide financial incentives to marry, especially if this would penalize the children of unmarried parents.

Policies that promote marriage as the best option for young parents can have unintended effects for partners who have experienced abuse, especially among TANF populations where its prevalence among adolescent parents is high.[35] When adolescents want to marry, they need help developing the knowledge and skills needed to sustain a marriage and delay another pregnancy.

No marriage can survive the ravages of domestic abuse, infidelity, alcoholism, drug addiction or repeated incarceration. Given the prevalence of these problems in the low-income population, promoting marriage will do more harm than good unless policy makers find a way to make low-income men better prospects for long-term relationships with women and children.[36] Marriage is difficult to sustain when more than half of mothers who leave welfare remain poor. Many value having children more than waiting for a "Mr. Right" for the following reasons:[37]

- They do not have enough money for a proper wedding.
- They cannot rely on a partner to settle down and provide support.
- Offspring from previous relationships disrupt current relationships.

Paradoxically in choosing unwed motherhood over marriage, adolescents also may be responding to cultural values that discourage early marriage.[38] The vast majority of adolescents want to marry some day, so emphasizing how childbearing dramatically reduces the chances of marriage may encourage avoiding pregnancy.

Unfortunately, the conservative right advocates marriage and the liberal left advocates family diversity. They cannot agree on polices that achieve both ends. The evidence indicates that helping all mothers and fathers—married and unmarried—to nurture their children is likely to have the highest payoff in producing stable families.[39]

Reducing unwed childbearing rates is a daunting task in the face of deeply held attitudes about having children and marriage. Marriage programs have little impact without an array of other resources.[40] Millions of children will continue to live in one-parent homes.

ONE-PARENT HOMES

Until the first part of the 20th century, one-parent homes were largely the result of the death of a spouse.[41] In the 1960s, most followed divorce when 80% of the public agreed that "a couple should stay together." By the 1980s, agreement with that statement dropped to 50%. Parents now feel less obliged to stay together for the sake of their children. Parental separation usually is painful for children but so is relentless conflict between their parents.

Currently, most parents are not single by death or divorce. According to the National Center for Health Statistics, the number of babies born to unwed women in their thirties and forties rose by 290% from 1980 to 2002.[42] Half of all children born in the United States will live in one-parent homes, primarily female-headed, at some point during their lives. More than half of those will live in poverty at least for a time and continue the cycle of family disadvantage. In 2003, 26% of homes with children were headed by mothers and 6% by fathers.[43]

During the past forty years, the greater financial independence of women contributed to the increase in one-parent homes encouraged by:[44] 1) the decline in family size, 2) the increase in divorce rates, 3) expansion of the service sector where most women are employed, 4) an increase in the women's earnings of women and 5) civil rights legislation. These trends improved both the occupations and earnings of women. As one-parent homes rose, crime rates went down and educational rates went up. Poor single mothers were committed to work and childrearing goals.[45]

The social policies of nations influence the well-being of children in one-parent homes.[46] Countries with low single-mother poverty rates have a combination of child allowances, guaranteed child support, unemployment assistance and housing allowances for low income families that benefit both one- and two-parent homes.

National policies regarding childbirth play an important role in family structures. In European countries with low birth rates, childbearing is encouraged. Russian mothers receive cash bonuses for giving birth, as well as child allowances and childcare subsidies.[47]

Without running an impossible experiment in which children were randomly assigned to different kinds of families, we do not know how children in one-parent homes would have fared if they had lived with two genetic parents. Most parents in one-parent homes raise their children successfully, however, their children have more problems than those raised in two-parent homes.

COMPARING OUTCOMES FOR CHILDREN LIVING IN ONE-PARENT AND TWO-PARENT HOMES

The majority of scholars believe that family structure matters for children.[48] One-parent homes are associated with a host of problems, especially if the parents are uneducated and unemployed.[49] Poverty forces mothers to rear their children in neighborhoods with high rates of unemployment, school dropouts, adolescent pregnancy and crime.

Kevin Lang, professor of economics at Boston University, and Jay Zagorsky, professor of economics at Ohio State University, found little evidence that one-parent homes caused by death affects children's economic well-being in adulthood.[50] However, a mother's death may reduce a girl's cognitive performance, and a father's death may lower a son's chances of marriage.

School Performance

Children who live in one-parent homes have lower academic achievement than those in two-parent homes.[51] Controlling for age, gender and grade level, secondary school students living in one-parent homes score lower on mathematics and science tests than children living in two-parent homes. Children in step-parent homes score somewhat higher than children in one-parent homes, but children who live with two genetic parents score the highest. Those who live with their mother and an unmarried partner score the lowest.

Children living with both genetic parents remain in school longer than children in one-parent homes. One study found that of children who completed the eighth grade, high school graduation rates were 90% for those in two genetic-parent homes, 75% for those in divorced-mother homes and 69% for those in unwed-mother homes.[52] Children with absent fathers are more likely to drop out of school than children who live with their fathers. In one study, 71% of children who lived with two genetic parents went to college compared to 50% of children living only with their mothers. Each additional year spent with a single mother reduces a child's educational attainment by half a year as does time spent in step-parent families.

Unwed Childbirth

Children who spend part of their childhood in a single-mother home are twice as likely to have sex at an early age than children who live with both genetic parents.[53] Daughters from single-mother homes also begin marital and non-marital childbearing at a younger age.

Whereas girls from two-parent homes have a 6% chance of having a child outside marriage by the age of 20, girls from single-mother divorced or unwed families have

11% and 14% chances respectively. Girls in stepfamilies have a 16% chance of unwed childbirth.[54]

Occupational Status

Growing up in a single-mother home and adult income are strongly linked.[55] In one study, children from high occupational status homes were less likely to be in high status occupations themselves if they came from a single-mother home. In another study, adults from single-mother homes were more likely to be unemployed and on welfare than those from two-parent homes.

Using occupational status as a measure of economic success, one study found that women who lived with both genetic parents at the age of 16 had significantly higher occupational status as adults than their counterparts who were living in other family styles.[56] Another study found that compared to children who grew up with both genetic parents, children who were raised apart from one of their parents earned $5,015 less in 2000.

Behavior Problems

Children in one-parent homes tend to be more immature and impulsive than those in two married-parent homes.[57] They are 72% more likely to show "at-risk" behaviors. The rates of domestic abuse also are higher among young than older single parents.

In a Baltimore study, 15–20% of all first grade students were seen as needing improvement in conduct, as compared with 30% of children living in one-parent homes.[58] A review of twenty three studies disclosed that all but three found that adolescents in one-parent and remarried homes were at higher risk for delinquency than those in married parent homes.[59]

Adults from single-mother homes report less self-respect and higher use of mental health services than adults from two-parent homes.[60]

SINGLE-PARENT FAMILIES BY CHOICE

Feminism as a movement to end sexist exploitation and oppression has empowered many women to choose sexual preference, marry or remain single, become a parent, pursue education and a career or combine these options.[61]

The organization *Single Mothers by Choice* is a support network for single women to have children without a relationship with a man.[62] Three quarters conceive with donor sperm. A single mother by choice typically is a career woman in her thirties or forties who decided to give birth or adopt a child, knowing she would be her child's sole parent at the outset. Her biological clock made her face the fact that she could no longer wait for marriage before starting a family. She became pregnant accidentally or from donor insemination, or she adopted a child. She seeks men as out-of-home social capital for her child.

FATHER ABSENCE

While over 90% of American children live with their genetic mothers at some time over the course of their childhoods, only about 50% live with their genetic fathers.[63] Children who do not live with their genetic fathers often are disadvantaged because of low income and poor relationships between and with their parents.[64]

Behavioral Effects of Father Absence

Although analyses of one-parent home outcomes include its effects, father absence has been specifically studied as well. A meta-analysis of the literature on father absence by the Princeton Center for Research on Child Wellbeing found lower levels of behavioral problems in adolescents living with their married genetic parents than with all other family styles.[65]

Growing up without two parents supporting each other are significant contributors to drug abuse and delinquency, especially when accompanied by poverty.[66] When fathers are absent, children may be less well monitored because their mothers need to work longer hours.

Children who live apart from their genetic fathers are more likely to use illegal substances and to be arrested.[67] Children below the age of 15 who live in a household without a father are 70% more likely to commit crimes and 28% more likely to use marijuana than children who live with both genetic parents. Children living apart from their genetic fathers are 19% more likely to smoke cigarettes than other children.

Children with behavior problems could well push fathers away, and children who are well behaved could draw them in.[68] But the behavior of parents likely has a greater effect on children than the behavior of children has on parents. Still, if fathers became more involved, their children's behavior problems may not decrease.

While children of divorced parents have more adjustment problems than do children of never-divorced parents, the divorce in itself may not be the cause.[69] Many of the problems seen in children of divorce can be accounted for by experiences in the years preceding divorce, such as marital conflict, violence and incompetent parenting.

When non-resident fathers maintain a high-quality relationship with their children some of the negative consequences of father absence can be attenuated. There is current interest in using social policy to strengthen the involvement of fathers with their families.[70]

Impact on Girls

When fathers are absent, girls lack opportunities to learn how to relate to males. A father-daughter relationship sets the stage for a girl's future romantic choices, shapes her sexuality and her sense of herself as a woman.[71] Developing an affectionate attachment with her father is an important experience as a girl works through the Electra complex in which she fantasies marrying her father and displacing her mother. By working through this process in actual experience with a father in her home, she comes to terms with the impracticality of this fantasy.

Without a father's dependable involvement in her life a girl lacks the modeling of adult male-female relationships and a tangible model of masculinity. Daughters need father figures who can be counted on, whether divorced or at home.[72] When they do not receive the attention and affection they desire from a father, they may seek such support elsewhere, predisposing them to early and unstable relationships with males. This is compounded when mothers are depressed. The following was written by 13-year-old Crystal for the National Center for Fathering:[73]

> I see my father a lot in my dreams but never does he turn around. I call for him, but he's just walking away. Every time I blow out the candles on my birthday cake, I wish that stranger would turn around and look at me. Maybe if he saw all the pain and suffering from living without him in my eyes, he would become a part of my life.

At the same time, if the relationship between father and daughter is too strong, a father may become the admired male in her life and fulfill the Electra fantasy in which she becomes his primary love.[74] When an incestuous relationship occurs, a girl suffers the consequences of sexual abuse, and her later life as a wife and a mother is adversely affected.

Impact on Boys

When boys have not formed solid identifications with their fathers, they may have emotional and behavioral problems that lead them to seek their absent fathers.[75] Understanding why they do so can help them become mature men. Acknowledging their own dependence on a father enables them to accept the dependence of others on them.

Sons and daughters abandoned by their fathers may blame themselves.[76] They may have difficulty developing and sustaining self-respect, forming lasting emotional attachments, recognizing their feelings and expressing themselves with their adult partners and children. They may focus on their fathers' faults to deny their need for a father. One boy said he could prove he did not need his father—before taking any action he would imagine what his father would do and do the opposite. He proclaimed: "I don't need anyone." Another boy on the verge of tears described his feelings about his absent father:[77]

> If my dad was still around, I wouldn't do so much dumb stuff. I'm pretty sure I'd be a good student. I'd have friends that were better for me. When I turn into a dad, I'm going to be different from my dad.

A boy's first identifies with his mother.[78] When a father is not available, he has difficulty resolving the Oedipal complex in which he fantasies marrying his mother and displacing his father. He cannot readily shift his identification from his mother to his father. This can lead to guilt over unresolved fantasies about his mother and repression of his masculinity.

On the other hand, many boys grow up successfully without fathers contradicting the stereotype that a boy inevitably suffers if raised without a man in the home. Peggy Drexler, a journalist, interviewed a group of "maverick moms"—relatively affluent and highly educated lesbians and single mothers by choice who were raising sons without fathers in San Francisco.[79] She found that the boys were socially savvy and generous, while passionate about sports and rough-housing with friends. The families she interviewed were on the fringe of society. Teachers did not accept their sons' drawings of their families, and peers teased them. Drexler sees these "maverick" moms as pioneering a new parenting style that rejects social judgments about family structure and gender stereotypes and stresses communication, community and love.

Father Fantasies

In their own minds, no boy or girl is without a father.[80] In the absence of fathers, they make up their own images. Even when disappointed or abused by their fathers, children may create images of loving fathers in order to bolster their own self-respect. Eleanor Roosevelt wrote about her love for her father in spite of his alcoholism and abandonment of her.[81]

When fathers are rarely or never seen, children depend on their mothers or other relatives for information about them. Boys and girls may feel that their fathers left home because they did not love them. One son put it this way: "A dad wouldn't leave a good kid, so it must have been my fault." If a mother speaks about an absent father realistically, a child is more likely to develop a positive father image. She may despise the father, but, if a father's problems can be understood, a child can develop a realistic image of a father. This also applies to absent mothers.

The Absent Father's Perspective

Absent fathers miss an important developmental experience themselves. Engaged fatherhood promotes a man's ability to understand himself, to empathically understand others and to integrate his feelings in intimate relationships with family members. Fathers are more likely to give back to their communities than childless men.[82]

The majority of absent fathers pay support and are in touch with their children.[83] Some may feel that mothers claim support for themselves, not their children. If mothers fail to accept or sustain father-child relationships, fathers can feel frustrated and victimized.

When fathers see themselves as victims whose rights are ignored, they become resistant and disengaged. Non-payment of child support can be seen as a father's defiance or a moral failing. A study of divorced, non-custodial "deadbeat fathers" revealed they agreed there were "bad" fathers but that meant persons other than themselves.[84] They accepted an obligation to contribute to their children's support, but deemed the amount or its terms to be unfair.

COHABITATION

Over the years, marriage has come to be seen less as an essential social institution for optimal childrearing and more as an intimate relationship between adults. This historic transition has taken place through piecemeal changes with little consideration of the social consequences of weakening the connection between marriage and childrearing.

The ethos of individualism has made unmarried cohabitation the life style of choice for many young people.[85] Formerly referred to as "shacking up" or "living in sin," cohabitation has become a common life style. In 1995, half of the women in their thirties had lived in a cohabiting relationship. Cohabitation usually functions as a substitute for being single, not for being married. Cohabitating couples are less likely than married couples to share and pool resources.

In 1994, two-thirds of the respondents under the age of thirty to the National Survey of Families and Households felt that unmarried sex, cohabitation and unmarried births were socially acceptable.[86] In 2001, 88% of young men and 93% of young women agreed that it is usually a good idea for a couple to live together before getting married in order to find out whether they really get along.[87] More than 50% of boys and girls now believe that having a child without being married is an acceptable lifestyle that does not affect anyone else.

Although children raised in stable, cohabiting-parent homes exhibit more behavior problems at age three than children raised in stable, married-parent homes, the difference appears to be largely due to differences in the background characteristics of the parents who choose cohabitation over marriage.[88] Once these personal factors are taken into account, children of cohabiting and married parents appear to be similar in terms of their behavioral problems. Children of cohabiting parents who marry after childbirth appear to be no better off than the children of cohabiting parents who remain unmarried.

On the one hand, these findings may be interpreted as indicating that marital unions are no more beneficial to children than cohabiting unions, as long as the union remains stable. On the other hand, marriages are more stable than cohabiting unions. In cohabiting families, children spend more time moving in and out of different family arrangements. The empirical fact that cohabitation does not ensure a stable marriage may be becoming more widely known.[89]

THE SCANDINAVIAN EXPERIENCE

Social progressives look to Scandinavia as a model for achieving family and child well-being.[90] If the United States would adopt Sweden or Norway's generous family benefits, they argue, we too could achieve similar low rates of child poverty, adolescent pregnancy and single parenthood. Social conservatives point to Sweden as a cautionary example of how generous social welfare policies weaken marriage and the family. But neither side tells the whole story.

Child poverty barely exists in Sweden, and adolescent birthrates are very low. Few babies are in daycare because mothers have one year of paid family leave following childbirth.[91] The Swedish marriage rate is one of the lowest in the world as divorce rates continue to rise for married couples. Sweden also leads the Western nations in cohabitation where breakups occur twice as frequently as in marriage.

The Swedish approach includes policies that many social conservatives would embrace, such as strict limits on abortion, a six-month waiting period before parents are allowed to divorce and a ban on *in vitro* fertilization for single women and on anonymous sperm donations. Both the United States and Sweden are among the developed nations with the lowest percentage of children growing up with both genetic parents. Despite these commonalities, the two societies are very different. Sweden is communitarian, ethnically homogeneous, socially cohesive and resolutely secular. America is individualistic, ethnically diverse and strongly religious.

Though Scandinavian family policies may be models for creating a more child and family-friendly society, we cannot simply adopt Scandinavian policies and achieve their results.

CONCLUSION

In the past, single parenthood usually resulted from the death of a parent or divorce. In recent decades, parenthood has been increasingly defined by choice and default. Single parenthood, cohabitation, divorce and remarriage have created a variety of parenthood styles.

Forty-six percent of the homes in the United States include children. Twenty-nine percent are married couples with children. Except for college-educated Americans, marriage continues to be less appealing. Individuals are marrying later and cohabiting more often than in the past.

Married people are generally happier, healthier and better protected against economic setbacks than people in any other living arrangements. Children living with both genetic parents attain higher education and income levels than children in one-parent homes.

We are on a trajectory in which one-half of all children will spend some time in one-parent homes. Most single parents raise their children successfully. However, one-parent homes are associated with poverty, dropping out of school, crime and welfare dependency—especially if parents are uneducated and unemployed. During the last decades of the 20th century, single mothers became political targets unfairly. Still, there is compelling evidence to show the benefit for children and society of having two involved parents even if they do not live together.

The stability of children's relationships with their parents is declining. Although children raised in stable, cohabiting-parent homes exhibit more behavior problems than children raised in stable, married-parent homes, the difference appears to be largely due to differences in the background characteristics of the parents who choose cohabitation over marriage.

There are strong currents operating against our integrative cultural values and scientific knowledge that affirm the need of children for the continuing love and nurturing of both parents for whom parenthood is their primary commitment. As the significance of marriage has declined, single parenthood by choice or necessity has become common. In this context, an adolescent girl who gives birth and does not marry the father no longer is a social misfit.

Chapter 5

Dysfunctional Social Policies and Services

Unless there also is a balance of economic power, the use of morality, reason, education, politics, and the law, in the end, will reinforce and serve the special interests of those with the most economic power.

Reinhold Niebuhr, 1932
Moral Man, Immoral Society[1]

Lust, greed and ambition often trump the common good. We pursue our own interests and prefer the status quo to change. But at times—when there is strong pressure to do so—we are guided by our "better natures" and try to address our social problems.[2]

Pressure to solve social problems usually comes when they are rising and lapses when they are waning. Downward trends in adolescent sexual behavior, pregnancy and childbirth tend to lull us into thinking we are effectively addressing these problems. In fact, these rates are much higher than in other developed countries and than we should tolerate in the United States. Most importantly, we do not recognize their connection to crime and welfare dependency.

The rebellion against tyranny that led to the Revolutionary War biased our political and legal systems toward protecting individual freedoms over common interests. Consequently, our political and legal systems make it easier for special interest groups to block action than to join others to solve our social problems. Similar forces block the effective delivery of resources that are fragmented into categories and are discontinuous.

FRAGMENTATION AND LACK OF CONTINUITY OF SERVICES

We break down social problems into categories. We crave the reassurance of labels. We see people as fitting into categories. This is easier than trying to understand their lives.

In the 20th century, a belief in objectivity and controlled experimentation created the social sciences so that scientific methods are now applied to social problems.[3] Specific problems are identified and the effects of specific interventions on them are measured. The separation of individuals into educational, mental health and social work diagnostic categories permits the illusion that problems have been identified and solutions found.[4] This belief that reductionistic interventions are consistent with prevailing living conditions has warped the social welfare field.

Just as science and higher education are divided into separate specialties, we approach each social problem as if is not connected with others. Because they do not address common underlying causes, separate, partial remedies often contribute to the very problems they are intended to solve. They pit advocates for each remedy against each other rather than foster cooperation between them.

Responses to social problems, such as poverty, child abuse, alcoholism, drug abuse and crime customarily separate an aspect of each problem as an entity unto itself, as if each one reflected a different cause requiring a different solution. Consequently, professionals concentrate on specific problems of individuals involved in each category, rather than on addressing the common underlying causes. Each problem area then competes with the others for attention and resources. As a result, remedial services and prevention programs focus on each social problem as if it is not related to the others. The status quo often is inadvertently maintained.

In this separate approach to each separate social problem, strengthening families and neighborhoods is replaced by service systems for each problem category. Personal relationships are replaced by professional services. "It's not my job" is a frequently heard response from providers of these categorized services.

The focus on specific problems shifts attention from the serious pursuit of greater social equality. Strengthening our families, neighborhoods, schools, communities and workforce would assure all Americans a similar, positive experience.[5] Good families produce good people. Good people create good families. Good neighborhoods support families. Good education produces skilled workers. Good employment creates self-sufficiency. Self-sufficiency produces good families. The sole focus on the specific problems of individuals has been detrimental for those who are poor, addicted, delinquent or mentally ill without thriving families, education or jobs.[6]

Because it emphasizes the technical skills of professionals, separating social problems into categories also shifts the responsibility for change from the recipients to the providers of services. It fosters the perception that professionals are the agents of change. This increases depending on professionals to intervene in individuals' lives. Accordingly, attention is diverted from individuals' responsibilities for their own actions and what they can do to help themselves and each other. Fragmented, discontinuous, ineffective and costly services result. However, the demand for all of these services does create jobs.

OUR SOCIETY'S NEED FOR PARENTAL INCOMPETENCE

The evolution of any complex society requires the development of ever more specialized competencies.[7] A farmer's competence in carpentry, plumbing and mechanics no longer is a viable model. Now competency in a service is based on the incompetency of one or hundreds or even thousands of other persons. Inevitably there is a point at which incompetence surpasses competence as the engine for economic growth. In a largely service-driven economy, incompetence is needed to provide employment. It increases the Gross Domestic Product.

Incompetent parents have given rise to millions of jobs in the social problem solving and crisis-responding systems, including law enforcement, education, social service, correction, court, mental health, health and prevention. All of these persons and their professions might feel threatened by reducing parental incompetence. In this context, inefficient systems protected from market forces that require accountability are "good for the economy." Thus, competent persons and incompetent persons are co-dependent.

Annother example of co-dependency occurs between industries and politicians in the relationship between products and cancer.[8] This was seen most notably with smoking in the 1998 Master Settlement Agreement between cigarette companies and state attorneys general. Because settlement payments to states depended on the solvency of the companies, states opposed high punitive damages. This kind of co-dependency is analogous to industries and politicians who question the importance of parental attachment bonding and breast feeding and promote rearing babies and young children in childcaring systems.

Incompetence also is sustained by the crisis-recoil nature of our political system that underlies our fragmented, discontinuous services.

THE POLITICAL CRISIS–RECOIL RESPONSE

When families and neighborhoods break down, the crisis–recoil response leads to public overreaction to the resulting crises followed by recoiling from their causes. This response adversely affects struggling families.[9]

The crisis-recoil response results in calling attention to social problems when rates are rising and disregarding them when rates are decreasing even though the problems remain significant. This is currently seen in the assumption that decreasing adolescent birth rates means they no longer merit special attention even if the numbers of babies born to adolescents increases because there are more adolescents.

Child Protection Policies

The crisis–recoil response is seen most clearly in removing neglected and abused children from their homes rather than strengthening their families.[10] The inevitable crisis in the availability of foster homes leads to seeking more foster homes and increasing foster care payments rather than addressing the family problems that necessitated so many foster homes in the first place.

Beneath these practices lies the failure of public policies to recognize that a child is not a free-standing person. A child is a part of a two-person, parent-child unit that depends on the integrity of the mediating structures of a family, a neighborhood, a school and a community. As a result, services that focus on individual children and that fragment families have been overdeveloped, and resources that strengthen families and build communities have been underdeveloped.

Child welfare services address a genuine need, however, practices that focus primarily on children often are ineffective and can be harmful. A child's death can result from refraining to remove a child from a violent family, but unnecessary removal of children from their homes breaks up families. Both extremes receive publicity and provoke calls for reforming the existing system. As a result, social service agencies under the direction of juvenile courts swing back and forth between "child safety" and "family preservation" policies. In either case, agencies overwhelmed by their caseloads have difficulty distinguishing between families that can and cannot respond to treatment while a child remains at home.[11] We need to shift the emphasis from *child* welfare to *family* welfare and adopt "family strengthening" policies.

Incarceration Policies

Another example of the crisis–recoil response is our punishment-based response to criminal behavior.[12] This approach leads to police intervention after crimes have been committed and to building more prisons in the belief that infusing more money into the penal system will control crime. The punishment and incarceration of an offender permits the public to believe that the crime has been resolved as the underlying causes are ignored. The United States has 1% of its population in prisons—5 times per capita as many as England and Wales and 9 times as many as France. On a given day in 1980, 1.8 million persons were in jail, in prison, on parole or on probation in the United States; in 2006, there were 7.2 million—four times as many.

In the wake of decades of overincarceration with little thought to the long-term consequences, released prisoners face major personal, social and employment challenges for which they have neither the ability nor the resources to overcome on their own.[13] Most return to their poor Black and Latino neighborhoods as hardened felons, who commit new crimes and spread sexually transmitted diseases.[14] They contribute to the instability of those neighborhoods and affect the health and safety of our cities. Former inmates were tracked for 3 years after their release from prisons in 15 States:[15]

- 68% were rearrested;
- 47% were reconvicted; and
- 25% were returned to prison.

Prisoners who are released directly from segregation have much higher recidivism rates than those who spent time in a regular prison setting before returning to the community.[16] Hans Toch, professor of criminal justice at the University of Albany, cautions:[17]

> Supermax prisons may turn out to be crucibles and breeding grounds of violent recidivism. . . . [Prisoners] may become 'the worst of the worst' because they have been dealt with as such.

The United States spends more than $200 billion annually on criminal justice functions, including nearly 5,000 adult prisons and jails where administrators must confront prisoner rape, gang violence, the use of excessive force by officers, contagious diseases, a lack of reliable data and a host of other problems. Solving these problems takes dedication and money. Some 750,000 persons work in U.S. correctional facilities.

The financial incentives to create and maintain jobs in prison communities run counter to rehabilitation.[18] For example, Youngstown, Ohio, has been able to compensate for the loss of a steel factory by the revenue generated by four prisons, two jails and two halfway houses.[19] An additional financial incentive exists in for-profit prisons where $40,000 to $100,000 is spent per inmate annually while we spend less than $9,000 per pupil in public schools. The profits of the private prison industry are increased by more prisons and more prisoners.[20]

Incarceration clearly does not rehabilitate most offenders, is not cost-effective and creates family instability that produces more young offenders—a sensible business plan for prisons, but a heavy burden for taxpayers. Community-based programs can keep offenders out of prison at much lower cost without disrupting families.[21]

THE INSTITUTIONAL ABUSE OF CHILDREN AND FAMILIES

The institutional abuse of children and youth usually is thought of as physical or sexual abuse occurring in residential settings, which does occur. However, it is inherent in all governmental and social institutions involved with young people and their families.[22] Unintended consequences occur when the lives of children are managed by impersonal systems.

Client-making rather than Self-sufficiency

Paradoxically, our underfunded service institutions may be too powerful. The state has the power to impose client status upon marginal citizens and compel them to remain in that position. Weak communities can be made even more impotent by service systems when the client-making process creates an artificial system of relationships. Service systems replace community participation with case management and replace relationships with services, creating what John McNight, professor of education and social policy at Northwestern University, calls a "careless society" dominated by ineffective institutions and burgeoning social pathology.[23]

A subtle form of the institutional abuse of children is illustrated by the fact that child welfare, mental health and legal agencies now occupy an established place in the American economy and are as dependent upon their clients as their clients are upon them. This does not mean that professionals in these agencies wish to promote the continuation of the problems they are supposed to solve. It does mean that the policies and procedures in their fragmented, institutionalized systems limit their activities to servicing, instead of preventing and solving, problems.[24] When that happens, the potential for individuals and families to help themselves become self-sufficient is obscured and often lost.

Juvenile Courts

Juvenile court judge Justine Polier called attention to the institutional abuse of young people by the juvenile court system.[25] Born of charitable impulses, juvenile courts were flawed from the outset. They never were able to become the envisioned guardians of troubled children. Because they were too closely modeled on charity that granted only what could be spared, they never had the resources or community support required to strengthen struggling families.

The extent to which the legal system can fail to resolve child custody and visitation contests and actually act against the interests of children is illustrated by *Morgan v. Foretich*. In this case, extensive litigation led to jailing a mother, hiding a child and relocation of mother and child in another country without resolution of the initial allegation of sexual abuse by the father.[26]

As a consequence of the failures of the juvenile justice system, the U.S. Supreme Court found it necessary in its 1967 *In Re Gault* ruling to protect children from the abuses of the institution that had been established to help them by insisting that the due process of law be followed in juvenile court proceedings.[27] The unintended result of that action was a tendency to further distance children from help, as procedural due process became the main concern of the courts. Confronted with heavier caseloads without the benefit of adequate resources, juvenile courts now are unable to help incompetent parents adequately and often cannot make a significant impact on the most serious juvenile offenders.

On the positive side, minors beyond the control of their parents and habitually disobedient or truant from school are considered "status offenders." Because punishing them as individuals was ineffective, the focus has shifted to strengthening their families.[28]

Child Welfare Services

The child welfare system's emphasis on child safety rather than strengthening families tends to punish parents rather than help them become better parents. Because child protective policies are reactive, neglected and abused children still grow up to be criminal and welfare dependent members of our society. The direct costs associated with their immediate needs and the indirect costs of their long-term and/or secondary effects total $94 billion annually.[29]

The Children's Bureau monitors state child welfare services through Child and Family Services Reviews designed to ensure that child welfare agency practices conform with federal requirements. The review completed in 2004 found that no state fully met federal standards and that most states fell significantly short.[30] Under the policy of "family preservation" without strengthening their families too many children are kept at home or returned too quickly. Or they are placed with grandparents or other kin who serve as foster parents but may not be competent parent surrogates.[31]

Universal home visitation for the parents of newborns would transform the child welfare system into a family welfare system by identifying struggling families and strengthening them as they are formed instead of waiting until they flounder.

THE LACK OF A COHERENT SOCIAL POLICY
FOR ADOLESCENT PARENTS

In 1987, the Committee on Child Development Research and Public Policy of the National Research Council concluded that the lack of a coherent policy in the United States toward adolescent pregnancy and childbearing contributed to the magnitude of the problem.[32] The Committee found that parenthood interferes with adolescents' development and opportunities in life. The primary goal of policy makers should be to reduce premature pregnancies.

Our usual approach to adolescent pregnancy is to direct solutions at the adolescents themselves and to advocate sex education, the availability of contraceptives, supportive education, welfare payments and expanded health care. None of these measures have an impact when adolescents deliberately choose to become parents.[33]

The challenge for society, professionals and parents is to find better ways to counteract self-defeating, premature parenthood. This can be done directly by inducing adolescents to change their behavior and indirectly by changing ambiguous social values and professional practices that promote premature parenthood. These ambiguities are evident in the gap between preventing adolescent pregnancies and supporting adolescent parenthood. The main reason for this dramatic reversal in attitude is the lack of holistic thinking about adolescence as a developmental stage in life and about realistic alternatives.

Adolescents are confused and stressed by bearing the full responsibility to make decisions regarding their pregnancies. Professionals and parents need to recognize their responsibilities to young people. We need to acknowledge the ways in which we give conflicting messages to them. We need to respect adolescence as a vital developmental stage in life and not expect adolescents to be capable of adult decision making. We need to help them find fulfillment in their lives and hope for their futures through realistic achievements other than parenthood.

When we enable adolescents to make self-defeating decisions, we actually reinforce the perception that we really do not care about them enough to give them guidance.

CONCLUSION

The downward trends in adolescent sexual behavior, pregnancy and childbirth tend to lull us into thinking that what we are doing now is effectively addressing these problems. We are not.

The crisis–recoil nature of our political system leads to overreaction to crises followed by recoiling from their causes. It underlies our fragmented, discontinuous services that adversely affect young people and their families. The crisis-recoil response of trying to prevent adolescent pregnancy and then supporting adolescent parenthood has self-defeating consequences for adolescent girls and boys, their babies, their families and society.

Our political approaches focus on categories of social problems. The partial remedies they spawn often contribute to the problems they seek to solve. They shift the focus from strengthening our families, schools and neighborhoods. In this separate approach to each social problem, families and neighborhoods are replaced by service systems for each problem category. Personal relationships are replaced by professional services.

The institutional abuse of children and youth usually is thought of as physical or sexual abuse occurring in residential settings. In a broader and more important sense, it is inherent in the operation of impersonal governmental and social institutions that affect young people and their families.

Because children do not vote and because families with children constitute a minority of the population, it is difficult for our political system to address their needs and problems—unless we open our eyes to the enduring crisis of adolescent parenthood.

Part 2

THEORETICAL FOUNDATION

Without a deeply held, commonly shared purpose that gives meaning to their lives and without deeply held, commonly shared, ethical values and beliefs about conduct in pursuit of purposes that all may trust and rely upon communities steadily disintegrate, and organizations progressively become instruments of tyranny.

Dee Hock
Birth of the Chaordic Age[1]

This section sets the stage for understanding and dealing with incompetent parents—the most preventable cause of our social problems.

Because of its complexity, ensuring that children have competent parents requires coherent theories. Ecological/transactional systems theory incorporates individuals and families within neighborhoods and communities in the fabric of their society and culture. Chaos/complexity theory helps us understand these interacting systems over time. It reveals how the chaos engendered by babies born without competent parents can affect us all—like a hurricane. It exposes how relying only on science to study and technology to solve our social problems deflects attention from our vital cultural values. It anticipates that our self-assertive social values will continue to be amplified in the public arena until the excesses they create are dampened by our integrative cultural values.

Legal principles reflecting cultural values about the rights of children, adolescents and parents are crystallized in laws that bring order to chaotic situations. The rights of children and adolescents derive from basic human rights. The rights of parents derive from their moral duty to care for the young. Minors are awarded adult civil rights and privileges through an age-grading process.

If all parents and all child-related institutions served children's developmental interests, the issue of parental rights would seldom be raised. These rights enable parents to discharge their responsibilities to their children and to society. They no longer are based on the presumption that children are the property of their parents.

The *parens patriae* doctrine justifies state intervention on parental authority. When family matters are brought into the legal system, the interests of children, parents and the state need to be balanced in order to determine the appropriate rule of law that applies to each case.

Chapter 6

Chaos/Complexity Theory

Our great weakness is the habit of reducing complex issues to the most simplistic moralisms. It has made it difficult for Americans to think honestly and to some purpose about themselves and their problems. We have acquired bad habits of speech and worse patterns of behavior, lurching from crisis to crisis with the attention span of a five-year-old. We have never learned to be sufficiently thoughtful about the tasks of running a complex society. What we need are great complexifiers, persons who will not only seek to understand what it is they are about, but who will also dare to share that understanding with those for whom they act.

Senator Daniel Patrick Moynihan, 1970[1]

A coherent theory is required to understand the ramifications of adolescent and dependent adult parenthood. But most of us have little patience with theories—even though beliefs (theories) routinely guide our own lives. We want facts, not theories, except, of course, when it comes to our own beliefs (theories). Still theories are needed to discover facts. Theories are especially important in resolving complicated social problems.

This chapter sets the stage for understanding and dealing with incompetent parents—the most preventable cause of our social problems. These problems are currently dealt with by ineffective, fragmented and discontinuous services at enormous financial and humanitarian costs to our society. Polarizing ideologies also block actions to improve the situation, ranging from claims that focusing on personal responsibility infringes on the privacy of the family and on individual rights to claims that focusing on the poor conceals a racist eugenic agenda.

We need to see the big picture in order to understand how to ensure that children have competent parents. Theories can organize our thinking about social problems that are deeply embedded in human nature and in our society, such as crime and welfare dependency. Theories can help us identify actions that can narrow the gap between *what is* and what *we agree ought to be*.[2] Theories (beliefs) also can obstruct understanding and resolving our social problems.

THE IMPORTANCE OF BELIEFS (PERSONAL THEORIES)

Our highly developed cerebral cortex seems to exist largely for belief-forming and decision-making purposes.[3] We form beliefs fast and firmly. We quickly lose insight into their origins. We become beholden to them and often adhere to them in the face of information to the contrary. Most of our moral beliefs and judgments derive from gut instincts hardwired in the brain. We often have an automatic reaction to a situation and then form a belief to explain why we feel the way we do.[4] Alexander Hamilton put it well when he said that human beings are:

> governed more by passion and prejudice than be an enlightened sense of their interest. A degree of illusion mixes itself in all the affairs of society.

Decisions about social issues are commonly made on the basis of three beliefs. First, the belief in individual freedom that permeates our society focuses attention on people as if we are free-standing rather than interdependent persons. It encourages the reductionistic theory that, if we focus on individuals involved in our social problems, we will find single causes. It encourages the belief that everything will be better if we just do one thing—what I advocate!

Second, the belief that an objectively verifiable universe will ultimately be understood with certainty by human beings encourages the belief that we will be able solve our social problems if we just do more scientific research.

Third, the belief that child development unfolds in a straight line fails to take into account how individual differences and changing environments amplify and dampen evolving life courses. It justifies standardized measurements of progress and overlooks "late bloomers."

As a result of these beliefs, efforts to relieve stress in our social systems usually suppress symptoms without altering the underlying causes.[5] An attempt to relieve one set of symptoms may produce short-term improvement but set the stage for long-term problems. Good ideas may be introduced at points in an evolving system where little leverage exists and fail.

Modern science recognizes that interdependence and uncertainty are inherent in all living systems and that theories, unlike personal beliefs, change in accord with new evidence. We do not live in an unchanging world that can be manipulated experimentally. We live in evolving physical and social systems from self-organizing body cells to self-organizing international networks. Our subjective mental life is expressed through our publicly observable behavior.[6]

Fortunately, the undulating evolution of civilization affirms that we can organize ourselves to solve human problems. We have done this by developing workable paradigms based on theories that deal with wholes rather than parts. We eradicated polio in the United States through a health system that found the cause and administered a vaccine through collaboration of innumerable individuals and systems. General Systems Theory explains that success.

GENERAL SYSTEMS THEORY

Models that integrate time and network relationships are essential for understanding human development and behavior.[7] In the 1940s, Norbert Weiner developed the concepts of positive and negative feedback systems in what he called cybernetics. A feedback loop connects an action to its effects on surrounding conditions that in turn amplify or dampen that action.

General Systems Theory, first proposed by Ludwig von Bertalanffy in the 1960s and elaborated by James G. Miller, holds that understanding living systems requires understanding the relationships between the components of a system and between that system and its environment.[8] It requires thinking in terms of relationships in the context of evolving, integrated wholes whose properties cannot be reduced to their parts.

Deep ecology founded by Arne Naess recognizes that all living beings are integral parts of their environments.[9] The field of *human ecology* was elaborated by Gregory Bateson and Urie Bronfenbrenner. Human ecology applies general systems theory to social problems in the context of the place in which a person lives with all of its human and environmental interactions.

Life course health development focuses on the timing and sequence of biological, psychological, cultural, and historical events and experiences that influence the health and development of both individuals and populations.[10] It is an adaptive process with multiple transactions between these contexts and human bio-behavioral regulatory systems during critical periods of life. It relates the internal worlds of human beings to their external worlds.

Urie Bronfennbrenner proposed an *ecological/transactional theory* to explain human development in 1979.[11] Since then it has been elaborated to incorporate child development; the family system; the individual and family within their neighborhood and community; and the individual, family and community within the larger societal and cultural fabric. The evolution of these interacting systems over time is the focus of chaos/complexity theory.

CHAOS/COMPLEXITY THEORY

The longings for order, perfection and certainty have deep roots in Western culture, but evolution compels us to admit the reality of disorder, imperfection and uncertainty. Classical science has been puzzled by the irregular, seemingly unpredictable side of nature. Disorder in the atmosphere and the oceans, fluctuations in wildlife populations, bodily rhythm oscillations and differing paths of child development have not had a coherent theoretical framework until the emergence of *chaos/complexity theory*.[12] This theory links our experience to our interactions in the world in which we are immersed through a complex web of nonlinear, interacting networks from which new patterns of complex order emerge. It incorporates General Systems Theory and the reductionism of classical science. It helps us make predictions by understanding how initial conditions set the stage for evolving transacting systems. It helps us understand why parenthood is not sufficiently valued in the United States; why some adolescents want to be premature parents and most do not; and why some children of adolescent parents thrive and most do not.

Chaos/complexity theory helps us understand how living systems work.[13] Instead of breaking things down into their components, it builds upward from simple initial conditions to more complex things as feedback in a system and between systems affects the systems' behavior. Fractal geometry (repeated similar patterns) helps us understand the interconnection of patterns in living systems. The structure and behavior (fractal) of a human cell is similar to the structure and behavior of a human being, which is similar to the structure and behavior of human groups. In the same way, the attitudes adolescents have toward sex and parenthood are nested in the attitudes of their families, their peers, their cultures and their society.

Chaotic Initial Conditions and Amplifying and Dampening Events

Chaos/complexity theory has enhanced our ability to understand how small initial events can have large repercussions in the weather in remote locations (popularly know as the "butterfly effect"). Small changes in temperature in an ocean at high risk of chaos can produce repetitive patterns (fractals) in weather that become hurricanes under amplifying circumstances. In the same way, adolescent pregnancy is a condition with a high risk of chaos that produces fractals that are amplified or dampened by influences on the lives of the adolescents, their babies, their families, their communities and society like miniature hurricanes. Figure 6.1 uses the genesis of hurricanes as a model for the repercussions of adolescent pregnancy and parenthood.

On the Edge of Chaos

Storms and adolescent childbirth can create chaos in their environments, but, paradoxically, being on the edge of chaos also can stimulate constructive reactions. The

Chaos/Complexity Theory	*Hurricanes*	*Adolescent Parenthood*
Pre-existing conditions	Water temperature above 80 degrees in the eastern Atlantic (high risk of chaos).	Pregnancy (high risk of chaos)
Precipitating conditions	Sahara dust storms. Winds converge at the same speed in the same direction.	Decision to become a parent
Initial event	Rainstorm under high pressure area. Earth's rotation spins the air.	Childbirth
Amplifying forces	High pressure area pumps air into storm. Heat transfer from water into air by spray.	Family, societal & cultural support
Dampening forces	Cooler water Landfall	Counseling, programs & adoption
Average annual U.S. cost	$5 billion (International Hurricane Research Center, Miami, FL)	$20 billion (See Chapter 28)

Figure 6.1.

"edge of chaos" also is the "edge of order." Mihaly Csikszentmihalyi, professor of psychology at Claremont Graduate University, sees optimal development as involving the "predictability of unpredictability" and the "unpredictability of predictability."[14] Jules Henry, who was a professor of anthropology and sociology at Washington University, put it this way:[15]

> Nature has destined man to move from one misery to another; but the record proves also that man has sometimes been forced by misery to enlightenment although he has never accepted it without a bitter fight.

Living systems, whether a human body, family, community or society are inherently unstable and are on the edge of chaos. They require the continuous inflow of energy to maintain themselves. The more complex a system, the more unstable it is. *Social systems from the family to society are inherently unstable and vulnerable to break down into chaos.* Constant effort is needed to keep these systems from breaking down, as anyone with a successful marriage knows.

Living on the edge of chaos with its inevitable uncertainty is difficult for most of us. It takes work to keep all of the systems in which we live from becoming chaotic whether it be our bodies, our families, our schools, our communities or our society. Unless we tend to the needs of our bodies and families, we jeopardize our personal well-being. Unless we strengthen and protect our families, social workers and courts must enter the lives of parents and children. Unless we have safe neighborhoods, our security suffers. Anyone who has seen a natural disaster or a riot knows how important the police and the national guard are when social order breaks down. Unless we vigilantly guard our liberties, we lose our freedom. Unless we protect our physical environment, our health suffers from toxic substances in degraded air and water.

Being on the edge of chaos can provide a strong motivation for constructive change.[16] The chaos created by adolescent pregnancy can be dampened by decisions based on the interests of all concerned or amplified by unrealistic decisions that can result in chaos.

Societies' cycles of social disorder are related to their crisis-recoil response pattern.

Cycles of Social Disorder

Human systems are held together by shared values that dampen chaos. Successful persons organize their lives around values to achieve their goals. Communities and societies are organized around values and laws. Without these values and laws, chaos ensues. In the political and economic spheres, civilization appears to be evolving toward increasing stability, although chaos constantly intrudes. As we enter the 21st Century, democracy and regulated capitalism are the favored choices for technologically advanced societies. However, cycles of social order and disorder are continually repeated over the course of generations.

In describing the cycles of social disorder, Émile Durkheim identified "anomie"—valuelessness—as so intensely uncomfortable that societies seek values to replace ones that foster disorder.[17] He traced the social disorder of the late 18th and 19th centuries to the disruptive effects of the Industrial Revolution. We now are in the throes of "anomie" as we adapt to the Information and Ideological Revolutions. We are awash in confusing information that leads us to fall back on polarized beliefs rather than thoughtfully resolve complicated problems.

More specifically, our society is in a phase of disorder in our families and schools. This is progress from a phase of community disorder in the 1960s and 1970s. But instability in the family lives of children is a major social problem now. Childhood poverty has increased. Classroom control and school safety have become as important as education, sometimes more so. The extension from urban ghettos into middle class schools and colleges of young people shooting others and the avoidance of more shootings by responding to warning signs reveal that significant numbers of our young feel hopeless, abandoned and enraged.

There is a growing sense that our society is out of touch with our basic cultural values that have kept it from degenerating into chaos. At the same time, we are distracted by chaos in the rest of the world reflected in clashes between cultures. In their book *The Fourth Turning*, historians William Strauss and Neil Howe see the United States as currently in a decisive era of upheaval in which our deteriorating society will be renewed by a resurgence of integrative cultural values—a crisis that occurs every 80 to 100 years.[18]

Charles Horton Cooley, a pioneer in sociology, knew that change can be dislocating but that enlightened public opinion can move society in a beneficial direction.[19] He laid the foundation for crisis intervention to strengthen families as a way to deal with the chaos of child neglect and abuse rather than by removing children from their homes. Such interventions are based on a theoretical model of parenthood that provides for the developmental needs and organizes the chaotic lives of children and adolescents.

A MODEL OF PARENTHOOD BASED ON THE DEVELOPMENTAL NEEDS OF CHILDREN AND ADOLESCENTS

Babies, children and adolescents need continuous "supplies"—*physical, psychosocial and sociocultural*—from their parents commensurate with their stages of growth and development.[20] Their development is impeded if there are deficiencies in these supplies. At the same time, children are not just passive recipients or victims. They influence their own physical and psychosocial environments from their earliest years. Adolescents who are parents have these developmental needs as much, or more, than adolescents who are not parents.

Physical Supplies

Physical supplies—food, shelter and opportunities for recreation—are necessary for growth and development and for the maintenance of health. They also include protection from bodily damage, such as by infection, trauma or toxic chemicals.

Psychosocial Supplies

Psychosocial supplies include stimulation of cognitive and emotional development through relationships with family members, peers and older persons in schools, neighborhoods and communities. Young persons need exchanges of love and affection, patterns of asserting and submitting to authority and participation in collaborative activities.

In healthy relationships, each person tries to satisfy the needs of the other in their respective social roles in line with the values of their culture. In unhealthy relationships, persons manipulate each other to satisfy their own needs.

Socio-cultural Supplies

The richer their cultural heritage, the better prepared young persons are to handle life challenges. The expectations of others in a community influence their actions and their feelings about themselves. If they are born into stable groups, their social roles provide them with opportunities for healthy personality development. If they are born into unstable groups, they may be deprived of growth-producing opportunities for success.

The unarticulated aim of childrearing in the United States is the balanced development of *both* children's and parents' potentials to function competently as responsible citizens. Childhood and parenthood are two sides of the same coin. Rewarding family relationships are as important for adults as they are for children. The family is the only institution that provides unconditional acceptance for both adults and children.

This model of the developmental needs of adolescents and their babies in the context of their families, society and culture is the basis for the organization of this book. It draws upon neuroscience as synthesized in *A Science-Based Framework for Early Childhood Policy*.[21] It highlights the differences between society and culture.

SOCIETY AND CULTURE

The terms *society* and *culture* often are used interchangeably, but they are different although interdependent. The difference between society and culture can be seen in the analogy of a tree. *Society* is like the leaves that carry on life processes that change with the seasons. *Culture* is like the trunk and roots that provide the underlying structure and nourishment.

The root of the word society is "companionship". A society is composed of networks, institutions and organizations.[22] Throughout history, societies have been formed to guarantee food and protection. Our economy provides for our material needs, and our governments provide security. Our society is shaped by the legislative and executive branches of our governments.

The root of the word culture is "cultivation". It refers to the human capacity to build continuity into societies by transmitting values, attitudes, beliefs and symbols of ethnic, religious and social groups to subsequent generations. Our culture evolves from the Declaration of Independence and the U.S. Constitution and is shaped by our judicial systems. It transmits a work ethic that develops human capital for society. Since every person has creative potential, the role of culture is to create a society in which human capital can be developed and mobilized.[23] Cultural values that stress openness and tolerance facilitate economic growth and democracy.

THE ORIGIN OF SOCIAL AND CULTURAL VALUES (*US/THEM* CODES)

Social and cultural values are based on *Us/Them* in-group and out-group codes.[24] *Us/Them* distinctions work automatically. We usually are not consciously aware of the *Us/Them* codes that shape our perceptions, beliefs and values.

Distinguishing between in-groups and out-groups has been essential for human survival. This capacity is based on primitive, biologically-mediated competitive urges to protect one's territory for physical survival and mating.[25] It is based on primitive brain circuits that give us gut feelings of "good" and "bad." The brain circuits important for learning and following rules—including the amygdala, temporal lobe, and prefrontal cortex—are involved in *Us/Them* codes.[26] They contain the values and customs we use to relate to other persons.

Stereotyped codes in our brains identify the group to which we belong. These codes tell us who we are in relation to other persons. We mark some people as for us (*Us*) and others as against us (*Them*). Whether one belongs to an *Us* or a *Them* group depends on one's perspective. My *Them* group can be your *Us* group. There actually is only one group—the *Us* group that needs to create a *Them* group to define it. *Us/Them* codes feel like they are based on facts about other people, but they really are based on our perceptions of others. They are grounded in instinctual self-centered narcissism and attachment bonding during early life. *Me/You* narcissism pits a child's wishes against a parent's wishes. This self-centeredness is dampened by *Me/You* attachment bonds formed in the first *Us* group of *Me* and *You* as the parent-child unit becomes *Us*. This instinctual bonding brings affectionate emotions into later *Us* group bonding.

A second instinctual basis for *Us/Them* is "stranger anxiety" in young children when they differentiate familiar persons from strangers. It brings fear of strangers (*Them*) who might harm *Us* into the *Us/Them* equation. The child retreats to the *Us* group in the face of the unknown.

The third instinctual basis for *Us/Them* is aggression that asserts *My* and *Us* interests in the struggle for survival. *Us* are seen as allies and *Them* are seen as competitors or in extreme as enemies that can be attacked and even killed.[27]

These three instinctual drives are the sources of emotions that place *Us* in a positive light and *Them* in a negative light. These emotions are evoked when symbols and signs are perceived by an *Us/Them* code that indicates a person is a *Them*. The evolution of *homo sapiens* in social group living has been possible because of *Us/Them* codes, emotions and behaviors. They make it possible for individuals to form family, community, national, religious, ethnic, cultural and athletic groups that advance the interests of *Us* in competition with *Them*.[28] *Us* groups are defined by values and symbols. *Them* groups have values and symbols as well since they are *Us* groups from the point of view of the members. From the point of view of an *Us* group, *Them* groups are usually seen as inferior. *Us/Them* codes define "pecking orders" between and within groups.

Together all of these instinctual forces link the security of individuals to the security of the group. The more secure individuals feel, the less reliant they are on *Us/ Them* codes. The less secure they feel, the more they rely on *Us/Them* codes. This means that within *Us* groups there are mechanisms that promote security, such as authority structures and practices that promote a sense of group identity. It also means that people who feel insecure have greater needs to identify with *Us* groups that provide security than do people who feel secure. The feeling that the *Us* group is "moral" and the *Them* group is not is deeply ingrained in human beings. Many of our feelings of right and wrong are actually feelings about *Us* and *Them*.

At the same time, the *Us/Them* code conceals the basic selfish nature of the *Us* group as it serves the selfish interests of its members. The underlying self-serving purpose of the group justifies destructive actions against *Them* under the guise of group loyalty and patriotism. When the *Us* is extended to communities and nations and manipulated by political motives, the *Them* can be dehumanized as enemies who do not deserve the fair treatment expected in the *Us* group.

Us/Them codes also influence small groups, such as families or peer groups. They account for the sudden shifts between affection, fear and aggression that characterize all human relationships. At one time, you can be an *Us*. When you and I differ, you can be a *Them*. For example, stable marriages are characterized by the dominance of *Us* feelings over *Them* feelings. Unstable marriages and divorce result when *Them* feelings become dominant.

Our *Us/Them* codes have a cost. Because we get emotional security from feeling we are part of *Us* easily—an external source—we can lose it easily. When our *Us* feeling is threatened, our emotions send up an alarm. If you are not one of *Us,* you are one of *Them*. A soldier in combat who runs away from the enemy faces the same fate as the enemy: capture or death. Emotional trauma—a physiological insult to the body— results from being rejected by *Us*. Especially intense feelings are evoked in adolescents by family and peer rejection.[29]

Us/Them perceptions are always under revision, responding to our shifting circumstances. To lock people into an *Us/Them* category, demagogical leaders try to freeze certain perceptions. With this reinforcement even as situations change, these perceptions can feel permanent—always right, as with patriotism. Following World War II, American attitudes toward the Japanese and the Germans took years to shift from a *Them* to an *Us* status. The Civil Rights movement still has not erased the feeling that Whites are *Us* and Blacks are *Them* and vice versa.

Politicians use *Us/Them* codes in order to garner support. They reinforce existing *Us/Them* codes or induce people to imagine a new category of *Us*. Social movements start by proposing new *Us* categories to persuade those who benefit from the old *Us* groups to join the new *Us* group. Our judgments usually are not made because we apply well-thought-out principles to a set of facts and deduce an answer. When we justify what we do, our reasons usually are rationalizations of what we intuitively decided to do. Much of what we believe is "right" reflects our *Us* group values, as in political partisanship.[30] For this reason, we can easily see what *Us* does as morally right and what *Them* do as morally wrong.

In general, *Us/Them* codes are used by groups and societies in constructive ways. Cultures gradually change from an old to a new mixture of *Us/Them* groups as they exchange perspectives. Fortunately, an *Us/Them* code does not own us. We own it like a control panel in our minds. We can decide whether or not to pull the levers.

SOCIAL VALUES AND CULTURAL VALUES

As different kinds of *Us/Them* codes, there is a fundamental tension between social and cultural values. That tension is reflected in human nature—the eternal struggle between the lust for riches and glory depicted by Homer on the one hand (social values) and the quest for truth and justice by Socrates on the other hand (cultural values). That tension is between individual survival instincts in lower brain centers that govern appetites and group survival instincts in higher brain centers that give rise to parent-child attachment bonds transmitted through families that foster the common good.[31] Through this process the capacity to act as *We* emerges by integrating *Me*s, as can be seen in hardwiring for competition and cooperation in fish behavior:[32]

> When two or three male Siamese fighting fish are in the same tank, they fight ruthlessly. When a dozen or more are together, they swim in a school.

Social Values

Social values deal with the short-term realities of daily life. They arise from society's contemporary life styles and pertain to individual survival issues of power and passion. Social values are strongly influenced by technology, because they are concerned with enhancing the comfort and power of individuals. They guide the transactions of organizations, businesses and governments. They are expressed through regulatory laws in the United States and fluctuate with the times. Those that reflect current tastes and fashions constitute the "pop culture."

The objectives of childrearing social values in the United States are to produce competent, competitive and productive consumers, who are educated and informed citizens. Thus, social values favor developing independent, ambitious adults who excel in material ways. But satisfying these needs can result in slighting our emotional and spiritual needs.[33]

Cultural Values

In contrast to social values, which fluctuate and are influenced by the "little picture" perspectives of individuals, cultural values reflect the "big picture" and evolve over generations in order to ensure the survival of a society. They deal with long-range issues. They reflect the traditions, customs and habits of groups of people. They are expressed in religious and secular forms of philosophy, the arts and literature. They support harmonious group living through reasoning about critical issues.[34] They are expressed in altruism based on our ability to empathize with the distress of another person and respond to that person. Because of their origins in innate moral proclivities selected through evolution for group survival, cultural values are enduring.

Morality is based on a genetically determined prefrontal cortex system that emerges during brain development.[35] It is expressed in thoughtful responses to social situations. A typical example is the "golden rule" found in most moral codes. Just as do languages, moral values differ between cultures. Still, humans are the consummate group-thinking, team-playing animal.

Jonathan Haidt, professor of psychology at the University of Virginia, describes five psychological foundations on which cultures construct their moral communities: avoiding harm to others, fairness, loyalty, respect for others and living in a sanctified rather than a carnal way.[36] The first two are prominent in the United States. Even though it can be destructive, morality usually reflects a human aspiration for decency and cooperation within and between groups.

Our pro-social behavior is influenced by culturally induced shame and guilt. Shame is based on our perception of how we look in the eyes of others and on who we are. It is an internal signal that we are violating an external value. Guilt is based on our internalized values and on what we have done. Currently, shame is losing its power as our capacity to see ourselves in the eyes of disapproving others diminishes.[37] Being nonjudgmental is popular now. Because they have not internalized the values of the dominant culture, some adolescents and adults do not experience shame and guilt in the way that most people do. The past shame and guilt associated with adolescent pregnancy and childbirth have been replaced by pride in some circles.

Self-assertive Social vs. Integrative Cultural Values

We live in an individualistic, self-assertive society. We tend to think of ourselves as separate persons making our own decisions and fulfilling our own ambitions. We search for personal well-being and contentment.[38] But most of us know that we depend on others—most notably on our families. Parents spend more time preparing their children for modern society and more time caring for their parents who are living longer. The individual is not the fundamental unit of our society—the family is. Each one of us belongs to a tangible or intangible family.

Michael Gilbert of the Annenberg Center for the Digital Future sees America as turning into a society of severely diminished men without distinctive roles and responsibilities and overburdened women trying to balance too many agendas.[39] Increasingly isolated, we are opting for freedom over permanence and marrying later if at all. Gilbert sees detachment from our cultural heritage as the culprit behind the marginalization of men, the overburdening of women and the failings of modern relationships. Still, he sees our cultural reverence for human life and the companionship bond as spawning rich moral possibilities.

Thomas Kuhn, professor of philosophy and history of science at the Massachusetts Institute of Technology, described paradigm shifts in science and technology that transform cultures, such as the invention of the wheel, electricity and computers.[40] Similar paradigm shifts occur because of events, such as abolishing slavery, child labor laws and civil rights legislation.

Our society needs a paradigm shift now from self-assertive social values to integrative cultural values. These self-assertive and integrative tendencies influence our thinking and our values. They underlie and resolve our cycles of social disorder. Fritjof Capra, a physicist and systems theorist, contrasts their opposing tendencies[41] (see Figure 6.2).

Self-assertive thinking is reductionistic and linear. Integrative thinking is holistic and nonlinear. Social values stress expansion and competition. Cultural values stress conservation and cooperation. In his book *All Together Now*, Jared Bernstein of the Economic Policy Institute vividly contrasts contemporary self-assertive social values (YOYO—You're On Your Own) with integrative cultural values (WITT—We're In This Together).[42]

The Interplay of Social and Cultural Values

In recent decades, self-assertive social values in the United States have stressed materialistic individualism. University degrees are seen as passports to well-paying jobs rather than as preparing leaders with cultural ideals.[43] For those who struggle to hold a job and raise a family, the free market has become a predatory institution. Market-based social values have replaced cherished American cultural values. Leisure has been sacrificed for productivity and family time for extra paid working hours. Many people feel that acquiring a new car and a new home are higher priorities than nurturing babies. Strong market economies can be dehumanizing.

Integrative cultural values that support committed human relationships and that support parenthood are currently eclipsed in the United States. Business for profit and working for money are adulated. However, this dominant emphasis on materialistic individualism has not fostered secure and fulfilling lives for most of our citizens. It has resulted in disappearing pensions, eroding health benefits, the time crunch faced by families and job layoffs.[44]

Unmodified self-assertive social values amplify chaos, as is seen in economic recessions. Integrative cultural values that dampen self-assertive values are essential to the survival of societies and dominate in the long range, especially when cultures absorb other cultures.

The survival of our society does not depend upon everyone being altruistic. Self-assertive, competitive social values enhance the survival of the fittest, and thereby the

Thinking		Values	
Self	Others	Social	Cultural
Self-Assertive	Integrative	Self-Assertive	Integrative
rational	intuitive	expansion	conservation
analytic	synthetic	competition	cooperation
reductionistic	holistic	quantity	quality
linear	nonlinear	domination	partnership

Figure 6.2.

group, as long as most individuals are guided by cultural values. Social values usually are implemented through governmental and commercial policies that cannot create the infrastructure of human relationships needed to ensure commitment to the common good. That depends on our mediating cultural institutions—families, religious groups and voluntary organizations.

The survival and prosperity of our society depends upon a critical mass of adults who are guided by our integrative cultural values and who are committed to the goals of the commonwealth. In order to insure its own survival, our society needs social values that reflect our integrative cultural values and that support rather than undermine its cultural institutions of which the family is the centerpiece. The problems created by adolescent parenthood highlight our society's dependence on competent parents who foster a sense of responsibility to others.

OUR CULTURAL VALUE OF RESPONSIBILITY TO OTHERS

People in the United States generally are seen as fair-minded and compassionate by the rest of the world. Our nation attracts immigrants from all corners of the Earth.

Alexis de Tocqueville observed in 1831 that European settlers in America were creating a society different from the one they knew in Europe. Communities were formed around citizens coming together to solve problems. In the absence of powerful governments, they found they had the power to solve their own problems. These citizen associations still shape our society.[45] At the same time, de Tocqueville considered Americans "empty-headed," in mortal dread of being different from their neighbors and lopsidedly preoccupied with making money and personal pleasures. He saw us as self-reliant without a need to help those outside our families or friends.

De Tocqueville's observation about our emphasis on self-reliance remains true. However, we are the most volunteer-oriented nation in the world. Volunteering our time and money gives many of us satisfaction. We try to solve social problems by compensating for the behavior of others. When motorists throw trash on our highways, volunteers clean it up. When parents flounder, mentors in schools or foster parents pitch in. We support adolescent parents.

In an effort to solve our social problems, we provide public services. But our willingness to pay for them waxes and wanes depending on whether or not we believe that people make responsible use of them.

Compassion vs Punishment

At times, we side with those who believe that government can solve our social problems. We have compassion for victims and even excuse their behavior. We provide welfare for the poor and income for the disabled. We provide after-school programs for working parents. When people need other kinds of help, we provide counselors, health care, legal services and specialized education. When we do this, some people expect and seek help from governments.

At other times, we believe people should be responsible for solving their own problems without government help. We emphasize punishment. We fine litter-bugs, remand juveniles to adult courts and send drug abusers to prison. When we do this, some people fear government.

The compassionate-punishment temper of the times can be measured by whether the rehabilitation of offenders or capital punishment is the dominant issue. But our swings between compassion and punishment have not produced the kind of society we want—a society in which individuals are free to pursue their aspirations and still are responsible for their actions. Neither compassion nor punishment ensures responsible behavior. Something is missing.

Personal Responsibility

The missing piece between compassionate helping and punishment is expecting personal responsibility. Responsible individuals are more likely to create the society we seek than individuals who expect help ("others will do it for me") or fear punishment ("others will do it to me"). Both the affluent and the poor can be responsible—or irresponsible—persons.

Our cultural value of personal responsibility needs to be clearly articulated through social disapproval and limit setting for irresponsible and self-defeating behaviors that have direct and indirect public costs in terms of money and resources. Irresponsible parents contribute to crime and welfare dependency. Smoking, obesity, alcoholism and drug abuse increase health care costs for everyone. Even compassion for the handicapped can foster dependency.

The motivation to be responsible depends upon knowing what society expects. For this reason, laws define the ages at which children and adolescents are capable of exercising mature judgment. Laws define mental competency to make important decisions. But we seldom set positive standards for responsible behavior outside of our schools for either children or adults, and respected models of responsible behavior are not visible. Instead, we are fascinated by irresponsible celebrities. We nourish fantasies of wealth by lotteries and gambling. We promote conspicuous consumption and credit card debt. We amass federal deficits. We are swayed by demagoguery. Neither adults nor children are sure what our society expects of them.

Why don't we make our cultural expectations for responsible behavior clear? One reason is that we bridle at being told what to do. Public expectations evoke the fear that government will run our lives. We also fear the reactions of people if we confront them with expectations. They might reject our efforts to help them. They might react violently or sue us. The result is indecisiveness and inaction in responding to irresponsible behavior.

Still, when pushed to the wall, we do draw upon our cultural values. The rude and disrespectful behavior of students has turned attention to the importance of civility.[46] Schools now provide character education. Parenting education focuses on prosocial values. We prosecute corruption in government and corporations.

We need to apply our model of the developmental needs of babies and adolescents to defining and monitoring the responsibilities of parenthood as a valued career.

DEALING WITH CHAOS/COMPLEXITY IN HUMAN DEVELOPMENT

Human beings have little or no influence on the course of hurricanes. We are similarly limited in our ability to predict and influence the course of human events. Although we cannot predict the future course of a particular person's life, we can identify desirable and undesirable influences at particular times in life.[47] We know that certain initial conditions in human existence are predisposed to adverse outcomes. We also know that there are key points in the development of human beings at which specific influences amplify or dampen human outcomes.

This book examines the significant times when amplifying and dampening influences can shape the course of the lives of adolescents and their babies.

CONCLUSION

Our social problems are currently approached without coherent theories through ineffective, piecemeal, uncoordinated efforts that result in fragmentation and lack of continuity of services at enormous financial and humanitarian costs to our society.

General Systems Theory incorporates the individual and family within a neighborhood and community in the larger societal and cultural fabric. Chaos/Complexity Theory helps us understand how these systems interact over time and how the chaos engendered by babies born without competent parents affects all of us. It exposes how our reliance on science to study and technology to solve our social problems deflects attention from implementing our cultural values. It anticipates that self-assertive social values will continue to be amplified until the excesses they create are dampened by our integrative cultural values.

There is a growing sense that contemporary society is out of touch with our basic integrative cultural values that can keep it from degenerating into chaos. We are distracted by chaos in the rest of the world. Still, there is a yearning for fulfilling family lives and fulfilling careers. Being on the edge of chaos in the lives of young persons can offer opportunities for change if we make a commitment to meeting the developmental needs of all of our children.

We need to shift from a helpless, compromising attitude toward adolescent parenthood—the prime example of parental incompetence—to one in which we offer hope and empowerment to vulnerable adolescents and their families before babies are born. Most importantly, we need to recognize that our charitable impulse to help the less fortunate can have unintended consequences when we support adolescent parents.

This book identifies a possible tipping point for a paradigm shift toward valuing parenthood as a life-long career in our society. Acting upon the simple fact that a minor cannot be a competent parent could lead to a paradigm shift from self-assertive social values that regard babies as the property of their genetic parents to integrative cultural values that regard babies as persons with developmental needs. This shift would go far toward resolving our social problems.

Chapter 7

The Rights of Babies and Adolescents

Each of our children represents either a potential addition to the productive capacity and the enlightened citizenship of the nation, or, if allowed to suffer from neglect, a potential addition to the destructive forces of the community.

Theodore Roosevelt
Special Message to Congress, 1909[1]

Children have come a long way from earlier centuries when they were seen as miniature adults. Childhood and adolescence are recognized now as unique stages of development in life.

Seeing a child as immature rather than as merely ignorant took shape in the eighteenth century under the influence of Rousseau and the Romantic poets.[2] The nineteenth century recognized the vulnerability of children, informing a wide-ranging "save the children" movement and ushering in the twentieth century as the Century of the Child.

The Civil War established the civil rights of individuals and led to a vision of the civil rights of children and the role of the state in American life. The Illinois Supreme Court decision *People v. Turner* in 1870 extended due process protection to minors and set the stage for juvenile courts that were expanded in the 1910s to administer cash disbursements to single mothers, a precursor of our current federal Temporary Assistance to Needy Families program.[3]

In 1900, the Swedish feminist Ellen Key published *The Century of the Child*. In Key's vision children would be conceived by loving parents.[4] They would grow up in homes where mothers were ever-present. This vision dominated most of the first half of the 1900s. The aim was to map out "childhood" in which children would acquire the "habit of happiness." This vision inspired the professional approach to childhood and adolescence through developmental psychology, child-centered pedagogy, child psychiatry and policy studies related to the young.

In the second half of the 20th century, a sense that childhood was disappearing arose.[5] The worlds of children and adults seem to be merging again. Better off materially than fifty years ago, children now are expected to be independent and to adjust to a variety of family styles. Adolescents especially are wooed as major consumers in our economy. Preparing the young for fulfilling lives is the theme of modern child-drearing.

Underlying these developments is recognition of the rights of minors that culminate in attaining most adult legal rights at the age of eighteen during late adolescence.

THE RIGHTS OF MINORS

Rights have two distinct but related functions: to protect a person's autonomy and to secure important interests.[6] The important interests underlying the "best interests of the child" principle are the right to protection from harm by others and by themselves and the right to care.

Beginning as babies, young persons lack the capacity and experience to marry, bring law suits or enter contracts without adult guidance until they reach a certain age. They are considered "minors" until they reach the age of "majority" and need custodial guardians, usually their parents. Since older adolescents are regarded as legal adults, the following discussion of rights is limited to early and middle adolescence when they are legal minors.

When babies and children were regarded as the property of their parents, they had no rights. Only their parents had rights. An important distinction exists between parental rights, which are legal *custodial* and *guardianship* rights, and minors' rights, which are moral *human rights* that flow from minimum standards of civilized behavior. Human rights include moral rights, civil rights and civil liberties that apply to all human beings.

Over the last century, minors have been accorded a series of civil rights and liberties based on their moral human rights.

The Moral Rights of Minors

Moral rights reflect cultural values that have an innate basis in human nature.[7] They express a sense of the common good that leads to an ethic of compassion for others. Emmanuel Kant said that each human being has dignity: "humanity must always be treated as an end, not merely as a means." To treat a person as a means is to use that person to advance one's own interests. To treat a person as an end is to respect that person's dignity and autonomy. This is important for the young who are vulnerable to oppression and exploitation by older persons.

The traditional view of minor's moral rights has come to be known as the "caretaker" view articulated in 1691 by the philosopher John Locke.[8] According to Locke, all humans are "born infants, weak and helpless, without knowledge or understanding." Therefore, parents were "by the law of nature under an obligation to preserve, nourish, and educate the children they had begotten." In Locke's scheme, parents have the right to make choices for their children:

> Whilst [the child] is in an estate wherein he has no understanding of his own to direct his will, he is not to have any will of his own to follow.

Moral rights impose a duty to actively help a person have or do something. For example, a minor's moral right to an education imposes a duty to provide that education.

Eglantyne Jebb, founder of the Save the Children Fund, began an effort to codify the moral rights of minors in 1922 in England in the *Charter of the Rights of the Child*.[9] That charter spelled out the moral right of all minors to be protected from exploitation; to be given a chance for full physical, mental and moral development; and to be taught to live a life of service. The League of Nations adopted it in 1924 as the *Geneva Declaration of the Rights of the Child*.

The moral rights of minors have been enumerated subsequently in a variety of organizational creeds, bills of rights for children and White House Conferences on Children in the United States in addition to declarations of the United Nations.[10] These rights are reasonable expectations that minors will be given whatever they require to grow into healthy and functioning adults. This is expressed in the basic premise of the United Nations Convention on the Rights of the Child that all human beings are born with the following inherent civil rights:

- to survival;
- to develop to the fullest;
- to protection from harmful influences, abuse and exploitation; and
- to participate fully in family, cultural and social life.

Whenever policy makers publicly express their hopes for newborns, they conclude in effect that minors have a moral right to competent parents and specifically to not live in foster care or institutions.[11] When persons make decisions on behalf of a child, they are acting as fiduciary guardians for the child. They are expected to put themselves in the position of the child and place the interests of the child above the interests of others and themselves.

In recent decades, the political emphasis on treating all citizens equally regardless of age and gender has obscured the fact that minor adolescents have special needs. As a result, many adolescents in the United States suffer today because efforts to help them treat them as adults and ignore two of their moral rights. The first is the right to have competent parents and to an education. The second is the right to be protected from acting in ways they would later regret.

Moral rights are not enough to protect minors from abuse and neglect. For this reason, certain moral rights of minors have become legal civil rights in the United States.

The Civil Rights of Minors

Civil rights derive from the seventeenth and eighteenth century reformist theories of human rights that supported the English, American and French revolutions.[12] They guarantee all citizens equal protection under the law regardless of race, religion, gender, age or disability; equal exercise of the privileges of citizenship; and equal participation in community life. Children are equal to adults in the sense they are entitled to as much respect as are adults.[13]

Moral rights became enforceable civil rights for adults only through great effort and vigilance. Even more effort and vigilance is required to enforce equally important civil rights for minors.[14] We now are poised for the first time in history to specify enforceable civil rights for minors in positive terms. These civil rights are based on their developmental needs and capacities not on their wishes.

Adult civil rights that apply to minors include freedom from racial and equivalent forms of discrimination; the right to life and personal security; freedom from slavery and involuntary servitude; and freedom from cruel, inhuman or degrading treatment and punishment. The U.S. Supreme Court recognized the relative incapacity of minors in 2005 and ruled that the execution of minors violates the cruel and unusual punishment clause of the Eighth Amendment.[15]

The gradual emergence of minors' civil rights in the United States began by treating them differently from adults in criminal law through juvenile courts. The first juvenile court was established in 1899 in Cook County, Illinois.[16] In the 1960s, because these courts were not adequately rehabilitating juveniles, the U.S. Supreme Court in *In re Gault* mandated due process to provide Constitutional protections but did not improve their abilities to help juveniles.

Minors' civil rights progressed from child labor, child neglect and abuse and education laws to the idea that children have rights to environments that give them reasonable opportunities to develop in a healthy manner. These include rights to adequate nutrition, housing, recreation and medical services, as well as love, security, education and protection against abuse and discrimination. This list does not include certain adult rights, such as the right to privacy, the right to confidentiality and the right to make their own choices on vital matters. All of this boils down to minors' civil right to competent parents.

Competent parenting actually is an enforceable civil right of minors because incompetent parenting is a cause for state intervention through statutory child neglect with the possible termination of parental rights. The U.S. Supreme Court in *Ginsberg v. New York* recognized society's interest in protecting minors from circumstances that might prevent them from becoming responsible citizens:[17]

> The state also has an independent interest in the well-being of its youth . . . to protect the welfare of children . . . safeguarded from abuses which might prevent their growth into free and independent well-developed . . . citizens.

Stated positively, minors have a civil right to nurturance, to protection and to make certain choices through age-grading statutes.[18] But the fact that parental rights are based on the right of minors to competent parents is not fully appreciated in courts and by the public.

Courts presume that parents have Constitutional rights to establish and maintain vital family relationships. Minors apparently do not.[19] A couple's decision to marry, a father's love for his child and a grandmother's wish to share her home with her extended family—all have been given Constitutional protection from governmental influence. Yet, the parallel need of minors for family intimacy have not been accorded the same protection. Although their interests often are said to be important in non-

Constitutional law and policies, minors occupy shadowy ground in Constitutional law that protects family privacy. The courts generally tend to defer to parental authority without considering the quality of family relationships from the children's perspective and the soundness of parental judgment. Legal rules governing decisions about children's relationships do not always require state decision makers to focus on the well-being of the affected children even though the "best interests of" or the "least detrimental alternative for" a child standards are widely applied.[20]

From society's point of view, the civil right of minors to competent parents is more important than adult rights to freedom of action because of the adverse consequences of incompetent parents for society. Adult rights benefit individuals and are the backbone of democratic societies. But minors' rights are more important for society. They are essential for the survival and prosperity of our society, which depends upon protecting and nurturing its young so that they become responsible citizens.

The Civil Liberties and Privileges of Minors

Civil liberties limit the power of the state to restrain or dictate the actions of individuals, such as speech and religious practice.[21] Civil privileges generally are accompanied by responsibilities that depend upon meeting certain criteria, such as registration to vote and obtaining a license to operate a motor vehicle.

Martin Guggenheim, professor at New York University Law School, points out the limitations of applying adult liberties to adolescents, such as the freedom of speech and the choice of religion, when they infringe on parental prerogatives.[22] Minors need restrictions of their civil liberties and privileges to protect them from their own mistakes, from the corrupting influence of others and to protect society from their actions. These restrictions are removed following an *age-grading* sequence that progressively grants minors adult liberties and privileges as they attain specific ages.

The age-grading of privileges is particularly important when the capacity to test competence is limited and the consequences of mistakes threaten the individual or others with substantial harm.[23] Age-grading statutes award liberties and privileges with accompanying responsibilities at certain ages, such as:

- choice in post-divorce custody and visitation matters,
- qualification for motor vehicle operating licenses and executing contracts,
- eligibility to vote,
- elibility to enter military service, and
- eligibility to marry.

Awarding these decision-making liberties and privileges generally is based on what a minor would see as appropriate looking back as an adult. Criteria for judging the maturity of an individual based on psychological research are generally regarded as insufficient to permit judges to make judgments about an individual minor's maturity. Therefore, the present system uses objective criteria, such as age, in spite of individual differences in rates of maturation.

MINORS' RIGHT TO COMPETENT PARENTS

None of us have a moral right to succeed. In fact, we have a "right to fail" unless our failure adversely affects other people. The serious failures of parents affect others, including their children and society, and fly in the face of the right of minors to competent parents. Accordingly, there is an exception to a person's freedom to fail when that person is a parent. Few would defend a parent's right to damage a child.

The legal right of minors to have competent parents derives from the fact that incompetent parents justify state intervention and the possible termination of parental rights. Because our society is paying an ever larger share of the cost of rearing, educating and treating neglected and abused children, we all have a financial stake in their welfare. Public decision making for children needs to take into account the interests of children and to acknowledge that parents usually protect those interests best. When parents' inabilities to do so are evident before childbirth, the state has an obligation to intervene in compliance with existing statutes to ensure that newborns have competent parents.[24]

Our society has an obligation to value parenthood enough to protect children's rights to competent parents and to enforce its expectations of parenthood. Whether or not childbirth by a minor was planned, the decision to rear a child should be based on a baby's right to a competent parent before that child is born. It should not be delayed until after childbirth when maternal and paternal instincts and ideologically based emotions compromise objective problem-solving and decision-making.

AGE OF MAJORITY

There is no national definition of the age of majority in the United States. Either state statutes or case law set that age. When adolescents reach the age of eighteen, they are considered to be an adult in all but two states, where the age of majority is nineteen. The age of eligibility to purchase alcohol and cigarettes may be as high as twenty-one.

There are two circumstances other than *age-grading* in which minors are awarded adult civil liberties and privileges. The first is the "mature minor" doctrine that awards specific privileges. The second is emancipation that awards some degree of legal adulthood.

The Mature Minor Doctrine

The Model Statute for Standards Relating to Rights of Minors defines "mature minor" in terms of specific privileges. For example, an adolescent over sixteen years of age who has sufficient capacity to understand the nature and the consequences of a proposed medical treatment for his or her benefit is a mature minor and may consent to medical treatment on the same terms and conditions as an adult.[25] The Standards do not deal with an minor's capacity to make decisions for another person, such as a minor's baby.

The mature minor doctrine allows health care providers to treat adolescents as adults based upon an assessment and documentation of the young person's maturity. Statutory guidelines, such as age, living apart from parents or guardian, maturity, intelligence, economic independence, experience and marital status are given.

Many states have granted adolescents over a certain age legal rights to treatment without parental consent for emergency medical care, sexually transmitted diseases, drug treatment, mental health care, pregnancy and contraception.[26] In Michigan, adolescents 14 and older may seek medical services, excluding pregnancy termination and the use of psychotropic drugs, without the consent or knowledge of the minor's parent or guardian. In Wisconsin, minors seeking pregnancy termination are required to have written consent from a parent, guardian, adult family member, or foster parent. However, minors may ask a court for a waiver, and clergypersons may petition a court on a minor's behalf. Some states authorize minor parents to give consent for the medical treatment of their children. However, the parents or guardians of minors are not liable for the costs of services received without their knowledge.

In this context, the limited legal privileges of adolescents are recognized by adoption agencies when a minor makes an adoption plan for a baby. Most adoption services require social workers to obtain a minor's consent to involve the parents or guardians in the adoption counseling process. If either or both genetic parents are minors, guardians *ad litem* may be appointed for each to implement their "best interests" in formulating and executing an adoption plan.[27] Because of the tendency to idealize the "best interests" of children, the "least detrimental alternative" has been suggested as a more pragmatic concept. It recognizes the fact that optimal alternatives may not be available.

Emancipation

Parents have a common-law duty to support and maintain their minor adolescents. The removal of a parent's duty to support a minor and of accompanying custodial guardianship is generally referred to as "emancipation" of the minor. Emancipation is a legal process by which minors can attain some degree of legal adulthood before reaching the age of majority.

States either have differing or no laws governing emancipation. The rights granted to legally emancipated minors may include the ability to make legally binding contracts, own property and keep their earnings.[28] A test for emancipation is whether adolescents are beyond the control of their parents and can demonstrate they can manage their own financial affairs.

States generally allow the emancipation of minors over the age of sixteen if it is determined to be in their "best interests" or if they have a valid marriage.[29] Emancipation may be total or limited to certain purposes. It may free parents from responsibility for an adolescent's debts but not for support. Fully emancipated minors are responsible for their own support.

Minors over sixteen generally may obtain a marriage license with the consent of their parents or guardians. If there is no parent or guardian, or if the guardian is an agency or department, the consent may be given by a court having probate jurisdiction. Most states have minimum marriage ages of at least sixteen with parental consent. The exceptions are Kansas and Massachusetts, which have twelve for girls and fourteen for boys and New Hampshire, which has thirteen for girls and fourteen for boys.[30] Marriage and entering military service have been held to be acts of self-emancipation.

A court may annul a marriage when a party lacked the capacity to consent to the marriage because of age, mental incapacity or infirmity; the influence of alcohol, drugs or other incapacitating substances; force or duress; or fraud.

PARENTAL NOTIFICATION OF A MINOR'S PREGNANCY

The dilemma created by a minor's pregnancy is revealed by the arguments for and against parental notification by professionals.[31] Underlying attitudes toward the professional obligation to notify parents of their minors' pregnancies is the dependent/independent nature of parent-adolescent relationships, which even under optimal circumstances are ambivalent. In fact, pregnancy often occurs when family relationships are strained, adding to the complexity of the matter. Unfortunately, the usual reaction of professionals and other adults to adolescent pregnancy is to take an adolescent's sometimes distorted perceptions of unworkable family relationships at face value, rather than to focus on improving those family relationships, even though that task may be difficult.

Arguments for Parental Notification

The case for parental notification includes the following concerns:

- Adolescents will terminate pregnancies during the first trimester without their parents' knowledge that they were pregnant.
- If a pregnant adolescent does not inform her parents, she cannot truly give "informed consent" to terminate or continue the pregnancy without realistic knowledge of her own capacities to be a parent and her family's ability and willingness to help her.
- Parents have legitimate interests in knowing about circumstances that affect them.
- Because parents are expected to be responsible for the care and nurturance of their adolescents, and in some states for their adolescents' children, they have a right to guide their decision-making and their behavior.

The argument for parental notification presumes a rational parental response to a minor's situation but provides for recourse through a court for minors who need protection in the event of a potential abusive parental response.

Arguments against Parental Notification

The main arguments against parental notification of a minor's pregnancy are:[32]

- There is no circumstance in which a minor's interests would be served by bearing a child when she does not want to do so.

- Parents might pressure an adolescent into a decision that would not be hers to terminate or to continue the pregnancy.
- Parents might act irrationally and harm the adolescent.
- The fear of parental notification might keep a pregnant adolescent from seeking family planning services or obtaining prenatal care.
- Minors have the same Constitutional right to privacy on sexual matters and to control over their bodies as do adults.
- Mandatory parental involvement may lead to risky terminations late in pregnancy.
- There is no persuasive evidence that laws mandating parental involvement improve family relationships or discourage adolescents from having sex.

The argument against parental notification presumes a possible irrational parental response but could provide for notifying them in the context of family counseling.

Parental Notification Statutes

The varying stances of state laws related to this issue illustrate how the relative merits of each of these positions have been applied.

In the 1970s in *Poe v. Gerstein* and in *Planned Parenthood v. Danforth*, the U.S. Supreme Court held that minors have a constitutional right to choose whether or not to bear a child.[33] The court pointed out that limiting minors' choices can only be justified when there is a "compelling state interest" in doing so. This compelling interest was recognized in 1990 in *Hodgson et al. v. Minnesota et al* and subsequently affirmed in *Ohio v. Akron Center for Reproductive Health et al.* when the U.S. Supreme Court held that states may require parental consent before a minor can terminate her pregnancy provided that she has access to overriding court approval. In 2006, the U.S. Supreme Court held in *Ayotte v. Planned Parenthood* that a New Hampshire statute requiring parental notification of an pregnancy termination would be unconstitutional when applied to minors for whom an emergency termination would be necessary to avert serious damage to their health.[34] Along this line, the Council on Ethical and Judicial Affairs of the American Medical Association concluded that, while minors should be strongly encouraged to discuss their pregnancies with their parents and other adults, minors should not be required to involve their parents before deciding whether to terminate their pregnancies. Because of political considerations and their own beliefs, some judges recuse themselves from minors' petitions for terminations.

Under current laws, a majority of states require parent involvement in an adolescent's pregnancy termination decision.[35] In the light of the two previously mentioned U.S. Supreme Court rulings that prohibit parents from an absolute veto of their daughters' decision to terminate their pregnancies, many states require the consent or notification of only one parent, usually twenty-four or forty-eight hours before the procedure. Several states allow grandparents or other adult relatives to be involved in lieu of minors' parents.

In effect, U.S. Supreme Court decisions reflect the expectation that judges would affirm minors' decisions to terminate their pregnancies even though they also give judges the power to exercise their moral convictions about termination and recuse themselves from certain cases.[36]

The politically sensitive nature of the termination of minors' pregnancies is illustrated by the following case in Florida:[37]

> A 13-year-old girl under state custody because she was maltreated by her parents asked her caseworker to arrange termination of her pregnancy as permitted by Florida law on the grounds that she was not old enough to assume the responsibilities of parenthood. Governor Jeb Bush obtained an injunction to block the pregnancy termination because a state statute forbids the Department of Children and Families from consenting to it. The Governor asserted that he was intervening to protect the girl's "best interests" and to prevent the loss of life. The state's psychologist testified that girls with a history of psychiatric problems could be at risk for a disorder called the "post-abortion syndrome." The presiding judge rejected the state's jurisdiction and argument and lifted the injunction with the comment that the state should have done more to help the girl before she got pregnant.

The small, but highly significant, number of girls who have been abused or are victims of incest need protection from their own parents. Minors have the option to petition a judge for permission to terminate a pregnancy when they do not want to involve their parents in all states except Utah.[38] To place this option in perspective, 16,000 terminations were performed on minors with parental permission in the twelve years ending in 1999 in Alabama. During that time, 200 were performed when judges bypassed parents. Reasons given ranged from not wanting to stress parents to fear parents would insist on carrying the pregnancy to term.

ESTABLISHING PATERNITY WITH MINORS

Some 150,000 babies are born each year to unwed parents at least one of whom is a minor. These parents cannot marry or bring a law suit without the permission of their parents.

Although some states allow minors to voluntarily acknowledge paternity without parental approval, many states require parents' permission for minors to do so. Because custody, visitation and support obligations are onerous responsibilities, it is reasonable to protect minor parents from entering these obligations without careful consideration. They might enter an ill-advised marriage. A boy might acknowledge a child who is not his offspring. A girl might sue to establish paternity with a male in order to leave her abusive family. Grandparent liability laws also can make paternal grandparents reluctant to allow establishing paternity of their minor son because they will be responsible for child support.

On the other hand, it is important for a baby to have genetic parentage determined. Otherwise, there might be a later proceeding to establish the paternity of another male when a child has become attached to a rearing father. Protections for minor parents and their offspring are appropriate to make sure that the interests of their babies are served.

The Center for Law and Social Policy suggests that states consider special rules for minor parents when establishing paternity means the father pays child support. Removing the fear of a support order might encourage low-income fathers to become involved in their children's lives. The Center differentiates between early, middle and late adolescents who are legal adults.[39] They recommend rigorous constraints on the youngest group and more options for the middle group. State laws on the age of majority, the age of sexual consent and the age of marriage generally reflect this kind of age differentiation. The younger the adolescent the more likely he or she will need guidance. Given the vulnerability of many young mothers and fathers, there is a need for professional guidance to help them choose the most appropriate route for paternity establishment, including the choice not to establish paternity in cases of rape, incest or domestic violence. States should help minors and their babies when criminal conduct has occurred.

STATUTORY RAPE

Statutory rape laws are designed to discourage the sexual exploitation of adolescents by adults.[40] They generally apply to sexual intercourse between an adult and a minor even with the minor's consent. Recent efforts to reform the welfare system and to connect adolescent childbirth with social problems have led many states to more strictly enforce statutory rape laws.

Forty-four percent of girls whose first sexual relationship is statutory rape give birth, compared with 26% of other sexually experienced girls.[41] Thirty percent of statutory rape offenders are male friends, and 60% are known to the girls. Despite declines in sexual experience among girls, there was no significant change in the overall prevalence of statutory rape at first sexual intercourse between 1995 (14%) and 2002 (13%). The younger the first sexual experience the more likely the partner is an adult. Of girls thirteen or younger at first sex, 65% experienced statutory rape compared to 53% of fourteen-year-olds and 41% of fifteen-year-olds.

The incidence of statutory rape is higher among adolescents who do not live with two parents, whose parents have little education and whose mothers gave birth as adolescents. They also are more likely than other sexually experienced girls to use alcohol and illegal drugs.

Boys also are subject to statutory rape by women.[42] Similar age patterns are found for males, although the percentages are smaller: 27% of those 13 and younger experienced statutory rape at first sex compared to 16% of 14-year-olds and 12% of 15-year-olds.

AGE OF CONSENT

State laws governing the age at which a minor is not deemed to be able to freely consent to sexual relations vary. In most states, the age is younger than 18.[43] If an adolescent is under that age, sexual relations with him or her is a crime, even if the older partner believed the relationship to be consensual. Most states distinguish young adolescents from middle adolescents. Mississippi, Hawaii and Georgia raised the age of consent from fourteen to sixteen.

Statutes regarding mandatory reporting of sexually active adolescents are complex and depend on the nature of the sexual contact, age of the adolescent and access to health care services. The Wisconsin statute illustrates this complexity.[44] Sexual intercourse with someone 16 or 17-years-old is a Class A misdemeanor and carries the same penalty as a fourth degree sexual assault. However, it does not fall under the mandated reporting requirement if a professional feels sexual intercourse was consensual. Some counties request that mandated reporters contact the Child Protective Service agency if they become aware of voluntary sexual relationships where the age differential exceeds a certain number, such as three years. Sexual contact or sexual intercourse with a person under 16 is a felony.[45] School professionals who believe a student under 16 has had sexual contact with another person and the student claims the sexual contact was consensual still must report this behavior to the county Child Protective Service agency. Reporting and enforcing these requirements is not assiduously pursued.

The case of Crystal and Matthew Koso illustrates how the attitudes of some families and communities contradict the age of consent and statutory rape laws:[46]

14-Year-Old Crystal Koso

In Falls City, Nebraska, Matthew Koso, 22, was charged with statutory rape of Crystal, 14-year-old mother of his baby, even though they were wed in Kansas that permits marriages of persons under seventeen. The Nebraska attorney general, Jon Bruning, accused Matthew of being a pedophile.

In Nebraska, as in many other states, intercourse between a 19-year-old and a 16-year-old is statutory rape even if the couple is married.

"We don't want grown men having sex with young girls," said Attorney General Bruning. "We make a lot of choices for our children: we don't allow them to vote; we don't allow them to drink; we don't allow them to drive cars; we don't allow them to serve in wars at age 13, whether they want to or not; and we don't allow them to have sex with grown men."

But Matthew's mother, Peggy, said she and her husband of 25 years were proud that their son did not disappear like so many deadbeat dads. "He's not always lived up to his responsibilities, but this time he will," Ms. Koso said. "He could have left, but he didn't."

Matthew and Crystal met when she was 8. He was in special education, graduated from high school in 2001 and joined the Marine Corps, but left after four months on a medical discharge.

The two became a couple, according to Crystal, when she was 12 and he was 20. A year later, Crystal's mother, Cecilia Guyer, who is divorced from her father, filed for a restraining order against Matthew.

Despite the court order, both mothers now say Crystal continued to go to the Kosos' home after school, sleeping over in Matthew's basement room on weekends. One afternoon when Ms. Guyer and her daughter were shopping at a second-hand store for a dress for an 8th grade dance, Ms. Guyer noticed that Crystal had stretch marks. The couple confessed, but said they were not interested in adoption. After consulting with a lawyer, they were married in a judge's chambers 18 miles away in Hiawatha, Kansas.

Mr. Bruning said he was shocked that more than 80% of the 250 people—most from outside Nebraska—who had contacted him opposed prosecution. Similar sentiment abounds in Falls City, where people say putting Mr. Koso in jail would most likely land his wife and child on welfare, an unnecessary double-burden for taxpayers. "They are trying to make a right out of a wrong," Mardell Rehrs, 67, said of the couple. "Give them a chance."

Paternity Establishment

State paternity establishment policies must take statutory rape into account.[47] If a minor parent seeking to establish paternity is a boy, it is likely that the mother also is a minor. However, if the minor parent seeking to establish paternity is a girl, there is a significant possibility that the father is an adult. The complexity of paternity establishment is illustrated by Marguerite who tried to use statutory rape as a means of involving her child's father in her life:

Sixteen-year-old Marguerite

Marguerite is just a few weeks shy of her 16th birthday. Her son Leson is two years old. Her mother, living in poverty and an unstable situation, kicked Marguerite out of the house when she became pregnant. Now Marguerite lives with a family friend, relying on welfare benefits and Food Stamps to support herself. She attends school sporadically.

Leson's father, Tomas, is in his early 20s. When Marguerite became pregnant at thirteen, 19-year-old Tomas said he would help care for the child. Despite occasional violence, Marguerite hoped the two would get married and start a family. As her due date came closer, he stopped seeing her. Now he lives nearby with a new, older girlfriend and has nothing to do with Marguerite or their child. A court-ordered paternity test revealed that he is the father. Still, Tomas has never paid child support.

Marguerite is hurt, furious, broke and alone raising her son. Her benefits may be cut off soon because the welfare law requires adolescent parents to live with a relative to be eligible for assistance. She needs help retaining her benefits and obtaining a child support order against Tomas. Unfortunately, even if an order is issued, it is unlikely that he will ever pay. Marguerite desperately wants Tomas brought to court for statutory rape. "All I really wish, is for the judge to tell him he was wrong for what he did to me and should help raise Leson. He shouldn't ignore me like nothing ever happened."

Intra-family Incest and Rape

Intra-family sexual abuse and domestic violence also must be considered in adolescent sexual relationships. Even if the mother is not an early adolescent, the possibility that incest or rape has led to the pregnancy exists. A relative or another male living in the household may be a baby's genetic father. In these cases, rather than seeking to facilitate paternity establishment, states need to provide avenues for the minor and her baby to escape an abusive situation.

Differential Enforcement of Statutory Abuse Laws

In some circumstances, criminal prosecution of statutory rape—not marriage—is indicated. Girls need protection from forced marriage. Sexually active girls 14 and under are particularly vulnerable to coercion and violence. They also are likely to have a significantly older partner, who may appear to the girl's family to be a good marital prospect even though she does not wish to marry. A minor mother might be coerced by her family to marry someone outside the family in order to conceal incest. She might also be pressured by an abusive partner to marry in order to avoid a statutory rape charge. The family of the statutory rapist may push him to marry in order to avoid prosecution. Judicial oversight is necessary to make sure that a decision to marry is free of coercion and not a way to avoid prosecution for criminal conduct.

The possibility of criminal action provides a deterrent effect. However, using the criminal justice system rather than social services in statutory rape situations may have unintended consequences. A criminal response is not designed to help the adolescent victims and can fail to deal with intractable issues underlying adolescent pregnancy.

Rigel Oliveri, professor of law at the University of Missouri, proposes differential enforcement of statutory rape laws. Instead of applying them to most offenders as criminals, Oliveri suggests increasing the penalties for the underlying abuse, exploitation and coercion that already constitute child abuse.[48] She proposes making the fact that a victim is a minor an aggravating factor in the underlying offense with increased penalties. For example, an offender in a domestic violence or rape case of a minor should have increased child support to help her complete schooling rather than incarceration.

Oliveri would bypass non-abusive, consensual relationships between adolescents over thirteen and young adults who are not in positions of authority over the adolescent. Her approach targets exploitative and dangerous relationships and is less susceptible to arbitrary or discriminatory application because its purpose is to prevent the abuse of adolescents. She hopes it will increase child support, which often is ignored when a statutory rape charge is made.

Oliveri's approach may discount the deleterious consequences that non-abusive, consensual sexual relationships with adults can have for adolescents. However, it is one thing to recognize sexual involvement with older men as a serious issue and another to make all such relationships serious crimes. Her proposal is pragmatic. Policy makers should consider revising statutory rape enforcement policies to make them more effective.

Balancing the Rights of Parents and Minors

The Century of the Child ended in unforeseen ways. The essence of childhood at the beginning of the century was its dependency. Competent parents respected this dependency by exercising parental authority judiciously.

In the second half of the century, parental authority actually declined. As a result, childrearing has become a matter of negotiation between parent and child with state and other agencies monitoring the process. In the past children were assumed to have capabilities we now rarely think they have because they were needed to help a family survive. In our efforts to give our children happy childhoods we tend to downplay their abilities to assume responsibilities and obligations.[49] Much present confusion about adolescence is caused by conflicts that can be stressful between adolescents' rights and their obligations to their parents. This highlights the minors' responsibility to accept legitimate parental authority and to cooperate with their parents.

Our tradition of individual autonomy has largely kept government out of the family. Elizabeth Bartholet, professor of law at Harvard University, points out that "family autonomy" really has been parental autonomy.[50] The law is moving in the direction of defining the limits of parental power. The Juvenile Justice and Delinquency Prevention Act of 1974 removed "status offenses" of incorrigibility and running away from juvenile delinquency. They now are regarded as resulting from the lack or inappropriate usage of parental authority rather than as solely from the adolescents themselves. The focus has shifted to therapeutic interventions with families. There also is a trend toward dealing with homeless adolescents' prostitution by providing "safe houses" with treatment resources rather than by using the criminal justice system.[51]

In some ways, the adolescent quest for independence represents a return to the time in which childhood did not extend beyond 14. The difference is that in earlier centuries persons were economically productive at the age of fourteen whereas now they have a minimum of four and possibly eight or more years before they become economically productive.

The shift in the balance of power from adults to children and adolescents has had emotional and economic repercussions. Parents now may look to their offspring for emotional support and give them excessive material goods that stress family finances. This shift in the balance of power extends to children and adolescents now having the right to bring legal proceedings against their parents—sometimes with justification. All of this has eroded parental authority with resulting frequent overindulgence of children and adolescents.

When family matters are brought into the legal system, the interests of children, parents and the state need to be carefully identified and balanced with each other in order to determine the appropriate rule of law that governs a specific case. The legal system should approach conflicts between them with openness and negotiation rather than antagonism and litigation.[52]

CONCLUSION

Children have come a long way from earlier centuries in which they were seen as miniature adults, and adolescence was not recognized. When children were regarded as the property of their parents, they had no rights at all. Now they have moral and civil rights.

Although parental rights derive from the Constitutional protection of the privacy of the family and individual liberty, they really are custodial and guardianship duties for minors. Minors' rights derive from human rights that specify the minimum standards of civilized behavior. They hinge on their right to competent parents.

There are two circumstances other than age-grading in which minors are awarded adult civil liberties and privileges. The first is the mature minor doctrine that awards specific privileges. The second is emancipation that awards adult liberties and privileges.

The gradual emergence of the civil rights of minors in the United States began by treating them differently from adults in criminal law through juvenile courts. Now juvenile courts follow due process procedures but still are limited in their abilities to improve juvenile behavior and family relationships.

Statutory rape laws are designed to discourage the sexual exploitation of minors. Recent national efforts to reform the welfare system and its connection with adolescent childbirth have led many states to enact stricter, and increase the enforcement of, statutory rape laws.

When family matters are brought into the legal system, the interests of children, parents and the state need to be carefully identified and balanced against each other in order to determine the appropriate rule of law that governs a specific case.

The legal system can help to ensure that the developmental interests of adolescents and their babies are taken into account in decision-making regarding parenthood prior to childbirth.

Chapter 8

The Rights of Parents

Today we may not blame parents for being largely instrumental in getting their boys and girls into trouble. But twenty or thirty years from now, we will have to point our finger against those parents who, because of neglect or ignorance, wittingly or unwittingly bring out the worst in their children.

David Abrahamsen, 1952
Who Are the Guilty? A Study of Education and Crime[1]

Most people assume that parents have rights that give them exclusive powers over their children. But specifying those rights only arises when things go wrong in families and child-serving institutions. When parents and child-serving institutions function well, the question of parental rights is seldom be raised.

Unfortunately for children, the emotionally charged issue of parental rights is important now. Parents compel state intervention when they neglect and abuse or dispute custody of their children. Minors give birth. Many child-serving institutions are dysfunctional.

Defining who is a parent can be complicated today.[2] With surrogate birthing and artificial insemination, the very meaning of "mother" and "father" is contested. Children can have as many as ten different legally recognized parents. By eliminating the ambiguous term "natural parent" from its rules for establishing a legal parent-child relationship, the Uniform Parentage Act encourages courts to focus on the precise relationship a female or a male has to a child. Is the relationship genetic, birth, functional, stepparent or adoptive?

In order to set the stage for thinking about parental rights, the evolution of the concept of individual rights merits consideration.

RIGHTS OF INDIVIDUALS

The idea that individual persons have certain rights springs from the vulnerability of human beings in the face of stronger forces.[3] The Declaration of Independence and

Constitution are based on the idea that the purpose of government is not to protect the elite, nor to facilitate greed or self-interest nor to promote a religious group's agenda. These documents led to our present government that guarantees certain inalienable human rights for all persons including the young. Contemporary talk about human rights in the United States usually emphasizes rights to benefits, overlooking the responsibilities that accompany rights.

The survival of all that is best in our society—individual freedom and the rule of law—depends on thriving families that rear children to become responsible citizens. Because of their responsibilities to their children and to society, parents need rights or prerogatives to protect and fulfill the human rights of their children.

PARENTAL RIGHTS

In the past, children have been treated as the personal property of their parents. Fathers even had the power of life and death over their children. To this day, the popular presumption is that children "belong to" their parents. But, since The Enlightenment of the 18th century, parenthood has been seen in the Western world as a contract between parents and society in which parents are awarded rights in exchange for discharging their parental responsibilities.

John Locke in the 17th century and William Blackstone in the 18th century held that the rights and powers of parents arise from their duties to care for their offspring.[4] They recognized that no society can survive without ensuring that its children grow up to be responsible, productive citizens. If there must be a choice, they held that it is more important to protect children than to protect adults.

The legal rights of parents to bear children, raise and guide them according to their beliefs is protected by the Constitution. Children also have the right to be raised by their parents without unjustified interference by the state. These rights in combination are called the *right of family integrity*.[5]

James Garbarino, professor of psychology at Loyola University Chicago, points out that these ideas about parental rights are influenced by personal and public views of child-parent relationships.[6] Are children:

- the private property of parents,
- members of families with no direct link to the state, or
- citizens with a primary relationship with the state?

Children as Private Property

Parental rights have become the most protected and cherished of all Constitutional rights.[7] They are based on the natural right to beget children and the likelihood that affection leads parents to act in the best interests of their children. The Constitution's Fourth Amendment protection of the privacy of the family and the due process clause of the Fourteenth Amendment have been interpreted as giving parents custodial guardianship of their children:

Amendment IV—The right of the people to be secure in their persons, houses, papers, and effects, against unreasonable searches and seizures, shall not be violated . . .

Amendment XIV—No state shall make or enforce any law which shall abridge the privileges or immunities of citizens of the United States . . .

The popular presumption that children are the property of their parents has been justified by the Fourth Amendment protection of the privacy of the home. A Parental Rights and Responsibilities Act was introduced in the 1995 Congress to create a Constitutional amendment that would specify absolute parental rights.[8] It did not gather support because the legal system already respects parental rights, and it would impede protecting children from neglect and abuse.

The Fourteenth Amendment has been interpreted to include the "right to reproduce" implying that a baby is the parent's property regardless of the parent's capacity to raise the child. This makes it possible to produce babies as intentionally designed persons without regard for their interests. In this vein, the competitive pricing of sperm and eggs according to the donor's characteristics, such as academic performance, athletic abilities and racial features, is a step toward making children commodities produced from marketable genetic material.

In spite of these interpretations, the legal system no longer considers children to be the property of their parents.[9] There is a genetic basis for the legal position that parents do not own their children. The genes we give to our children are not our own. In the process of reproduction, our own genes mix with others. Our genes have a life of their own beyond our control extending back through previous generations and into successive generations. We are only temporary custodians of our own genes and of our children.

Mary Lyndon Shanley, professor of political science at Vassar College, holds that an individual's right to reproduce and a parent's wishes cannot be the primary foundation of family law. The primary focus must be on children's needs and interests.[10] The parent-child relationship is one of stewardship. Parental authority involves responsibilities beyond parental wishes.

Our legal system is based on the principle that no individual is entitled to control the life of another human being whether an adult or a child.[11] Guardians of incompetent adults have a guardianship, not an ownership, role. They are agents for incompetent adults rather than owners of them. In the same way, the childrearing rights of parents are of two kinds: 1) the right to the physical custody of a child and 2) the guardianship right to make decisions on behalf of a child. These rights are based on the interests of a child.

Children as Family Members

Children generally are regarded as members of families with no direct link to the state. The concept of parental rights is a product of traditions and Constitutional precedents that endow birth and adoptive parents with special rights for their children.[12]

Parental rights are legal parental prerogatives based on the moral and civil rights of children to have the nurturance and protection of competent parents. They really are custodial and guardianship duties.[13] Parents are presumed to be in the best position to decide how to raise their children without undue interference by the state. Without a voluntary or involuntary forfeiture of parental responsibilities, the state cannot remove children from their parents' custody in order to seek a "better" home for them.

Children as Citizens

Two trends have moved regarding a child exclusively as a family member to validating a child as a citizen. The first is the growing emphasis on the rights of children to be able to develop their potentials without being neglected or abused. The second is the progressive limitation of parental control, as seen in child neglect and abuse laws, child labor laws, mandatory education laws, adolescent health care policies and parental responsibility laws. When parents do not fulfill their responsibilities to their children, child welfare services intervene, and a governmental agency assumes custody of the children. At that time, children's primary relationship is with the state that has assumed custodial guardianship.

Like other guardians, parents have legal prerogatives to make decisions in the interests of their children.[14] Society generally defers to their authority. Society's challenge is to encourage parents to act in the interests of their children rather than in their own selfish interests. Toward this end lawmakers rely on persuasion and education to help parents fulfill their obligations unless child maltreatment is suspected or demonstrated.

THE PARENT-SOCIETY CONTRACT

James Dwyer, professor of law at William and Mary University, affirms that parental rights do not have a direct basis in the Constitution.[15] The emergence of rights for children reflects this position as our society has progressively limited the control parents have over their children's lives.

Dwyer endorses the Enlightenment view that persons who conceive and give birth to babies enter into an implicit contract with society to raise the children to become responsible citizens. This "parent-society contract" provides a strong moral imperative for public efforts to ensure the safety and quality of life of the resulting child because a contract implies mutual obligations. Both parents and society are accountable to each other.

Government's role in this "parent-society contract" is reflected in debates about:

- ensuring child well-being—Is it an entitlement? A privilege? A tool for social control? *The trend is to view it as an entitlement.*
- adolescent childbirth—Who has guardianship of a minor's baby? *Strictly speaking, no one, but relatives and government policies support minor parents by default.*
- child financial support—Is financial responsibility for a child purely a private matter or a public responsibility? *Both. Federal and state laws mandate childrearing benefits in addition to child financial support from parents and sometimes grandparents through governmental agencies.*

In the "parent-society contract," government plays a vital role in supporting parents in rearing their children and preventing child neglect and abuse. State and local governments aim to provide schools and safe neighborhoods to support childrearing. They provide health insurance, tax deductions and benefits and welfare benefits to eligible parents.

Parents really do not need specifically defined rights. They have prerogatives that flow from their children's rights to nurturance and protection. Unfortunately, these parental prerogatives and children's rights do not fit well in contemporary society.[16] There is little room for accommodating the interests of parents in workplaces. When children are lost in supposedly temporary foster care, their right to competent parents is not fulfilled.

Public policies must recognize that children have a right to be cared for by persons with an enduring commitment to parenthood.[17] Public policies also need to recognize that in the "parent-society contract" society is responsible for ensuring that parents have access to essential childrearing resources.

The parental rights debate would be resolved by a paradigm shift from children as their parents' property to parenthood as a career. Parenthood is the "parent-society" contract with prerogative rights derived from nurturing a child and advocating that child's interests.

Being the mother or father of a child does not necessarily mean that one has the parental custodial and guardianship rights of parenthood. A minor can be a mother or father without having custodial guardianship rights. One remains a mother or a father after parental rights have been terminated and other parents have assumed the roles of motherhood and fatherhood.

THE RIGHTS OF MOTHERS

The laws of every state give the woman or girl who conceives and bears a child automatic recognition as the legal mother of the child. Giving birth follows an already formed relationship during pregnancy.[18] These laws reflect a strong bias in favor of birth mothers, especially those who have cared for and formed a relationship with their babies. This is complicated now by surrogate birth mothers who are not genetic mothers.

The state rarely challenges genetic/birth maternity unless there are compelling circumstances, such as when a pre-birth parental-unfitness petition is filed. In such cases, the baby is placed in state custody at birth with the intention of rehabilitating the genetic/birth mother. This intent often is not realized as illustrated by women who gave birth in prison: 40% of their babies were placed with others when the mothers were released.[19] Of those babies, 51% went to grandparents, 31% to relatives or friends, 11% to foster care and 7% to the father.

Women and girls who give birth are free to decline parenthood by voluntary revocation of their parental rights through a Termination of Parental Rights proceeding so that an adoption plan can be made.[20] Involuntary termination of parental rights can be initiated after reasonable efforts to reunite parent and child have failed. Parental rights also may be terminated automatically under extreme circumstances, such as previous involuntary terminations or murder of a sibling. Third parties, such as foster parents, can petition for termination of parental rights in some states.

THE RIGHTS OF FATHERS

Unlike maternity that does not need it, substantial Constitutional guidance has been provided for states in attributing paternity.[21] States must insure that males have the opportunity to seek paternity. A genetic connection and a relationship, or at least an effort to establish one, with the child is a necessary condition for Constitutional protection of a paternity claim.

In order to claim parental rights, males must register with putative father registries in most states within varying time frames in order to participate in decisions affecting children.[22] Agencies are required to notify putative fathers of adoption plans made by mothers. At the same time, questions arise about the feasibility of making fathers aware of their need to register.

In child-support situations where genetic fathers do not want to acknowledge fatherhood, state agencies try to establish paternity through genetic testing, other biological evidence or acknowledgement by the mother or the male alleged to be the genetic father.

A father's genetic tie to a child can be overridden when a child's interests are determined to be better served by a father who is married to the mother and who has established a relationship with the child. In *Michael H.* the genetic father of a child produced in an adulterous relationship was denied paternity in favor of the father who actually had raised the child.[23]

THE LIABILITY OF PARENTS

The common-law doctrine of parental immunity has maintained that, absent willful and wanton misconduct, children may not sue their parents for negligence within the scope of the parental relationship.[24] However, incest is a criminal offense outside of parental immunity.

Most states and courts are beginning to define the liability of parents for damage to a child. As long ago as 1963, in *Zepeda v. Zepeda*, a child sued his father for having caused him to be born out of wedlock.[25] Although that suit was unsuccessful, it raised the persisting issue of a child's legal right to be wanted, loved and nurtured—in essence to be competently parented.

Children have successfully sued their parents for negligence and have brought actions against third parties who alienate one of their parents from the family. In 1992 in Orlando, Florida, 11-year-old Gregory Kingsley legally "divorced" his mother so he could be adopted by his foster parents.[26] Because minors cannot be sued, virtually all states allow victims to file civil suits against parents for damage caused by their children.

THE *PARENS PATRIAE* DOCTRINE

The most significant fact justifying state involvement in children's lives is that they do not choose the families into which they are born. The opportunities families can provide for their children also are not equal.[27]

The civil rights of minors in the United States are based on the *parens patriae* doctrine, which justifies state intervention on parental authority as a part of the "parent-society contract."

Parens patriae is Latin for "father of the people." The doctrine grants the inherent power and authority of the state to protect persons who are legally unable to act on their own behalf. It gives state courts the power to intervene to protect the "best interests" of dependent persons whose welfare is jeopardized. It gives state courts the ultimate power to terminate parental rights.

The *parens patriae* doctrine is based on three assumptions:[28]

- Childhood and adolescence are periods of dependency requiring supervision.
- The family is of primary importance in the supervision of children and adolescents, but the state should play a role in their education and intervene when the family fails to provide adequate nurturance, moral training or supervision.
- When parents disagree or fail to exercise their authority, the appropriate authority to determine a child's or an adolescent's interests is a public official.

State Interventions on Parental Authority

The *parens patriae* doctrine enables the state to compel parents and minors to act in ways beneficial to society, but it never presumed that the state would assume parenting functions.

A shift from the primacy of the rights of parents to the primacy of the "best interests" of children has been gradually emerging in our courts for two principal reasons:

- Recognizing the human rights of children through child neglect and abuse statutes that define the developmental needs of children for nurturance and protection.
- Recognizing that the well-being of society depends upon children being educated and not being exploited.

A 1985 decision by the Supreme Court of Canada made a child's welfare the paramount consideration in disputes between genetic parents and third parties. In *King v. Low*, the Court stated that although the claims of genetic parents were to receive serious consideration, they must give way to the best interests of their children when the children have developed close psychological ties with another individual.[29] This view is taking hold in American courts as well.

Our legal system distinguishes between what parents can do to themselves and what they can do to their children. For example, they may refuse essential medical treatment for themselves, but they usually are not allowed to do so for their children. They also are not permitted to physically harm their children or to allow children to physically harm themselves.

Legal sanctions against parents can be used when they do not respond to persuasion and education. However, except in life-threatening emergencies, children cannot be removed from their parents without a hearing in a family or juvenile court.

Parents who fail to provide a minimum level of care, who abandon their children or who fail to provide supervision can be found guilty of neglect. Parents who physically, emotionally or sexually abuse their children can be found guilty of abuse. A child usually must be placed under state supervision for a period of time before proceedings that terminate parental rights may begin. Parents who have been convicted of a serious crime, who abuse drugs or alcohol or who cannot meet return conditions when their children have been removed from their care can be found to be unfit. When persons cannot be persuaded or educated to become competent parents, the termination of parental rights with a permanent placement, usually adoption, takes place.

The Liability of the State

In spite of the *parens patriae* doctrine as the basis for the "parent-society contract," the liability of the state if it does not protect minors has not been clearly defined.

In 1989, the U.S. Supreme Court ruled in *DeShaney v. Winnebago County Department of Social Services* that the state is not required by the Fourteenth Amendment to protect the life, liberty or property of its citizens against invasion by private actors:[30]

> Joshua DeShaney suffered brain damage from repeated beatings by his father at the age of four. As a result Joshua was expected to remain institutionalized for life. The U.S. Supreme Court rejected arguments that the state had a duty to protect Joshua because it once placed him in foster care and later because social workers suspected he was being abused by his father but took no action. It held that only "when the state takes a person into its custody and holds him there against his will" does the Fourteenth Amendment due process clause require officials to take responsibility for the individual's safety and well-being. At the same time, the Court did not rule out the possibility that the state acquired a duty to protect Joshua under tort law.

In a similar way, an appellate court in California upheld a local court's dismissal of a suit by a 17-year-old boy who alleged damage by mismanagement of his adoption as a newborn:[31]

> At the age of 17, Dennis Smith filed a complaint against the Alameda County Social Services Department alleging the Agency was liable for damages because it failed to find an adoptive home when his mother gave him to the Department for the purpose of adoption shortly after his birth. The Agency placed Dennis in a series of foster homes, but no one adopted him.
>
> Dennis claimed that the Department negligently or intentionally failed to take reasonable actions to bring about his adoption. Therefore, he was deprived of proper and effective parental care and guidance and a secure family environment. Dennis alleged that this caused him mental and emotional damage.

The dismissal of Dennis' complaint was upheld in appellate court on a number of grounds, including the difficulty in directly linking damage to Dennis to the Alameda County Social Services Department's failure to arrange for his adoption. Significant other grounds were that the proposed liability would not reduce future harm to others and that it would impede the proper functioning of agencies that operate under budgetary constraints. The court implied that liability could result with more convincing linkage of early life experience and later outcomes.

In contrast with Dennis Smith's case, Cook County, Illinois, settled a claim out of court by an 18-year-old boy that he had been damaged by the negligence and incompetence of county social workers. In this case, the linkage between professional practices and damage to Billy Nichols apparently was made effectively:[32]

> In December of 1981, attorneys for the State of Illinois and Cook County paid $150,000 in an out-of-court settlement of a suit of a former dependent child, Billy Nichols, who had been entrusted to the child-welfare system and later as an adult sued the county social service agency for the negligence of social workers that kept Billy dependent and unfit to live in society.
>
> On September 19, 1960, Billy and his seven-month-old sister were abandoned by their mother and found eating garbage behind a skid-row mission in Chicago. Billy's age (approximately five) was a mystery, and his speech was unintelligible. He was sent to an institution for the retarded in Michigan for four years. After a subsequent stormy foster-home placement, he was placed in Cook County's juvenile security prison for nearly three years, although the superintendent repeatedly petitioned the court to remove him.
>
> In 1969, a legal aid lawyer, Pat Murphy, filed a class-action suit to release dependent and neglected children from prison on behalf of Billy. At 14 Billy was transferred to Elgin State Hospital, where he ran away ten times and was committed to the Illinois Security Hospital at Chester at the age of 18. Three years later Attorney Murphy intervened to enroll Nichols in a psychiatric program for two years, until he was jailed for car theft.

Law suits continue to be advanced in an effort to redress the adverse impact of foster care on individuals, such as a 2008 suit against the Florida Department of Children and Families.[33] There is a trend to use class action suits to force improvements in child welfare services. For example, a class action suit was filed in 1993 in Wisconsin by the American Civil Liberties Union and the Children's Rights Project, Inc., against Milwaukee County and the state for failing to adequately protect children.[34] In response, the duties and authority of child welfare services were transferred from the county to a state Bureau of Milwaukee Child Welfare.

THE RIGHT TO BE A COMPETENT PARENT

To say that a parent has a right to be competent may stretch the notion of rights too far. However, the logic for the right to be a competent parent in our society is compelling.

First of all, by definition the child-parent unit is irreducible. One half of the dyad is a parent and one half is a child. The interests of children and the interests of parents are inseparable and both derive from a child's goal of responsible citizenship. When parents face dangerous environments, poverty, unemployment, illness and mental incapacities, their children inevitably face the same problems in addition to the risk of incompetent parenting. Therefore, if children's interests are to be fulfilled, the interests of parents also must be taken into account. If children have a moral right to be competently parented, then parents have a moral right to be competent if possible. If this rationale is not enough, there are at least two more.

The second rationale is that the integrity of society itself depends upon competent parents. Incompetent parents threaten the stability of society and incur enormous public costs. Therefore, to become a competent parent when possible deserves the status of a right.

The third rationale is that human beings have a genetic predisposition toward being competent parents in order to ensure the survival of our species. The goal of the human reproductive cycle is parenthood, not just procreation. Conceiving and giving birth to a child initiate parenthood as the fruition of the developmental stages of childhood, adolescence and adulthood. In the most fundamental sense, competent parenthood fulfills the role of a woman or a man in the reproductive cycle. Therefore, in order to preserve the human species and our society, individuals have a right to fulfill their reproductive potentials if they choose to do so and to become competent parents if possible.

CONCLUSION

If all parents and all child-serving institutions served their children's developmental interests, the issue of parental rights would seldom be raised.

Parental rights are no longer based on the presumption that children are the property of their parents. Parental custodial guardianship rights enable parents to discharge their responsibilities to their children and to society in a "parent-society contract" that provides a strong moral imperative for public efforts to ensure the safety and quality of life of children.

The laws of every state give the woman or girl who conceives and bears a baby automatic recognition as the legal mother of the child even though the girl as a minor cannot logically have custodial guardianship rights for her baby. States have rules for identifying legal fathers.

The civil rights of minors in the United States reflect the *parens patriae* doctrine, which justifies state intervention on parental authority.

Parents who fail to meet specified conditions can have their parental rights terminated to permit making an adoption plan for the child. Most states have set aside the parental immunity doctrine so that children now may sue their parents under certain circumstances.

A shift from the primacy of the rights of parents to the primacy of the "best interests" of children has gradually emerged in our courts.

Parental rights really are prerogatives in the context of the responsibilities of parenthood.

Part 3

THE HUMAN DEVELOPMENTAL PROCESS

Children are expensive . . . it used to take one income to raise a family, it now takes two. Then again the experience of having children—however irksome, expensive, wearying and career-hampering it may be—is also thrilling and delightful and full of continually changing fascinations. A child lifts the heart and gives meaning to life.

Paul Johnson
British historian[1]

The first step in understanding how the lives of young people can go awry is to examine their developmental needs and the influences that amplify or dampen the natural drift of their lives toward chaos.

The notion that all babies need is feeding, diapering and being kept warm is prevalent in popular thought and public policies. The facts that babies are interacting, learning human beings and that their development as human beings depends on forming enduring attachments with their parents is not fully appreciated in our society.

A human being is a complicated self-organizing system that includes self-organizing internal subsystems, especially the mind. Human nature is interwoven with nurture as behavior influences biology. The evolution of the brain depends upon communication between the minds of a parent and a child.

Adolescence is a time for preparing for adulthood by experimenting socially, growing physically and maturing emotionally. It is a developmental stage to be fully lived and enjoyed. Adolescents need competent parents as much as younger children do—even more so because of their vulnerability to risks that permanently alter their lives.

The transition from adolescence to adulthood is both exciting and stressful. Adolescents need the guidance and financial help of stable families in order to make this transition successfully. They also need mentors and education to help them gain the knowledge and confidence they need to succeed in life. Unfortunately, many young people find themselves facing adulthood unprepared, unsupported and dispirited.

Two vital aspects of parenthood are commonly overlooked. The first is that parenthood is a developmental stage in the life cycle. The second is that the readiness for parenthood follows completion of the adolescent stage of life. Achieving the ability to assume responsibility for one's own life as an adult is a prerequisite for assuming responsibility for the life of another person. Conversely, premature parenthood interferes with adolescent development and exposes a baby to high risk.

Chapter 9

Developing Human Relationships: Attachment Bonding

No society can long sustain itself unless its members have learned the sensitivities, motivations and skills involved in assisting and caring for other human beings.

Urie Bronfenbrenner, 1976
The Ecology of Human Development[1]

Babies usually are seen as objects to be adored and cared for—not as persons. This view makes it possible to overlook the facts that a difficult birth and time in intensive care are traumatic for newborns.[2] It makes it possible to ignore the babies while pre-occupied with the crisis of adolescent childbirth, including establishing paternity. It makes it possible to ignore the connection between baby-parent love and loving adult relationships in later life that are based on the same brain circuits.[3]

The notion that all babies need is caregiving in the form of feeding and diapering prevails in popular thought and public policies. The fact that they are interacting, learning human beings has not taken solid root in our society. Babies analyze and re-spond to sounds. They stop eating to listen to something. When they hear other babies cry, they usually cry with them. They may stop crying on hearing a recording of their own voice—suggesting they recognize themselves.

We now know that newborn babies are persons in every sense of the word. They gaze deeply into their mothers' eyes like lovers, called *en face* socializing. They closely observe their mothers. They are upset when their mothers wear expressionless masks in experiments. They are upset when their mothers are depressed. The fact that their development as human beings depends on forming enduring attachments with their parents is not fully appreciated, in part because other activities compete with parenthood.

ATTACHMENT BONDING SYSTEMS

Building on the work of Charles Darwin, historians, archeologists and anthropologists have defined the evolution of the human emotional capacity for attachment bonding, cooperation and altruism from early life.[4] Animal research even suggests that bonding between mother and baby is encoded through the alteration of genes rather than the usual memory process. This capacity tempers self-assertive individual survival drives with integrative species-survival drives.

Competition, territoriality and tribalism rooted in fear of predators and based in the lower brain centers (the limbic system) served early humans well. But the limbic system is short-sighted and does not favor species survival.[5]

While competition is a key motivator in human affairs, cooperation is equally important. The viability of both interpersonal relationships and market economies depend upon our virtuous nature.[6] Higher brain centers evolved to permit species survival through the reproductive advantages of attachment bonding between parents and children and persons living in intimate groups. These trust-inducing advantages contributed to the evolution of neurological attachment bonding systems influenced by the hormones oxytocin in females and pitressin in males.[7]

Attachment bonding begins before birth. Research on lifetime health records reveals that characteristics in later life are affected by our experiences in the womb.[8] A classic example was seen in the retarded growth of women who were fetuses during the Dutch Hunger Winter of 1944-1945 and later gave birth to smaller babies themselves.

Babies are social beings predisposed to attachment bonding. They can form close relationships, express themselves forcefully, show preferences, form memories and influence people from the start.[9] They show evidence of thinking when they reach out, give an inquisitive look, frown or scream in protest, gurgle in satisfaction or gasp in excitement. They listen intently to their mothers' voices, which they readily distinguish from other voices. They engage in complex activities that integrate their senses and enable learning.

John Bowlby's ground-breaking theory of attachment bonding borrows from cybernetics—the study of how mechanical and biological systems self-regulate to achieve goals while their external and internal environments change.[10] Attachment theory begins with the idea that two basic goals guide young children's behavior: safety and exploration. A child who stays safe survives; a child who explores develops the intelligence and skills needed for adult life. These two needs often oppose each other, so they are regulated by a cybernetic "thermostat" that monitors the level of ambient safety. When safe, a child explores and plays. But when safety is uncertain, a switch is thrown leading to fear and withdrawal. The attachment bonding process permits children to internalize images of their caregivers. Children mature by internalizing working models of their caregivers that become self-regulating "thermostats."

There are four components of the human attachment bonding system.[11] The first is the *succorant bonding system* present at birth. It extends from infancy into adolescence and seeks bonding with parents. The second is the *affiliative bonding system*, which emerges during childhood and continues into adulthood where it sustains friendships. The third is the *sexual bonding system*, which becomes prominent after puberty, continues through adult life and fosters romantic relationships. The fourth is the *nurturant bonding system*, which also flowers after puberty, continues throughout life and fosters bonding to a child and intimate relationships between adults. Development of the *nurturant bonding system* builds on the *succorant* and *affiliative* systems that depend, in turn, on having had the experience of being nurtured.

The capacities for each of these bonding systems are present during early life and emerge more fully at successive levels in human development. Each system is based on human needs that persist throughout life. The purpose of these bonding systems is to ensure the survival of individuals so that they can produce progeny and continue the species. Many people lead full lives without participating in the reproductive cycle, but the evolutionary purpose of their interpersonal bonding systems is reproduction, not just companionship and sexual gratification.

The stability of family relationships depends upon dampening self-assertive individual-survival drives expressed through the succorant and sexual bonding systems by integrative species-survival drives expressed through the affiliative and nurturant bonding systems.

Succorant Bonding System

The succorant bonding system that seeks caregiving is essential for the physical survival of babies. Without attachment bonding, babies fail to thrive and even die as has been seen in orphanages. Templates for the readiness for succorant bonding to mother and father images appear to be genetically programmed in humans.[12] The precursor for human maternal attachment can be seen in mammals that seek out their mother immediately after birth. Their capacity to identify their mothers is based on prenatal experience in the mother's womb. Lacking prenatal experience, human babies have a genetic basis for perceiving a father, but not a specific male.

Mothers who give birth to babies have a deep attachment to the human beings who were in their bodies.[13] The placenta produces progesterone that helps sustain the pregnancy and contributes to changes in estrogen and progesterone levels that "prime" a mother to respond maternally. During the birth process itself, further hormonal changes, particularly oxytocin, produce the muscle contractions in childbirth. Oxytocin also has an opiate-like, soothing effect, preparing the mother for nurturing her baby. Her brain and hormones respond to birth by activating feelings of love and tenderness. In the nursing process, a mother's blood pressure decreases as calming oxytocin suffuses her and her baby through her milk.[14]

Prenatal exposure to the mother's voice and odors prime a newborn to respond preferentially to a birth mother in the succorant bonding process.[15] Babies have their mothers' antibodies for a period of time after birth. Human babies recognize the sight, sound, smell and touch of their mothers, but they apparently do not recognize their fathers' voices. On the other hand, both mothers and fathers do appear to be able to differentiate their own newborns from other newborns in a nursery solely by touching their babies' hands.

At first, attachment bonding is unidirectional as a baby seeks succorance. Over time working models of the parent are encoded in the child's brain, and images of the baby are encoded in the parent's brain. A baby's distress triggers caregiving instincts in the mother. A baby's drive for succorance is reinforced by the nurturant actions of the person to whom the baby attaches. Oxytocin is the affectionate glue between baby and parent. It also is secreted under stress, causing a desire for succorance.[16]

Nurturing instincts are designed to insure that mothers are devoted to the care of their babies. After birth, her baby is the center of a mother's life. Physical transformations within her body continue after birth. Nurturing her baby produces hormones and inscribes new pathways in her brain that lower the threshold of stimulation needed to elicit maternal responses. Breastfeeding releases oxytocin with a relaxing effect. Within days a mother can pick out her own baby's clothes by smell alone. Elevated prolactin levels produced by her baby's sucking intensify her feelings of protectiveness.

Without DNA testing, fathers have no way of being certain about their parentage other than what they believe to be true. Still, prolactin levels in men living with pregnant women go up over the course of pregnancy, as do cortisol and to some extent estradiol levels.[17] Testosterone levels drop in men shortly after birth. The more involved they are in nurturant bonding with their babies, the more likely their testosterone will continue to drop. This might reduce male behaviors that divert them from nurturing, such as competing with other males. A fully attached father can be more committed to his baby's well-being than a weakly attached mother.

Affiliative Bonding System

The affiliative bonding system favors cooperative behavior essential for the survival of the species. Also referred to as "reciprocal bonding," affiliative bonding builds on succorant bonding in babies and nurturant bonding in their parents.[18] It goes beyond a child's instinctive quest for security and a parent's instinct to possess and protect. It involves a range of dimensions that include intimacy, shared humor and positive emotions. It probably is based on a "mirror" neuron system that underlies an empathic awareness of the feelings and desires of others. Congenital deficiencies in this system, such as in autism, impede affiliative bonding.

A child succorantly attaches *to* a caregiver. A child affiliatively bonds *with* a caregiver, and a parent nurturantly bonds *with* a child. Initial succorant attachment seeks affiliative bonding. However, babies do not become affiliatively bonded with genetic mothers and fathers who do not intimately interact with them.

Babies and children form affiliative bonds with adoptive parents who nurture them. Children who discover they have been adopted have socially conditioned reactions to that information, but they do not automatically shift their bonding relationships from their adoptive parents to their genetic parents. Life experience creates affiliative parent-child bonding.

A deep emotional bond with blood relatives is not based on genes. It is based on reciprocal affiliative bonding that takes place through child-parent and sibling relationships. Affiliative attachment bonds are imprinted in the brain. Adoptive parents are the "real" parents of adopted children because of their shared affiliative bonds.

Affiliatively bonded adults and children build evolving images in each other's brains. They sense and respond to each other's needs for interaction. Reciprocal interactions with responsive caregivers develop a child's capacity for higher mental functions, empathy, compassion and resilience.[19]

The Developing Mind

A human being is a complicated self-organizing system that includes self-organizing subsystems, including the central nervous system—the seat of the mind.

The development of the brain depends upon communication between the minds of parent and child.[20] It occurs through observation and interaction with more knowledgeable members of the culture. Connections between two minds involve an energetic resonance in which information freely flows between two brains. This can be exhilarating. Rather than following predetermined steps, a child's mind evolves toward increasing complex patterns (fractals) guided by amplifying and dampening internal and external structures. Internal structures include synapses between neurons that form memories, beliefs and attitudes. External structures include human relationships and environmental conditions.

Stable mental images (fractals) are formed as working models as babies interact with caregivers. For example, a baby and mother recognize each other's faces and smile. Positive feelings are associated with being with the mother. Working models of such situations are "attractor states," meaning they organize behavioral responses around that situation. A baby's secure feeling when with the mother is an "attractor state."[21]

Emotions are attractors that organize behavior around mental images of feelings, attitudes and beliefs. Babies form images of their parents' behavior as their developing minds are shaped by their parents' minds. Positive images and emotions acquired through interacting with attachment figures during early life enhance the development of self-regulating brain structures.[22]

A child learns to regulate emotional states in response to parental constraints.[23] The orbitofrontal cortex plays an important role in emotional regulation that is especially sensitive to face-to-face communication. It operates as a "clutch" that disengages the sympathetic nervous system (the "accelerator") and activates the parasympathetic system (the "brakes"). This is why eye-contact between parent and child facilitates setting limits. The meaning of the word "no" is conveyed more effectively with eye-contact than by shouting across a room. This is the basis for the maxim in setting limits with young children: "Use your feet instead of your mouth."

As time progresses, learning that a child's wishes are not automatically gratified and that a child's mind and a parent's mind are separate is necessary for a child to learn self-control and modulate behavior and emotional states in pro-social ways. The clash of separate minds and wills is an essential element in mental and social development. Experiments with monkeys suggest that mildly stressful experiences that do not exceed a child's coping ability enhance the development of brain systems that regulate emotional, neuroendocrine and cognitive control.[24]

The world of symbolic meaning in play opens the door to awareness that one has a subjective experience—a mind of one's own. Play enriches personal growth and the capacity for enjoyment and creativity in later life. Symbols involved in play crystallize children's ideas, so that ideas can be thought and thought about. When children understand they and others have independent minds, they acquire their own distinctive minds.[25] They expand their creative imaginations. Then the insight dawns that the child is one among others. From this time on, a child can think about other people as individuals with subjective experiences of their own. At this point children take off into the realms of society and culture. Young children who passively view television may be less imaginative and empathic than those who engage in creative play.[26]

Affiliative Attachment Styles

When it has developed, the affiliative attachment bonding of children is classified as secure, insecure-avoidant, insecure-resistant, ambivalent or disorganized.[27] Attachment bonding in itself does not differentiate unhealthy from healthy relationships. The strength of a child's need to form succorant attachment bonds in spite of adverse experiences was revealed in a study that classified almost one-half of abused children as securely attached to their maltreating parents.[28] Although attachment insecurity in early life contributes to unhappiness in later life, it apparently does not directly cause clinical disorders unless combined with other risk factors.

Attachment styles emerge gradually over time.[29] A child with a particular temperament makes bids for nurturance. A mother with a particular temperament responds, or does not respond, based on her mood, how overworked she is or what childrearing expert she has been reading. Children with sunny dispositions with happy mothers are likely to develop secure attachment bonding, but a dedicated mother can overcome either her own or her child's less pleasant disposition and foster secure attachment bonding as well.

A parent's capacity to respond to the emotional and mental states of a baby is the foundation of secure attachment bonding. These mutually attuned experiences allow a baby to develop a reflective capacity that creates an internal sense of cohesion and interpersonal connection.[30] Over time children build up what Bowlby called an "internal working model" of themselves, their mothers and their relationships. This self-organizing model (attractor state) provides a sense of security when a mother is not present.

Most children make a transition from patterns of personal distress to modulated expressions of concern for the welfare of others.[31] This is facilitated during the second year of life when children learn the meaning of "no." Parents who are empathic set firm limits and emphasize the rights and welfare of others have children who show high levels of pro-social and compassionate behaviors. Genetic differences in sociability also play a role. In adverse environments, such as a chaotic family life, child maltreatment and parental mental illness, children may become frightened or angry and lash out or turn away from others. In steeling themselves against their own pain, they become inured to the pain of others.

Sexual Bonding System

The sexual bonding system appears early in life in the form of the Electra and Oedipal complexes based on fantasies in which girls replace their mothers and marry their fathers and boys do the same with their fathers and mothers.[32]

Romantic love evolves during adolescence to direct human mating and reproduction through three brain networks that govern lustful craving and romantic passion: the hypothalamus, caudate nucleus and prefrontal cortex.

Lustful Craving

Lustful craving is the basic motivation to seek sexual union with a partner. It is mediated by the lower brain centers in the hypothalamus, the site of appetites essential for individual survival and for reproducing the species. Lust does not automatically result in romantic passion or the urge to attach to a mating partner over time.

Lust's capriciousness may be a part of nature's plan. Lust enabled our ancestors to follow two complementary reproductive strategies in tandem.[33] If a male had one mate and two children and secretly gave a female from a different band two more young, he would double the number of his descendents. Likewise, a female who had a mate and became involved with another might bear the latter's baby and acquire extra food and protection for her children.

Oxytocin floods the brain when two people are in skin-to-skin contact producing a soothing and pleasurable effect. The biggest rush of oxytocin—other than during birth and nursing—comes from sex, especially if it includes cuddling, touching and orgasm. Many of the same circuits involved in baby-parent bonding are activated.[34]

Romantic Passion

Romantic passion—the elation and obsession with "being in love"—focuses courtship on one individual at a time, thereby conserving precious mating time and energy. It emanates from the motor of the mind, the caudate nucleus.

When romantic passion is reciprocated, the brain reacts with positive emotions, such as excitement, pleasure and anticipation. Regions of the pre-frontal cortex plan tactics, calculate losses and gains and register one's progress toward the goal—emotional, physical, even spiritual union with the beloved.

Passionate love's symptoms overlap with those of heroin (euphoric well-being) and cocaine (energetic euphoria).[35] Passionate love involves the release of dopamine and puts one at risk of "addiction" to the beloved. As with drug addiction, the brain reacts to a passion-induced surplus of dopamine, develops neurochemical reactions that oppose it and restores its own equilibrium. At that point, tolerance sets in. When an addicting drug is withdrawn, the brain is unbalanced in a negative direction. When one's passion is spurned or thwarted, the brain reacts with negative feelings, such as despair, depression and rage similar to withdrawal from heroin or cocaine. Except in pathological emotional states that do resemble drug addiction, passionate love eventually wears off.

Nurturant Bonding System

The nurturant bonding system is first seen in caregiving impulses in young children. It is fully expressed in parenthood and adult companionship that fulfill the reproductive cycle essential for the survival of the species.

Romantic passion does not necessarily turn into nurturant attachment. They are two separate processes and have different time courses. Under the influence of oxytocin, nurturing attachment grows slowly over time as lovers rely upon, care for and trust each other. A metaphor for passionate love is fire. For nurturant love, it is a growing vine that intertwines two people. This is seen in enduring parent-child and marital relationships. Nurturant attachment motivates staying with a partner long enough to rear the young.[36] At the same time, it can bring pain when disrupted. The desire for nurturant attachment generally is stronger in females than in males.

Homo sapiens is a social species, full of emotions finely tuned for loving, helping, sharing and otherwise intertwining our lives with others. There are as many ways to have enduring companionship attachments as there are couples, but being willing to compromise with and tolerate a partner and to nurture each other underlies them all.

QUALITY OF FATHER RELATIONSHIP

Most children have warm relationships with their fathers; some receive inconsistent support; some are adversely affected by their fathers' behavior; still others lose their fathers early in life. Some children have high levels of involvement with males other than their genetic fathers, such as grandfathers and uncles.

Fathers can provide emotional support to the mothers of their children and participate in the care of the children whether or not they live with the mother. One study found that mothers who are supported in breast-feeding by their husbands continue to breast-feed their children longer than those who do not receive such support.[37] Fathers also can offer children links to their extended families and community resources.

A father's nurturing behavior and overall parenting style early in a child's life outweigh the influence of his gender.[38] Fathers are more likely to engage children in physical and stimulating play interactions, while mothers tend to spend more time in verbal activities.

US/THEM MEMES

The feelings associated with relationships that are not based on attachment bonding are based on the genetic capacity to form *Us/Them* codes and are culturally transmitted through behavioral and feeling patterns called *memes*.[39]

Our perceptions of our genetic relatives are based more on learning than on genes. There are biological mechanisms for feelings associated with the perception of genetic ties even though there is no genetic connection. They are based on the brain circuits that mediate *Us/Them* feelings and behaviors. These circuits evolved to create protective family and tribal relationships necessary for survival. Our tribal forbearers relied heavily on the perception of genetic ties to unite them in identifiable groups. As time went on, the disadvantages of mating with close relatives became evident and reinforced the need to identify genetic kin. An example of how kinship feelings can be evoked by abstract information is when a person learns of a DNA connection to another person and experiences a "visceral feeling."[40] This *Us/Them* feeling is not equivalent to the feelings associated with attachment bonding. It is based on a meme.

Us/them meme feelings can be shifted away from people as our perceptions of them change. For example, friendships shift depending on how attitudes between people evolve. Marriages endure because of nurturant bonds that develop between couples not because of romantic or affiliative feelings or *Us/Them* meme codes.

The emotions involved in genetic and adoptive kinship are based on attachment bonding not on genes or *Us/Them* memes. As adopted children and their parents well know, their mutual love is based on attachment bonding to each other not on their genes.

RESILIENCY

Genetically and experientially individual differences appear to play a role in children's resiliency under adversity. Avshalom Caspi, professor at the Institute of Psychiatry in London, and his colleagues found that a variation of a specific gene appears to promote resilience to adverse experiences in early life, including child abuse.[41] This finding was confirmed by Joan Kaufman, a professor of psychiatry at Yale University. Another study found an association between child maltreatment and mental health problems in males with another genotype. [42]

Still, babies need nurturing environments that facilitate attachment bonding to activate genes that influence resiliency. In this sense, parents act as genetic engineers when they know what to expect from their children; how to discipline constructively; and how to manage anger and stress.[43] Free exploratory play, not programmed activity, is the key to optimizing the resiliency of babies and young children.

CONCLUSION

The notion that all babies need is caregiving in the form of feeding and diapering prevails in popular thought and public policies. The facts that babies are interacting, learning human beings and that their development depends on forming enduring attachments with their parents are not fully appreciated in our society.

Parental investment in offspring reflects genetic attachment bonding potentials of children and parents that emerge when brought out by appropriate life experiences.

Four components of the human attachment bonding system have been described: the succorant, affiliative, sexual and nurturant bonding systems. The capacities for these bonding systems are present during early life and flower at successive levels in human development. Their purpose is to enhance the survival of individuals so that they can produce progeny and ensure the survival of the species.

A human being is a complicated self-organizing system that includes self-organizing subsystems, especially the human mind. The development of the brain depends upon communication between the minds of parent and child. Babies internalize "working models" of their parents so that their developing minds are shaped by their parents' more mature minds.

Competent parenthood rests upon attachment bonds between child and parent that promote self-respect, self-confidence and resiliency in dealing with the vicissitudes of life.

Chapter 10

Adolescent Development

I would there were no age between sixteen and twenty-three, or that youth would sleep out the rest; for there is nothing in the between but getting wenches with child, wronging the ancientry, stealing, fighting . . .

William Shakespeare
The Winter's Tale.[1]

In 1904, the psychologist G. Stanley Hall first described adolescence as "the elongated hiatus between childhood and adulthood."[2]

Adolescence is recognized in all cultures as starting with puberty and extending for increasing lengths of time as societies modernize.[3] As the cutting edge of the next generation and a significant factor in our economy, adolescents inevitably affect our society through the ever-changing "pop culture." They are equal or superior to adults in their physical and mental agility. When treated like adults, they usually rise to the challenge.

The image of adolescence as tumultuous is by no means universal.[4] However, when trapped in a disadvantaged peer culture, committing a crime or becoming pregnant can be seen as ways for adolescents to declare adulthood.

Most children enter adolescence with self-regulation skills, relationships with prosocial peers and adults and positive beliefs about themselves. They have a far lower risk for behavior problems than children who already are struggling.[5] However, even for the latter, a trend away from risky behavior occurs in the late teens as knowledge and decision-making skills grow.

The adolescent brain can learn and amass more knowledge than at any other time in life. Still, adolescents are "diamonds in the rough." Each one has a compelling need to "be me." Dramatic physical changes occur as they form their own identities and become increasingly independent from their families. They need stimulating music and activities to organize maturing brain circuits. They need to learn how to deal with powerful emotions—love, hate, envy, jealousy, greed and discouragement. They need to be silly and audacious with a minimum of adverse consequences as they experiment with new roles. As they try to be more than they are, they fear they are less than they are. Unfortunately, experimentation can lead to actions with enormous consequences, such as pregnancy, injury and even death.

Adolescence is an intensely personal experience with many pathways to adulthood as each adolescent seek answers to the questions: How do I fit in? What can I do? Each one "reinvents the wheel" as she or he encounters the realities of life for the first time.

Looking back on her adolescent years, K.L. Hong wrote:[6]

> When I was a junior in high school, I guess I looked pretty normal on the outside. On the inside, though everything was awful, and I was terribly unhappy. School seemed pointless. Nobody, it seemed, understood me. My parents didn't seem to understand me. They fought with each other, and we often fought over what I was wearing. I just endured and did the best I could.

With adult understanding and guidance, adolescence usually is an enjoyable stage of life.[7] However, how young people traverse the path to adulthood is strongly associated with the socio-economic status of their parents. Disadvantaged adolescents often live in unstructured worlds fraught with disappointments, failures and deprivations. Their aspirations often are high, but they lack opportunities and abilities to achieve them on their own. For them the American Dream can be an American Nightmare. How adolescents are perceived by society matters.

THE CULTURAL AND SOCIETAL PERCEPTION OF ADOLESCENCE

From the cultural and societal points of view, adolescence is a vital stage of development in both indigenous and modern societies. Most indigenous societies have two rites of passage to adulthood.[8] The first pubertal rite marks the individual's readiness to enter training for adulthood. The second marks the individual's formal entrance into adulthood. Ironically, indigenous societies usually do not equate puberty and adulthood, whereas the current trend in the United States does, as reflected in calling adolescent girls "women" and adolescent boys "men."

In the United States, the perception of adolescence as an immature phase in life was reflected in three innovations that began in the late nineteenth century:[9]

- Child labor legislation that specified working hours and conditions for minors.
- Compulsory education between six and sixteen.
- Juvenile courts for persons under eighteen.

Adolescents are easily misunderstood either by expecting too much or too little of them. This is especially true in our "adolescent society" that adulates the audacious, self-centered, adolescent behavior of celebrities. Many adults have not mastered the developmental tasks of adolescence and would rather look and act like adolescents than accept the responsibilities of adulthood. The pop culture is rife with sexual and violent themes. It emphasizes reacting to the present rather than planning for the future. This climate amplifies rather than dampens the inherent immaturity of adolescents, especially those without solid moorings in their families.

Whether from the biological, psychological or social points of view, adolescence is an inevitable developmental stage in the life cycle rooted in the maturation of the brain. It cannot be by-passed or eliminated by wishing, education, legislation, child-birth or parenthood. In fact, it now has an earlier onset and a delayed ending in modern societies.

THE ONSET OF PUBERTY

Over the last century, young people entering puberty at earlier ages have found entry into adulthood delayed by the increasing complexity of modern societies.[10] In 1970, the average age at first marriage was 21 for women and 23 for men. In 2000, it was 26 for women and 27 for men.

Female Puberty

Contemporary girls in nomadic tribes on the African savanna are active, intermittently fed and lean. They begin menstruating around the age of 16.[11] In the 1980s, the median age of menarche for the Melanesians in New Guinea was between 15 and 18. In contrast, in industrialized nations the average age of menarche now is 12.

In Northern Europe from 1900 to 1970, the average age of menarche dropped from 15.5 to 13.5. In the United States it shifted from 14 to 12.5 over the same time span.[12] Although the ability to conceive may not occur for one to three years after its onset, the earlier onset of menarche has made pregnancy possible at younger ages.

Menarche is just one milestone in a complicated developmental process involving physical growth and psychological changes that result from hormonal and brain development.[13] The uterus usually does not reach full adult size until the completion of physical growth. More importantly, the maturation of the parts of the brain that control sexual drives is not completed until 18 to 20 years of age. Sex hormones activate drives controlled by immature brains during adolescence.

In the past in the United States, the onset of puberty before the age of 9 was linked to hypothyroidism.[14] Now 15% of White and 48% of Black girls show the early signs of puberty at the age of 8 with normal thyroid functioning. The onset of early sexual characteristics in girls is a significant event, signaling physiological and psychological changes of profound importance. Before they have outgrown doll houses, many young girls are now faced with confusing mood swings, hormonal changes and sexual attention that accompany physical maturation.

If girls are unhappy with their bodies, menstruation becomes a particularly unsavory event, known as the "curse" and incites concealment.[15] The way that girls experience their bodies at the first menstruation can have a strong impact throughout their lives, especially on how they feel about themselves as sexual beings.

Early puberty has negative implications for girls' mental health and quality of life.[16] They tend to have early sex, low IQs, increased risk of pregnancy, short birth spacing, increased psychological stress, poor mental health and behavior problems. They also have higher rates of drinking, smoking, depression, sleeping problems and suicide.

Male Puberty

Boys are starting puberty earlier as well.[17] By the age of 9, 58% of Black boys and 30% of White and Latino boys start genital development. The onset of ejaculation usually occurs between 13 and 15.

A study of high school boys found that those who matured earlier than their classmates were more likely to drink and smoke and were twice as likely to have substance abuse and disruptive behavior problems.[18] They also tended to have lower self-respect, poorer coping skills, miss more days of school and be more likely to attempt suicide.

Explanations of Earlier Pubertal Onset

A number of factors contribute to the earlier onset of puberty: [19]

• Increased prevalence of obesity accompanied by depression.
• Soy, beef and dairy products containing chemicals that mimic estrogen.
• Hormone-containing pesticides.
• Socioeconomic stressors.
• Stressful family conditions.
• Genetic variations.

Patricia Draper and Henry Harpending, professors of anthropology at the University of Nebraska and the University of Utah respectively, proposed that early menarche might be a useful reproductive strategy in stressful environments or when male parental investment is low.[20] Father-absent girls seem to reach menarche earlier and are more attracted to the faces of babies than father-present girls, suggesting a greater attraction to parenting.

Although visible external changes in the body are the most prominent signs of adolescent growth, the most important developing organ system is the brain.

ADOLESCENT BRAIN DEVELOPMENT

The cerebral cortex is a thicket of nerve cell branches crisscrossing and touching billions of times. The density of these contact points rises meteorically between birth and age two and remains at 50% above the adult level until puberty.[21] Most of the connections arising after birth are chaotic random hookups awaiting the amplifying and dampening influences of experiential stimulation. Everything heard, seen, tried, learned, thought, tasted and felt by a child brings order to the chaos of the brain and creates patterns of functioning neural network images (fractals).

Adolescent behavior and emotions reflect brain development but they also influence the developing brain. Stress creates hypersensitivity in dopamine-producing neurons. Stimulating environments produce neuronal connections.

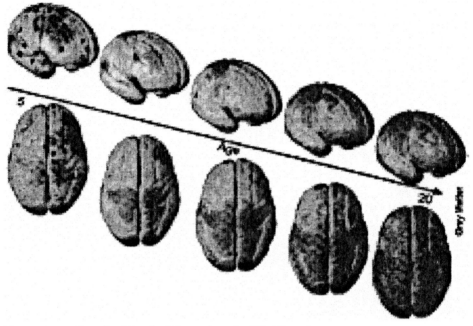

Figure 10.1.   Growth of Cerebral Cortex into the Third Decade.

Modern imaging techniques reveal that the brain develops irregularly. Every brain function seems to have its own timetable. Motor and sensory brain areas involved in spatial orientation, speech, language and attention mature early. Areas involved in executive functions continue to mature into the 20s.

The brain overproduces neurons at first. This process is known as *blossoming*. Experience causes certain neurons to fire. As they fire, the connections get stronger. The branches that do not fire wither and disappear. This process is called *pruning*. It reduces the density of synapses by about one-third during the first four years. The window of opportunity for learning the meaning of different sounds is open the widest in the first three years. One of the strongest predictors of a child's reading ability is the amount of conversation between caregiver and child during the first three years of life.[22]

A second wave of blossoming peaks in the prefrontal cortex at around eleven or twelve. This can produce dramatic changes in personality as the process of pruning follows in response to brain circuit usage.[23]

An appetite for adventure, a predilection for risks and a desire for novelty and thrills reach high levels for adolescents. They are drawn to music videos that bombard the senses. They flock to horror movies and exciting rides at amusement parks. Although these patterns are evident in most adolescents to some degree, individual differences range widely. For some, activating strong emotions and an affinity for excitement can be subtle and easily managed. For others, these inclinations can lead to impulsive decisions and reckless behavior.

The pubertal brain is ready for a NASCAR race but has the brakes of a Model T.[24] Adults use the rational part of the brain to interpret emotional expressions, whereas adolescent rely on gut reactions. Misreading emotional cues can lead adolescents to misjudgments and violence or withdrawal. The more they are encouraged to think before they act the stronger brain circuits that control impulses become. True to the use-it-or-lose-it principle, adolescents who are not held accountable for controlling their impulses have difficulty developing that skill later.

Adolescents gradually acquire reasoning and problem solving skills that facilitate coping with stressors and challenges.[25] Yet, during this period of resilient health, burgeoning energy and new-found capabilities, there is a dramatic increase in death and disability: high rates of serious accidents, suicide, homicide, aggression, violence, alcohol and illegal drugs use, emotional disorders, sleep disturbances and the consequences of risky sexual behavior.[26] Behind this paradox lie brain changes and "raging hormones."

Hormonal Development

Brain maturation changes three principle hormone systems emanating from the hypothalamus—the master hormone control center.[27]

The first system is activated by testosterone-like hormones and cortisol from the outer parts of the *adrenal glands* on top of the kidneys. They usually begin to rise between the ages of 6 and 9 and steadily increase for more than a decade, peaking in the early 20s. This system contributes to changes in skin (including acne), as well as the growth of pubic and underarm hair and unpredictable responses to stress.

The second system is activated by growth hormone released from the *pituitary gland* at the base of the brain. Growth hormone contributes to physical growth and has powerful effects on the neurotransmitters norepinephrine, dopamine and serotonin. Norepinephrine is the energizer hormone and prepares the body for its fight-or-flight response. Dopamine is the "feel-good" neurotransmitter. Serotonin stabilizes moods. A lack of serotonin can make one feel depressed or aggressive.

The third system is activated by a cascade of hormones that activate the *ovaries and testes* and produce high levels of estrogen, progesterone and testosterone in both boys and girls. Boys can have five to seven surges of testosterone daily during puberty so that some become emotional powder kegs.

The relationship between these systems varies with individuals. Once hormones begin surging they affect serotonin levels, which are important in regulating moods and arousal. Dopamine increases one's capacities to learn in response to rewards.

Branching neurons in the prefrontal cortex change their architecture in order to meet cognitive and emotional challenges. They enable reasoning, planning and understanding long-term consequences of actions. They follow a trajectory relatively independent of the physical changes of puberty and continue to show refinements long after puberty.[28] By the end of the 20s, the profile of neuronal networks reaches an adult pattern, and the number of connections reaches a steady state that persists until old age.

Individual differences in rates and patterns of brain development are influenced by genes.

Genetic Influences on Development

Genotype is the inheritable information carried in the cells of all living organisms. The manifestations of the genotype in the body and behavior are in the *phenotype*. Relationships between genotype and phenotype are contingent on environmental experience and random mutations in cells during the developmental process. Individual fingers do not have the same fingerprints (phenotype) even though their cells have the same genes. Although identical twins have virtually identical genotypes, their phenotypes are not identical. Studies of identical twins affirm the importance of life experiences in determining personality development and behavior. [29] All of this is because genetic expression in the phenotype is determined by internal and external environmental influences. In general, genes determine less than 50% of an individual's traits.

Genes are like lines in a computer program acting autonomously with IF and THEN capacities. IF they are turned on, THEN they build a specific protein. They are turned on and off by regulatory proteins that tie the whole genetic system together. Rather than acting in isolation, most genes act as parts of elaborate networks in which the expression of one gene is a precondition for the expression of the next. Genes are the dominant factors in gender differences.

Gender Differences

Gender differences in attitudes, thinking, abilities and behavior vary widely so that some females are like males on these traits and vice versa. Inflated claims about gender differences can have undesirable costs in the workplace and in relationships. Still, it is possible to generalize about gender differences in brain development.

Janet Shibley Hyde, professor of psychology and women's studies at the University of Wisconsin-Madison, reviewed forty-six meta-analysis reviews of the literature on gender differences and found support for the *gender similarities hypothesis*, which holds that males and females are similar on most, but not all, psychological variables. [30] Gender differences can vary substantially at different ages and depend on the context in which measurements occur. Physical aggression is much and verbal aggression somewhat greater in males. Males have strikingly greater incidences of masturbation and casual, uncommitted sex.

Louann Brizendine, professor of psychiatry at the University of California-San Francisco, summarized advances in neuroimaging and neuroendocrinology that supply insights into how female and male brains function differently. [31] Every brain begins as a female brain. It only becomes male about eight weeks after conception, when excess testosterone shrinks the communication center, reduces the auditory cortex and makes the part of the brain that processes sexual impulses twice as large. In later life, different levels of estrogen, cortisol and dopamine can cause females to be more stressed than males.

Structural, chemical and functional variations have been documented in the brains of males and females.[32] The cerebral cortex reaches maximum thickness by eleven in girls and twelve in boys. The following areas of the brain generally are larger and mature earlier in females than males:

- Hypothalamus—earlier puberty and more sensitivity to hormone fluctuations.
- Prefrontal cortex—controls impulses, making females more patient.
- Insula—makes females more sensitive to emotional cues.
- Anterior cingulate cortex—makes females more prone to anxiety.
- Hippocampus—makes female emotional memory stronger.
- Corpus callosum—enhances collaboration between right and left hemispheres.

The amygdala is smaller in females making them less likely to take risks and fight. Females seem to link the analytic left brain with the intuitive right brain more readily and to process information more rapidly and accurately than males. Males tend to focus one hemisphere on a given task. When shown pictures of fearful faces, adolescent girls register activity on the right side of the brain, like adults. Boys use both sides, a less mature pattern of brain activity.

Boys' testosterone levels are much higher than their estrogen and progesterone levels. The combination of a tendency toward aggression brought on by testosterone and poorer verbal skills caused by slower development of the left brain leads many boys to have difficulty in school and to misbehave when frustrated. The net result is that boys may struggle to keep up with girls academically. As a result, females now outnumber males on college campuses.[33]

Female and male brains process the same emotionally arousing material differently. Females tend to process the central aspects and males more the details. Females are more attuned to auditory and males to visual learning. Girls chat with eye contact. Boys make contact indirectly while walking, shooting baskets or driving in a car. Boys tend to be less empathic with others and more adept at analyzing systems than girls.

Juvenile male chimpanzees battle to establish and maintain their places in a hierarchy and to avoid appearing weak. The same evolutionary imperative can make it difficult for boys to thrive in school when they try to "act tough." William Pollack, professor of psychology at Harvard University, described "The Boy Code":[34]

- Show no fear.
- Avoid the honor roll.
- Stick to sports.
- Whisper to other boy-coders about sexual exploits you've never had.

The extreme outcomes of the Boy Code are: bullying, low grades, delinquency, sexual violence and low self-respect in boys suffocating in "toughness armor."

Males are more likely than females to suffer from slow mental development, attention deficit disorders, stuttering, enuresis, encopresis, sleepwalking, autism and dyslexia.[35] Adult males far outnumber females in trans-sexuality, sexual perversions, alcoholism and drug addiction. Estrogen and progesterone spikes increase girls' risk for depression.

THE DEVELOPMENTAL TASKS OF ADOLESCENCE

The most important developmental tasks of adolescents are learning how to:

- Accommodate the growth of their bodies, emotions, urges and fluctuating moods.
- Relate to parents and siblings and fit into their social worlds.
- Identify their strengths and weaknesses and establish their unique self-identities.
- Accept responsibility for their actions and inactions.
- Develop a work ethic for school and other responsibilities.
- Deal with peer pressures and figure out their own values.
- Deal with attraction to risky behavior and plan for their futures.

Different aspects of maturation progress at different rates during adolescence, including height, weight, body proportions and sexual organs. Individual differences in the growth rates of brain functions are reflected in the abilities to think, reason, plan, strategize, understand the consequences of actions and control behavior in reliable ways. Some 13-year-olds are more mature in one or more of these aspects than some 18-year-olds.

THE DEVELOPMENTAL STAGES OF ADOLESCENCE

There are three peaks of brain maturation during adolescence: at 12, 15 and 18. These peaks define the early, middle and late stages of adolescence.[36]

Early Adolescence

During *early adolescence* from 12 through 14, young persons are preoccupied with accommodating bodily changes and learning how to cope with newly acquired sensations and skills. They turn to others for mirroring and acceptance that provide self-validation. They are sensitive to criticism and vulnerable to encouragement to take risks. Boys grow facial and pubic hair, and their voices deepen. Girls grow pubic hair and breasts and start menstruating. They may worry about these changes and how they are regarded by others. They become more independent as they develop their own personalities and interests. They focus on themselves, alternating between high aspirations and lack of confidence. Moodiness and short tempers accompany less affection shown toward parents. Anxiety may rise as schoolwork becomes more challenging.

Middle Adolescence

During *middle adolescence* from 15 through 17, young persons are preoccupied with exploring intimate relationships with other people. At the same time, sexual urges encouraged by contemporary social values thrust boys and girls into sexual encounters before they have an opportunity to become fully familiar with their own bodies, their own feelings and their cultural values. Many middle adolescents assume pseudo-adult facades and engage in adult behaviors in efforts to quickly shed the trappings of childhood. As a result, they are vulnerable to seduction, exploitation and betrayal, especially for those who are temperamentally or psychologically inclined to form intense relationships.

Late Adolescence

Late adolescence flowers from 18 through a variable number of succeeding years. The central issue is settling on one's identity in realistic social roles and in choosing a life style and a career. During this time access to opportunities for education and for employment is vital. Ideally, this stage is a "psychosocial moratorium" in which adult commitments are delayed until individuals can find niches in society compatible with their needs and abilities.[37]

DECISION-MAKING SKILLS

Mental development during adolescence includes situation analysis, conceptual thinking, goal setting, problem solving and deferral of immediate gratification for long-term gain. When with friends, a 16-year-old boy or girl, who can use adult logic and understand the consequences of their actions, can make reckless choices that a 9-year-old sibling would say were "dumb." Although able to understand that an action is wrong, an adolescent's emotions can hijack thoughtful decision-making because the prefrontal cortex is not fully developed.[38]

Key areas of the adolescent brain, especially the orbitofrontal cortex that controls higher order skills, are not fully mature until the third decade of life. As the world gets more complex, school becomes more difficult and social relations become more obtuse, adolescents may have passion but not mature judgment.[39] In making choices involving risk, adolescents do not engage the higher-thinking, decision-and-reward areas of the brain as much as adults do.

There is a clear distinction in decision-making skills between adolescents under and over 15. Awareness of the importance of the future consequences of one's actions and seeking appropriate advice progressively increases after 15. However, a study of 12th graders found that only half regarded future consequences and obtaining advice as important in their decision making.[40] They are especially prone to the fallacious gambler's belief that winning is more likely than losing.

Fantasy and reality interplay in the developmental process.[41] Children and adolescents who are heavy viewers of action television shows and frequent violent video or computer game players are more likely to show higher levels of aggression and disruptive behavior than those who do not. At the same time, videogames in moderation can be useful mental exercises. They force making fast decisions, prioritizing objectives and working with abstractions. Imaginative play through live or electronic interactions can enhance creativity.

Adolescents are capable of extraordinary intellectual, athletic and artistic accomplishments. They are full of promise, energy and caring that can be tapped to contribute to their communities. They show remarkable spurts in intellectual development and learning. But neurologically they are not adults. Because of the immaturity of the prefrontal cortex, most adolescents do not have the adult capacity to make sound judgments when confronted by complex situations and strong impulses. These limitations need to be considered in life-course-altering decisions, especially when they involve the life of another person, such as a baby in continuing a pregnancy and entering parenthood.

Insights about adolescent brain development can be used unfairly. If viewed as neurologically immature, adolescents might be denied making appropriate decisions. Immature brain development also might be used inappropriately to excuse minors for criminal behavior.

IQ, EQ AND SQ

Adolescent development occurs along three lines regarded as reflecting intelligence.[42] The best known is the Intelligence Quotient (IQ), which is strongly related to genetic inheritance and education. More important are the EQ (Emotional Intelligence) and the SQ (Social Intelligence) that are genetically determined as an aspect of temperament but are strongly influenced by life experiences. EQ involves the ability to monitor and discriminate between one's own and others' feelings and to use this information to guide one's thinking and action. SQ refers to the personal and social skills involved in relationships and work.

IQ is measured by tests composed of items related to abstracting, cognitive and visual-motor abilities calibrated to age. EQ can be measured to a degree by tests, but is calibrated to adult standards and is best measured by the way people live their lives, such as: [43]

1) Awareness of emotions:
   a. Knowing when one's judgments are based on feelings.
   b. Feeling shame and guilt.
2) Understanding one's emotions:
   a. Why am I feeling this way?
   b. How do emotions affect my behavior?
3) Ability to control and regulate emotions:
   a. Control arousal level so it does not interfere with performance.
   b. Persistence in the face of frustration and temptation.
4) Ability to use emotions to enhance one's performance.

Psychologist Daniel Goleman points out that the most important function of the brain beyond survival of the individual is to navigate the social world.[44] He describes social intelligence (SQ) as having two components: *social awareness* and *social facility*.

Social awareness extends from instantaneously sensing another's state to understanding complicated social situations. It includes:

1) Empathy: Feeling with others; sensing nonverbal emotional signals.
2) Attunement: Listening with full receptivity to another person.
3) Empathic accuracy: Understanding another person's thoughts, feelings and intentions.
4) Social cognition: Knowing how the social world works.

Social facility builds on social awareness to allow smooth, effective interactions with others. It includes:

1) Synchrony: Interacting smoothly at the nonverbal level, from smiling and nodding at the right moment to orienting one's body to the other person.
2) Self-presentation: Presenting oneself effectively.
3) Influence: Shaping the outcome of social interactions by soothing and encouraging others.
4) Concern: Caring about other's needs and acting accordingly.

A 40-year longitudinal study of boys—two-thirds from welfare families and one-third with IQs below 90—found that IQ had little relation to how well they did in the rest of their lives.[45] Their abilities to handle frustration, control emotions and get along with other people (EQs and SQs) were more important. A study of Ph.D. graduates in science in their early seventies found that social and emotional abilities were four times more important than IQ in determining their professional success and prestige.[46] EQ and SQ are as, or more, important than IQ for success in workplaces that require communication skills and teamwork.

IDENTITY DEVELOPMENT

One's identity evolves throughout life, but its critical foundations are laid during childhood and adolescence. Babies discover their bodies, young children discover their minds, older children discover their aptitudes, adolescents discover their personalities and young adults discover their careers. All of these discoveries interact and contribute to our sense of ourselves—our identities. Our identities are shaped by our cultural values and by our social roles that have expanded exponentially because of technological advances and life style options.

To grow up and fully know ourselves is challenging. Whether we recognize it or not, each of us is poised between two existential fears: 1) being unknown and unseen with our anguish and our joys unnoticed and 2) being known so completely that we are painfully exposed.[47] This is seen in an adolescent's needs for both attention and privacy. The telephone and the internet resolve this dilemma—intimate communication without complete exposure.

Guilt and Shame

Internalizing the actual and imagined views others have of us shapes our identities. Guilt and shame are vital emotions that reflect these internalized views. Guilt occurs when we have done something that violates the internalized values of our conscience. It gives rise to the feeling "I have *done* something wrong." The prospect of guilt makes it possible to avoid antisocial behavior. It can deepen our relationships when we are forgiven.[48]

Shame is based on our imagined reactions others have to us. It produces the feeling, "I *am* wrong or unworthy."[49] The prospect of shame enables us to avoid the disapproval of others.

Guilt and shame are weak or absent in people without effective consciences and empathy for others. When they are repressed or denied, they contribute to clinical depression.

One's True Self

The most important developmental task of adolescence is forming an identity based on one's true self. Inner directedness is the predisposition to follow one's own judgment and conscience rather than calculations of external approval. It flows from the true self, which is one's genetically and experientially determined potential in contrast to our false selves that we more or less deliberately present to others. Just as ancient Greek actors wore masks (*personas*) while performing, we wear false-self masks we have learned to show to others in our social roles. They are generally adaptive but can work against us when they obscure our true selves.

In order for adolescents to discover their potentials in their true selves, they need the freedom to explore their strengths and weaknesses in close relationships with peers and adults unencumbered by adult responsibilities. For this reason, legal age-grading that gradually awards adult privileges and responsibilities is in the developmental interests of adolescents. It permits them to experiment within manageable limits. Conversely, assuming adult responsibilities prematurely interferes with fully discovering one's true self and self-fulfillment.

Sexual Identity

Adolescence is a time for trying out different social roles. Establishing one's sexual identity during adolescence is a challenge for both boys and girls. Surges in testosterone and estrogen result in intense sexual fantasies and curiosity accompanied by "wet dreams" in boys and masturbation by both boys and girls.[50]

As adolescents sift through their dating opportunities, they acquire knowledge about themselves and others and develop likes and dislikes.[51] The challenge for maturing adolescents is to work out ways of respectfully handling their sexual urges so that future possibilities for mature nurturant-bonded companionship are not impaired.

These developmental imperatives frustrate educational and clinical efforts that assume that adolescents will use sexual information and contraceptives wisely. Egocentricity and impulsiveness are at their peak even in well-integrated adolescents.

Adolescent "Crushes"

The story of Romeo and Juliet has moved audiences for centuries:

> A young guy notices a girl at a party. Immediately smitten, he showers compliments on her. She plays coy but finds the boy appealing. Romantic feelings kindle quickly. On the basis of one brief meeting and a brief conversation, each cannot stop thinking about the other. They manage a secret late-night rendezvous. Passionate feelings accelerate at a feverish pitch. They are willing to spurn friends and family, disregard dangers and act as if being together is more important than life itself—even though they just met four days before and barely know each other. They tragically die together.

This story reveals the brain's "high and low roads" for integrating emotions and reasoning.[52] Both are connected to the reward system in the amygdala of the brain. When the amygdala receives signals from the prefrontal cortex, the reasoning part of the brain, we control ourselves. This is the "high road." But the amygdala also receives signals directly from sensory regions of the cortex that bypass the prefrontal cortex. This is the "low road." It is irrational, powerfully emotional and difficult to control. The "low road" can engulf lovers in unthinking, uncontrolled emotions and actions.

Romantic love appears to be based on a biological urge separate from sexual arousal and long-term attachment. It is closer to drives like hunger, thirst or drug craving than to emotional states. According to Helen Fisher, professor of anthropology at Rutgers University:[53]

> When you are in the throes of this romantic love it's overwhelming, you are out of control, you are irrational. When rejected, some people contemplate stalking, homicide, suicide. This drive for romantic love can be stronger than the will to live.

Brain activity in romantic love is similar to that of cocaine.[54] Falling in love elevates dopamine, which explains the euphoria. It elevates norepinephrine accounting for a racing pulse and sweaty palms. It decreases serotonin resulting in a roller coaster of emotions. Most adolescent crushes are not long lasting.

Attachment Hormones

Boys tend to view girls as sex objects. Girls tend to focus on the relational aspects of sexual attraction, such as spending time together and conversing.

For girls, the hormone associated with loving relationships and forming intimate bonds is oxytocin, which is also involved in childbirth and nursing.[55] It makes many adolescent girls fond of cuddly objects and babies. Meanwhile, it prepares them for long-term relationships. For boys, the attachment hormone is vasopressin. As levels of vasopressin rise, boys and men are more apt to become protective and attentive to their partners' needs.

Adolescent Attitudes toward Sexual Relationships

In our exhibitionistic society, sex is a commodity and sexual conquests a sport. The separation of pleasure from the reproductive purpose of sex has led to the contemporary scene in which "hooking up" permits sexual interactions without commitment. The result is the dehumanization of the most intimate human relationship and interference with developing a mature sexual identity as a partner and as a parent.

These attitudes ignore the vital importance of committed intimate attachments. Freud was misunderstood by those who thought he promoted uninhibited sexual expression. To the contrary, psychoanalysis emphasizes the importance of conscious awareness and control of sexual fantasies and impulses. It reveals how inner psychological conflicts and consequent developmental aberrations can trap persons in immature sexual behavior.

Typical adolescent beliefs about sexual relationships were described as fables by John Mitchell, a developmental psychologist. Several that apply to adolescent parenthood are:[56]

> No adolescent fable has more significance than the fable which asserts that "I" will not become pregnant. It is bolstered by the invulnerability fable (others become pregnant, but I will not), by the uniqueness fable (my love is so unique it could not result in an unwanted outcome), and by egocentric idealism (if I do have a baby it will be perfect, as will my relationship with it). The pregnancy fable is reinforced by fidelity (the impulse to bond) and particularization (the belief that one's love is caused solely by one's partner). All of these experiences take place when a girl is experiencing her sexuality in a richer and more profound way than ever before, when she is searching for her own sexual identity, and when she is trying to figure out the emotional peculiarities of her boy friend. Thus, adolescents believe that they are unlikely to suffer the negative consequences of their actions, and hence take risks that adults would not.

Mitchell also calls attention to the self-centered attitudes characteristic of adolescence:

- The belief that those to whom I am attracted are attracted to me as well.
- Criticism is implicitly interpreted as an attack and is rejected.
- A sense that I am entitled to special benefits and rights.
- Humiliation and anger when others do not treat me as a special person.
- A keen and thoughtless tendency to divide people into *Us* and *Them* groups.

Fortunately, most adolescents grow out of these immature attitudes. Exuberant adolescent sexual experimentation is not a characteristic of adult maturity.

ADOLESCENT IDEALISM

Adolescents are susceptible to high idealism and deep disillusionment when their ideals are disappointed.

The *ego ideal* is an ideal image of oneself that determines what kind of life we live. Rooted in infantile self-centeredness, the *ego ideal* of most adolescents is based on fantasies of a perfect world and involves identifying with celebrities. This gives them a sense of immortality and certainty that persists to a degree throughout life in many persons. Collectively, adolescent idealism can foster religious or political revolutions or even war.

Eventually, adolescents realize that pursuit of the perfect *ego ideal* is not practical and temper their *ego ideals* with more realistic aspirations for themselves. The closer they come to fulfilling these realistic aspirations, the higher their self-respect. The more they fall short, the more inclined they are to consciously or unconsciously feel shame and worthlessness.[57] Fantasy images in the media and in computer games reinforce the illusion that a childhood *ego ideal* can be fulfilled. Adolescents can be confronted with crushing disappointments in later life.

MORAL DEVELOPMENT

Moral values play vital roles in amplifying and dampening human behavior. We all are a baffling mixture of good and evil and of cooperation and selfishness. Nothing is more evil than war, which is made possible by the cooperation and selfless sacrifice of individuals who share opposing political and moral points of view. We often make what we define as moral judgments without considering fairness, human rights and ethical values.

Parents are central in the moral development of their children. Their responses to their children's transgressions and their explanations of the reasons for rules and expectations facilitate moral development.[58] The same principles apply to school personnel and moral education curricula.

A combination of Lawrence Kohlberg's theory of moral development that emphasizes justice and Carol Gilligan's theory that emphasizes caring is useful.[59] These stages of moral development are relevant to an adolescent's decision to enter parenthood. Adolescents vary in their levels of moral development from the preconventional to the postconventional levels.

Preconventional Level

At this level, an adolescent makes judgments on the basis of what is liked and wanted and what is disliked or hurts oneself. There is no concept of rules or of obligations independent of one's wishes. The decision to enter parenthood is based on what "I want now."

Age Range	Stage	Issues
	Preconventional	
Birth to 9	Selfish	Avoid punishment and shame. Gain rewards.
9 to 20	Transition from selfishness to responsibility to others.	
	Conventional	
	Self-sacrifice is good.	Gain approval & avoid disapproval. Duty & guilt.
	Transition from being good to empathy with others.	
	Postconventional	
20+ or never	Pursue the common good.	Human rights & justice. Personal morality.

Figure 10.2.   Kohlberg & Gilligan Stages of Moral Development.

Conventional Level

Desirable behavior is defined by stereotypes about what is acceptable in an individual's life experience. The decision to enter parenthood is based on the approval of a family or peer group or on a sense of duty to take responsibility for the consequences of conception.

Post-Conventional Level

The individual defines moral values and principles on the basis of empathy with other persons and respect for their dignity. The decision to enter parenthood is based on the best interests of the adolescent, the baby, the family and society.

RISK TAKING

Adolescents need to make choices on their own before they are fully mature so that they can learn how to take responsibility for their own lives. Franklin Zimring, professor of law at the University of California, describes adolescence as the "learner's permit" stage of life.[60]

Adolescents need to be able to experiment without suffering adverse long-term consequences. Unlike their affluent counterparts, poor adolescents who experiment in risky behaviors—crime, drug addiction, alcoholism, sexually transmitted diseases and pregnancy—suffer consequences that often close doors that can never be reopened again. They are given little margin for error in negotiating the developmental tasks of adolescence.

Still, adolescents are attracted to risks that trigger exciting arousal or anxiety.[61] Their turned up dopamine systems heighten motivations that are not sufficiently balanced by the orbitofrontal cortex. Genetic and temperamental factors explain why some adolescents participate in activities because of risks and some in spite of risks. Others avoid risks altogether.

The combination of elevated sensation seeking and attraction to risk leads adolescents to try activities that can be dangerous to themselves and to others. They tend to assess health risks to be lower than is realistic, especially when combined with an easygoing "party" attitude. Their actions can have consequences that foreclose their options in life: accidents can kill and disable; delinquency can become criminality; and sexual behavior can result in pregnancy.

The 2005 national Youth Risk Behavior Survey indicated that 71% of all deaths among 10 to 24-year-olds result from four causes: [62] motor-vehicle accidents, other injuries, homicide and suicide. During the 30 days preceding the survey, high school students engaged in following behaviors: 10% had driven a car or other vehicle when they had been drinking alcohol; 19% had carried a weapon; 43% had drunk alcohol; and 20% had used marijuana. During the 12 months preceding the survey, 36% had been in a physical fight and 8% had attempted suicide. They are four times more likely than older drivers to have accidents. More than 9 adolescents die each day of injuries caused by motor vehicle accidents. A number of highway safety advocates call for "black boxes" to monitor young drivers.

Adolescents' Need for Advice and Guidance

The boundaries of adolescence have become more blurred at both ends, increasing the challenges of an inherently unstable time in life. As puberty occurs at earlier ages, preparing for adult roles has become more complicated and prolonged.

Most adolescents understand the consequences of risky behavior but are prone to disregard them.[63] Traditional programs that appeal to adolescents' rationality are inherently flawed, not because adolescents fail to weigh risks against benefits, but because they tend to weight immediate benefits more heavily than risks when making decisions. They need higher levels of stimulation than adults to achieve the same feelings of pleasure or excitement.

Fortunately, adolescent passions can be aligned in healthy ways. Passion motivates the highest levels of human endeavor: for ideas and ideals; for beauty; to create music or art; and to succeed in sports, business or politics. One of the most important challenges for parents, teachers, clinicians and political leaders is enlisting adolescent passions for the common good. Unfortunately, these passions can be harnessed by leaders like Hitler and Bin Laden.

Ned Hallowell, psychiatrist and author, emphasizes the importance for adolescents of connectedness to the past, to family and to neighborhood and community.[64] Too many adolescents relate exclusively to peers and do not know how to relate to adults. The most vulnerable adolescents need mentoring from parents, teachers, coaches and other adults.

In our confusing and seductive social climate, it is evident that adolescents need parents who set limits and show they really care about them. The most frequently heard reason adolescents use for staying out of trouble is "My parents wouldn't like it." Without feeling that "I have parents who care about what I do," adolescents are highly susceptible to peer pressures that can be contrary to their interests. Put another way, adolescents need advice that helps them restrain their impulses. We cannot expect them to deal wisely with situations they have never encountered before. Parents, mentors and professionals have an obligation to share their expertise and wisdom with young people.

Adolescents need protection from making choices that will irreversibly change the courses of their lives and preclude options they should have as adults. Childbirth permanently changes a girl's body. It alters the range of her experiences in growing through adolescence. If he takes responsibility for the child, an adolescent father's development is altered as well. These facts become apparent when one asks what would an adolescent parent's life have been like without parenting responsibilities?

Unfortunately, surveys indicate that even in families with two parents only half of adolescents talk with their mothers and only one-quarter talk with their fathers about their concerns.[65] Parents' attitudes and interactions with their children wax and wane in response to social conditions and events such as 9-11. After September 11, 2001, 80% of men and 91% of women with children said they would like to spend more time with their families. A year later, those percentages dropped to 35% for men and 41% for women; 7% of women said they would like to spend less time with their families.

Because of the lack of communication between adolescents and parents, the pressure on societal institutions to assume parental functions is increasing.

THE LACK OF OPPORTUNITIES FOR ADOLESCENTS

The most important reason to restrain our immediate urges is the prospect of benefits if we do so. Adolescents who believe that success in school and avoiding pregnancy will prepare them for attractive jobs behave differently than those without hope for the future.

The lack of opportunities for social and economic advancement was recognized as contributing to unrestricted procreation long ago. During the early 1800s, the English economist and demographer T.R. Malthus attributed the rapid increase in the population of Ireland to the English subjugation of Irish Catholics, who, seeing no escape from their lowly condition, "spent their lives proliferating."[66] He pointed out then that no one would plan for the future unless "they believed that their industrious exertion would benefit them."

Steven Rose, professor of biology and neurobiology at the University of London, notes that the genetic/medical/psychiatric approach to antisocial behavior can deflect attention from societal, educational and parental deficiencies by focusing on adjusting the minds of individuals rather than their physical and social environments.[67]

An increasing number of adolescents who grow up in environments with few material assets and world-expanding experiences feel the future holds little promise for them. They do not see themselves as gaining from completing high school. They become alienated and hedonistic when they cannot imagine achieving long-range goals by present-day self-restraint. Having financial assets and property can foster awareness of one's personal stake in the future consequences of present actions, an awareness that is lacking for people without those assets.[68]

CONCLUSION

Adolescence is a developmental stage to be lived fully and enjoyed. Dramatic physical changes are occurring as adolescents form their own identities and become independent from their families. With adult guidance and understanding, adolescence usually is a relatively enjoyable stage of life in spite of its stormy reputation.

The earlier average onset of menstruation at 12 has made pregnancy possible at earlier ages. The capacity to procreate is present long before the cognitive, emotional and social maturity required for parenthood in our society. The maturation of the brain is not complete until the third decade of life.

The most important developmental task of adolescence is forming an identity based on one's potential true self. In order to do so, adolescents need to be able to act experimentally without suffering adverse long-term consequences. Unlike their affluent counterparts, poor adolescents have little margin for error in negotiating the developmental tasks of adolescence.

Because of the immaturity of the prefrontal cortex, adolescents do not have the adult capacity to make sound judgments and to plan effectively when confronted by complicated situations and strong impulses. These limitations in weighing the consequences of life-course-altering decisions need to be considered, especially when decisions involve the life of another person, such as a baby by continuing a pregnancy or entering parenthood.

The moral development of adolescents progresses from a stage in which the decision to become a parent is based on what "I want now" to what is in the "best interests" of the adolescent, the baby, the family and society. Parents, mentors and professionals have an obligation to share their expertise and wisdom with young people.

Adolescents need competent parents as much as younger children do—even more so when their abilities to permanently alter their lives are taken into account. Our society must respect adolescence as an essential developmental stage in life that precedes parenthood and that is compromised by premature childbearing and childrearing.

Chapter 11

Emerging Adulthood

Not only does democracy make men forget their ancestors, but it also clouds their view of their descendants and isolates them from their contemporaries. Each man is forever thrown back on himself alone, and there is danger that he may be shut up in the solitude of his own personal interests.

Alexis de Toqueville
Democracy in America, 1840[1]

In our culture, adulthood ideally means productive citizenship and readiness for parenthood. But when adulthood begins no longer is clear. When adolescent parenthood is supported by our society, the meanings of both adulthood and parenthood are unclear.

This chapter places adolescent parenthood in perspective by offering an overview of the transition from late adolescence into adulthood in contemporary mainstream society.

In the 1950s, most adolescents finished high school, entered the work force and started a family. Now becoming economically and psychologically independent by the early 20s is uncommon. The choices posed by new freedoms and responsibilities can be overwhelming for adolescents sheltered by some twenty years of schooling, often beginning in early childhood.[2]

Late adolescence is called *emerging adulthood* by Jeffrey Arnett, a professor of human development at the University of Maryland. It is the self-focused age of exploring possibilities when hope flourishes or is disappointed.[3]

Young people grow up with varying degrees of structure and enter a uncertain world of diversity and experimentation. The job market and social life are more fluid than in the past.[4] As they move into their mid-twenties, many extend their education, postpone career choices and yearn for the companionship that buffered adolescence. One-third between 22 and 34 still live at home with their parents—a 100% increase over the last 20 years—often because of student loan and credit card debts.[5]

GENERATION Y

Generation Y ("millennials") composed of young people born between 1982 and 2003 is the demographic echo of the Baby Boomers (1945-1964) who with Generation X (1965-1981) are their parents. They are nearly a third of the population and will dominate the next generation.[6]

Generation Y reflects the sweeping changes in American life over the past 20 years. For many of their parents, spanking was out and boosting self-esteem was in.[7] They have been driven to organized activities. They are multi-taskers with computers, cell phones, music downloads and instant messaging. Many are plugged-in citizens of the global community, but many have unrealistic online relationships. According to a Pew Survey, 42% talk with their parents every day. Their common traits are: confident, team-oriented, conventional, pressured and achieving.

Generation Y is changing our society. It has affected school construction, college enrollments, product development and sales and media content. It is the largest, healthiest and most cared-for generation in American history.

Neil Howe and William Strauss in *Millennials Rising* believe that generation Y will usher in a return to civic duty resembling the World War II generation.[8] The number of volunteer hours they put in rose by nearly 14% from 2002 to 2005. This is confirmed by Morley Winograd and Michael Hais in *Millennial Makeover*, who see them as collaborative problem solvers benefiting from self-organization through computer technology and internet communication. At the same time, Jean Twenge, professor of psychology at San Diego State University, sees Generation Y as self-important and vulnerable to disappointment:

> We enjoy unprecedented freedom to pursue what makes us happy. But our high expectations and an increasingly competitive world have led to a darker flip side, where we blame other people for our problems and sink into anxiety and depression. When we hit young adulthood we face an enormous mismatch between what we expect and what we actually get.

High school seniors' ambitions do appear to outpace what they are likely to achieve.[9] A 2004 survey of almost 50,000 college students found that 45% had felt so depressed it was difficult to function; 63% had felt hopeless at times. An American College Health Survey in 2007 found that 76% of college students felt "overwhelmed" while 22% were sometimes so depressed they could not function; 44% engaged in binge drinking.

In 2000, the Harvard dean of admissions encouraged the "fast-track generation" to take time out from school, to:[10]

> step back and reflect, to gain perspective on personal values and goals, or to gain needed life experience in a setting separate from and independent of one's accustomed pressures and expectations.

Melvin Levine, professor of pediatrics at the University of North Carolina, calls attention to another side of Generation Y.[11] Because they have been rewarded for participation not achievement, they lack a realistic sense of their strengths and weaknesses. When they enter their first jobs, they expect to be told how well they are doing. They focus on the immediate rather than the long-term. They have difficulty delaying gratification and are easily bored.

All of this raises questions about defining adulthood and whether or not it matters.

THE LEGAL DEFINITION OF ADULTHOOD

Culture strongly influences the definition of adulthood. Even in the 1990s, most Hmong girls in Laos married within two years and boys within four years after the onset of menstruation.[12] As in other indigenous societies, a Hmong boy's ability to marry required a level of achievement, such as making a first kill on a hunt or developing skills to provide for a family.

Most modern societies base legal adulthood on reaching a specific age without requiring a demonstration of readiness for adulthood. In the United States, legal adulthood usually is achieved overnight at 18 with all of its privileges except for the purchase of tobacco and alcohol.

The legal transition from childhood to adulthood is described in unflattering terms. In legal language, adulthood comes after a sequence of ages that remove "the disabilities of infancy" and grant special liberties and responsibilities.[13] For example, each state has an age and testing-based process for obtaining a license to drive a motor vehicle.

THE TREND TOWARD DELAYING ADULTHOOD

The number of people in their 20s and 30s who would qualify as functioning adults based on completing their educations, leaving home and beginning their vocations has decreased significantly.[14] Marriage no longer signifies adulthood. The criteria for adulthood in 2004 were:

- accepting responsibility for one's actions,
- making independent decisions, and
- becoming financially independent.

The book *On the Frontier of Adulthood* suggests three reasons for delayed adulthood:[15]

- *Longer education.* 14% of the population completed high school in 1910. In 2000, 70-83% did so. The percentage completing college rose from 3% to 25%.
- *Longer time living with parents.* In 1900, only 41% of male and 46% of female White sixteen-year-olds were attending school and living with their parents. In 2000, those percentages increased to almost 90%.[16]
- *Delay in marriage and family formation.* At 19-20, 10% of females and 5% of males

are married; 7% of females and 4% of males have children.[17] American and European females leave home later and are likely to cohabitate before marriage.

THE DEVELOPMENTAL TASKS OF EMERGING ADULTHOOD

The transition from adolescence to adulthood is both exciting and stressful.[18] Trying to "take hold of some kind of life" describes the overarching developmental task of emerging adulthood. Although most young people succeed in this task, many have difficulty functioning in adult roles. The stress of transitioning into adulthood may overwhelm those already having difficulties in adolescence, although some improve as previously unavailable opportunities arise.

Adolescents need the guidance and financial help of a stable family, mentoring adults and educational experiences to help them gain the knowledge, skills and confidence they need to succeed in modern life.[19] Most are surrounded by employed adults and are exposed to mainstream occupations. Some are surrounded by unemployed adults and antisocial models.

Having vocational goals is not enough to ensure a smooth transition into productive adulthood.[20] Opportunities and sheer luck determine what a young person can do. Self-respect, ambition, enthusiasm, curiosity and optimism translate into successful life outcomes. However, a person can be optimistic and have high self-esteem because of concrete accomplishments or because of expecting little of oneself, as William James pointed out over 100 years ago.[21] High self-esteem can reflect complacency and low ambition. Boring and inadequate schooling also can dampen curiosity and lead students in the direction of cynicism and disinterest.

Melvin Levine calls attention to emerging adults who have not learned how to deal with their own weaknesses and to exploit their strengths.[22] They need self-awareness, understanding of the working world, basic mental tools and the ability to relate to other people effectively. One way to learn working skills is to encourage young people to take part in activities that create a "flow state" in which they are so absorbed that they feel at one with the activity.[23] When in "flow," we feel greater levels of enjoyment, happiness, motivation and self-respect. We can experience "flow" when challenges are within our abilities and when we have positive outlooks.

Most emerging adults want satisfying and enjoyable work. Most want to live a personally fulfilling life while doing some good for others. Unlike previous generations, they are not constrained by gender-prescribed rules for relationships. At the same time, finding a compatible partner has become more difficult. Twenty-five percent are unmarried by the age of 30.[24]

MARKERS OF WELL-BEING DURING EMERGING ADULTHOOD

The transition to adulthood provides new roles and opportunities for young people. For most, well-being tends to increase during this period. But some young people who functioned well in the structure of high school fall apart.

Monitoring the Future Study

The University of Michigan Monitoring the Future Study showed that in general well-being was higher for those 19-20-year-olds who were not married, did not have children and were in college.[25] Forty-three percent were thriving as defined by graduating from a two- or a four-year college. By the age of 26, forty-one percent were financially independent with all their financial resources supplied either by themselves or by a spouse; slightly more than half were thriving in their romantic lives with success defined as being married or engaged (whether cohabiting or not) and not being divorced; and about 20% of those who had high levels of well-being during their senior year in high school were doing much worse.

According to the Michigan study prosocial activity in the 10th grade predicted lower substance use and higher self-esteem and an increased likelihood of college graduation.[26] Performing arts participation predicted more years of education as well as increases in drinking between ages 18 and 21 and higher rates of suicide attempts and psychologist visits by age 24. Sports participation predicted positive educational and occupational outcomes and lower levels of social isolation but higher rates of drinking. The Study suggested that emerging adulthood is a time of experimentation that ceases once adult roles are assumed. See Figure 11.1.

Michigan Study of Life Transitions

The Michigan Study of Life Transitions examined the relationship between high school identity groups and later life.[27] Twenty-eight percent identified themselves as Jocks, 40% as Princesses, 12% as Brains, 11% as Basket Cases, and 9% as Criminals. Through the age of 24, the Brains had the highest education levels; the Jocks had the highest mental health levels; the Criminals had the lowest education levels; and the Basket Cases had the lowest mental health levels. See Figure 11.2.

Out of School, Unemployed Adolescents

As long as chances for middle-class achievement are unevenly distributed, disadvantaged adolescents will deviate from the mainstream. The weak link between educational

Life Arena	Percentage Thriving	Percentage "Making It"	Percentage Floundering
Education	43%	36%	21%
Employment	28%	58%	14%
Financial Independence	41%	29%	29%
Romance	51%	32%	16%
Leisure	32%	47%	21%
Healthy Lifestyle	28%	57%	16%
Citizenship	40%	45%	15%
Religion	29%	45%	26%

Figure 11.1. How 26-Year-Olds Were Doing on Key Developmental Tasks.
Source: University of Michigan Institute for Social Research, 2002.

Categories	Graduated College	Seen a Psychologist	Attempted Suicide
Brains	49%	18%	3%
Princesses	36%	21%	11%
Jocks	30%	6%	6%
Basket Cases	29%	25%	14%
Criminals	17%	20%	12%

Figure 11.2. High School Identity Groups and Later Life.
Source: Barber, Bonnie L., et al (2001) *Journal of Adolescent Research* 16: 429-455.

institutions below the college level and potential employers leaves most young people without guidance or support in seeking positions in the labor force.[28]

Many young people find themselves facing adulthood unprepared, unsupported and dispirited. An estimated 3.8 million adolescents between the ages of 18 and 24 are neither employed nor in school—roughly 15% of this population.[29] The ranks of these non-engaged young adults grew by 19% between 2000 and 2003. For many the transition to adulthood is a time of fear and frustration. A significant number of these adolescents have neither the skills, supports, experience, education nor confidence to successfully transition to adulthood.

A large share of these adolescents come from minority and low-income families. Their lack of preparation makes it difficult to secure good jobs. Their odds of being incarcerated or victims of crime are high. They are likely to continue living in high-poverty areas and are unlikely to become reliable providers for their own children.

NATIONAL SERVICE AS A RITE OF PASSAGE

William James was a physiologist, physician, psychologist, philosopher and advocate. With Oliver Wendell Holmes, John Dewey and others he formed the Metaphysical Club that helped shape the intellectual agenda for the 20th Century.

Deeply moved by our Civil War and European wars, James wrote "The Moral Equivalent of War" for the Association for International Conciliation in 1910.[30] He saw men as inheriting "all the innate pugnacity and all the love of glory of his ancestors. Showing war's irrationality and horror is of no effect on him. The horrors make for fascination. War is the *strong* life; it is life *in extremis* . . ."

To harness young men's impulse for war, James suggested conscription for public service as an "army against injustice." He wrote:

> The military ideals of hardihood and discipline would be wrought into the growing fibre of the people . . . no one would remain blind, as the luxurious classes now are blind, to man's relations to the globe he lives on. . . Through hard work men would get the childishness knocked out of them and come back to society with healthier sympathies and soberer ideas.

James' candor may be too much for contemporary ears, but the idea of public service following high school has been advocated during the last decade. Senators John

McCain and Evan Bayh urged that September 11, 2001, be a call to service to give our young people a way "to claim the rewards and responsibilities of active citizenship." They hoped that public service would become a rite of passage for young Americans.

Many adolescents are at loose ends. Consider this incident:

> Three adolescents from affluent homes knocked over 32 headstones in a cemetery in Largo, Florida, and were found cutting themselves and drinking each other's blood. They said that they were not enacting a Satanic or goth ritual—they were just relieving boredom.

Adolescents are exposed to enticements to serve themselves—buying, eating, reading, watching, listening, playing video games or competing—more than to serve others. Academic and athletic competition can relieve boredom, foster character development and build teamwork, but they do not inspire helping the less fortunate.

The noted psychologist Erik Erikson called attention to the late adolescent developmental need for a "psychosocial moratorium"—a timeout to find one's purpose in the world.[31] For most young persons that world is limited to where they grew up or to their college campuses. Many enter college burned out after high school years packed with college-level courses, test preparation classes and after-school activities. No wonder there is a strong tendency to "live it up" when away from home.

College courses in themselves do not meet the need for a "psychosocial moratorium." Extracurricular activities can do so. Perhaps the lack of personal fulfillment, in addition to lack of money, contributes to the fact that up to 50% of college and technical school students drop out before obtaining a degree, although most return later. Many are unprepared for college work. Many suffer personal or family crises. Many are bored. Many have high aspirations and know what to do, but fail to do it.

A survey of 15 to 25-year-olds revealed that 80% favor expanding programs through which they could give a year of public service and earn money for college.[32] They could be matched with community and national service organizations through the USA Freedom Corps. The accomplishments of remunerated Peace Corps, VISTA, AmeriCorps, Teach For America and unremunerated private programs attest to the value of public service to both recipients and volunteers. 250,000 Americans have served one-to-two-year stints in AmeriCorps since 1994. They receive a stipend and college financial aid. Like veterans returning from World War II, they are serious, goal-directed students.

Youth Service America (YSA) is a resource center that partners with organizations committed to increasing the quality and quantity of volunteer opportunities for young people, ages 5 to 25, to serve locally, nationally and globally.[33] Founded in 1986, YSA's mission is to strengthen the effectiveness, sustainability and scale of the youth service and service-learning fields. YSA envisions a powerful network of organizations committed to making service-learning a common expectation of all young people. The International Association for National Youth Service brings together youth service organizations across the globe.[34]

William James and Erik Erikson were right. Young people can find purpose in life through "a war against injustice." They need encouragement and opportunities to do so. Many schools now require community service for graduation from high school.

CONCLUSION

In the United States, legal adulthood usually is achieved on one's eighteenth birthday. However, less than half of emerging adults are thriving as defined by graduating from either a two-year or four-year college or being financially independent.

The transition from adolescence to adulthood is both exciting and stressful. Adolescents need the guidance and financial help of a stable family in order to make this transition successfully. They also need mentoring adults and educational experiences that help them gain the knowledge and confidence needed to succeed in life.

Unfortunately, many young people find themselves facing adulthood unprepared, unsupported and dispirited. A large share of these disconnected adolescents come from minority and low-income families. They are the most likely to become parents and thereby add to the challenges of emerging adulthood.

In order to increase the number of college and technical school graduates, we need to promote stable homes so children can develop the self-discipline they need to succeed in school. We need to improve our schools and expand mentoring programs and support groups. We need to help young people make informed decisions so they can obtain the most appropriate education and training.

A strong youth service movement would foster citizenship, knowledge and the personal development of both affluent and disadvantaged young people. They could find purpose in life through service to others without prematurely assuming the responsibilities of parenthood.

Chapter 12

Parenthood as a Developmental Stage in Life

It would be easier if we could get the age of reproduction to mesh with the age of reason.

Ellen Goodman
Syndicated Columnist, 2005[1]

An 8-year-old outwits burglars in the movie *Home Alone*. A 10-year-old can explain the intricacies of a computer to an adult. A 12-year-old can get a baby-sitter license from the Red Cross. Why can't a 16-year-old enter parenthood?

In the popular view, especially among people who have never been parents, parenthood simply is caring for children like baby-sitters do. Parenthood seldom is clearly recognized as the developmental stage that complements childhood and follows adolescence in the life cycle.

Parenthood meets the needs of parents as well as children. It satisfies parents' biological drives to procreate and nurture. It fulfills both parents' and children's needs for intimate relationships. These rewards of parenthood are more readily appreciated by parents who had good relationships with their own parents than by those who did not.

Parenthood is hard work. Like any career, it expands one's perspective, knowledge and skills. Unlike other careers, it is a financial cost—$10,000 a year for each child in the United States—rather than a source of income.[2]

Parenthood is responsibility for the life—custodial guardianship—of another person. A baby is a person. There is no greater responsibility in life. The prerequisite for assuming responsibility for the life of another person is the capacity to assume responsibility for one's own life. Readiness for parenthood logically follows adolescence.

THE DEVELOPMENTAL PHASES OF PARENTHOOD

Parenthood involves more than knowledge about child development and parenting skills.[3] It is custodial guardianship of a child as that child and parent grow together.

143

Most parents raise their children successfully without consciously experiencing the developmental phases of parenthood, as is the case with other life stages.[4] They enhance their coping skills, altruism and self-respect as they revive and work through unresolved developmental issues in their own lives. Parents who successfully master these challenges achieve new levels of psychological and emotional maturity as do their children.

Parenthood progresses from egoistic to integrative phases as described by Carolyn Newberger, professor of psychology at Harvard University:[5]

Phase 1: *Egoistic*
Parents are self-focused and see their children as extensions of themselves.
Phase 2: *Conventional*
Perspectives shift from self-centeredness to childrearing beliefs drawn from traditions, experts and age-related norms.
Phase 3: *Individualistic*
Children are viewed as unique individuals.
Phase 4: *Integrative*
Parents learn and mature with their children in their families, communities and society.

Most parents intuitively meet the challenges of each phase. Many need help in learning how to grow with their children. Some need education and clinical treatment in order to be able to function as competent parents. A small but critical number are unable to function as competent parents at all—typically adolescents and dependent adults.

THE READINESS FOR PARENTHOOD

In spite of the rhetoric inveighing against adolescent pregnancies, our society devotes little attention to readiness to assume the responsibilities of parenthood. Dependent adult and young adolescent childbirths from unplanned and planned pregnancies generally are accepted as facts of life. The presumption is that these parents will learn to handle parental responsibilities.

Most of the literature about adolescent pregnancy and parenthood does not distinguish between minor and adult adolescents. Late adolescents are legal adults in most matters. Whether or not a parent is a legal minor or an adult is an important issue when childbirth occurs.

CAN ADOLESCENTS PLAN REALISTICALLY FOR THE FUTURE?

Giving birth to a baby does not produce an adult brain or eliminate the developmental issues of adolescence. John Mitchell, a developmental psychologist, calls attention to romanticized notions that can hide elementary facts about adolescent development:[6]

Romanticizing adolescence blinds us to the adolescent's capacity for life-diminishing choices. Romantics refuse to tally the teen suicides, runaways, juvenile sex trade, prisons, broken mothers, damaged infants, and abusive fathers. In order to mature, the natural talent of youth must be aimed and trained.

Because of their stage in life, many adolescents are wishful thinkers, who lack a future orientation because of their sense of invulnerability and their attraction to risks. They are easily swayed by the belief "it can't happen to me." This omniscient and omnipotent flavoring of adolescence underlies the attitude "I don't care about that now" in spite of knowledge that cigarettes, drugs, noise and steroids produce diseases, addiction, hearing loss and shorten life. These developmental characteristics are not removed by pregnancy or parenthood. Babies and young children need protection from these characteristics of adolescent parents.

Adolescents who become pregnant have difficulty envisioning alternatives and reasoning about the consequences of childbirth. This point is illustrated by the following conversation I had with a fifteen-year-old White girl from a middle-class family:

> Doctor: I'm told that the test results show that you are pregnant.
>
> Patient: My boyfriend and I knew it because the condom broke.
>
> Doctor: What do you plan to do?
>
> Patient: I'm going to have my baby and keep it. My boyfriend will drop out of school to support us.
>
> Doctor: Do you think that you are old enough to raise a child?
>
> Patient: No. I certainly wouldn't try to get pregnant.
>
> Doctor: Then how is it that you plan to raise this baby?
>
> Patient: Oh, it was an accident. Besides I don't like school, and I can get money to live on. I know a lot of kids who are doing it.

Most adolescents who become pregnant are unprepared for decision-making and other responsibilities involved in parenthood. Mature adolescents are likely to recognize that they are not ready for parenthood and terminate their pregnancies or make an adoption plan for their babies.

Is There a Biological Right to Parenthood Regardless of Age?

In the United States, there is a strong emphasis on the reproductive freedom of women.[7] The U.S. Supreme Court described the right to procreate as a "basic liberty" in *Skinner v. Oklahoma.* This has been interpreted as establishing a right to procreate.[8] The political right may oppose pregnancy termination and urge girls to continue to childbirth. The political left may hold that minor adolescents have the right to procreate when physically able to do so.

GirlMom.com describes itself as a "politically progressive, left-aligned, pro-choice, feminist" web site that supports young mothers of all backgrounds in their struggles for reproductive freedom and social support. It holds that adolescents are socially conditioned to believe that they are irresponsible. This creates a self-fulfilling prophecy in which adolescent parents believe that they cannot parent well and, therefore, they do not. Adolescent parenthood is not a crisis; the crisis is that adolescent parents do not receive enough support.

Kristin Luker, a professor of sociology at the University of California-Berkeley, points out that adolescents have raised healthy children throughout human history.[9] She holds that when good prenatal care and nutrition are available, the adolescent years are the best time to have babies from the physical point of view. Luker believes: "the jury is still out on whether or not adolescents make 'bad' parents." Sara Ruddick, professor emeritus at New School University, hopes that the youngest mothers will have all of the resources to which all mothers are entitled.[10]

These viewpoints reflect a widely held belief that parenthood, as is procreation, is a right rather than a privilege. These views conflict with the moral and legal principle that a child is not the property of the genetic parent. From the moral point of view, parenthood is not an entitlement awarded by procreation. It is earned by nurturing a child, as adoptive parents well know. From the legal point of view, the rights of genetic parents are custodial guardianship rights that can be defined and revoked in accordance with child neglect and abuse laws.

Is the Genetic Parent Always the Best Qualified to Raise a Child?

Generally, a genetic parent is in the best position to raise a child. This principle guides the family preservation movement in social work and is affirmed by fetus-mother bonding throughout pregnancy and breastfeeding after childbirth. But possessing the judgment, skills and economic wherewithal required for parenthood in our complicated society is more important than the capacities to conceive and give birth. Recognizing these facts leads genetic mothers and fathers to make adoption plans for their babies.

Is Alienation of Adolescent Mothers and Their Parents Irreversible?

Some adolescent mothers say they cannot live with their parents who have mistreated them. This statement often is taken at face value in the absence of evidence of neglect or abuse and without taking the inherent conflicts between adolescents and their parents into account.

The most humane and efficacious approaches to troubled family relationships around adolescent pregnancy are counseling and family therapy. Unfortunately, they often are not available to those who need them the most. Even when available, the pain involved in resolving family conflicts may interrupt treatment that would have been successful if pursued to its conclusion. There is an urgent need for counselors for pregnant adolescents and their families.

LEGAL AGE FOR MARRIAGE

In most states minors over 16 may obtain a marriage license with the consent of their parents or guardians. Kansas and Massachusetts specify 12 for females and 14 for males. New Hampshire specifies 13 for females and 14 for males.[11] If there is no parent or guardian, or if the guardian is an agency or department, consent may be given by a court. Marriage and entering military service can be acts of emancipation.

Most European nations make 18 the minimum marriage age.[12] In Malta, people may marry from the age of 16, although paradoxically the age of consent for sexual intercourse is 18. In Turkey, the legal age for marriage is 17 for both girls and boys. In Portugal, the age of majority and for marriage is 16. In Ireland, a court may authorize the marriage of minors under 18 years under certain conditions.

Decision-making that leads to adolescent parenthood can be flawed and is an appropriate concern for public policy.[13] In this view, immaturity renders a minor incapable of giving truly informed consent in deciding to marry or to become a parent.

THE DOUBLE STANDARD

Franklin Zimring points out that our acceptance of low-income adolescent parenthood while we encourage middle-class adolescents to choose pregnancy termination or an adoption plan reveals a double standard.[14] Ageism, sexism and racism contribute to this double standard.

Most adolescents who become pregnant realize that it is unwise for them to enter parenthood. But they often do not receive reinforcement of this wisdom from their families, professionals and society. To deprive adolescents of the procedures involved in informed consent—the most important of which is insuring that they fully understand the consequences of their actions—is an abrogation of parental and professional obligations to them. It violates the responsibility of professionals to do no harm.

Title XX of the Public Health Service Act specifies necessary services for Adolescent Family Life Demonstration Projects that include adoption counseling and referral services; education on the responsibilities of sexuality and parenting; and counseling for the immediate and extended family members of the eligible person.[15] This model should be available to all pregnant adolescents.

CONCLUSION

Two vital aspects of parenthood are commonly overlooked. The first is that parenthood is a developmental stage in the life cycle that progresses though egocentric, conventional, individualistic and integrative phases.

The second is that the readiness for parenthood follows completion of the adolescent stage of life. Achieving the capacity to assume responsibility for one's own life as an adult is a prerequisite for assuming responsibility for the life of another person.

Controversies arise over whether or not pregnancy and childbirth in themselves promote maturity; whether or not everyone has a right to parenthood regardless of age; and whether or not genetic parents are always the best qualified to raise a child.

In the past, preparation for parenthood took place through families. With loosening family ties and family strife in the United States, preparation for parenthood now often must come from educational and clinical sources.

In order to ensure that children have competent parents, parenthood must be recognized as a developmental stage in life that follows adolescence and as an essential complement of childhood.

Part 4

THE DYNAMICS OF
ADOLESCENT PARENTHOOD

. . . Causing the existence of a human being is one of the most responsible actions
in the range of human life. To undertake this responsibility—to bestow a life which
may be either a curse or a blessing—unless the being on whom it is to be bestowed
will have at least an ordinary chance of a desirable existence, is a crime against that
being.

John Stuart Mill
On Liberty, 1859[1]

Following the hurricane analogy, the initial conditions that set the stage for adolescent
childbirth (tropical storm) are followed by a swirl of events and patterns that can ultimately directly and indirectly affect our entire society. The short-term and long-term
effects are most keenly felt by the adolescents themselves and by their children.

A number of cultural, social and psychological factors amplify or dampen adolescents' choices to become parents. Adolescent parenthood may appear to be a rational
choice for a poor girl faced with limited economic opportunities, peer pressure or fear
of losing a boyfriend. Having a child can give her purpose in life.

However, most girls who give birth and decide to become parents are vulnerable
emotionally, psychologically and developmentally. They have been physically, sexually or emotionally abused—or all three. They are prone to depression and risky sexual behaviors. The burdens of childrearing add to these traumata.

Adolescent fathers have received far less attention than adolescent mothers but are
equally important. They are unlikely to be in a position to provide financial, emotional
or other parental support for their children.

Fatherlessness is now approaching parity with fatherhood as a defining feature of
American childhood. When fathers do not fulfill their appropriate roles, the chances
of maladjustment in their children increase.

The crisis of adolescent childbirth draws society's attention to supporting the girl as
a mother rather than to her own and to her baby's developmental needs. The fact that
there are two young persons with developmental needs usually is not taken into
account.

The offspring of adolescent parents are the prototypical sources of habitual criminals, welfare dependency and adolescent parents who continue the cycle. At least one in three of the daughters of adolescent mothers become adolescent mothers themselves and are trapped in later life by the interwoven strands of men without jobs; women without husbands; children without fathers; and families without money, hope, skills, opportunities or resources that might help them escape from poverty.

Chapter 13

Choosing to Be an Adolescent Parent

If receiving attention and support at home and school can motivate adolescents to become mothers, what might the same attention and support do for them before they become pregnant?

Evelyn Lerman
Teen Moms, 1997[1]

Women who wait until they have established careers may have difficulty becoming parents. In contrast, some girls intentionally and unintentionally easily become parents.[2]

In order to understand why adolescents choose childbirth instead of pregnancy termination or an adoption plan, a look at rational choice theory is in order.

RATIONAL CHOICE THEORY

Rational choice theory holds that virtually all decisions are rational from the perspective of the persons making them.[3] "Rational" means reasoning from a premise in logical steps that may appear illogical to an observer and be logical (rational) to the person holding the premise.

Three principles can be applied to decision-making:

- We make decisions thoughtfully in ways that *we and others regard as rational*. Our behavior is forward-looking and consistent over time within the constraints of our capacities, resources and opportunities. We decide to marry, have children or divorce by comparing the benefits and costs of each alternative.
- We make decisions thoughtfully in ways that *we regard as rational, but others regard as irrational*. The premise that life begins at conception appears irrational to those who believe that life begins in the uterus. A psychotic person acts logically from a false premise based on a delusion or hallucination. Crime may be more lucrative than legal employment. Rational thought processes also can be based on lack of experience, as can be the case with adolescents.

- We make decisions *intuitively without a conscious thought process*. Athletes make split-second decisions correctly and incorrectly. We often act on impulse or emotion without a thought process because we "feel like it." After we act, we may wonder why we did it. Still, these intuitive decisions can serve our interests, particularly if based on previous experience with a situation.[4]

Even with our rational choices, we all make mistakes. Their impact on us depends on our margin for error. Those of us with personal, family, economic and social resources have a large margin for error. Those of us without these resources have little margin for error. For them mistakes in judgment can lead to adverse consequences: pregnancy, addictions, arrests, fatal accidents, homicide and suicide. Rational decision-making can be self-defeating.

MOTIVATIONS TO BECOME ADOLESCENT PARENTS

There are a number of cultural, social and psychological initial conditions that predispose adolescents to choose to enter parenthood. When a pregnancy is unplanned, a girl may decide to become a parent because she:[5]

- is frightened by the prospect of terminating her pregnancy;
- does not acknowledge her pregnancy early enough for termination;
- does not have access to termination services; or
- believes terminating a pregnancy is against her religion.

Adolescents who choose to become pregnant usually follow a premise with a logical thought process even though an observer may disagree with the premise and its conclusions.

Adolescent parenthood can be a rational choice for poor girls faced with limited economic opportunities, peer pressure or fear of losing a boyfriend. Having a baby can lead to greater organization of her life. She can gain adult status and still depend on her family.[6] She can obtain public assistance. 16-year-old Melanie, who gave birth while in a homeless shelter, said:

> Well, I came to New York and got put into the system . . . so then I was drinkin' and fightin' and um everything . . . and I needed a change and so I knew . . . unless I had something in my life that I could love or felt good about or something that I need to work toward. . . I would continue . . . I would continue doing the same thing.

Comments from adolescents during their first prenatal health care visit in Providence, Rhode Island, about their first pregnancies included:[7]

12-year-old with intended pregnancy: "Gonna get your own family and stuff."
14-year-old with unintended pregnancy: "I will have more responsibilities in my life. I will have to be more mature."

18-year-old with unintended pregnancy: "I think that it will keep me away from doing bad things like drinking and doing drugs. It will make me be more responsible and I'll learn how to depend on myself more."

15-year-old with unintended pregnancy: "The good thing is that I have someone to live for."

15-year-old with unintended pregnancy: "There's not too many good things. Except now I'm gonna have a huge responsibility and have to love and care for something. To me that's a good thing."

Cultural Factors

In some cultures, adolescent childbearing is accepted and even encouraged. When childbirth occurs, families assist adolescent parents in childrearing, or a marriage ensues creating a family within an extended family. Immigrants from these cultures may continue these customs until acculturation occurs in the United States.

The view is held by some that poor minorities have babies at young ages to hedge against higher infant mortality and to secure childrearing help while their extended family members are healthy.[8] This view sees early childbirth as a way to bolster minority populations and increase political power. It regards limiting minority adolescent childbirth as a form of ethnic eugenics.

The decline of marriage as a cultural expectation also affects adolescent childbearing.[9] Marriage can be seen as unconnected with parenthood. Marriage is reserved for couples who are financially secure. In this view, marriage can wait until later but not motherhood:

> Marriage was the last thing on 16-year-old Jewell's mind when she became pregnant in high school.[10] Her older sister, a single mother herself, all but begged her not to start down the same hard path. "I had been thinking about it for a long time," Jewell said. "I just wanted something that's mine, that I could love. I just wanted a baby, just wanted one. Even though I wasn't working, I didn't have my own place, whatever—I still wanted a baby."

There also are subcultures in which pregnancy termination is not acceptable. Boys or men and girls who conceive unintended pregnancies are duty bound to marry and establish a family or to support a girl as a single parent. Continuing pregnancy to childbirth is an honorable outcome, although a "shotgun marriage" may ensue.

Societal Factors

Daniel Patrick Moynihan called attention to the social phenomenon of defining deviance downward so that behaviors previously defined as unacceptable become normal.[11] This belief enables girls to become inured to hardship when adolescent parenthood is defined as normal. The image of the female bearing the pain and burden of childbirth and childrearing can be extended to the image of females as compensating for the irresponsibility of males.

Pregnancy and childbirth are challenges for some girls. Unlike other challenges, a baby brings emotional, status and financial benefits. Welfare support can be regarded as a form of public scholarship for them to complete their educations and training. Working to be good mothers enhances their self-respect.[12]

Far more than their middle-class counterparts, disadvantaged girls are likely to see terminating a pregnancy as wrong and childlessness as unfortunate. Having a baby rather than a career promises a human connection in a world where trusting relationships are scarce.

Still, most socio-economically disadvantaged girls and boys do not become parents. Some disadvantaged groups have a tradition of adolescent parenthood. When they move up the socioeconomic ladder, they relinquish this tradition.

A survey of disadvantaged 15- and 16-year-old girls revealed that 13% of Black, 9% of Latino, and 5% of White girls definitely would consider having a child out of wedlock. 20% more in each category said that they might.[13] In another survey, 85% of White and 70% of Black disadvantaged adolescent mothers said they wanted their babies after they became pregnant.[14]

Discouraged, disadvantaged adolescent girls are the most likely to desire to become pregnant. Motherhood seems to offer a chance for respectability in a squalid world. The girls take pride in setting themselves apart from mothers who "don't take care of their kids." Ruth Horowitz, Professor of Sociology at New York University, observed that most participants in a Chicago program for adolescent mothers would buy only new clothes because they were embarrassed to be seen in a Goodwill Store buying used garments:[15]

> On the day I went to a second hand store with five of the participants, no one bought anything because the clothes looked "old and nasty."

Affirming the importance of exposure to role models, such as adolescent parents, an elegant study of 10- and 15-year-olds in Chicago revealed that exposure to violence is causally related to violent behavior.[16] Being exposed to firearm violence almost doubles the probability that an adolescent will perpetrate serious violence over the subsequent two years. This finding has implications for role modeling of adolescent parenthood as well. Older adolescent mothers and fathers strongly influence younger adolescents to become mothers and fathers.

The Role of Fathers

Girl's motivations to become mothers occur in the context of predatory, usually older, males with the sexist attitude that the responsibility for contraception lies with females. They may disdain contraception that interferes with their own pleasure and convenience. The girls gain acceptance by emulating admired peers or by pleasing a boy friend.

The book *Promises I Can Keep* describes interviews with Black, White and Latino adolescent mothers in the poorest neighborhoods of Camden, NJ, and Philadelphia.[17] Girls as young as 14 simply wanted to have babies. They spoke about the "joys of motherhood." Their boyfriends often said to them: "I want to have a baby by you."

The euphoria of birth may suddenly resolve the tumultuousness of the previous nine months. Even if a father has urged his girlfriend to terminate the pregnancy or claimed the baby is not his, branding her as a "cheater" or 'whore", he may feel a powerful bond with his newborn and vow to mend his ways. The mother usually is eager to believe his promises. Still, despite these young couples' resolve to stay together, most separate before the child is three years old.[18]

Although 75% of boys in a Sexually Transmitted Disease clinic sample said they had no plans to get someone pregnant in the next 6 months, 56% said that there was at least some likelihood that they would do so during that time.[19]

All of these considerations raise questions about psychological motivations to become adolescent parents beyond cultural and societal factors.

Psychological Factors

A number of psychological factors can motivate a girl to become a mother.

Identity as a Parent

The choice to become a parent despite the obstacles that lie ahead is a compelling demonstration of maturity for some girls. Extreme loneliness, struggles with parents and peers, depression, despair, school failure, drugs and a general sense that life has spun out of control are compensated for by the purpose, validation, companionship and order that babies bring to their lives. Giving birth and caring for a baby satisfies maternal instincts. These girls may believe that a baby has the power "to solve everything." In a Boston study, school-age mothers believed their lives were enriched by childbearing.[20] Some said that the birth of their child persuaded them to give up drugs or to stop "running the streets." In spite of poor schools and little contact with churches and neighborhood organizations, these mothers had relatively high self-esteem enhanced by having babies as their role models did.

However, decades of research have shown that high self-esteem can reflect overconfidence and does not correlate with success in school or later life.[21] Mature adults realize that knowing "who I am" does not come easily and that life is a process of self-discovery. Adolescents discover the different parts of themselves by experimenting with different roles and skills. Resulting confusion, uncertainty and failure can lead to defensive denial in the form of appearing to be certain and confident. Boys are particularly likely to act "macho" rather than reveal uncertainty and weakness. This uncertainty can be relieved by assuming the identity of a mother for girls or of a father for boys.[22]

> 16-year-old Devon said, "I need some little mes (children). I got a reputation to hold up, but, I can't see myself being with one woman every day."

Being a parent is an identity that appeals to adolescents who have little else to strive for. A baby can give them a sense of control over another person and themselves.

Egocentricity

All of us are driven by a *self-centered cluster* of instincts and emotions governed by lower centers of our brains.[23] They are vital for individual survival. We must satisfy hunger and thirst and fend off predators. The *other-centered cluster* in the higher centers of our brains is vital for species survival. We must mate and become attached to and care for others in families and beyond for the survival of our society.

Merging of self-centered and other-centered drives occurs as young persons learn to postpone gratification and tolerate frustration of their wishes. The adolescent tendencies to feel invulnerable and all-knowing are remnants of the self-centered narcissism of babies. If self-centeredness is not tempered, adolescents retain the omnipotent, omniscient attitude of toddlers:

- I want to be the center of attention.
- I am right. You are wrong.
- I don't need to listen to you.
- I want what I want now.

The ability to delay gratification is vital for success in life.[24] Adolescents who lack self-discipline often resort to self-deception and self-indulgence when they encounter challenges that elicit discomfort. They overeat, use drugs and alcohol and resort to sex to assuage painful feelings. They use body-piercing and tattoos to overcome their insecurities.

Children who receive the love and limits needed to develop self-discipline relinquish their extreme egocentricity and become adolescents who can cope with the challenges and disappointments of life. For example, a young homeless mother, Casey, belatedly acknowledged that she was unprepared for motherhood as she asked herself, how did I become homeless?[25]

> I could say it's my husband's fault because he lost his job and became violent so I had to quit my jobs. Or I could say I didn't have enough money to pay the rent and bills. What I have learned is that the real reasons for my homelessness were a lack of education, a lack of financial planning, a lack of resources, and an unwillingness to make sacrifices in my life.

Immature Judgment

Adolescent girls tend to underestimate their chances of becoming pregnant and parents.[26] The immature judgment of adolescents is exemplified by 16-year-old Jody:

> One Saturday morning, I woke up feeling sick to my stomach. I hadn't gotten my period. I thought I can't be pregnant—we always used condoms. I went to Planned Parenthood and found out I was. I was so overwhelmed by the thought of having a baby and being a mom that I forced myself to not think about it. When I was four months pregnant, I finally called and made an appointment to get an abortion. But by the time the date came, my boyfriend and I didn't know how much it would cost, and I didn't go. I didn't tell my parents. When I was eight months pregnant, my mom sat me down and asked if there was

something wrong with me. I told her I was just upset because I'm gaining weight and can't get it off. I started worrying about my health—and the baby's—since I hadn't seen a doctor. Finally my dad asked if I was pregnant. I burst into tears and nodded. I was just so relieved to finally have the truth come out. A year later my boyfriend and I broke up. I live with my parents. Being a single mom is really hard, working and going to school full time. I really regret not turning to my parents sooner for help.

Psychiatric Disorders

Adolescents who have not developed sufficient self-discipline experience frustration easily when they cannot have their own way, fail or are unable to control others. They are prone to depression when their vulnerability is exposed. Instead of working through stressful experiences, they shut them out of conscious awareness and experience chronic stress.[27] Sexual gratification relieves their anxiety and depression. A baby relieves their loneliness. Self-justification is one way they avoid anxiety and depression associated with their decision to become parents. It allows them to believe that becoming parents was good for them.

Two studies showed that girls and boys who exhibit high levels of risky sexual behaviors are prone to depression.[28] A twenty-year study of Black girls disclosed that those who suffered from depression were more likely to become parents than those who did not. In a Baltimore study, 49% of predominantly Black, low-income 12 to 18-year-old girls had a subsequent pregnancy within two years with depressive symptoms in 46% contributing to that outcome.

Adolescents with the greatest risk of developing significant psychiatric disorders are those with attachment disorders and unresolved trauma or grief. They are not able to sustain a sense of self-continuity across the past, present and future or in relationships with others with whom they tend to be controlling and aggressive.[29] They are at risk of post-traumatic stress disorders and delinquency related to community and family violence. Forty to seventy percent of adolescent mothers report a history of sexual abuse.

ADDICTION AS A MODEL FOR SELF-DEFEATING ADOLESCENT PARENTHOOD

The addiction model can be applied to understanding and managing adolescent pregnancy and parenthood when they result from persistent behavior in the face of harmful consequences.[30] Addicts are unable to resist immediate self-defeating rewards, even when they want delayed self-enhancing rewards. They discount future consequences of their behavior.

Addiction Dynamics

Drug and alcohol addictions cut like a deadly scythe through adolescents mowing down 10% or more, some for a few years, others for their lifetimes. Addiction underlies the façade of "normal" adolescent drinking and drug "experimentation."[31]

Addiction also underlies the intergenerational cycle of adolescent parenthood. Adolescent parents may not be addicted to drugs or alcohol, but the concept of addiction is relevant in understanding compulsive sexual behavior that alleviates painful feelings or fulfills fantasies, as is characteristic of alcoholics and compulsive gamblers. The addiction model is especially relevant for girls with multiple pregnancies and with concomitant drug and alcohol addictions.

Drug addiction ultimately reduces addicted persons to helpless spectators of their own self-defeating behavior. Repetitive generations of adolescent parents are helpless spectators of their own self-defeating behavior. Peter Blos, a pioneer in adolescent psychoanalysis, described repetitive, compulsive behavior as a self-defeating attempt to master adverse life experiences that can be based on an unconscious wish to hurt or punish oneself.[32]

Most adolescents who become pregnant are vulnerable persons with anxiety, depression and little self-respect.[33] Pregnant 15- to 25-year-olds are more likely to use illicit drugs and smoke cigarettes than older women. Boys and girls who are vulnerable to drug abuse and gang membership are likely to become adolescent parents. They resort to sex, drugs and alcohol as adaptive behaviors. In this sense, pregnancy and parenthood also are adaptive for them.

Like drugs, sex provides immediate gratification and relief from stress. For girls, sex can fulfill fantasies of being loved by a partner and possibly by a baby. For boys, sex adds a sense of power to immediate gratification by controlling females and by producing progeny.

Addiction is reinforced by a combination of physical, emotional and environmental elements. Parents and siblings often have enabling relationships with their drug-abusing adolescents.[34] Similar co-dependency is seen in families that foster adolescent parenthood. Peers model drug and alcohol addiction, and they model pregnancy and parenthood.

Addiction Management

The basic assumption in the management of addiction is that an addict can make constructive choices in a supportive environment. The addicted person is torn between an appetite for a drug and reasons for not indulging.[35] People recover from self-defeating addiction to the extent that they:

- believe that an addiction is hurting them and wish to overcome it;
- feel able to manage withdrawal and life without addiction; and
- find sufficient alternative rewards to make life without addiction worthwhile.

The addiction management model is relevant to the extent that an adolescent's pregnancy has deep, compelling roots in the repetitive cycle of adolescent parenthood. It can serve as a guide in handling self-defeating behavior.

Integration of the steps of Alcoholics Anonymous with cognitive-behavioral techniques is relevant to managing denial and depression in adolescent pregnancy and parenthood.[36] Thoughts, such as "I can't, I have to and I'll try," result in feelings of hopelessness, worthlessness and failure. In contrast, using cognitive-behavioral therapy with pregnant adolescents in a supportive environment can develop self-affirming attitudes to replace defeatist thinking with "I can, I'm choosing to and I'll do my best." This can provide a basis for wise decision making.

CONCLUSION

Adolescent parenthood may be a rational choice for girls faced with limited economic opportunities, peer pressures or fear of losing boyfriends. Having babies can lead to greater organization of their lives, especially in supportive cultural and social environments.

When tempering of self-centeredness does not occur during childhood, adolescents retain the omnipotent, omniscient attitude of toddlers. Their inability to fully anticipate the consequences of their actions destines many to repeat the cycle of premature parenthood, educational failure, health problems, welfare dependency and crime they have observed in their own families and neighborhoods.

Most girls who decide to become parents are vulnerable emotionally and developmentally. They have been physically, sexually or emotionally abused—or all three. They are prone to depression and exhibit high levels of risky sexual behaviors. The burdens of childrearing are added to these traumata.

The addiction model can be applied to repetitive generations of adolescent pregnancy and parenthood to highlight their deep roots and to guide handling self-defeating behavior. Parents, siblings and peers can have enabling, co-dependent relationships with their drug-abusing adolescents and with their adolescents who are parents.

The complicated causes and consequences of adolescent parenthood call for identifying and applying dampening influences through counseling pregnant adolescents and their families.

Chapter 14

Profiles of Adolescent Parents

The musical *West Side Story* depicts an adolescent girl and boy
hoping that, "somehow, there is a time and place for us."

West Side Story[1]

This chapter is devoted to typical examples of girls and boys who choose to enter parenthood for reasons other than following cultural traditions of early marriage.

ADOLESCENT MOTHER PROFILES

Categories of adolescent mothers were proposed by Herbert Quay, former professor of psychology at Northwestern University:[2] 1) achieving an identity through motherhood; 2) seeking the affection of a baby; 3) seeking pregnancy to precipitate marriage; 4) unintentional outcome of relationship; 5) taking responsibility for a pregnancy; and 6) gang life style.

1) Achieving an Identity through Motherhood

The first group is of girls who are gratified by attention from males. They have few chances to explore options in life. Many are sad and angry because they did not have fathers who devoted time and attention to them.[3]

When they become pregnant, they choose to give birth. Motherhood promises them a pathway to personhood and gives them an identity and status. They believe they are creating better lives for themselves by having a baby.

Tanisha

16-year-old Tanisha felt isolated in school. She met a boy who was the only person who ever said she was beautiful. They had sex.

If I didn't do it with my boyfriend, then he wouldn't love me? My life could get harder, or I could get pregnant. Because you don't care about yourself so if it happens to me, who cares? I'm half-dead anyway, emotionally.

Later a pregnancy test was positive. She thought her life was over. She called her boyfriend. He asked if she was sure the baby was his.

I don't remember answering him. I think I got very sarcastic and did not speak to him after that.

Tanisha told her mother when she was three months pregnant. They cried and became closer than they ever had been.

I'm staying away from guys at least until June. I'm having a boy, Isaiah. His name means "saved by God." I couldn't have gone through with the pregnancy without God. My family is fighting over him. I really am somebody now.

Her mother agreed to help raise Isaiah while she finished high school.

Tiffany

Nineteen-year-old Tiffany was referred to a psychiatric clinic because she had neglected her three-year-old daughter. She said:

Damion and me knew I could get pregnant, and he had condoms, and I had those pills, but you know how it is, we were young and so much in love that we didn't use them. We talked about getting married, but he couldn't get a job, and he started drinking more. My baby was so cute, and I felt so important because I had her, but she cried a lot, and then she had to have her own way all the time. It was just too much for me so I started using and drinking.

2) Seeking Affection from a Baby

Girls in the second group seek a baby as a source of love rather than as a growing person to nurture.[4] Because they did not bond sufficiently with their own parents, these girls usually are not prepared to form solid attachment bonds with their own babies.

Brook

Brook was 16 when she gave birth to a baby boy:

When I got pregnant nobody was really mad at me, but my mother and grandmother wanted me to have an abortion. But they had babies when they were kids too so I didn't listen to them. I decided to have my baby because I feel so lonely. You have somebody to love, somebody to love you, and somebody to talk to. This is my child, and nobody can ever take him away.

3) Seeking Pregnancy to Precipitate Marriage

Girls in the third group seek pregnancies in order to precipitate marriage and escape from difficult lives in their own families.[5] They are troubled adolescents who repeat intergenerational cycles of family conflict. Pregnancy also can be an act of rebellion against overly strict parents.

Eloise

At the age of 20 Eloise described what happened in her life:

> I hated my stepfather. He sexually abused me, and my mother did nothing to stop him. She blamed me for making up lies. I had to get out of there. I left off the pill for a while without telling my boyfriend hoping that I would get pregnant, and then he would marry me. I did, but he didn't. As soon as he found out, he didn't want to have anything to do with me. They finally got him for child support, and me and my 3-year-old get along on welfare.

4) Unintentional Outcome of a Long-term Relationship

The fourth group is composed of girls who are careless with birth control in long-term relationships with males in which unintentional pregnancy occurs. Marriage accompanies childbirth. Three-fourths of these marriages end in divorce.[6]

Casey

> Sixteen-year-old Casey and her boyfriend Corey were friends since entering high school. They were with each other constantly and occasionally slept together in his mother's home. When Casey spent time with others in school, Corey was jealous. They planned to get married later. When Casey became pregnant, Corey supported her and was present at their daughter's birth. They married and set up housekeeping. Both found jobs. As Corey spent more time with his friends and resented his parental responsibilities, Casey ultimately obtained a divorce.

5) Taking Responsibility for Being Pregnant

An increasing number of girls reject pregnancy termination as an option. They view becoming a parent as the honorable resolution of the mistake of pregnancy.[7]

Alex

When asked why she wouldn't choose to terminate her pregnancy if she faced the choice, 15-year-old Alex pointed to responsibility and regret.

> I think abortion is not natural, and you need to deal with the mistakes you've made in a responsible way. As much as it would affect my life and take away a lot of the opportunities I would have had, I think it would open up a lot of other doors for me, and probably make me more mature than going to college and having a career would. I would use birth control, but if something happened, I would probably accept the responsibility by

having the child. I see abortion as a regret. Years later I would think, "that could have been the sweetest little child, and I missed out."

6) Gang Life Style

Girls who relate or belong to gangs are prone to pregnancy.[8] In order to be accepted by, or to become members of, gangs, they endure homelessness, betrayal, the separation of incarceration and the insidious damage of poverty. They seek excitement and find troubled boys whose gang activities lead to spells in prison. This outlaw life style with "gangsta" glamour, drug dealers and street corner society is graphically described in *Random Family*.[9]

Some girls and women are attracted to "bad-boy" types as captured in the lyric of the Waylon Jennings song—"Ladies love outlaws like babies love stray dogs"—and in the life of serial killer Gary Gilmore glamorized in Normal Mailer's book *Executioner's Song*.[10] The pop culture's adulation of male violence and unstable families create girls who seek power in a world that has granted them none by joining males who both depend on and dominate them.

Angela[11]

Angela grew up in Chicago's gangland. Her father was a drunk. She had her first baby at 17, dropped out of high school and had two more in quick succession. She didn't have a diploma or a job. The man she loved, Greg, was making good money selling cocaine. Once, when he went out without feeding the kids, she tried to shoot him. Unlike most adolescent parents, they stayed together, but by the time their eldest child entered school Greg was arrested, and Angela was unable to pay the bills. She moved to Milwaukee where she could get welfare, an apartment and have money left over.

Angela ultimately was a survivor. Repeating her family's long-standing pattern, her daughter Kesha got pregnant by a 14-year-old boy who abandoned her. Kesha dropped out of school and moved in with a 24-year-old boy friend, who was living with his mother. Angela urged her to end the pregnancy, but Kesha wouldn't hear of it. "It's wrong to kill a baby. If you're grown enough to have sex, you gotta take responsibility." At 19 she had her second child.

ADOLESCENT FATHERS

Adolescent fatherhood has received less attention than adolescent motherhood. Most adolescent fathers are not centrally involved with their children, but a few are the primary parent.

Adolescent Fathers with Little or No Involvement in Childrearing

Adolescent fathers generally are poorly educated and economically disadvantaged.[12] A study of adolescent fathers in Houston, Texas, revealed that 69% were school dropouts; 73% were unemployed; 40% had substance abuse problems; and 30% had committed a felony. Less than half had declared paternity for their children. They did not want substance abuse counseling, child support services or help in obtaining a GED.

Fathering a child may be just one event on a continuum of antisocial behaviors. Some clearly intend to impregnate girls.[13] In one survey, 40% of boys ages 15-19 agreed that "getting a girl pregnant makes you feel like a real man." Fifty-one percent agreed that they often receive the message that sex and pregnancy are not "big deals."

Seven percent of all adolescent boys are fathers, with higher rates for inner-city Black (22%), Latino (19%) and White adolescents (10%).[14] They tend to be two to three years older than the adolescent mothers. They often continue an intergenerational pattern of adolescent childbearing, welfare dependency and low educational achievement. They may live with their children sporadically, but most do not pay child support even with vigorous enforcement.

Interviews with a group of Black adolescent fathers revealed that pregnancies often complicated long-term relationships with the mothers.[15] They seemed confused about the conflict between adolescent perspectives on dating and adult perspectives on committed relationships. They lacked the interpersonal skills needed for negotiating parenthood responsibilities.

The question of a genetic factor emerges whenever anti-social behavior occurs. A gene associated with an increased risk of male adolescent criminal behavior appears to only be significant when interacting with psychosocial factors and does not cause this behavior in itself.[16]

Adolescent Fathers Involved in Rearing their Children

The common stereotype is that adolescent fathers shirk their responsibilities because they do not care about the welfare of their offspring.[17] The Fragile Families and Child Wellbeing Study found that one year after birth adolescent mothers reported that 75% of the fathers who had a romantic relationship with them were present at the birth and had at least weekly contact with their children. Forty-seven percent reported that marriage was almost certain. The survey did not include fathers who had little or no contact with the mother around the time of birth.

Some adolescent fathers do assume major childrearing responsibilities:

Brian

Seventeen-year-old Brian, a "baby daddy," said:

> If I tell someone I have a child, they ask me if I still am with the mother. I don't like that in the sense that they believe that I was there, had my fun, a child came out of it and that was it. That's not how it happened.

Brian lives with his mother but still is involved with his son's mother, 16-year-old Elaine. They have been inseparable since eighth grade. Their 14-month-old son lives with Elaine, but she and Brian share responsibility for him. Brian continued:

I can't brush it aside in my head saying that it's just an accident. I can't forget about it. Not like my father forgot about me. I know that when I was growing up, my dad wasn't around a lot. I would not want my son to feel the same exact way. I wanted to be pretty much what my dad wasn't. Be there.

Adoption was never an option Brian considered. His mother was pregnant at 16, and her parents made her give up the baby—his sister—who would be 8 years older than he was.

My grandparents threatened to kick her out if she didn't give her child up for adoption. My mother has been searching for her for most of my life. Before my son was born, I didn't care about school. Now? Someone else depends on my success. The better I do in life, the better he will be able to do as well. He'll have a role model to look up to. I never did.

Information for Adolescent Fathers

Unlike adolescent mothers for whom the answer is obvious, adolescent fathers must find out if they are parents of particular children. Ultimately, a child deserves to have information about paternity as well. The web site, Teen Fatherhood FAQ, offers practical advice about determining paternity through blood type and DNA matching.[18]

Courts regard adolescent fathers as entitled to know their genetic children and to participate in their lives. Either they or their parents are responsible for the support and care of their children. If they are non-custodial parents, they must pay child support. They can be involved in their children's lives and make decisions presumably in the "best interests" of their children.

The pressure to marry when an unwanted pregnancy occurs can be overwhelming but there are important legal ramifications that genetic fathers must know. Under common law, a child born to parents who are legally married at the time of birth is presumed to belong to the husband who then has the parental rights of a genetic father.

Fathers cannot force mothers to terminate a pregnancy or make an adoption plan for their children, but they can relinquish their parental rights. They can make a custody and child support arrangement with a court. If a father believes that a mother is neglecting or abusing their child, he has a responsibility to report it. Conversely, if a mother believes that a father is harming a child, she has a responsibility to request court action to stop or limit access to the child.

CONCLUSION

There are six typical adolescent mother profiles. The most common is achieving an identity through motherhood. Other profiles are seeking a baby as a source of love; seeking pregnancy in order to precipitate marriage and escape from a difficult family life; consummating marriage in a long-term relationship with a male in which unintentional pregnancy occurs; taking responsibility for the mistake of pregnancy and becoming a parent as the honorable resolution; and trying to make a family with gang members.

Adolescent mothers tend to be girls with complicated problems, who may initially see having a baby as more appealing than finishing high school or employment.

The needs and interests of adolescent fathers receive insufficient attention. They are unlikely to be able to provide financial, emotional or other parental support for their children. Fathering a child may be just one event in a continuum of antisocial behaviors. Some clearly intend to impregnate girls.

Chapter 15

The Impact of Parenthood on Adolescents

> . . . people having the most children are the ones least capable of supporting them.
>
> *Philadelphia Inquirer*, 1997[1]

In 1987, a Committee of the National Research Council concluded that adolescent parenthood is a handicap for adolescents because it interferes with their development and their opportunities in life.[2] It recommended that the primary goal of policy makers should be to reduce adolescent pregnancies. It urged young people to postpone sexual intercourse until they are capable of making responsible decisions regarding their personal lives and forming families.

When adolescents assume the responsibilities of childrearing prior to their readiness for parenthood, the courses of their lives are drastically altered. Their freedom to develop as adolescents is curtailed. Their emerging independence is compromised. Pregnancy and childbirth alter girl's bodies before they have fully developed physically. Having a second child sets them on a life course that becomes increasingly difficult to alter.

On the other hand, parenthood can have maturing effects on adolescent attitudes, motivation and skills. In a broader sense, natural selection in evolution favors people who reproduce.[3] The sooner reproduction begins, the more progeny for our species.

This chapter aims to place the impact of parenthood on adolescents in perspective.

MATURING EFFECT OF PARENTHOOD ON ADOLESCENTS

The Healthy Teen Network is a national organization founded on the premise that adolescents can make responsible decisions about sexuality, pregnancy and parenting.[4] It holds that adolescents can be effective parents when they have culturally relevant and developmentally appropriate information and support. It believes that it is unfair to exclude adolescent mothers from public benefits available to adult mothers. Some adolescents do mature rapidly after childbirth, especially those who are legal adults. The cessation of drug abuse has been reported.[5]

Biological Maturation

Successful reproduction in mammals demands that mothers become attached to and nourish their offspring. Pregnancy and birth in rats promote growth in lower brain centers that govern behaviors affecting the survival of their offspring, but rat mothers are not better than virgin counterparts at other tasks.[6] Although this implies that similar growth occurs in lower centers of the human brain, rearing a human child is more complicated than rearing a rat.

During human pregnancy, the ovaries and placenta produce extra estrogen and progesterone. They appear to enlarge hypothalamic neurons that regulate basic maternal responses, as well as neuronal branches in the hippocampus that govern memory and learning. The hypothalamus and pituitary gland secrete oxytocin that triggers birth contractions, prolactin that stimulates the mammary glands and endorphins that ease birth pains. Oxytocin also stimulates the growth of neurons in the hippocampus, lactation and maternal behavior.

Pregnancy and childbirth stimulate maturing of brain centers that govern behaviors affecting the survival of offspring. However, other parts of the brain do not mature more rapidly.[7]

Maturing of Attitudes and Motivation

A significant minority of all adolescents (boys 15%, girls 12%) say they would be pleased with a pregnancy.[8] Of sexually active 15 to 19-year-olds, 23% percent of boys, 17% of girls and 31% of mothers with one child say they would be pleased with a pregnancy.

Some adolescent mothers believe that having a baby changed their lives for the better. Three 17-year-olds said:[9]

- I have to be responsible now. I have to care about what I do. I can't hang out with stoners. They're childish, and I have to be grownup.
- I have to take care of my baby or Child Protective Services will take him.
- Being a mother didn't really change my life. I never did anything before. I didn't have a lot of friends, so it's not too different now except that wherever I go, my baby goes too.

Resiliency

Adolescents have varying degrees of resilience related to individual differences in temperament.[10] The areas of the brain that control attention, impulse-control and thinking are more active in resilient adolescents than in those who are not.

Longitudinal studies consistently point to positive traits that enable resilient young people to accommodate long-term exposure to poverty, mental illness and physical disability.[11] They are able to seek and cultivate positive relationships; have positive school experiences and verbal skills; and have a positive outlook on life. These characteristics act as protective shields that help them cope with adverse circumstances by building relationships with adults, refusing sexual advances, avoiding high-risk situations and negotiating the use of birth control. Supportive family and community resources also favor positive outcomes.[12]

Resilient mothers in one study were achieving at grade level when they became pregnant.[13] They received support from the fathers, were socially competent and involved in a variety of school and other social activities. They were prepared for their maternal roles and had adaptive parenting attitudes, adequate knowledge and appropriate expectations of their babies.

From Adolescent Parenthood to Professional Careers

A survey of Black professional women who became mothers between the ages of 14 and 19 and had received public assistance found that:[14] 86% were motivated to provide a better life for their children; 89% found a mentor and networked with others with similar goals; and 56% received financial support from their families and mentors. One woman said:

> I would listen to my theme song, *Ain't No Stopping Us Now*. It was empowering. I sang it in my head . . . you're not going to stop me!

Even when confronted with racism and sexism, their strong spiritual beliefs inspired them to persevere and achieve their goals. Most obtained vocational training and jobs that offered advancements. Some had college degrees. They strongly believed that short-term sacrifices produced long-term gains as they moved out of poverty. One recalled:

> I had to learn to live on a very tight budget, which meant carefully planning meals, sewing my children's clothes and buying carefully at resale shops.

These women also had times when they resorted to self-defeating behaviors including drug and alcohol abuse, social isolation, involvement in dysfunctional relationships, eating and sleep disorders and workaholic and perfectionist behaviors. They sought help for these problems.

They pointed to the strengths of their ancestors, and spoke of how they learned to deal with obstacles and adversities from them. One recalled:

> I witnessed women in my family overcoming barriers all of the time. Using "your wits" bargaining and "one-step ahead" strategies were in my heritage.

Another study found that in spite of experiencing depression as adolescent mothers, women who pursued goals, experienced deep connections to others, exercised self-direction and possessed self-respect found high levels of well-being in their fifties when they had stable marriages along with educational and career satisfactions.[15]

STRESSFUL LIVES BEFORE AND AFTER PARENTHOOD

Many of the negative outcomes for adolescent mothers are related to disadvantaged environments and conflicts with peers, parents and siblings, especially when they are depressed.[16]

Stress and Adolescent Mothers

Adolescent girls who are trapped victims of abuse, disappointing love affairs, poverty and powerlessness often have stress-related disorders. They lack self-esteem, dignity, self-respect and hope for different lives. They are prone to conceive and give birth.

Beginning in 1984, the Notre Dame Project in South Bend, Indiana, and Aiken, South Carolina, followed pregnant adolescents (70% were 17 or younger) recruited from girls who sought educational, medical or social services, thereby excluding the most at-risk adolescents.[17] They manifested signs of socio-emotional and behavioral adjustment problems, insecure social supports, low IQs (63% below 90) and insufficient readiness for parenting. Six months after the birth of their first child, their parenting was characterized by less than optimal attitudes and knowledge, high stress and behavioral problems. Five years into the study they showed multiple problems, including anxiety in 63%, depression in 34% and mild mental retardation in 7%.

The Chronic Stress Response

Our stress-response system allows us to cope with potential threats to our well-being.[18] It involves the interaction of genetic, physiological, psychological and environmental factors. The stress response initially is adaptive and restorative. Short-term stress evokes the fight-flight response that helps the body adapt to stressors. Stress hormones (corticosteroids) are used to treat inflammation. However, long-term stress throws regulatory systems out of balance and adversely affects the development of the brain and the body.

Stress affects all body systems, especially the endocrine and immune systems. People with excessive stress in their early lives, such as living in poverty and bearing the burdens of childrearing, show earlier aging, more depression, suicide, substance abuse and an earlier decline in both physical and mental functioning than those who have not.[19] Experiencing significant stress as a child also causes long-term activation of the stress response so that weaker stressors produce stronger responses. Adolescents with insecure or disorganized relationships have high stress hormone levels when they are frustrated.

The stress response begins deep in the brain where the hypothalamus alerts the adrenal gland medulla through the autonomic nervous system.[20] The adrenals answer immediately by pouring out adrenalin for the classic fight-flight response. Next the hypothalamus secretes corticotrophin releasing factor, which moves through specialized blood vessels to the pituitary gland, which in turn produces adrenocorticotropic hormone that travels through the blood stream to the adrenal cortex. The adrenal cortex secretes cortisol into the blood stream. It replenishes energy stores depleted by the adrenalin rush. It also increases activity and hunger. Too much adrenalin results in surging blood pressure and can damage blood vessels.

Prolonged stress has adverse effects on adolescents' health and learning in school. In the short-range, cortisol mobilizes energy and increases appetite. Too much cortisol prevents insulin from stimulating muscle to take up glucose and enhances the storage of fat. In the long-range it causes obesity, premature puberty, diabetes, atherosclerosis, muscle wasting and bone thinning. In the short-range, it enhances but in the long-range suppresses immunity. In the short-range, it enhances attention and memory. In the long-range, it impairs memory by causing the loss of nerve cells in the hippocampus. It weakens the ability of the hippocampus to perceive that something is not genuinely stressful and prevents the stress response from shutting off. Long-term stress delays adolescent development by impeding the adaptability and growth of the brain.

Twelve-Year-Old China

The reality-based novel *Broken China* gives insight into the attitudes, judgment and vulnerability that create stress in adolescent girls:[21]

> Twelve-year-old China gave birth to Amina. During her pregnancy she felt that her baby was imprinted in her: "Her name was written in each chamber of my heart." She could not bear the thought of an abortion because, "A mother who buries her child buries herself."
>
> China's mother was 17 when China was born. She managed to get a GED and worked as a beautician until she died of cancer. Thereafter, China lived with her wheel-chair-confined Uncle Simon, who did not advise her about whether or not to become a parent because he saw that advice had not worked with her mother. China sporadically attended school and never expected Amina's 15-year-old father to do anything. "We had a baby together. Both of us messed up, but I'm the one that got stuck. I had her, he didn't."
>
> Amina died of an undiagnosed heart disease at the age of 2 when China was 14. China was induced to pay $7,000 on credit for the funeral and spent the next several years as a strip teaser to pay off the debt. When she discovered that the funeral director also owned the strip tease club, she was angry, but, "I was the one who decided to go to work at the club."

IMPACT OF PARENTHOOD ON ADOLESCENT DEVELOPMENT

A girl who becomes a mother and a boy who becomes a father are deprived prematurely of opportunities to socialize with peers, to develop skills and hobbies and to make career choices. A girl cannot form a complete sense of her own body image when the physical changes of childbearing occur before her own body has fully matured. On the other hand, if she desired a pregnancy and receives support, she may well take pride in her pregnant body.[22]

The fact that babies require care 24 hours a day for 7 days a week and are not always cute, happy and playful is not in line with the expectations of adolescents. In addition, the fluctuating moods and interests of adolescents add to their frustrations with childrearing. When their babies have developmental problems, they may well be over-whelmed.

An adolescent mother's search for her own identity may intrude on parenting re-sponsibilities.[23] Her views of herself and her child are likely to be egocentric. She is likely to have poor problem-solving skills and stressful relationships with her own mother, partner and baby. She is likely to be disorganized and fail to seek help.

Adolescent fathers also need to master the developmental challenges of adoles-cence.[24] Cultural norms and social contexts influence their decisions regarding being sexually active, using contraception and pregnancy outcomes.

Adolescent parenthood need not preclude experiencing aspects of adolescent de-velopment. Under optimal circumstances, an adolescent mother may not be excluded from other roles, such as student, worker, girl friend, wife and daughter.[25] When rela-tives assist in caring for her baby, an adolescent can be a mother and remain an ado-lescent in some respects. However, she is not free to experiment with the full range of social roles and opportunities involved in adolescent development.

IMPACT OF PARENTHOOD ON THE MOTHERS' EDUCATION

Respected studies reveal differing pictures of the educational impacts of adolescent motherhood on high school graduation or its equivalent rates. One study found that 70% of adolescent parents dropped out of school but did not track those who re-turned.[26] A review of the literature in 1987 and in 1997 revealed that about 30% of adolescent mothers failed to complete high school or its equivalent.

Center for Impact Research

A Center for Impact Research survey in 2000 found that in Chicago and Atlanta one-fourth of minor mothers were not in school and one-half were not on track with their educations.[27] In Atlanta, only one-half of mothers over the age of 18 who were not at-tending school had a high school diploma or GED.

Adolescent Family Life Survey

The Adolescent Family Life Survey in Cook County in the 1980s of adolescent moth-ers 17 and younger who received welfare revealed that 30% left school before or shortly after childbirth. Of the 70% remaining in school, 47% had obtained a high school diploma or a GED at the age of 19. Of the entire original sample, 33% had a high school diploma or a GED.[28]

The Robin Hood Foundation Study

The Robin Hood Foundation commissioned seven coordinated teams of the nation's leading scholars to study the connection between adolescent parents and social prob-lems.[29] The teams compared adolescents who had their first babies at the age of 17 or younger with mothers who delayed their first births until the ages of 20 or 21 in 2000. The studies separated the differences between these two groups attributable to age and to background factors such as ethnicity, socioeconomic class and parental education. They also accounted for motivation, self-esteem, peer-group influence and community impact.

The teams found that 70% of those who became mothers when 17 or younger had not completed high school compared to 20% for those who became mothers at 20- and 21. They spent four times more of their young adult years as single parents. Half of these differences were deemed to be due to adolescent childbearing and half to background factors.

The Notre Dame Study

Although none of the adolescent mothers in the Notre Dame study said they regretted having their children, a common theme was that they wished they had waited longer. Fifty-five percent of the original sample was evaluated after three years. When their children were 3- and 5-years-old, these adolescent mothers tended to be undereducated, underemployed and to have additional children.[30] Only 18% of the adolescent mothers were regarded as living successful lives in all areas by meeting the needs of their children, continuing to pursue their own educational and career development and establishing constructive social relationships.

IMPACT OF PARENTHOOD ON FATHERS

The fathers of adolescent mothers' children are an average of two to three years older. By 19, 15% of all Black males had fathered a child in 1994; the corresponding rates for Latinos and Whites were 11% and 7%, respectively.[31]

In one study, adolescent fathers, who were one third as likely to become active parents as were girls, finished an average of 11 years of school by the age of 27 compared with 13 years of school by their counterparts.[32] They tended to be poor and often continued an intergenerational pattern of adolescent childbearing, low educational achievement and crime. They may have lived with their children sporadically, but their child support contributions were low even with vigorous enforcement because they lacked financial resources. Becoming an adolescent father may spur greater delinquency.

Still, the Robin Hood Foundation estimated that fathers who do not marry adolescent mothers have incomes sufficient to offset as much as 40-50% of the welfare costs of adolescent mothers and their families.[33] More rigorous paternity establishment and child-support enforcement could provide financial gains for children and taxpayers.

The need of adolescent fathers for counseling often is overlooked.[34] The birth of a child they conceived can be a crisis for them as well as for the mothers. They may experience anxiety, guilt, depression and low self-respect, which create barriers to staying involved with their children. Abandoning their children is a way to alleviate these emotional burdens.

CONCLUSION

One view holds that adolescents can be effective parents when they have culturally relevant and developmentally appropriate information, parenting education and support.

The fact that some adolescent parents with personal, family, community and financial assets overcome personal and social obstacles and achieve success and satisfaction in later life supports this view. However, the evidence is clear that parenthood is fraught with problems for most adolescents and their children and families. Today's adolescent parents faced with increasing educational and employment demands may fare worse than previous cohorts of young parents.

Prolonged stress before, during and after childbirth has adverse effects on adolescents' health and learning in school. It contributes to premature puberty, obesity and diabetes.

A girl who becomes a mother and a boy who becomes a father are deprived prematurely of opportunities to socialize freely with peers, to develop talents and hobbies and to make career choices. A girl cannot develop a complete sense of her own body image when the physical changes of childbearing occur before her body has completely matured.

Respected studies reveal differing pictures of the educational impacts of adolescent motherhood with high school or equivalent graduation rates between 30% and 70%. The Notre Dame study found that 18% of the adolescent mothers could be regarded later as living successful, self-fulfilling lives.

The fathers tend to be poor and older. They often continue an intergenerational pattern of adolescent childbearing, low educational achievement and crime. They may live with their children sporadically, but their child support contributions are low even with vigorous enforcement since they lack financial resources.

Research does not suggest that parenthood has benefits superior to those attained from completing adolescent and career development without childrearing responsibilities.

Chapter 16

The Impact of Adolescent Parenthood on Children

When a baby is born to a mother who has not yet grown up herself, both mother and baby are likely to have limited futures and to place substantial burdens on society.

Lisbeth B. Schorr & Daniel Schorr
Within Our Reach[1]

Having a baby may not greatly affect the life courses of disadvantaged adolescent mothers whose opportunities already are limited. However, their babies' opportunities in life are greatly diminished.[2] Children of adolescent parents are more likely to experience school failure, delinquency, homelessness, early childbearing, welfare reliance and incarceration than those born to adults.

How much of the negative effects of adolescent parenthood on children is related to a mother's age and how much is related to socioeconomic disadvantage are not easily separated.[3] Arline Geronimus and her colleagues compared first cousins born to sisters, one of whom had an adolescent birth and the other did not. They did not find that children born to adolescent mothers had lower cognitive test scores than children born to older mothers. They construed this finding to mean that the age of a mother does not critically influence child development.

An analysis of a 20-year study estimated that maternal characteristics accounted for 21%; family factors 32%; and both together for the remaining 47% of the effects of adolescent childbearing on offspring.[4] Other studies found that when family structure and socioeconomic status were controlled, the effects of the mother's age remained important. The ages of adolescent mothers and their life circumstances influence the development of their children.

PRENATAL HEALTH

Experience in the womb shapes the brain and lays the groundwork for personality, temperament and cognitive development.[5] Fetuses are attuned to their mothers' feelings and actions. The quality of fetal life may influence susceptibility to coronary artery disease, stroke, diabetes, obesity and a multitude of other conditions later in life.

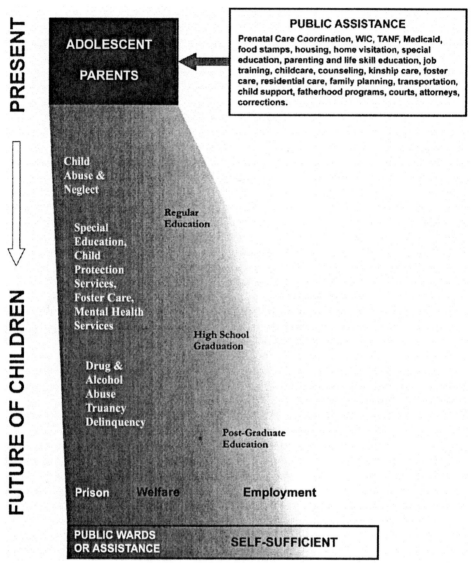

Figure 16.1.   Socioeconomic Status of Children of Adolescent Parents.

The 1996 Robin Hood Foundation report, *Kids Having Kids*, and other sources found that compared to older mothers the children of adolescent mothers were:[6]

- less likely to receive adequate prenatal care;
- twice as likely to have a preterm birth;
- 50% more susceptible to infant mortality;
- 50% more likely to have low birth weight and developmental problems;
- at higher risk of infanticide; and
- twice as likely to have health problems and higher health care costs.

MATERNAL SUBSTANCE ABUSE, SMOKING AND HIV

Adolescent mothers are at risk for smoking, alcoholism and drug abuse. The effects of prenatal exposure to cocaine, methamphetamine, ecstasy and nicotine can be seen in low birth weights of their babies, behavior disorders of their toddlers, cognitive and behavior problems in their school-age children and vulnerability to drug usage in their adolescents.[7] The additional medical costs of a drug-exposed baby in intensive care can exceed $250,000. Expenses for a developmentally delayed child through the age of eighteen can reach $750,000.

Mother-to-child transmission of Human Immunodeficiency Virus in the United States has decreased dramatically since its peak in 1992 but continues to occur among Black adolescents.[8]

ATTACHMENT BONDING

An adolescent mother's lack of capacity for nurturant bonding because of her immaturity places her baby at risk for a variety of developmental problems, including insecure and disorganized attachment bonding. A study of poor adolescent mothers revealed that only 30% of their children were securely attached to their mothers at one year of age and 41% at five.[9]

The Notre Dame project found that delegating parenting to grandmothers made it less likely that adolescent mothers would securely bond with their own babies.[10] Children who do not form secure attachment bonds with their mothers have difficulty relating to other persons in later life. They have low levels of oxytocin and vasopressin that mediate affectionate relationships.

POVERTY AND CHILD NEGLECT AND ABUSE

The poverty rate in later life for children of adolescent mothers is twice that of children of older single mothers.[11] Higher poverty levels are correlated with child neglect and abuse.

Two studies found that the children of poor adolescent mothers are five times more likely to be neglected or abused than those of poor mothers over 20 and 17 times more likely than children born to mothers over 22.[12] Up to 51% of all abused children had adolescent mothers.

The children of young adolescent mothers are over twice as likely to be placed in foster care during the first five years of life than those born to 20 and 21-year-old mothers.[13] After controlling for other risk factors affecting these outcomes, delaying a birth from 17 or earlier to 20 or 21 would lower the foster care placement rate for these children by a third, while neglect and abuse would fall by almost 40%.

Neglect and abuse can damage the developing brain.[14] Just as the body needs nutrition, the brain needs nurturing human interactions to grow.

EARLY CHILDHOOD DEVELOPMENT AND SCHOOL PERFORMANCE

In the Notre Dame Project that did not include the highest risk adolescent mothers, the physically normal children at birth showed increasing problems at 1, 3 and 5 years, including insecure attachments, low IQs, language delays, visual-motor difficulties, emotional problems and behavioral disorders.[15] By the age of 3, less than one third were performing at age level with even less at the second grade level. At age 8, 70% of the children had academic difficulties, and nearly 40% met criteria for learning disabilities or mild mental retardation.

Children born to mothers 17 and younger begin kindergarten with lower levels of school readiness than children of older mothers.[16] Children born to 18 and 19-year-old mothers do not do much better. The most pronounced differences are observed when children born to mothers 17 and younger are compared to those born to mothers over 22.

Compared to children of older parents, children of adolescent parents are two to three times less likely to be rated "excellent" by their teachers and 50% more likely to repeat a grade. They are two to three times more likely to run away from home. They are less likely to graduate from high school. One third become adolescent mothers themselves.[17]

Children born to 18 and 19-year-old mothers do not perform much better in school than children of mothers 17 and younger.[18] This suggests that delaying births into the later adolescent years would not result in notable improvement for these children. Possible factors offsetting the older age advantages might be that a child born to a young adolescent is more likely than a child born to an older adolescent to live with a grandparent or other relative so the adolescent mother can attend school. Older adolescent mothers also are more likely to be married at the time of their children's births (almost one-third compared with 12% of mothers 17 or younger). Their marriages usually are unstable, exposing their children to conflict and violence. Older adolescent parents also may live with unrelated adults where their children are nearly fifty times more likely to die of inflicted injuries than children residing with two genetic parents.[19]

A twenty-year follow-up study of low-income Baltimore families in the 1980s documented the consequences of the stresses of adolescent childbearing.[20] The preoccupations of those adolescent mothers with their own developmental struggles during their children's formative years bore significant costs for their children. Long-term outcomes were poorest for those whose own parents had low-levels of education or a history of welfare dependency and for those who had two or more additional children within five years of the first child. As in other studies, one-third of the Baltimore offspring bore children as adolescents and had bleaker educational and employment prospects than their own mothers and were less likely to marry.

Of children born to adolescent mothers 17 and younger in the mid-1970s and early 1980s, only 66% earned their high school diploma by 22 compared with 81% of children of mothers whose first birth was at 20 or 21.[21]

INCARCERATION

The sons of adolescent mothers are more likely to become violent delinquents than sons of older mothers and more than twice as likely to enter prison than the sons of 20 to 21-year-old mothers.[22] During the same time period, the sons of adolescent mothers spend an average of .57 years in prison, over 2.5 times longer than the sons of women whose first birth was at 20-21.

RELIGIOSITY

One study assessed the impact of religiosity on the socioeconomic and behavioral outcomes of adolescent mothers and their offspring.[23] Mothers high in religiosity had higher self-respect and lower depression scores, exhibited less child abuse potential and had higher educational attainment than low religiosity mothers. Children with more religious mothers had less emotional and behavioral problems at the age of 10 than those of low religiosity mothers.

FATHER ABSENCE

Adolescent parenthood usually is associated with father absence.[24] A meta-analysis of the literature on father absence from the Princeton Center for Research on Child Well-being found lower levels of behavioral problems in adolescents living with their married genetic parents than those in all other family structures.[25] Children who live apart from their genetic fathers perform less well in school than children who live with both genetic parents.

CONCLUSION

The offspring of adolescent parents are a major source of habitual criminals, long-term welfare dependency and adolescent parents who continue the cycle. Whether these outcomes are due to the ages, personal characteristics or life circumstances of adolescent mothers is more of academic than practical interest.

Compared to older mothers, adolescent mothers are more likely to receive inadequate prenatal care, to have low-birth-weight babies with heightened risk of developmental problems and to have children with health problems.

Children of adolescents are at high risk for difficulties stemming from violence in their parents' lives and from neglect and abuse in their own lives. They begin kindergarten with lower levels of school readiness than children of older mothers. They are more likely to repeat grades in school, drop out of school and engage in delinquent behavior.

At least one in three of the children of adolescent mothers are trapped in later life by the interwoven strands of men without jobs; women without husbands; children without fathers; and families without money, hope, skills, opportunities or effective services that might help them escape from poverty. Still, the majority of the children of adolescent mothers and fathers ultimately do become at least marginally self-supporting adults. But they will never know what their lives would have been like if their parents had not been adolescents.

The burden of proof lies with advocates for supporting adolescent parenthood to show that it is in the interests of their babies, the mothers, their families and society.

Part 5

FAMILIES

Liberals emphasize social policy but are criticized for ignoring values. Conservatives emphasize values but are criticized for avoiding social policy

Senator Daniel Patrick Moynihan, 1987
Family and Nation.[1]

The initial conditions of the families of adolescent parents play crucial roles in decisions their daughters and sons make to become parents. The crisis of adolescent childbirth often evokes a sense of helplessness in family members and in professionals that can amplify its impact on emerging life patterns.

Adolescents who live in conflict-ridden families without supportive relationships often are trapped victims of abuse, disappointing love affairs, powerlessness and poverty. They often have stress-related disorders. They are the most likely to choose to become parents.

The number of children being raised by relatives has increased dramatically over the last twenty-five years. The typical family unit for adolescent parents is an adolescent mother, grandparent, her baby and often her siblings.

Relatives are safety nets that keep children out of the formal foster care system. Grandparents and other relatives caring for children face health concerns as well as childrearing burdens. In states with grandparent liability laws, grandparents are required to support the children of their minor parents.

Chapter 17

THE FAMILIES OF
ADOLESCENT PARENTS

You are the bows from which your children as living arrows are set forth.
The archer sees the mark upon the path of the infinite, and He bends you
with His might that his arrows may go swift and far.
Let your bending in the archer's hand be for gladness;
For even as He loves the arrow that flies,
so He loves also the bow that is stable.

Kahlil Gibran, *The Prophet*[1]

Half of our personalities and minds are preordained by genes. The other half is influenced by life experience.[2] Peers, schools and the media strongly influence the language, fashions and behavior of adolescents, but families shape their characters. In general:

- Over three-quarters of all parents have close relationships with their adolescents.[3]
- Adolescents with strained family relationships are more likely to become parents than those with stable families.[4]
- Sons and daughters repeat cycles of family conflict.[5]
- The prominence of economic disadvantage in the lives of adolescents who become parents distracts attention from underlying problems in parent-child and sibling relationships.[6]

FAMILY RELATIONSHIPS

Our society idealizes families. But family life is a crucible for both painful and joyous emotions and behavior. In our families, we can hurt each other in ways we would not dare to do elsewhere. Harsh words, blows, betrayal and desertion hurt most keenly. But love, compassion and compromise in family life bring rewards unavailable elsewhere.[7]

Family strength is measured less by the love exchanged and more by the ability of family members to accommodate each other's anger and personal peculiarities.

Members of thriving families are not always mutually supportive, but they deal with life's problems together.[8]

In addition to affection, family relationships include hostility, jealousy, envy and rivalry.[9] When family members lack self-control, these emotions are especially likely to be acted upon. Parents can foster maladaptive behavior in their own offspring. Some parents derive covert satisfaction from seeing their adolescents go through the same hardships they experienced. Parents can envy successful offspring and knowingly or unwittingly sabotage their progress.

Children are imbued with hostility by rejecting and harsh parents.[10] Insecure attachment bonding with parents leads to a lack of social skills, weak self-control, anger and aggressive behavior. In contrast, secure attachment bonding inspires confidence and hope.

Parents influence their children by expressing and modeling their values. However, modern parents tend to be guides and teachers rather than limit-setting role models. This can undermine the foundation of a child's character. Children need to press up against the authority of their parents as a stable foil and be constrained. Then they can internalize their parents' values so that they become their own and form a solid independent identity. When they oppose their parents and win or when their parents gratify their wishes, children do not internalize cultural values through their parents. They incorporate the doubts and insecurities of their parents and pass them on to the next generation. Their physical and emotional well-being is jeopardized when their parents do not use authority effectively.[11]

Parental conflict has both positive and negative effects on children.[12] It is not whether parents fight with each other that matters. It is how they fight. Children benefit from witnessing conflict and its resolution and by parents agreeing to disagree. In contrast, violent hostility or withdrawal without conflict resolution by parents often fosters similar behavior in their children.

The hidden complexity of family relationships is illustrated by parents who use their children perversely. The most obvious example is incest. A less obvious example is when a parent's hostility evokes a child's hostility. This response permits the parent to act violently toward the child. Without conscious intent, the parent's violence exposes the parent to prosecution for child abuse thereby satisfying the parent's hidden self-destructive impulses.[13]

FATHER ABSENCE

The absence of fathers in early life puts girls at risk for early sexual activity and adolescent pregnancy by making them more vulnerable to influences outside of their families. Daughters who do not have contact with their fathers are 53% more likely to marry as adolescents; 111% more likely to have children as adolescents; 164% more likely to be a single parent; and 92% more likely to divorce if they marry than daughters in two-parent homes.[14]

Two long-term studies followed girls in the United States and in New Zealand that have the highest and second-highest rates of adolescent pregnancy among developed nations.[15] Girls whose fathers left their families before the age of six had the highest rates of both early sexual activity and adolescent pregnancy, followed by those whose fathers left at a later age. When other factors that could have contributed to early sexual activity and pregnancy, such as behavioral problems and life adversity, were taken into account early "father-absent" girls were five times more likely in the United States and three times more likely in New Zealand to become pregnant than were girls whose fathers were present in their homes. This may be in part because of the daughters' greater exposure to their mothers' dating.

PHYSICAL AND SEXUAL ABUSE

Adolescent pregnancy is strongly linked to previous neglect and abuse. Conceiving a pregnancy is more common among abused adolescents (13% to 26% for girls and 22% to 61% for boys) than among non-abused adolescents (8% to 10%).[16] Some girls become pregnant because of incest, sexual abuse or contraception sabotage. Others live in unsafe situations where they are exposed to sexual advances. They may experience emotional or psychological damage that makes them especially vulnerable to coercive or violent partners when they leave home. They may be depressed and self-medicate with drugs or alcohol.

From another perspective, 40% to 70% of adolescent mothers report a history of sexual abuse. As many as 80% were in violent, abusive or coercive relationships just before, during and after their pregnancies.[17] The perpetrators also are likely to have been sexually or physically abused as children and to be repeating a cycle of violence. Boys are exposed to abuse and family violence at rates similar to girls. They are prone to higher pregnancy and sexually transmitted disease rates, including HIV infection, and to perpetrating violence in their own families.[18]

Sexual abuse can lead to earlier sexual debut, more sexual partners and an increased risk of violence. Sexually abused adolescents have experienced the violation of their most intimate boundaries. This can create a sense of powerlessness in relationships and make them less likely than their non-abused peers to use contraception.

FAMILY STRESS-RELATED DISORDERS

Adolescents who live in conflict-ridden families without supportive relationships are especially at risk for stress-related physical, emotional and mental disorders.[19] Their family experiences interact with genetically-based vulnerabilities and produce anxiety and depression; impaired emotional and social functioning; and self-defeating health behaviors, especially smoking and substance abuse.

FAMILIES AND POVERTY
AS CAUSES OF ADOLESCENT PARENTHOOD

Ronald Mincy and Susan Weiner of the Urban Institute found that poverty is less influential than the characteristics and behavior of her own parents in an adolescent girl's chances of becoming pregnant.[20] Studies of the effects of poverty must take into account the possibility of unmeasured causal factors. For example, parental mental illness or disability may be the key factor contributing to adolescent childbirth in a poor family.

Five hundred families were studied in a deteriorating neighborhood in southwest Philadelphia where schools were dysfunctional and parks unsafe.[21] The majority of these families were functioning reasonably well, considering that close to 50% were living in or near poverty. Most of these parents, both single and couples, differed little from middle-class parents in their aspirations and the energy they devoted to childrearing. Overall the beneficial effects of parents' education outweighed the detrimental effects of economic hardship. Good parenting was more common than good neighborhoods, good schools, and good social services.

Greg Duncan, professor of education and social policy at Northwestern University, and Jeanne Brooks-Gunn, professor of child and parent development at Columbia University, found that family structure was the most important determinant of school behavior problems and unwed childbearing.[22] Opportunities for learning, warmth of parent-child relationships and physical conditions of the home were the most important contributors to positive outcomes.

CONCLUSION

Peers greatly influence the language, fashions and behavior of adolescents, but parents shape the character development of their children for better and for worse.

Adolescents who live in conflict-ridden families without supportive relationships are trapped victims of abuse, disappointing love affairs, poverty and powerlessness. They often have stress-related disorders.

Healthy families are crucibles of conflict and irrationality. Children benefit from witnessing conflict resolution. But the hidden complexity of family relationships is revealed by parents who use their children for perverse purposes. The most obvious example is incest. A less obvious example is when a child is unconsciously induced to act out a parent's own self-destructive urges.

Father-absent girls are more likely to experience adolescent pregnancy than are girls whose fathers are present in their homes. Sons abandoned by their fathers may have difficulty developing and sustaining self-esteem and forming lasting emotional attachments with adult partners and their children.

Young children who have been abused may have significant emotional problems in later life. Sexually abused adolescents are predisposed to premature pregnancies.

Families play crucial roles in whether or not adolescents become parents and enter parenthood.

Chapter 18

The Impact of
Adolescent Parenthood on Families

A credible family policy will insist that responsibility begins with the individual, then the family, and only then the community, and first the smaller and nearer rather than the greater and more distant community.

Senator Daniel Patrick Moynihan
Family and Nation 1987[1]

The planned birth of a baby is a celebrated event. Unexpected pregnancies can be greeted with anticipation and joy. But adolescent childbirth, even when desired, is a disruptive crisis with profound repercussions for the adolescents, their families, schools, communities and society.

The impact of adolescent pregnancy and childbirth on families often is not taken into account. The families of adolescent parents play crucial roles in, and are deeply affected by, decisions their daughters and sons make to become parents. They play vital roles in dampening or amplifying the short- and long-term outcomes of adolescent parenthood.

REACTIONS TO ADOLESCENT PREGNANCY

Adolescent pregnancy stirs up emotional reactions in family members that are not easily resolved. Parents, siblings and grandparents may experience anger, disappointment and even joy as they cope with the pregnancy. Termination of the pregnancy may be encouraged or opposed.

Some families endorse the parenthood of their daughters and sons. When her baby is desired by her family, an adolescent mother can attain an elevated position. Even when this is not the case, adolescent mothers and their families often are reluctant to consider adoption. Their families may feel that adoption is a sensible option, but parting with their babies is too painful a prospect for them and their daughters to be seriously considered.[2] The fact that an adolescent can delay parenthood and have children later is not persuasive for them. They feel that they must care for their adolescent's child, who would be lost to the family by adoption.

In some subcultures, the families of adolescent parents willingly take on parenting. They may see adoption as genocide by cutting children's ties to their cultural roots:

> One grandparent was indignant when adoption was raised as a possibility for two of her grandchildren whose mother was addicted to drugs. The grandmother likened placement for adoption to placement on the block in slave trading. She felt that adoption destroys Black families like slavery did.

Although potentially uniting families, the discovery of pregnancy also causes conflicts. A school teacher described the following experience:

> Fourteen-year-old Alyson, one of my former students, showed up on my steps in the middle of the night. After her father whipped her with a belt, he told her not to come home again and disowned her. The welts and bruises on her back were appalling. She is going to have a baby. She is not a kid who I thought would end up in this mess. She is bright and kind of sweet. My phone call to her home elicited the response, "We have no child by that name."

IMPACT ON SIBLINGS OF ADOLESCENT PARENTS

Thirty-nine percent of adolescent mothers and 48% of adolescent fathers live in households with one or more siblings.[3] Younger siblings of adolescent parents are up to six times more likely to become pregnant as adolescents than those whose sisters are not parents. One study found that 50% of younger siblings of adolescent parents were sexually active, compared to 24% whose older siblings were not parents.[4] Another study found that having an adolescent, childbearing sister fosters sexual activity more than just having a sexually active sister.[5]

Compared with the mothers of never-pregnant adolescents, one study found that the mothers of adolescent parents monitored and communicated less with their other children and were more accepting of adolescent sex after their older daughter gave birth.[6]

THE ROLE OF RELATIVES IN RAISING MINOR'S CHILDREN

The number of children being raised by relatives has increased dramatically over the last 25 years. More than six million children—nearly 9% of all children—live with grandparents (4.5 million) or other relatives (1.5 million).[7] Almost 40% of these children are being raised solely by their grandparents or other relatives with no genetic parents present. One study found that 28% of adolescent mothers were not active parents or did not live with their children.[8]

In 2004, over 40% of all grandparents had some degree of responsibility for their minor grandchildren.[9] Sixty-two percent of grandparent-headed households consist of a grandmother alone, 18% of whom live in poverty. More than 10% of all grandparents raise a grandchild for at least six months with most providing lesser amounts of care for three years or more.

Living with Grandparents

Eighty percent of adolescent mothers live at home one year after giving birth.[10] The basic family unit usually is an adolescent mother, grandmother, baby and often siblings.

Grandparents become parents for their children's offspring as they continue to parent their own children when they have the energy and financial resources to do so.[11] They usually expect their daughters to assume parenting responsibilities but also encourage them to participate in adolescent activities and complete their educations.

When their own mothers care for their babies, adolescents' dependency on their mothers can be fostered. Over reliance on grandmother support can interfere with an adolescent's completion of her development as well as her acceptance of maternal responsibilities. Living with one's parent also can lead to conflicts and interfere with parenting both generations.[12]

Some grandmothers are distressed when their daughters want to take their children with them when they leave home. These grandmothers feel that their grandchildren belong to them since they essentially raised them.

THE IMPACT OF REARING ADOLESCENTS' CHILDREN ON RELATIVES

Relatives may well shoulder unanticipated burdens when they raise their minors' children. They may be working or living on fixed incomes. Many have had debilitating family events. They are confronted with regulations and laws that were not designed to accommodate relatives raising children, such as live in housing that prohibits children.

An Illinois survey found that about a quarter of grandmothers continued working when they assumed care of their grandchildren.[13] Another quarter stopped working. Many rearranged their work schedules, changed jobs or made other accommodations. Two-thirds were caring for grandchildren with emotional or behavioral problems. Eighty percent had one or more health problems; one-third were depressed. They reported that the children often thought about their parents, which was emotionally stressful for their grandchildren and for themselves. One said:

> I can take them to school, I can feed them, clothe them, and their minds' on their parents.

It was particularly challenging for children and grandmothers when the genetic parents were in and out of their homes. One said:

> The child's mother came back occasionally so I ended up with him . . . and it was very hard, very, very hard on him because he felt abandoned; he went through 6—yeah 6 months—with his crying every night.

In three-generation families, an adolescent mother's responsible relationship with her mother is most important in predicting positive outcomes. When this is not the case, adolescents can become disengaged from their own children, creating problems for their parents.[14]

The demands of childrearing may be harmful to the physical and emotional health of relatives, who may need mental health services themselves.[15] The stress of caring for young children, accompanied by their own health difficulties, can be overwhelming for older grandparents and relatives and result in a variety of stress-related illnesses.

Grandparent health problems are aggravated when grandchildren pose behavioral and health problems.[16] Stressful family relationships that often accompany relative care can create emotional problems for the grandparents as well as the children. Grandparents caring for their grandchildren are twice as likely to become depressed as the general population.

Grandparents raising grandchildren with little social support and financial problems experience high levels of stress.[17] They may have less contact with family and friends and experience marital dissatisfaction as well. This is especially the case when a grandchild's parent is addicted to drugs or alcohol.

Grandparents tend to downplay their own health problems. Still, their health affects their grandchildren. In one study, 49% of grandchildren in which both their parents and their grandparents were depressed had some form of psychopathology.[18] A study of Latino grandparents rearing their grandchildren in New York City found poverty rates three times and poor health and depression rates twice as high as those of grandparent caregivers nationally.[19]

Many contemporary grandmothers are reluctant to accept parenting roles. They resent being forced into parenting again because they have their own lives to lead. One grandmother, who was the third of four living generations of adolescent parents, said:

> Something has to be done about this terrible epidemic of teenage pregnancies. My mother and I got by because there weren't so many drugs around, and life was simpler then, but I want my grandchildren to go somewhere in this world and not be left behind like I was.

In the book *Random Family*, a grandmother said to her daughter with two children:[20]

> I haven't gotten nowhere because, from being a mother, I became a mother again for my grandchildren. Honey, the boys that are growing up now, it's only for your pussy. A girl has to be smart now. Study. Be somebody. So when you become somebody, you don't have to have this straggly shit on your lips, sitting on your ass, to see if they could support you. You should support yourself. They respect you, because they know they could lose you right there and then. You don't need them, you understand?

LEGAL LIMITATIONS OF RELATIVE CAREGIVERS

Grandparents and other relatives do not automatically have custodial guardianship of their grandchildren and are confronted with numerous barriers in the realms of housing, education and health and mental health care.

Housing

Relatives often have difficulty accommodating babies in their residences. Senior housing may not allow children. These families struggle to find affordable homes that will accept children. This was dramatically illustrated by Clearwater, Florida, grandparents who were threatened with eviction if they cared for their son's children while he was stationed in Iraq.[21]

Education

In order to enroll children in school, many school districts require proof of legal custody or guardianship, which relatives do not have. Most states have residency requirements to prevent abuses, such as by a child living with a grandmother during the week because her district school has a better football team than the parents' school district.

Health and Mental Health

Relative caregivers often are unable to give consent for medical, dental and mental health services. Unless a relative caregiver has adopted a child, many private insurance policies do not allow the caregiver to include the child. Public programs, such as the Children's Health Insurance Program and Medicaid may require that caregivers have legal custody or guardianship of the children in order to give consent for their medical care.

ESTABLISHING A LEGAL RELATIONSHIP WITH MINORS' CHILDREN

Relatives can establish legal relationships with children in their care, but many do not want to do so, hoping that the children will be raised by their parents in the future. To obtain guardianship of the children, they must bring a legal proceeding against the parents. In *Moore v. City of East Cleveland* and in *Troxel v. Granville*, the Supreme Court acknowledged that grandparents have limited constitutional protections.[22]

When grandparents assume parental responsibilities for their grandchildren, they need legal assistance to obtain custody or guardianship in order to access public benefits, school enrollment and health insurance for the children.[23] If contested, these proceedings can be lengthy and difficult emotionally for everyone. A court must determine the fitness of both sets of parents and the "best interests" of the child. These proceedings can strain fragile family relationships.

Grandparents can obtain legal prerogatives through procedures that vary from state to state: parental power of attorney, legal custody and legal guardianship. Gerard Wallace, a family law attorney, outlined the legal options for relative caregivers.[24]

Parental Power of Attorney

Most states have provisions for a Parental Power of Attorney or a Delegation of Parental Authority that can be made by the legal parents of a child. This gives relatives the right to act on behalf of children placed in their care, such as for school enrollment or medical care. In New York, a limited Parental Power of Attorney grants persons having the responsibility for caring for their children temporary authority to make decisions for them.[25]

Legal Custody

Relatives or other caregivers may petition courts for the physical custody of children. A court assumes guardianship of the child or leaves guardianship with the parent.

Physical custody means that a parent cannot remove a child at will from a relative's custody, but, in custody disputes, a preference for parental reunification places legal custodians at a disadvantage. To gain custody of grandchildren, grandparents must present evidence that the parents are unfit. The strongest evidence is that the parents physically or sexually harmed a child. When a parent leaves a child with another caregiver for an extended period of time, some states deem this to be sufficient reason to grant custody to the non-parent caregiver.

Depending upon state laws, physical custodians do not have the authority to make decisions for children in their care. Washington state allows relatives to consent to medical and mental health care.[26] In other states, courts may make special provisions for necessary authority. Relatives usually are well advised to petition a court for both custodial and guardianship rights.

Legal Guardianship

To obtain legal guardianship in addition to custody, relatives must have a "placement plan" which outlines: 1) the reasons for placement with the relative, 2) visitation and contact plans between the parents and the child, 3) the duration of the guardianship, 4) who will support the child and 5) any other agreements regarding the child. A court must approve the plan and any changes in it, including return of the child to the parent.

Guardianship includes all parental prerogatives. Many states have standby guardianship laws that enable parents and guardians to name a guardian in their stead upon their incapacity or death.[27] Both legal custodians and guardians can obtain TANF child-only grants.

Legal custodians and guardians have access to more resources than informal caregivers in states where kinship care programs provide additional services and higher stipends when relatives assume care of children because of neglect or abuse.[28]

Maine and South Carolina award "de facto guardianships" to adults who have cared for a child under the age of 3 for six months and for one year for a child 3 years or older when there is a lack of consistent participation of a parent.[29] Any time after a legal proceeding by a parent to regain guardianship of a child has begun cannot be included in the required minimum period. Indiana, Kentucky, Oklahoma, Texas and Minnesota have similar laws.

KINSHIP CARE

Kinship care is rooted in ancient cultural practices. The term "kinship care" was defined by the Child Welfare League of America in 1974 to recognize Black kinship networks as: [30]

> . . . the full time nurturing and protection of children who must be separated from their parents by relatives, members of their tribes or clans, god-parents, step-parents, or other adults who have a kinship bond with a child.

In 2002, 2.3 million children lived with relatives without a genetic parent present in the home.[31] Seventy-eight percent—1.8 million—were privately placed with relatives without child welfare agency involvement. The remaining .5 million were publicly placed in kinship care through an agency. In 2002, 18% of children in public kinship care lived in poverty, down from 35% in 1997; 31% of children in private kinship care lived in poverty. Public kinship families may be eligible for more resources than private, but resources usually are inadequate.[32]

Children are in kinship care because their parents have significant problems, such as drug and alcohol abuse, child abuse and/or neglect, abandonment, poverty, mental illness, incarceration or abandonment. These children may suffer from problems, such as depression, attention deficit disorder, fetal alcohol syndrome, learning disabilities, or anti-social conduct.

According to a report by the Center for Law and Social Policy and other studies, children in kinship care experience greater stability and have fewer behavior problems than children in foster care.[33] These children may have been less troubled in the first place. Kinship care also maintains cultural traditions and reduces racial disparities.

Relatives providing public kinship care are eligible for federal matching funds to states that provide foster care through the Temporary Assistance to Needy Families Program (TANF). States ordinarily do not impose work requirements or time limits on kinship caregivers who receive child-only TANF grants that are less than foster parent stipends.

In 1997, the federal Adoption and Safe Families Act required states to ensure kinship caregivers were licensed foster parents in order for states to receive reimbursement for foster care payments through Title IV-E.[34] Federal, state and local benefits are available to non-foster kinship families, but many do not access them, sometimes to avoid scrutiny of their families.

KINSHIP FOSTER CARE

In the period leading up to termination of parental rights proceedings, a child is placed with a temporary custodian. This may be a grandparent or other relative, a friend or a foster parent appointed by the court. If a grandchild has been living with a grandparent, that grandparent has a particularly strong case to continue the arrangement. If grandchildren are old enough, statutes may permit consideration of their wishes.

Some states provide full foster parent certification for relatives, who receive the same level of financial assistance as do non-kin foster parents. Kinship foster parents are not free to make parental decisions except as specified by a state agency or court. The financial benefits of kinship foster care may support a family. The training, monitoring and services provided to kinship foster parents and their children are less than for traditional foster parents.[35]

Becoming a foster parent does not confer legal custody. The children remain in the legal custody of the state until the court deems that parental rights must be terminated. At that point, the children may be legally adopted. When a state has legal custody and guardianship of children, relatives are at higher risk of losing children than are genetic parents because they are not afforded the same rights and protections.

Many states offer subsidized guardianship to kinship foster parents who leave the foster care program but who continue to support children.[36] In 2006, 36 states provided limited financial support for children who are under the legal custody of relatives.

In the United States, the care of children is not seen as a social responsibility carrying adequate public benefits, such as child-rearing allowances, health coverage and respite care, for whoever performs the task. If all parents including kinship caregivers were equally eligible for such benefits, state custody and foster care often would not be necessary.[37]

KINSHIP ADOPTION

Kinship caregivers are less likely to adopt children than are foster parents. This may be due to reticence to terminate a relative's parental rights, particularly when the caregiver is a child's grandparent.

Grandparents may petition a court for adoption. If it is considered to be in a child's "best interests," the adoption may be granted. Grandparent age is a factor in the decision. If a grandparent is in good health and has a close relationship with the child, the court is more inclined to rule in a grandparent's favor.

Although adoption may be advantageous for a child, it may be detrimental to the finances of adoptive relatives since their income will be deemed available for the support of the child and may eliminate receiving a child-only TANF assistance grant. Adoptive parents, like genetic parents, may be eligible for public assistance only if their total family income falls below 185% of the poverty level.[38]

Kinship adoption can be tailored to specific circumstances.[39] Parental rights are recognized as a package of responsibilities and prerogatives that can be divided between divorcing parents or between the state and parents of children in foster care. Kinship adoption following partial termination of parental rights could create a new parental relationship, while leaving in effect some aspects of the genetic parent-child relationship, such as visitation and access to school records. A kinship adopter could become the child's permanent legal parent, while the genetic parent could remain a non-custodial parent with specific prerogatives.

If a grandchild is adopted by someone else or is in foster care, grandparents may be given visitation rights if it would be in the "best interests" of the child. Grandparent visitation rights do not necessarily prevent either genetic or adoptive parents from moving to another state.

LIABILITY FOR SUPPORT OF A GRANDCHILD

A grandparent ordinarily does not have a duty to support a grandchild, except when rearing the grandchild. However, some states make grandparents liable for child support.[40] A parent of a minor son for whom paternity has been established is responsible for maintaining his child. The Personal Responsibility and Work Opportunity Reconciliation Act of 1996 enables states to enforce paternal and maternal grandparent support of a child of minor parents.

In states with grandparent liability laws, all of the grandparents of a child of their minor parents have an equal obligation to support the child.[41] A court may prescribe the proportion each of two or more of the grandparents must contribute to maintain the minor parent and child.

Termination of Grandparent Support Obligation

The complicated lives of minor parents create situations in which grandparents' liability can be terminated. For example, the parent of an adolescent who is the victim of adjudicated rape resulting in childbirth is not responsible for the maintenance of her child. In other instances, a 17-year-old girl was held to be emancipated by voluntarily living apart from her parents, who had no control over her activities, and a minor was deemed emancipated when she moved into an apartment with her boyfriend, set up housekeeping and had a child.[42]

Grandparent Support Obligation Not Terminated

A grandparent support obligation was not terminated for a grandfather when his daughter was dependent upon her mother for financial support and continued to reside with her mother.[43]

Another grandfather was ordered to pay child support to the grandmother, his former wife, for support of their minor daughter, who moved in with her boyfriend and later bore a child and was declared emancipated by a trial court and less than a year later returned to her mother's home with the baby.[44]

Another grandfather was ordered to continue to pay child support because his 19-year-old daughter was not gainfully employed; had not left her mother's home; and was still subject to parental control and guidance.[45]

Restitution from a Son or Daughter

After a minor parent attains the age of 18, a grandparent who has cared for a grandchild may petition for a court order to compel reimbursement by the son or daughter for the amount of maintenance provided for the grandchild by that grandparent.

POLITICAL CONSIDERATIONS FOR GRANDPARENTS

The difficulties grandparents face when their grandchildren need their help has led to forming support organizations, [46] such as the National Committee of Grandparents for Children's Rights and GrandFamilies of America. The Grandfamilies State Law and Policy Resource Center is devoted to education about state laws and legislation. It assists exploring policy options to support relatives and children in their care in and outside the child welfare system.

Patricia's experience illustrates the need to improve social service practices:[47]

> Patricia's daughter dropped off her baby boy at her parent's house, said goodbye and disappeared for nine months. She was in and out of the child's life until shortly before his third birthday. Child Protective Services failed to notify Pat that her daughter had given birth to another son who had been placed in foster care and had been adopted by another family.

The obstacles faced by kin who want to care for children are related in part to inconsistent statutes, regulations and case law. Some generalizations are possible. All states protect parental autonomy and are reluctant to terminate a parent's rights, but they try to use kin to care for children who are abused or neglected. Grandparents need to be represented in the political arena to ensure that their interests are protected.

CONCLUSION

The families of adolescent parents play crucial roles in, and are deeply affected by, decisions their daughters and sons make to enter parenthood that either dampen or amplify its impact. They often pitch in to help raise their adolescents' children.

The typical family unit for adolescent parents is an adolescent mother, grandparent, her baby and her siblings. Younger siblings of adolescent parents are prone to repeat the adolescent parenthood cycle.

The number of children being raised by relatives has increased dramatically over the last 25 years. Relatives are a safety net that keeps children out of the formal foster care system. In states with grandparent liability laws, grandparents have an obligation to support the children of their minor parents.

Grandparents and other relatives may well be shouldering unanticipated burdens when they undertake raising their grandchildren. Many contemporary grandmothers are becoming less willing to accept parenting roles. They face health concerns as well as childrearing burdens. Difficult family situations that often accompany children's transition to their relatives' care can create emotional problems for the grandparents as well as the children.

Relative caregivers need a continuum of resources, such as financial support; access to medical care, childcare and schooling; respite care; and support groups. Legal procedures are available to give relatives prerogatives they need to raise adolescents' children: parental power of attorney, physical custody and legal guardianship.

Some states provide full foster parent certification for relatives who want to become foster parents. Grandparents also may adopt grandchildren.

Public policies and practices should encourage the responsible actions of relatives who step in and care for children.

Part 6

NEIGHBORHOODS AND COMMUNITIES

Instead of embedding our children in webs of sustained adult relationships, we segregate them from the wisdom and experience of adults, raising them in neighborhoods, institutions, and communities where few know their names. Instead of fully investing in their growth and education as the promise of the future for society, we send them to underfunded, understaffed, and sometimes inattentive schools, child care centers, and after-school programs. Then we wonder what went wrong when yet another youth crisis or tragedy hits the headlines.

Peter L. Benson, 2006
All Kids Are Our Kids[1]

Neighborhoods and communities play vital roles in adolescents becoming parents. They amplify and dampen the problems that emerge in the lives of all of those affected.

Social class is the most important correlate of adolescent parenthood and of previous neglect, abuse and attachment disorders.

Two opposing paradigms dominate our thinking about poverty. The first is that poverty results from systemic factors. The second is that poverty results from individual factors. The interplay of both is needed to explain poverty in the United States.

The argument that adolescent childbearing does not cause poverty is valid to the extent that poverty breeds attitudes and behaviors that lead to adolescent childbirth. Still, most girls living in poverty do not become pregnant. The behavior of their own parents is more important than being poor. The birth of a child in a poor family obviously increases the number of people living in poverty.

Peers strongly influence how adolescents behave away from home and the nuances of their language and fashions. Previous maltreatment and mental health problems increase the risks of early sex for girls and drug dealing for boys. Adolescents are oversensitive to the damaging effects and undersensitive to the warning signs of alcohol abuse and smoking addiction. Dating abuse is an epidemic for adolescents, who are ill-informed about the long-term effects of abusive behavior.

The majority of gangs in the United States are peer groups that offer marginalized adolescents a cause greater than themselves that awards security, power and status. Gangs are firmly embedded in the illegal economy of poor neighborhoods and are a growing challenge for our society. Gang members have higher rates of adolescent pregnancy and parenthood than non-gang members. Because of their high levels of incarceration, especially for males, gang members contribute significantly to the number of children in fatherless and motherless homes.

Chapter 19

Social Class and Adolescent Parenthood

. . . the future of a society may be forecast by how it cares for its young.

Daniel Patrick Moynihan, 1986[1]

The fantasy that wealth is within the reach of everyone, if only by winning a lottery, obscures the importance of social class in America. Even those with little chance of attaining it may aspire to the high standard of living enjoyed by most Americans and adulate the wealthy.

The importance of social class also is obscured by the fact that economic status is not its only determinant. Education and occupation are important as well. Low incomes do not lower the social class of clergypersons or community workers. Still the most relevant determinant of social class is income.

Intriguingly, many of us prefer to believe that we do not have social classes. The most important division in our society is seen as race rather than social class.[2] Some sociologists say the concept of social class is meaningless because people move upward and downward.

SOCIAL CLASS IN THE UNITED STATES

The social class into which they are born does have lifetime consequences for babies.[3] Whether or not they remain in that social class depends on their individual traits, family-facilitated opportunities and luck.

James Heckman, professor of economics at the University of Chicago, points out that our society waits too long to compensate for birth into a social class that destines a child to become a criminal or welfare dependent.[4] Crime is extremely expensive—costing us $1.3 trillion a year. Heckman notes that growth in the quality of our labor force is slowing because so many children do not have the opportunity to become productive citizens. At the current rate, fewer college graduates will be added to our work force in the next than in the last twenty years.

201

But Richard Weissbourd of the Harvard Graduate School of Education challenges labeling children "at risk" solely because of their social class.[5] The families into which they are born are more important. There is no strong evidence that increasing parental income in itself positively affects the school readiness of children.[6] Each child's life evolves uniquely in both poor and affluent families. Still, at a time when education matters more than ever before, success in school is determined by how much parents can invest in their children. Affluent families can facilitate their children's progress. However, their children may not appreciate how fortunate they are. Some seem to have been "born on third base but believe they have hit a triple."

A more useful way than income of assessing the importance of social class is through its relationship to *social capital*—a set of factors, such as trust, reciprocity and cooperation, among members of a social network. Social capital includes supportive interactions within and among families, neighborhoods and communities. States with higher social capital have lower adolescent pregnancy rates as with other problems, such as child abuse, violence, mortality, infectious disease, cardiovascular disease and even the common cold.[7] Over the past three decades, social capital has played a greater role in life outcomes than race in the United States.

In the 1980s, it seemed that the grandchildren of the wealthy and the poor would be on nearly equal footing at the beginning of the 21st century. This has not occurred, but there has been movement in this direction. A 2005 *New York Times* poll revealed that 45% of respondents said they were in a higher class than when they grew up, but 16% said they were in a lower class.[8] Overall, 1% described themselves as upper class, 15% as upper middle class, 42% as middle class, 35% as working class and 7% as lower class. A 2007 Pew survey found that two of three Americans have higher incomes than their parents, but one third are falling behind.[9] Only 6% of children born to parents at the bottom make it to the top.

In spite of upward mobility, America is becoming compartmentalized as the wealthy increasingly isolate themselves. Charles Murray, a fellow at the American Enterprise Institute, described our "custodial democracy" in which the mainstream walls off and subsidizes the underclass as defined by criminality, unwed parents and workforce dropouts.[10] Our "custodial democracy" expects that a portion of the population will not function as citizens. Accordingly, we provide homeless shelters, welfare and more prisons without dealing with underlying causes.

Developing social capital requires thought and planning so that families become nurturing centers of life; neighbors perform neighborhood functions; and children grow up understanding the necessity and dignity of productive work. It requires thinking about which of our values are more important—our self-assertive social values or our integrative cultural values.

Thinking about these things calls attention to our large underclass living in poverty in the midst of our affluence.

THE NATURE OF POVERTY

Most Americans do not understand the nature of poverty.[11] We do not know that one-fifth of our population is either in or precariously close to falling into poverty at any point in time.

The distance between top and bottom incomes has increased dramatically in the United States. In the 1980s, the ratio between the incomes of people in the top 5% to those in the bottom 5% was 6 to 1.[12] In 2006, that ratio was more than 200 to 1. The wealthiest 1% have 20% of our entire nation's pretax income.

Between 1966 and 2001 average wage and salary income kept pace with productivity growth, but half of the income gains went to the top 10%, leaving only half for the other 90%.[13] Income distribution is skewed to the top 1% consisting of celebrities and corporate executives. This increase at the top combined with de-unionization, immigration and free trade pushing down wages at the bottom led to our unprecedented gap between the wealthy and the poor.

Defining Poverty

In 1964, the Office of Economic Opportunity defined poverty in terms of the amount of *money income* needed for a subsistence budget.[14] This definition does not include income from food stamps, housing subsidies, the Earned Income Tax Credit and Medicaid. The Census Bureau's *disposable income* definition of poverty includes income from these sources.

With both *money income* and *disposable income* criteria, poverty thresholds are set at the same levels across the nation in spite of variations in the cost of living. Poverty rates also do not distinguish between the temporary income loss of middle class families and the long-term hardships of chronically impoverished families.

Poverty Statistics

In 2004, using the *money income* definition the prevalence of poverty was estimated to be 13% (39 million persons). Using the *disposable income* it was 10%. (30 million

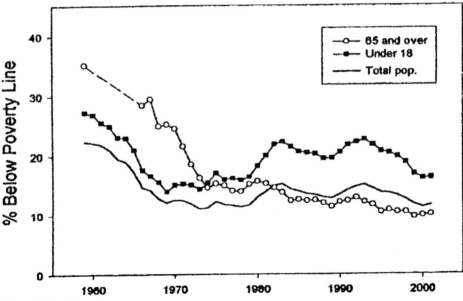

Figure 19.1.   Poverty.

persons) Using the *money income* definition, 18% of children under 18 were below the poverty line in 2005. Using the *disposable income* definition, the child poverty estimate in 2004 was 13%.[15]

Although poverty rates have been falling since highs in the 1960s, the actual number of children living in poverty is rising because of our increasing population. The number of families with incomes at or below 50% of the poverty line is rising as well.[16] Another estimated 5 to 10% live precariously close to the poverty line. Fifty seven million Americans, including 21% of the nation's children, are near poor with incomes between $20,000 and $40,000. The number of Americans living in severe poverty reached a 32-year high in 2007 (16 million).

In 2005, persons of all ages living in poverty using the money income definition were: White—11% (25 million), Asian—11% (1.4 million), Latino—22% (9.5 million) and Black—25% (9.3 million). Children under 18 living in poverty were: Asian—11% (.3 million), White—14% (7.8 million), Latino—28% (4 million) and Black—35% (3.9 million).[17] The Black poverty rate dropped from 55% in 1959 to 22% in 2000. The poverty rate of female-headed families dropped from 50% in 1959 to 42% in 2004.

Thirty percent of the poor reside in central cities, 40% in suburban areas and 30% in rural areas.[18] Over 30 rural counties in 11 states have poverty rates higher than the poorest large cities.

The Federal Interagency Forum on Child and Family Statistics uses the following indicators of economic security for persons under the age of 18:[19]

- Living with at least one parent employed full time annually—78%.
- Covered by health insurance—89%.
- Families reporting housing problems—37%.
- Food insecure—19%.

Causes of Poverty

Two paradigms dominate our thinking about poverty. The first is that poverty results from systemic factors that prevent people from raising their standard of living. The most important are the inability of our labor market to provide enough decent paying jobs for all families and our ineffective safety net. Poverty results from failings in our competitive economic system based on maximizing profits that leads businesses to pay the lowest possible wages.[20] In one-parent families, parents must work and raise children themselves. Females have lower wages than males. The growing earnings inequality, the changing nature of work, the instability of households, increased immigration, population diversity and inadequate anti-poverty polices all contribute to the intractability of poverty.

The second paradigm is that poverty results from a lack of adaptive personality traits—punctuality, hygiene, industriousness, deferral of gratification—that interfere with employment.[21] Adaptive intelligence is distributed in a bell-shaped curve so that half of the population is below average and half of the population is above average in coping abilities. Moving out of poverty-ridden neighborhoods is easier for those who have self-discipline and are adaptable. The less organized and adaptable remain in poor ghettos.

Poverty results from both systemic and individual factors. Mary Corcoran, professor of social work at the University of Michigan, concluded that research shows increasing the income of poor families will not suffice without improvements in social capital—families, neighborhoods, schools and workplaces.[22]

POVERTY AND THE QUALITY OF LIFE

When poor persons receiving government benefits are seen wearing expensive shoes, shopping in convenience stores and being overweight, it is difficult to generate compassion for them. This attitude is reinforced by the fact that many people move out of poverty.[23] Racial animosities also operate in public attitudes and economic institutions.

In fact, hardships accompanying poverty have adverse effects on health and well-being. Although the material circumstances of persons defined as poor have improved over the past four decades, social disorder and crime still accompany high levels of poverty.[24] The graphic in figure 19.2 depicts the multiple repercussions of living in poverty.

Day-to-day life in poverty was described by an 18-year-old-boy living in a two-parent home in an urban ghetto:

> Our apartment's been broken into three times, my bike's been stolen, my dad's been mugged and had his car ripped off, my little brother has been held up for lunch money, and I can't tell you how many times my mother's been threatened by drunks or junkies when she comes home from work. You hear gunshots at least twice a week and sirens a lot more.

Increasingly, the working poor live with insecurity.[25] Their buying power is eroding; the health care gap is widening; unions have lost influence; low-wage immigrant workers are in the labor market; and childcare costs are high. Two trends plaguing low-wage workers are: 1) high-cost lending scams and 2) the absence of affordably

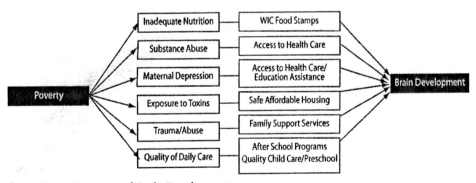

Figure 19.2.   Poverty and Brain Development.

priced merchandise in low-income neighborhoods. They pay higher prices than mid-dle-class Americans for necessities. In 2007, a gallon of milk cost $5 at an accessible shop and $3.50 at a distant supermarket.

Health and Mental Health

At a time of extraordinary advances in health care, social class differences in health and life span are widening.[26] Low social class contributes to poor health, which leads to lower social class. Of Western nations in 2003, the United States had the greatest discrepancy between expenditures on health care (first) and life expectancy (29th). The lack of access to health care, unhealthy life styles, exposure to risk and chronic stress contribute to obesity, cardiovascular disease, depression and diabetes. For ado-lescents, depression is the most important.

The prevalence of obesity is more than 50% higher in older adolescents living be-low than those above the poverty line.[27] When their "junk food" diets do not contain essential vitamins and minerals, brain development is affected. Malnutrition saps the energy of children in school.

Environmental exposure to toxins—lead, pesticides and solvents—is heightened for people living in poor urban neighborhoods. The direct effects on pregnancy are in-creased risks of miscarriages, preterm deliveries and low-birth-weight babies. Lead accumulated in a mother's bones can be delivered to her fetus, affecting brain devel-opment.[28]

The first ecological study of mental illness in Chicago in the 1930s found that adults and children with psychiatric disorders remained in ghettos compounding their disad-vantaged status over time. This has been confirmed by recent research.[29]

Happiness

Happiness is a barometer of success in achieving our goals. It can be defined as an emotional state that feels good, such as contentment, love, joy and satisfaction. Un-happiness includes fear, anxiety, sadness and hatred. A genetically determined set point for happiness likely explains individual differences in happiness.[30]

Happiness is irrelevant when survival is at stake. Still happiness is relevant when we see poor people who seem happy and wealthy people who seem unhappy.[31] The simplest kind of unhappiness is caused by extreme poverty, but high income does not assure happiness. People living in poverty become happier if they have enough money to cover the basics in life. Beyond that their expectations usually rise with their in-comes. Those with above average incomes are comparatively satisfied with their lives but may be tense and may not spend much time in enjoyable activities. In the last fifty years, the general happiness of the population has not seemed to increase in the United States in spite of increases in standards of living.

We are the happiest when we are totally immersed in challenging tasks closely matched to our abilities.[32] This helps explain why some of the most happy people have little in the way of material possessions. Those who are able to connect with and help other people are the happiest. A civic sense, social equality and control over our own lives constitute the triangle of happiness in society. Satisfaction comes not only from personal pleasures and from civic engagement and spiritual connectedness, hope and charity. It also comes from selfless acts of kindness.

The emotional impact of poverty depends on one's perception of one's status. Being relatively poor in a rich country can be stressful even when one's income is high compared to world standards. Some families regarded as living in poverty in the United States now would be considered middle class by 1971 standards.[33] In 2001, 91% of poor people owned color televisions; 74% owned microwave ovens; 55% owned VCRs; and 47% owned dishwashers.

Popular definitions of happiness in our society appear to be based on material possessions rather than on inner peace. Paul Stiles, an entrepreneur who did not find happiness in business success, sees the "free market" as a "Jekyll-and-Hyde" creature that creates material prosperity at a heavy price.[34] The unbridled rule of the market opposes our national creed of "equality and opportunity." In a "marketocracy" there are only winners and losers. This contributes to stress, the breakdown of families, the vulgarization of our pop culture and the decline of morality in a winner-take-all society.

Michael Marmot, Professor of Epidemiology and Public Health at the University College London, argues that income, heath-related behavior and genes are all important determinants of health but that wealth is less important than autonomy—having control over your life—and full participation in one's life's opportunities.[35]

THE ROLE OF POVERTY IN ADOLESCENT PARENTHOOD

A sense of little control over one's life contributes to poor adolescents' feelings of anxiety and despondency. Their crowded schools offer little individual attention and inadequate teaching. When they expect low incomes and dangerous lives, they have high birth rates.[36]

Does Poverty Cause Adolescent Parenthood?

Kristin Luker, professor of sociology at the University of California-Berkeley, holds that poverty causes adolescents to have babies.[37] She does not believe that adolescent childbearing causes poverty. She believes that postponing pregnancy does not lessen adolescents' discouragement nor make them more advantaged. Low skill levels, discouragement and disadvantage are there before and after childbirth.

Luker attributes whatever suffering the children of adolescent mothers experience to poverty and discouragement not to their mothers' immaturity. She suggests that the high fertility medical costs of older women are greater social problems than adolescent parenthood.[38]

Luker's conclusion that adolescent mothers would be disadvantaged with or without childbirth was shared by Thomas Whitman and colleagues who conducted the Notre Dame Parenting Project.[39] They concluded that most Project adolescent mothers would be in the same situation—school failure, personal instability, abuse and negative visions about their futures—even if they did not become pregnant.

Ruth Turley, a professor of sociology at the University of Wisconsin-Madison, analyzed a nation-wide sample of 3- to 16-year-olds and found that the age of their mothers in itself was not the primary factor in their disadvantaged status.[40] She suggests the focus should be on inherited attributes and contextual settings, such as divorce and poverty. Although maternal age symbolizes such factors in mothers' background, Turley believes it is not the culprit in the disadvantages of their children.

Some feminists point out that a focus on adolescent motherhood ignores the systemic causes of poverty.[41] They believe that adolescent girls have the right to choose parenthood. They believe that the public debate about adolescent motherhood perpetuates negative stereotypes. Some raise the possibility that adolescent pregnancy prevention reflects a eugenic bias against minorities—even that it represents genocide.[42]

Luker and some other experts believe that welfare benefits do not encourage adolescent pregnancy.[43] They base this on the facts that welfare benefits are higher in European countries where adolescent childbirth is much lower and that states with the lowest benefits in the United States have the highest adolescent birth rates. But these comparisons do not take into account cultural differences between these countries and states and the decrease in welfare roles in the United States when benefits were shifted from an entitlement based on the number of children to an eligibility status based on employment. Since Aid to the Families of Dependent Children that increased benefits with more children was replaced by the Personal Responsibility and Workforce Opportunity Reconciliation Act of 1996 that does not, adolescent childbirths already dropping because of contraception and pregnancy termination continued to decrease.

While a substantial proportion of adolescent mothers were economically disadvantaged and behind in school before giving birth, careful research controlling for background characteristics reveals that adolescent parenthood is associated with a greater likelihood of dropping out of high school, lower economic productivity, higher poverty and greater reliance on public assistance, as well as single parenthood.[44] This underscores the strong connection between adolescent parenthood and many other social problems. Delaying childbirth may not increase an adolescent mother's opportunities in life, but it will delay public costs for her support, and there will be no maternal educational costs. If children were not born to parents who are not ready and able to care for them, our nation would see a significant reduction in a host of social problems.

The argument that adolescent childbearing does not cause poverty is valid to the extent that poverty fosters attitudes and behaviors that lead to adolescent childbirth. However, the birth of a child in a poor family obviously produces one more person living in poverty. Conversely, the decline in adolescent birth rate during the 1990s was a factor in reducing child poverty during those years.[45] The adolescent birth rate peaked in 1991, and since then fell by 30% as the child poverty rate fell by 23%. If adolescent birth rates had not declined after 1991, almost 1.2 million additional children would have been born to adolescent mothers by 2002, increasing the number of poor children by 460,000.

A flaw in the argument that poverty causes adolescent parenthood is that most girls living in poverty do not become parents. A survey of 15 and 16-year-old poor girls, who were underachieving in school, revealed that only 5% of White, 13% of Black and 9% of Latino girls definitely would consider having a child out of wedlock. 20% more in each category said that they might.[46] In Madison, Wisconsin, 31% of girls ages 15–17 living in poverty were mothers as were 21% in Milwaukee in 2003.[47]

The argument that the age of an adolescent mother does not matter overlooks the fact that no one has demonstrated that adolescent childbearing is preferable to not becoming a parent. It reflects a double standard in which affluent adolescents are encouraged to avoid pregnancy while poor adolescents are supported in repeating the cycle of adolescent childbirth. Two-thirds of the offspring of adolescent mothers do not have children as adolescents. But one-third do, and that amounts to millions of repetitions of the cycle of adolescent parenthood.

Saul Hoffman, professor of economics at the University of Delaware, points out that reducing early parenthood will not eliminate the powerful effects of growing up in poverty and disadvantage. But it is a strategy for widening the pathways out of poverty or, at the very least, not compounding social disadvantage.[48]

LACK OF SOCIAL CAPITAL AS A CAUSE OF ADOLESCENT PARENTHOOD

The majority of poor parents try to raise healthy, successful adolescents, and most feel they are doing well as parents.[49] Yet they do so in the face of multiple challenges in their communities and society. Most have little support beyond their immediate family.

Lower class neighborhoods have less of the *social capital* that helps middle class families raise adolescents. Parents who can select their neighborhoods prefer those with high social capital in the form of good schools, services and neighbors. Poor families must rely on themselves to manage their families in dangerous neighborhoods. Ninety-one percent of children from high social capital neighborhoods are involved in out-of-school-time programs, compared with 51% of children from low social capital neighborhoods.[50]

Low social capital in the form of high rates of violence, drug use and unemployment in inner-city neighborhoods place many adolescents at risk of limited life opportunities and early death. They grow up with little or no parental guidance. Their parents may be under the influence of alcohol or drugs or overwhelmed by working several jobs. They are surrounded by media images that treat sex partners as objects with no enduring commitment and glorify violence, whores, pimps and unprotected sex.[51]

Low social capital is a crucial determinant of adolescent parenthood. Black, Latino and White adolescent girls living in socially disorganized, poor communities without family planning services have an increased likelihood of early pregnancy. As many as 60% of adolescent mothers live below the poverty level and upward of 80% turn to welfare for support following the birth of their first child.[52] Fifty-five percent of all welfare recipients gave birth as adolescents.

Mental Health and Segregated Schools

People living in the underclass commonly adopt the debased image mainstream society has of them. Mental health problems increase the risks of early sex for girls and drug involvement for boys.[53] Poor mental health diminishes adolescents' aspirations and hopes for their futures and predisposes them to unhealthy and dangerous behaviors.

Jonathan Kozol visited nearly sixty inner-city schools and reported in 2005 that conditions had grown worse for children since the federal courts began dismantling the landmark ruling in *Brown v. Board of Education*.[54] Segregation of Black children has reverted to a level that the nation has not seen since the 1960s. Kozol concluded that inner-city children have little knowledge of the world in which middle-class children live.

The Unavailability of Reliable Men

The collective absence of fathers from families and neighborhoods reduces the supervision and monitoring of adolescents and makes them vulnerable to risky behavior.[55]

The lack of two-parent homes in ghettos is directly related to marriageable men disappearing from the inner city along with manufacturing jobs. More than 40% of poor men who have a child outside of marriage have been in prison or will be by the time the baby is born. Nearly 50% lack a high school diploma, and 25% have no jobs.[56] Women are understandably reluctant to marry men with prison records, drug addiction and quick tempers. They may hope that the birth of a baby will tame them. Sometimes it does lead to "maternity ward conversions." However, by the time the child is three two-thirds of these mothers are on their own again.

LACK OF PURPOSE AND MEANING IN LIFE TRANSCENDS SOCIAL CLASS

In spite of their advantages, many middle and upper class adolescents share the lack of meaning and purpose in life characteristic of disadvantaged girls who chose to become parents. Although most adolescents have attainable goals in their lives and pursue their education and career development methodically, a significant number are adrift. They resort to alcohol, drugs and high-risk activities to relieve their ennui.

Sixty percent of all 8th graders complete high school and go on to college or trade school from which 29% graduate.[57] Put another way, 22% of those who enter college drop out after the first year. Only 49% complete a bachelor degree in four years. Each month 49% of all full-time college students binge drink, abuse prescription drugs and/ or abuse illegal drugs. When these behaviors are coupled with casual "hooking up," middle and upper class adolescents have outlooks resembling those of lower class girls and boys who become parents. However, college cultures and peer groups are not conducive to parenthood.

THE INTRACTABILITY OF POVERTY

Professionals and volunteers often are disappointed when they find they cannot assume that poor persons would live differently if they had a choice.[58] Some persons living in poverty seem to prefer their freedom to express their personalities and their intense emotional experiences over middle class life. Moreover, alcoholism, lack of motivation and drug addiction are extremely difficult to change. Even acquiring wealth itself can be stressful: [59]

The acquisition of immense wealth by a lower class person does not insure success or happiness in life as illustrated by Mack Metcalf and his estranged second wife, Virginia Merida, who shared a $34 million lottery jackpot. Years of struggle gave way almost overnight to limitless leisure, big houses and lavish toys. Metcalf died from stress-related alcoholism a few years later.

The intractability of poverty is revealed in the barriers to employment found in the Milwaukee TANF Applicant Study.[60] Three of four participants reported at least one barrier to employment four years after entering the Study, including being disabled; caring for a family member with a disability; being in fair or poor health; having an alcohol or drug problem; lacking a high school diploma or GED; being involved in an unsafe or physically abusive relationship; or having a mental health problem. Two in five reported two or more barriers, and more than one in five reported three.

APPROACHING POVERTY BY BUILDING SOCIAL CAPITAL

The greatest threat to our way of life does not come from terrorism but from the poor seceding from our mainstream institutions—our schools, workplaces and laws.

Lawrence Mead, professor of political science at New York University, points out that our nation's greatest resource in dealing with poverty is not its wealth but the civility that has undergirded our politics since the Founding of our nation.[61] The widespread poverty in the United States is unwise, unjust and intolerable. Lisbeth Schorr, Harvard social analyst, shows how solutions lie in building social capital by strengthening families through creating adequately paying jobs, buffering the economic consequences of family changes, building individual and community assets, providing a sensible safety net and devising an equitable tax structure.

Linking Benefits to Responsibilities

Seymour Lipset, former professor of public policy at George Mason University, pointed out that in the face of inequality Americans usually opt for policies that offer more opportunities rather than the redistribution of wealth.[62] Isabel Sawhill, a Brooking Institution Scholar, and former Senator John Edwards argue that those who finish high school, delay child bearing and make a good effort to support their children should not be poor. Sawhill believes that the work requirements of the Personal Responsibility and Work Opportunity Reconciliation Act of 1996 positively affected poverty rates.[63] She adds that educational, training and treatment programs need to surround employment that rewards persons adequately for their productivity.

Annual Cash Grants

In his seminal 1984 book *Losing Ground,* Charles Murray sparked national debate by arguing that the Great Society social programs of the 1960s failed to help the poor and actually made things worse.[64] In his 2006 book *In Our Hands,* he offers a radical solution for poverty. He sees welfare as a dead end, stripping life of fulfilling choices and responsibilities.

Murray would eliminate all federal, state and local level income transfer programs—including Social Security, Medicare, Medicaid, welfare and corporate subsidies—and would substitute an annual cash grant of $10,000 for life beginning at age twenty-one.

However, the evidence suggests that simply giving people money would not produce a dramatic improvement in the physical health, mental health or development of children.[65] More effective are targeted programs that provide education, nutritional supplements, medical care, early childhood education and housing. Cash benefits now are available through the Earned Income Tax Credit to more than 22 million families at a cost of $38 billion in 2006.

Individual Development Accounts might be more effective than cash grants in encouraging low-income persons to save through government matching their savings.[66]

Self-fulfillment in Work

Greed can fuel a 24/7, "always-on" pace of life. Stress, anxiety, burnout, self-medication and other forms of psychological injury have replaced physical injuries as contemporary workplace hazards. According to Richard Florida, professor of public policy at George Mason University, societies that build the most efficient means for harnessing human creative energy though self-fulfillment in work will move ahead of those continuing to make a fetish of greed.[67]

Self-fulfillment is replacing financial gain as the primary motivator for work. When basic needs have been met, intrinsic rewards from work are more effective in motivating people than extrinsic rewards.[68] Increasing numbers of people have come to value intrinsic or creative opportunities over simply making money. The job qualities most highly valued are those that involve challenges, responsibility and tangible satisfactions from accomplishment.

Community Building

An inner-city ghetto is comparable to a developing nation in many ways. The social dislocation is so massive that it requires federal support on a significant scale if it is to be meaningfully addressed.[69] We cannot expect values and norms to change radically in the absence of major improvements in social capital. Character education is not enough. To achieve changes in adolescent sexual attitudes and behavior, especially in their decisions about pregnancy, and childbearing, it will be necessary to substantially modify their environments, to provide them with educational incentives, to enhance their career opportunities and to increase their access and exposure to mainstream values and life-styles. Community building cannot take place unless people have homes that give them a sense of permanency and a stake in creating a positive social climate in their neighborhoods. When groups believe they need each other, they can overcome their prejudices and join programs that foster interaction and cooperation.

In theory, our free market system permits parents to choose where they live and where their children go to school. In fact, these choices are constrained by economic and social opportunities. Public schools in urban ghettos are conspicuously inept at engaging parents in their children's education. We need to rethink ways of building publicly and privately funded recreational institutions, such as YMCA, YWCA and Boys and Girls Clubs, to stabilize communities and support overburdened parents.

ADOLESCENT PREGNANCY AND PARENTHOOD IN SWEDEN AND SOUTH KOREA

Sweden and South Korea offer contrasting examples of how social capital in the forms of affluent class hope for the future and of lower class traditions minimize adolescent pregnancy and parenthood.

Sweden is an affluent nation without the underclass seen in the United States.[70] It also ranks much lower than the United States in rates of adolescent pregnancy and parenthood despite having one of the world's most generous family welfare policies. Swedish young people delay parenthood because they want to complete their educations, find vocations and enjoy leisure without being encumbered by childrearing. Their culture fosters commitment to the common good rather than individualism. They have hope for the future through access to free college education, employment, childrearing allowances and parental leave benefits.

South Korea is an example of a society in which integrative values also outweigh self-assertive values. It is a lower class society, yet it ranks much lower than the United States in adolescent pregnancy and parenthood rates.[71] The major reason is the Korean reluctance to accept sexual relations outside of marriage. Most young people prefer marriages with parental consent. However, cohabitation and premarital sex are rising with urbanization and Westernization.

The United States does not need to emulate Sweden nor South Korea to benefit from their experiences. In both of these contrasting cultures, integrative cultural values counter balance self-assertive social values. This can happen in the United States as well. An example of applying integrative cultural values in private business is the way in which Ikea, a Swedish company with 30 stores in the United States, provides family benefits for its 11,000 employees.[72]

CONCLUSION

Social class is the most important correlate of adolescent parenthood. Compared to other children, boys and girls who grow up in poverty are more likely to experience neglect and abuse and have attachment disorders. They are more likely to have developmental disorders with consequent school failure. They are more likely to lack self-discipline and self-respect.

More children in the United States are born in disadvantaged environments than forty years ago. In 2004, using the *money income* definition an estimated 13% of the population lived in poverty. Eighteen percent of children under 18 were below the poverty line in 2005. Thirty percent of the poor reside in central cities, 40% in suburban areas and 30% in rural areas.

Two opposing paradigms dominate our thinking about poverty. The first is that poverty results from systemic factors. The second is that poverty results from individual factors. Both paradigms are needed to explain poverty in the United States.

The argument that adolescent childbearing does not cause poverty is valid to the extent that poverty fosters attitudes and behaviors that lead to adolescent childbirth. However, without additional income, the birth of a child in a poor family increases the number in poverty. Reducing adolescent parenthood removes the public costs of raising poor adolescents' children and of their educations now. It reduces poverty in the future by breaking the cycle of adolescent parenthood. The argument that the age of a poor mother does not matter overlooks the fact that no one has demonstrated that adolescent childbearing is preferable to not becoming a parent.

Poverty is less important than the behavior of her own parents in influencing an adolescent girl's chances of becoming pregnant. Research has not shown that increasing the income of poor families will suffice without increasing their social capital.

If the privileged one-third of our society continues to be dominated by self-assertive social values and to separate themselves from the bottom one-third, our social and economic conditions will continue to stagnate or deteriorate. Parenthood will continue to be attractive to some adolescents. Mobilizing our integrative cultural values to build social capital could transform our society.

Chapter 20

Peer Influences on
Adolescent Parenthood

Inside of me there are two dogs, one evil and one good. The evil dog and the good dog fight all of the time. Which dog wins? The one I feed the most.

Native American parable[1]

Parents determine where children live and shape their character development. They have less influence on their children's choice of peers.

Judith Rich Harris, a writer of college textbooks, reviewed the research and affirmed that peers strongly influence adolescents' language, fashions and behavior away from home.[2] But peers play a modest role in adolescent life outcomes compared to family influences.[3] Adolescents with close relationships with their parents who set clear expectations for them are less likely to be influenced by their peers than those who do not.

Peer socialization often starts in day care, gathers momentum in same-gender groups and reaches its height in adolescent cliques.[4] Peers transmit pop cultural norms and promote conformity. Antisocial peer groups foster rebellion against mainstream values. Sensitivity to their appearances in the eyes of peers underlies the power of peer pressure in adolescents' lives.

SENSITIVITY TO PEER PERCEPTIONS

Sensitivity to what other people have and how they view us has been documented in every culture surveyed.[5] A desire for the material things and qualities possessed by peers begins in early childhood, peaks during adolescence and persists to some degree throughout life.

Adolescents typically want to be popular, fit in with the crowd, be attractive and avoid the harsh spotlight of peer judgment.[6] Their self-images are shaped by their perceptions of how they are perceived by peers. Bringing one's self-image into line with reality rather than to these confusing, circular perceptions of others' perceptions of oneself is a challenge for adolescents.

215

Girls tend to be especially sensitive to feeling they are being judged by others.[7] They tend to internalize frustration and aggression and take it out on themselves more than do boys. The feeling of being negatively judged by others involves the same neurological mechanisms as physical pain. As 16-year-old Cheryl said:

> Why are girls so mean and snooty? Why do they hurt each other so much? I rarely see boys talking about each other behind their backs. It seems that everything we do today is extreme. Good sense seems locked in a closet.

Cliques are exclusive groups, such as jocks, nerds, techies, drama types, skaters, kickers and gangstas. They contribute to the pleasures and the discomforts of adolescent life. Exclusion from a clique can be devastating for vulnerable adolescents.

When adolescents lose hope for the future, they withdraw or rebel, resulting in a downward spiral of self-confidence, family conflict, academic apathy and risk-taking behavior. The fear of exposing one's flaws and of parental reactions often prevents adolescents from seeking help for these problems. They may use sex to relieve anxiety and depression.[8]

ADOLESCENT SEXUAL INTERCOURSE

Adolescent sexual behavior is strongly influenced by peer values and behavior.

Epochs of Excess and Restraint

Throughout recorded history, the sexual behavior of adolescents has fluctuated between eras of excess and restraint. Recent decades have witnessed widespread excesses so that it appears we may be entering an era of restraint.

Premarital sexual activity was common in 15th and 16th century England. Puritans in England reacted against that behavior. Most colonial American women apparently married in their early 20s when the age of menarche was 17 or 18.[9] Premarital births apparently rose from 10% in the seventeenth century to nearly 30% in the second half of the 18th century. Waves of religious revival swept across the United States in the early 19th century, and sex outside of marriage was condemned once again. This negative view of premarital sex was reinforced by physicians, who regarded sexual activity as hazardous for physical development. In the late 19th century when the average age of menarche probably was 15, less than 5% of 14 to 19-year-olds were documented as married in Massachusetts.

Although Kinsey's surveys in the 1940s and 1950s suggested that less than 25% of adolescents under 20 had sexual intercourse, retrospective surveys of women who were adolescents during that time revealed that the vast majority actually had experienced intercourse by that age.[10] The rate of adolescent childbearing reached a peak after World War II in 1957 for 15 to 19-year-olds. However, adolescent pregnancy did not appear to be a major social problem then because most girls either gave birth in maternity homes with an adoption plan, or they quickly married the fathers. Since married women were expected to stay at home then, early marriage was not seen as disrupting a girl's life.

Age of First Intercourse and Partners

Sexual activity now begins during the middle school years for both boys and girls. Boys especially feel pressure to engage in sexual behavior because "everyone is doing it," to prove their "manhood" and more recently from sexually aggressive girls.

Thirty-five percent of 8th through 10th graders in twenty Missouri schools indicated that they had sex.[11] Fears of pregnancy and AIDS were the most frequent reasons given for not having sex followed by feeling unready for sex and waiting for the right person.

The median age of first intercourse for males was 16 in 2005.[12] Of adolescent girls in 8th to 12th grades, 31% had intercourse by 15 and 45% by 16. Seventy-nine percent of boys describe their first sexual relationship as romantic, compared with 89% of girls.

Prevalence of Sexual Intercourse

Adolescents in the United States continue to have pregnancy, birth and sexually transmitted infection rates that greatly exceed those of adolescents in other developed countries.[13]

In 2007, the National Youth Risk Behavior Survey reported that 48% of both boys and girls had sexual intercourse by the 12th grade compared to 54% in 1991.[14] No longer can it be said that most high school students have had sexual intercourse ("everyone does it"). Most say that sexual intercourse is "against my religion or morals." Black boys (63%) are more likely than both Latino (55%) and White boys (41%) to have had sexual intercourse. Black girls are more likely (57%) than White (46%) and Latino girls (40%) to have had sex intercourse.

Frequency of Sexual Intercourse

In 2005, 34% of high school students reported having sexual intercourse with more than one person during the previous three months.[15] Boys were slightly more likely than girls to feel pressured to have sex (82% vs. 79%). Girls said romantic partners exert the most pressure, while boys said pressure was most likely to come from other boys. Eighteen percent of high school-age boys reported having four or more sexual partners in their lifetime, down from 23% in 1991. For girls, the percentages were 11% in 2005 and 13% in 1991. Thirteen percent of White, 21% of Latino and 39% of Black male high school students had four or more sexual partners.

Ages of Sexual Partners

Girls are more likely than boys to have had an older first sexual partner. In 2002, 81% of girls had a partner who was at least one year older than they were at first sexual intercourse, compared with 46% of males.[16] Twenty-four percent of girls had a sexual partner who was three to four years older than they were at first sexual intercourse, compared with 5% of boys. An additional 13% of girls and 3% of boys had a partner who was five or more years older. More than one in four babies born to mothers between 15 and 17 are fathered by someone five or more years older.

Prevalence of Contraception

Adolescents use contraception inconsistently. Surveys report contraception usage by 15 to 19-year-olds ranging from 28% to 80% with percentages somewhat higher for boys than girls and higher for Whites than Blacks, who are higher than Latinos.[17] For sexually experienced adolescents, having sex with an older person is associated with reduced use of contraception and a greater risk of a pregnancy.

Research on adolescent brain development reveals that young adolescents are not prepared to make decisions about sex and contraception.[18] Much of the failure to use contraception is not due to the lack of knowledge or availability, but to its inconvenience. Some boys say they would be embarrassed to buy condoms in a drugstore. Others say that using a condom reduces their physical sensations. Boys agree that girls influence the decision to use contraception more than boys.

Geography of Sexual Behavior

The National Longitudinal Study of Adolescent Health found that suburban public high school students have sex more and pregnancy less than urban students:[19]

- 43% of suburban 12th graders and 39% of urban 12th graders have had sex with a person with whom they did not have a romantic relationship.
- 14% of suburban 12th grade girls and 20% of urban 12th grade girls have been pregnant.

There are regional variations in sexual behavior. For example, the percent of Wisconsin high school students who reported never having had sexual intercourse rose to a high of 63% in 2003 and decreased to 55% in 2007.[20]

Sex without Intercourse

The reduction in adolescent sexual intercourse partly reflects a trend toward oral sex as an alternative.[21] More than half of high school boys and girls have engaged in oral sex. Although oral sex reduces most sexually transmitted diseases, Chlamydia, human papillomavirus, herpes and gonorrhea infections have increased in part through oral sex and mutual masturbation.

Attitudes toward Sexual Intercourse

Over two-thirds of adolescents say they have talked with a parent at least once about sex.[22] Ninety percent of boys from 12 to 19 say it is important for them to receive a strong message that they should not have sex until they are out of high school. Nearly equal percentages of boys and girls (81% vs. 84%) say that sex should only occur in a committed relationship.

Boys are more likely than girls to think that it is embarrassing to admit that they are virgins (24% vs. 14%). Among sexually active adolescents, boys are less likely than girls to wish they had waited longer before having sex for the first time (55% vs. 70%). A double standard is revealed when 91% of 15 to18-year-old girls and boys say that girls get bad reputations from having sex while only 42% believe that boys do.

Boys are less likely than girls to say their decisions about sex are influenced by what their parents might think; by what they have learned in sex education; and by what their religion says about sex. Boys are more likely than girls to agree with the statement, "sex is something that just happens" (33% vs. 17%).

Attitudes toward Adolescent Pregnancy

The overwhelming majority of boys (84%) and girls (88%) say they would feel upset if they caused a pregnancy.[23] Girls are more likely (61%) than boys (51%) to report that they would be *very* upset if pregnancy occurred. While 59% of White boys would be very upset if they got their partner pregnant, only 38% of Latino and 36% of Black boys would feel that way. Forty-nine percent of Latino and 51% of Black girls would be *very* upset if they got pregnant, compared to 66% of White girls. A significant minority of all adolescents (15% of boys and 12% of girls) say they would be pleased with a pregnancy. However, 23% of sexually experienced boys and 17% of sexually experienced girls say they would be pleased with a pregnancy; 31% of adolescent mothers say they would be pleased with another pregnancy.

A Seventeen/Candie's Foundation survey revealed that 70% of adolescent girls said that having a plan for their futures would help prevent unplanned pregnancies; 48% thought they might become pregnant in the next five years; 67% had friends who became pregnant as adolescents; 67% were more worried about sexually transmitted diseases than pregnancies.[24]

Melinda

Melinda Robertson became pregnant at the age of 15 after her first sexual intercourse. She describes the realities of her life as an adolescent mother in her book *Motherhood: What You Don't Know* in an effort to prevent adolescent parenthood.[25] At the same time, her successful negotiation of high school might be an inspiration for adolescent mothers as well.

Timken Senior High School

At Timken Senior High School in Canton, Ohio, which has an abstinence only sex education program, the pregnancy rate is higher than the national rate.[26] In the fall of 2005, Timken High began offering a class called Pregnancy Life Skills in which pregnant girls and mothers learn prenatal care and child development. Sixteen-year-old Courtney said:

> Being pregnant at Timken is no big deal. Some girls think its cool, like it'll get them attention and make them more popular. At Timken you're a nerd or a geek if you're still a virgin.

Seventeen-year-old Jessica, a mother of two children, put it this way:

> I wasn't embarrassed when I found out I was pregnant. People made me feel good. My friend Heather was so sweet. She rubbed my tummy. One of my teachers said that she got pregnant at sixteen; everything would be okay.

Eighteen-year-old Monica said:

> I've been crying every day and every night. I keep on blaming myself for being six months pregnant. I worry about starting classes at Timken Senior High School with a bulging belly and am planning an adoption.[27]

Joanne, mother of 8-months pregnant 16-year-old Raechel, said:

> Timken's abstinence-based sex education program is not enough. It's time to take the blinders off and realize that these kids are having sex. If we have to, just give them condoms. Raechel does not fit the mold some think pregnant adolescents come from. She has straight As. We were constantly checking on her. She plans to return to the 10th grade after completing an adoption. Many students are sexually active and need more information about birth control. It can happen to anybody no matter who you are, not just bad girls.

Gloucester, Massachusetts

In the 2007-2008 school year, seventeen girls 16 or younger in Gloucester, Massachusetts, became pregnant—four times the typical rate. According to the *Gloucester Daily Times* a number of these girls had chosen to become pregnant.[28] Others tested at the school-based clinic were disappointed when their pregnancy tests were negative.

SOCIETAL INFLUENCES ON SEXUAL BEHAVIOR

Sexual behavior is strongly influenced by broader social values and practices and by the social skills and activities of individual adolescents.

Conflicting Societal Messages about Sex

The conflicting messages about sexual activity in the United States leave many young people perplexed and misinformed.

The societal encouragement of adolescent sexual intercourse is reflected by the phrase "sexually active." This implies that exercising self-restraint is being "inactive or passive," negatively valued attributes in our achievement-oriented society. Referring to adolescent girls as "women" and adolescent boys as "men" to avoid offending them also fosters a premature sense of attaining adulthood. Our double standard discourages girls' but offers a "wink and a nod" at boys' sexual activity.

Most importantly, adolescent attitudes about sexual behavior mirror those of many adults who deny that values restraining sexual activity are an appropriate component of childrearing at all. In his book *The Modernization of Sex,* Paul Robinson, professor of history at Stanford University, described sexual activity as simply a physical act, like eating or riding a bicycle and denied that values, other than good manners, apply to sexual activity.[29] This belief underlies much of the commercial advertising and entertainment directed at adolescents.

In this view, since adolescents are sexually active, they are entitled to contraception. Since they are entitled to contraception, they are entitled to be sexually active. If they do become parents, they are entitled to public support. This circular thinking is based on the assumption that sexually active adolescents are "mature minors." However, mature adolescents are the most likely to choose to not be sexually active and to not become parents if pregnant.

Parental religious beliefs apparently weakly influence adolescent sexual behavior. Adolescents with parents who hold strong religious beliefs are somewhat less likely to have sex before the age of 18 (41%) than their peers whose parents do not (48%).[30] They are more likely to be involved in social activities, particularly church affiliated.

The American Psychological Association Task Force on the Sexualization of Girls reported that the excessive sexualization of girls has negative effects on cognitive functioning, physical and mental health, sexuality, attitudes and beliefs.[31] It is linked with eating disorders. Unfavorably comparing one's body to sexualized ideals undermines comfort with one's own body and causes shame, anxiety and depression. Its societal effects may include an increase in sexism; fewer girls pursuing careers in science, engineering and mathematics; increased sexual harassment and violence; and increased demand for child pornography.

The mixed messages adolescents receive and apparent adult helplessness result in many adolescents feeling that adults are out of touch with them.

Lack of Conversational and Social Skills

The lack of conversational skills, especially for boys, induces sexual activity. Although adolescents have a developmental need to talk to peers as they explore themselves and the world around them, many have not learned how to communicate their thoughts and feelings in face-to-face relationships. This deprives them of the authentic feedback they need from peers. It also predisposes them to relate to others on a physical rather than a conversational level.

> In a focus group meeting of Black high school boys, "player" was used to refer to sexually active boys. They acknowledged that players' talk with girls was sexy. "What else is there to talk about?" They described girls who invite sex with boys and men. They said the media encourages sex. They saw poverty and "messed up" families as creating a lack of hope for the future.

"Hooking up" or having "recreational" sexual intercourse is an impulsive experience that replaces social interactions. In this context, adolescents do not learn to integrate sensual pleasure with the intimacy and commitment of mature sexuality.[32] Especially for girls, casual sexual activity can result in a loss of self-respect and a distorted concept of their own feminine worth.

DATING ABUSE

Dating abuse is a silent epidemic. Adolescents lack awareness of how to handle abusive situations, seek help and terminate such relationships. They are ill-informed about the long-term effects of abusive behavior. Peer rejection can lead a girl to seek sexual partners to gain their acceptance. Intense dating can facilitate having a number of sexual partners.

Verbal, Emotional and Physical Abuse

One in three adolescents reports knowing a friend who has been physically injured by a partner. One in four girls says she has been in a relationship where she was verbally abused by her partner, and 13% report physical abuse. In a 2003 survey, the percentage of girls and boys in grades 9 through 12 who reported being victims of physical dating abuse to adults were: White 7%, Latino 9% and Black 14%.[33]

We all have sadistic and masochistic thoughts and urges at times. We are most likely to vent these impulses on people close to us. These sadistic impulses become abusive when they are based on a need to dominate someone else. Abuse is perpetuated by a masochistic partner with low self-respect. Emotional abuse includes possessiveness, jealousy, unrealistic expectations and isolating a person from friends and family. Verbal abuse includes degrading comments, name-calling and minimizing accomplishments.

Because of their inexperience, adolescents have difficulty managing complicated feelings, conflicts and decisions in their relationships. They may interpret jealousy, possessiveness and abuse as signs of love. Many adolescents regard emotional and verbal abuse as normal in relationships. Fifteen-year-old Lauren put it this way:

> I didn't think I was being abused because he wasn't hitting me. I stayed with him because I couldn't see anything physical that he was doing wrong to me. I thought the torment I felt must be all in my head.

Adults also may not take adolescents seriously when they describe abusive relationships. Parents may minimize their emotional reactions and erroneously expect them to break up easily.[34]

Although girls are more likely to be the victims of dating abuse, boys are subject to abuse as well. Abusive girls tend to attract abusive boys. A girl may have the fantasy that she is the only person who can rescue a boy. She makes excuses for his behavior. They play out mutually abusive behavior in their relationship. Jill Murray, a marriage and family therapist, cites the following signs that girls and boys are in abusive relationships:[35]

- Before she started dating this person, she had more friends.
- His grades declined after he met his partner.
- She cries a lot or seems very sad.
- He has become more secretive.
- She carries a cell phone constantly so she won't miss his calls.
- He makes excuses for his partner's behavior.
- She misses him terribly when they are not together.
- He is jealous of other people in her life.
- She is less involved in activities than she used to be.
- He often makes fun of her, but says he is kidding.
- She changed her appearance to please him.
- She has bruises she can't explain.

Most dating abuse occurs in steady relationships. Some abusers become more violent when they fear a relationship breakup.[36] Sixteen-year-old Madison said:

> I started trying to break up with him. But he would come to me crying, "I love you. I'll never hurt you again." When I'd see him cry, I'd remember his softness and gentleness. When his crying didn't work, he threatened to hurt me and my friends and my Mom. He even threatened to commit suicide.

The Stockholm Syndrome in which captives submit to captors can be a model for abusive relationships.[37] In it an abuser controls a victim who cannot escape. Isolated from others, the victim must turn to the abuser for nurturance. Small kindnesses reassure the victim, who denies rage at the abusive side of the abuser.

In some subcultures, domestic and economic roles make women emotionally and financially dependent on men. Girls are socialized to believe that they cannot have a full life without a partner.[38] They believe they are fortunate to have a man who will let them love him. Adolescents are particularly susceptible to these views, as 15-year-old Megan said:[39]

> I never told anybody about what he did to me because I was ashamed. I didn't want to talk about it. I had nightmares about it. I tried to hide it from Mom.

To foster healthy relationships among adolescence, the Centers for Disease Control launched a nationwide campaign *Choose Respect*.[40] The *Ending Violence* curriculum for Latino/a students encourages early intervention for dating violence.

Sexual Abuse

A flagrant blind spot exists in our view of sexual relations between minors. We may prosecute an adult who has sexual relations with a minor and ignore the equal, if not greater, hazards of adolescent boys and girls having sexual intercourse. In most states, an 18-year-old's sexual intercourse with a 14-year-old is a crime, but a 17-year-old's it is not.

About 20% of all adolescent girls report they have had unwanted sexual experiences with one-third of them describing it as rape.[41] Seventy-four percent of sexually active girls younger than 14 and 60% of those younger than 15 had unwanted sex. Eighteen percent of all females in the United States have had an attempted or completed rape; of these, 22% were younger than 12 when they were first raped, and 32% were between the ages of 12 and 17. Unwanted sex occurs in 40% of Black adolescent sexual relationships, often due to fear of the partner's anger if denied sex. A girl's history of sexual abuse, conformity to peer influences and having either authoritarian or permissive parents predict susceptibility to unwanted sexual advances.

Two-thirds of undergraduate female college students have encountered some type of sexual harassment.[42] The Ms. Project on Campus Sexual Assault found they have a four times greater chance of being raped by someone they know than by a stranger. Thirty-eight percent were 17 or younger at the time of their first assault. 75% of men and 55% of women involved in acquaintance rapes reported using alcohol or other drugs prior to the incident.

The Ms. Project found that more than 50% of high school boys and 42% of high school girls believe that it is acceptable for a male to physically force a female to engage in intercourse.

CONCLUSION

Parents determine where their children live and shape their character development, but they have less influence over their children's choice of peers. Peers strongly influence children's behavior away from home, their language and their fashions.

Cliques powerfully influence adolescent behavior. Sensitivity to the qualities and perceptions of other people is inherent in adolescence. One of the risks of this sensitivity is losing hope for success and withdrawing or rebelling with a downward spiral of family conflict, academic apathy, self-confidence and risk-taking behaviors.

The sexual behavior of young people fluctuates between eras of excess and restraint. The excesses of recent decades appear to be yielding to an era of restraint, although the biological pressure to engage in sexual activity now begins during the middle school years.

The overwhelming majority of boys and girls believe it is important for them to receive a strong message that they should not have sex until after high school and that sex should only occur in a long-term, committed relationship. When adolescents do not receive these messages from their families, they are exposed to our society's confusing combination of permissiveness, prudishness and double standards about sexual issues.

Sexism is reflected in an epidemic of dating abuse among adolescents, who are ill-informed about the long-term effects of abusive behavior. Younger sexually active adolescents are especially vulnerable to coercive sex. They lack clear direction from peers and adults for seeking help for handling abusive situations.

Peer influences are crucial in determining the sexual behavior of adolescents and resulting pregnancies and parenthood. Still, parents have more influence over their adolescents than they realize.

Chapter 21

Gang Influences on Adolescent Parenthood

My own personal view, as a magistrate, is that our society intervenes far too late in the process of antisocial behavior as this develops in children. It is much easier, and more viable, to make rules in the home and at school and enforce these, than to try rehabilitation programs on adults whose lives have been ruined by society's unwillingness to get involved until it is too late for the life habit of crime to be reversed.

Magistrate Sybil B.G. Eysenck, 1989[1]

Most gangs in the United States are composed of adolescent boys and are spawned by conditions in urban ghettos.[2] They are centers of neighborhood social and political life embedded in the illegal economy. They have internet links through "netbanging" and even prison linkages.

An estimated 731,500 adolescents in more than 21,500 gangs were active in the United States in 2002. Every city over 250,000, and most over 100,000 have gangs.[3]

Gangs include childhood-onset and adolescent-onset delinquents.[4] Childhood-onset delinquents have incompetent parents and cognitive, emotional and behavior disorders. These qualities are less prominent with adolescent-onset delinquents. The male-to female ratio is 10 to 1 for childhood-onset but only 1.5 to 1 for adolescent-onset delinquency.

HISTORY OF GANGS IN THE UNITED STATES

Street gangs originally were formed for survival purposes by children of the same ethnic background who had been abandoned or lost by their immigrant parents.[5]

In the 19th century, criminal gangs in our large cities resulted from the lack of jobs. Irish immigrants formed the first gangs in The Five Points in New York City. A gang called the Fourty Thieves battled the Bowery gang so intensely that the U.S. Army was called to intervene. Before the Civil War, New York City's gangs easily plundered businesses and homes.

After the Civil War, New York City had Jewish, Italian, Black and Irish gangs. Chinese gangs appeared in California. By 1870, Philadelphia had over 100 gangs. In the early 1900s, gangs appeared across the nation.

By the mid-1920s, there were over 1,300 gangs following ethnic lines in Chicago with more than 25,000 members. Over two million Mexican imigrants flooded California pursuing the American dream. Some adolescents became Pachuco gang members and wore "Zoot suits."

During World War II, over half a million Puerto Ricans arrived in the United States. Most settled in New York City and contributed to the greatest gang era in history. During the 1950s, gang fighting rose to an all time high across the country, usually over girls or turf. Gang murders rose as drugs entered the scene. Female gangs with strong ties to male gangs formed.

The 1960s saw a decline in gang activity. Attention shifted to Vietnam, the Civil Rights Movement and Hippies. By the early 1970s, gangs made headlines again. Expansion of the drug trade produced a new form of turf control. Gang wars now resemble guerilla warfare with rooftop sniping and drive-by shootings.

CURRENT STATUS OF GANGS IN THE UNITED STATES

The 2005 National Gang Threat Assessment revealed several new trends in gang activity and migration.[6] Latino gang membership is growing, especially in the Northeast and South. Gangs are more sophisticated in their use of technology and computers in crime. They recruit in elementary, middle and high schools because minors receive lighter sentences when convicted of crimes. In Florida, the average ages of gang members varies from 16 to 25. In Hernando County almost half of gang members are between 10 and 15.[7]

As gangs expand their territories across the country, they bring crime, violence, babies and children. They enter neighborhoods previously gang-free or come into deadly conflict with existing gangs. An example of the spread of gang violence across the United States occurred in 2006 in Raleigh, North Carolina, a city not known for gang activity, when a boy was killed by a rival Bloods gang member in a drive-by shooting simply for wearing the Crips gang color.[8]

New immigrant populations isolated by language barriers and lack of employment are vulnerable to gang activity. Latino gangs flourish by providing their communities with support and protection. On the other hand, Asian gangs often victimize other Asians who are afraid to report crimes. Only about one-fifth of Asian gang members apparently belong to Asian gangs.[9] The others belong to more inclusive gangs

Public denial of their existence contributes to the increase in the number, size and strength of gangs. Outward signs of gang affiliations are becoming less visible as gangs hide from law enforcement. This allows gangs to maintain drug networks with anonymity. In some cities, large gangs are being replaced by small, loosely organized gangs of young men who commit violent offenses before breaking up or ending up in prison.[10]

Gangs are a growing challenge for our society. New forms of violence enhanced by the media, advances in communication and dysfunctional families in suburbs combine to produce the "new affluent gangsters," who may be the next wave of criminality.

MOTIVATION TO JOIN GANGS

Gangs are a result of marginalized adolescents' need to identify with a cause greater than themselves to achieve status, security and power. This readiness to bond reflects the *Us-Them* code. A few strangers on an airplane, an athletic team or an infantry platoon can quickly develop *Us* feelings and sometimes ferocious solidarity against outsiders.[11] Bonding with athletic teams permits participants and fans to express aggressive urges in a socially acceptable way. Gangs offer even more direct ways to act out aggressive urges.

The "three Rs" of gang culture have been described:[12]

- *Reputation:* A "rep" applies to the gang and to each member. Having the most "juice" (illegal drugs) gains the most status.
- *Respect:* "Gangbangers" seek status for themselves and their gang. Often to join, one must be "jumped in" by a beating followed by bonding as a "family."
- *Retaliation/Revenge:* Many confrontations between gangs result from drug deals or territorial infringement and revenge for previous attacks.

Loyalty to a gang analogous to patriotism is seen in the willingness to endure suffering in service of a gang. Gangs are particularly attractive to adolescents who have not formed solid attachment bonds with their own families and have been physically or sexually abused. A gang becomes their family. The solidarity of a gang compensates for depressive feelings and provides an outlet for anger and hatred. The values, codes and trappings of gangs give members a sense of belonging, power and superiority over others. Adolescents feel like "men" and "women." They gain protection and financial benefits, but they do not fully appreciate the hazards they face.

Children as young as eight are lured into gangs and commit acts of violence like older, street-wise members. Some parents may not realize that their children are engaged in gang activity. Other parents do not discourage and may even encourage gang involvement.

Financial gain alone does not explain participation in gangs. Average earnings by gang members are only a little higher than legitimate wages.[13] The intrigue of drug dealing and the prospect of future riches are more important than current income.

GANG IDENTITIES

Many gangs are divided into *sets* or *cliques*.[14] Sets usually apply to Black gangs and cliques to Latino gangs. The Bloods and Crips are the most widely recognized Black gangs with hundreds of sets. Bloods ("Be Loyal or Otherwise Die") usually align with the People Nation, and Crips (Community Revolution In Progress) usually align with the Folk Nation.

Clothing is the primary form of gang identification. Growing out of the "grunge" look of the hip-hop culture with its "attitude," baggies and shaved heads, gang attire has become popular with upper and middle-class White adolescents.

Gangs use graffiti to mark their "turf," to advertise status and power, to declare their allegiance to the gang and to boast about criminal activities. Innocent residents can be subject to gang violence by the mere presence of graffiti in their neighborhood.[15]

Gang members seek advancement in a gang but not in the rest of the world. If they advance in their gang, they are proud social outcasts. If they advance in society, they lose status in their gang and possibly even their lives.[16]

GANG VIOLENCE

Gang membership usually is a transient adolescent phenomenon, but it can have profound consequences. From the earliest days of gang research by Frederic Thrasher in the 1920s, the evidence is clear that gang members are more extensively involved in violent delinquency than other young people.[17] As bullies, they likely came from homes where they learned aggression is the way to get what they want.

Aggressive behavior is an instinctual defense against threats to our vital interests as individuals and as groups. Sadistic aggression is a product of distorted instinctual drives and is not socially significant unless it is endorsed by a group or nation. People can overcome inhibitions against hurting others when victims are seen as inferior or as enemies. Drugs and alcohol lower inhibitions as well. The prejudices of a group legitimize violent behavior: [18]

> Billy Ammons and Brian Hooks, both 18, and Tom Daugherty, 17, were convicted of first-degree murder in the 2006 fatal beating of Norris Gaynor, a homeless man. The attackers were White, and the victim was Black.

The U.S. Army guards who abused prisoners at Abu Ghraib in Iraq were acting in a social context that permitted and reinforced sadistic behavior.

GANGSTA RAP

Ghetto life is protrayed in rap videos that define the young, poor and disaffected as oppressed.[19] Gangsta rap is built around the image of the strong "hypermacho" male, who asserts his dominance and demands respect as a brave, countercultural criminal raging at mainstream society. He dominates women. He rebels against oppression and feeds strained race relations that can escalate gang violence.

Gangsta rap is an imaginary outlet for most young people, but for many it leads to prison. It clearly undercuts efforts to help males assume the responsibilities of parenthood.

After a spate of rapsters shootings in 2005, rap engagements were cancelled in Las Vegas, Nevada. The Nevada State Gaming Control Board now holds casino licensees accountable for violent incidents.[20]

HELLS ANGELS AND SKINHEADS

White motorcycle gangs like Hells Angels have existed in California for decades. These gangs are considered organized crime rather than street gangs.

In the late 1980s, the Skinheads were identified as the primary source of White street gang violence in California. They are racist gangs and usually are not turf oriented nor profit motivated. Their crimes range from vandalism and assault to murder. Generally, targets of their crimes include non-White, Jewish, homeless and homosexual individuals. The ages of both male and female Skinhead gang members vary from the early teens to mid-20s. They have graffiti and hand signs, including the letters "W" and "P" for White Power and the Nazi salute. Tattoos include swastikas and the letters SWP for Supreme White Power. They are associated with White supremacy groups, such as the Ku Klux Klan and the White Aryan Resistance.

FEMALE GANG MEMBERS

Three-fourths of gangs apparently have female members. In juvenile correctional institutions, about half of the boys and girls acknowledge gang membership.[21] Many Gangs have auxiliary female units, but few exist as autonomous gangs. Generally gang life for female members usually means being exploited by male chauvinism.

Many female gang members ran away from abusive families, including sexual abuse. Joining a gang can assert independence from cultural and class constraints as well. In one study, gang members became mothers at ages from 13 to 27. One quarter had their first baby by 17; half by 19; and three-quarters by 22.[22] An example of a gang mother in Madison, Wisconsin, is:

> Eighteen-year-old Kari Tha bought the bullets used in a shooting that wounded three people in August, 2005. She had a 2-year-old son and was pregnant at the time of her sentencing in October, 2006.

GANG PARENTS

Both boy and girl gang members are more likely to engage in sexual behavior that results in pregnancy than their non-gang counterparts. In one study of those in juvenile confinement, 40% of the girls had been pregnant one or more times, and 55% of the boys had conceived a pregnancy.[23] Some 42% of the boys and 19% of the girls first willingly had sex before the age of twelve. 100% of the boys and 98% of the girls had sex before the age of 17. These girls are twice as likely as boys to have had a sexually transmitted disease.

The Rochester Youth Development Study followed boys and girls from 13 to 22.[24] Of the male non-gang members 15% reported impregnating girls, whereas 32% of the short-term and 47% of the long-term gang members did so. Twenty percent of the non-gang members were fathers, whereas 22% of the short-term and 55% of the long-term members were fathers. Forty percent of non-gang member females became mothers compared with 61% of the gang members. Gang members contribute significantly to children in fatherless and motherless homes.

GANG PREVENTION PROGRAMS

The increase in gangs over the last two decades led to forming the National Youth Gang Center in the Office of Juvenile Justice and Delinquency Prevention to assist policymakers, practitioners and researchers in reducing adolescent gang involvement. Prevention programs range from diverting adolescents from joining gangs to interrupting gang formation. A variety of diversion strategies have been employed, including community organization, improving living conditions, early childhood programs, school-based programs, local clubs and after-school programs.[25] The *YouthRising* program is sponsored by Youth Service America and the Office of Juvenile Justice and Delinquency Prevention. It offers grants to engage high-risk and gang-involved youth in volunteer service. The 10,000 Men Campaign in Philadelphia is an example of proactive community action to deter gangs.

Formed in 1995, the Chicago Project for Violence Prevention (CeaseFire) takes a public health approach to violence prevention.[26] It relies on outreach workers, faith leaders and other community leaders to work with adolescents at high risk of violence by intervening in conflicts or potential conflicts and promoting alternatives to violence. It includes public education to change attitudes and behaviors toward violence.

CONCLUSION

The majority of gangs in the United States are composed of marginalized adolescents who seek a cause greater than themselves to gain status, security and power.

Gangs are particularly attractive to adolescents who have not formed solid attachment bonds with their own families and have been physically or sexually abused themselves. A gang becomes their family.

Gangs are firmly embedded in the illegal economy of poor neighborhoods. They may be linked to prison gangs and play a significant role in neighborhood social and political life. They are a growing challenge for our society. Latino gang membership especially is growing in the Northeast and South. Gangs are becoming sophisticated in the use of technology and computers to perpetrate crimes.

Prevention programs range from diverting adolescents from joining gangs to interrupting gang formation.

Gang members have higher rates of adolescent pregnancy and parenthood than non-gang members. Because of high levels of incarceration, gang members contribute significantly to the population of children in fatherless and motherless homes.

Part 7

CULTURE

Puccini's opera *Madama Butterfly* tells the tragic story of a 15-year-old Japanese geisha, Cio-Cio-San, the bride of U.S. Navy LT Pinkerton, who abandons her. While she remains faithful, he returns three years later with his American wife. Cio-Cio-San gives up the son she had with Pinkerton and commits hari-kari while the *Star Spangled Banner* plays in the background.

Giacomo Puccini, 1904
Madama Butterfly[1]

Cultural factors can shape the nature and intensity of evolving problems by dampening or amplifying the degree of adversity in any parent's life, but they are particularly influential for adolescents.

The developmental goals of adolescence are the same in all cultures—to prepare young people for responsible roles in their society. However, biological, societal and some cultural pressures in the United States encourage rather than discourage adolescent parenthood.

In many urban and rural areas, Black extended families have supplanted nuclear families that prevailed prior to the 1950s. These extended families are available to support adolescent parenthood.

Latinos in the United States emigrated at different times from over twenty countries, each with their own culture and motivation for coming to the United States. The traditional culture of Mexican-American families accommodates adolescents who marry and have children.

Generalizations about American Indians are fraught with exceptions because of differences between tribes. American Indian adolescent parenthood generally is higher than the national rate and usually is accepted by extended families. Unemployment is high on most Indian reservations as is resulting poverty.

In Islam, both males and females are expected to be chaste and to seek fulfilling relationships in marriage. In Islamic law, marriage is a civil contract rather than a sacrament and can occur at an early age. Growing numbers of Muslim women interpret the Qur'an in non-patriarchal ways.

The Hmong culture has a history of resistance, accommodation and transformation as an ethnic minority, first in China, then in Laos and now in the United States. Hmong immigrants have achieved significant progress since their arrival in the United States over thirty years ago while they maintain some of their marriage traditions.

Chapter 22

Cultural Influences
on Adolescent Parenthood

> The central conservative truth is that it is culture, not politics, that determines the
> success of a society. The central liberal truth is that politics can change a culture and
> save it from itself.
>
> Senator Daniel Patrick Moynihan[1]

Adolescence is the proving ground for the core functions of any society—socialization
and reproduction. From indigenous to modern societies, sexual and aggressive urges are
socialized by cultural values and traditions.

Virtually all cultures recognize that the capacity to conceive and bear children precedes the capacities required to enter adulthood. Incest taboos, pubertal circumcision
and rites of passage into adulthood delay childbirth in indigenous societies until their
young are deemed able to assuming the responsibilities of parenthood. Eastern cultures have family-arranged marriages for adolescent girls. Western cultures try to prevent adolescent pregnancies.

These cultural traditions are being challenged in developed countries by human
evolution that is moving toward earlier childbearing as adulthood is postponed far beyond puberty. Menarche now averages around twelve in the United States and is trend-
ing downward. Yet, adolescents are expected to postpone sexual intercourse until a delayed adulthood or to use contraception to prevent pregnancy in the face of strong
pressures to be sexually active.[2] In this context, adolescent parenthood can be seen as
a response to accelerated physical development, to frustrations created by delayed
adulthood in our society and to subcultural practices.

A girl's desire to become a parent may be consistent with her personal desires and with
her immigrant or indigenous cultural tradition that supports adolescent parenthood.

IMMIGRATION IN THE UNITED STATES

Immigrants come to the United States for a variety of reasons including joining families already in this country, employment opportunities and political persecution. Our

foreign-born population includes naturalized citizens, lawfully present aliens and un-documented aliens. Over a third are naturalized citizens.[3] Estimates of the undocu-mented immigrant population range from seven to eleven million, comprising up to 30% of the foreign-born population.

Children in immigrant families are the fastest growing segment of our nation's chil-dren.[4] One in five children in the United States has an immigrant parent. During the 1990s, the number of children of immigrants grew seven times faster than children of native-born parents. Ninety-three percent of these children were born in the United States and are U.S. citizens. By 2015, children of first generation immigrants are pro-jected to rise to 30% of the school population.

In 2004, the foreign-born population in the United States was at an all-time high: 34 million comprising nearly 12% of the population. Half of all foreign-born persons in the United States arrived in the last fifteen years. Yet in historical terms, this pro-portion of foreign-born is not exceptionally large—it rose to 15% during the early 1900s and fell to below 5% in 1970.

Recent immigrants to the United States are more diverse than in earlier decades. In the 19th and early 20th centuries, the majority were European. In the late 19th Century, French Canadians migrated south to mills in New England, supplanting Irish immigrants. Since the 1960s, Latin American and Asian immigrants have come in un-precedented numbers.

Today's immigrants speak many languages and are more dispersed across the nation than in previous decades.[5] In the West and Southeast, the foreign-born population in-creased by more than 100%—in some states more than 200%—during the last decade. These new receiving communities often lack support networks for immigrants.

The population projection for 2010 is as follows: White 65%, Latino 15%, Black 13%, Asian 4% and other 3%.[6] Minorities are expected to be almost half of the popu-lation by 2050.

ASSIMILATION AND ACCULTURATION

Assimilation is the process of merging into a host society. Acculturation is the process of adopting a host culture's values, symbols and language.[7] Assimilation is more im-portant than acculturation for successful adaptation to a society. People can strongly identify with their original cultures as long as they assimilate as productive citizens.

Generalizations about cultures have limited value because individual differences are inherent in any culture. Although often regarded as unchanging, cultures evolve as they come into contact with other cultures.[8] Change takes place because individuals find it to their advantage to do so. The history of America from the beginning has been a blending of European, Native American, African and Asian cultures all of which have created a distinctive American culture.

Assimilation

The United States has reinvented itself as an American society by absorbing new eth-nic groups. This ability has had a huge impact on creativity and economic growth from the Industrial Revolution to the high-tech growth of Silicone Valley.[9] Nearly 25% of all our scientists and engineers, 40% of engineering professors and more than 50% of Ph.D.s in engineering, computer science and the life sciences are from foreign countries. Communities with higher levels of diversity have better economic growth rates than homogeneous communities.

Groups whose presence is welcome are likely to experience a smooth transition through assimilation and acculturation to the middle class. They want to learn English, obtain citizenship, learn American history and become involved in American politics.

Groups whose presence is not welcome often assimilate in the underclass, bringing them into conflict with mainstream society.[10] In between are those for whom community resources facilitate social and economic mobility. Even if a group is resented by the mainstream, the support of others in the same group can be a source of strength.

Acculturation

Acculturation can be *unidimensional* or *bidimensional*. Unidimensional acculturation occurs along a linear continuum from non-acculturated to complete acculturation. In bidimensional acculturation, significant elements of the original culture are maintained while incorporating aspects of the new culture.[11]

Unidimensional Acculturation

European immigration to the United States during the late 19th and early 20th centuries was largely unidimensional with almost complete assimilation and acculturation through intermarriage between cultural groups.

Immigrants who came before the 1920s followed different paths at different paces and ultimately reached relatively equal socioeconomic positions even though there was initial resistance to acculturation.[12] They came from oppressive regimes and became Americanized on their own terms. Many southern and eastern European immigrants were not considered to be White. Immigrants from Southern Italy also had a negative view of schooling:[13]

> In Southern Italy, schools were maintained by the upper classes at the expense of the peasants. Few peasant children went beyond the third grade. On arriving in the United States, Southern Italian immigrant parents saw schooling as a challenge to their parental control and way of life.

Every immigrant group has some people who do well by moving out of the ports of entry and others who remain in ghettos. Immigrants from Asia have higher educational and occupational aspirations than many U.S-born Latinos, Blacks and Whites and assimilate and acculturate rapidly. Some immigrant groups experience better mental health than U.S.-born persons.[14] Others' mental health deteriorates as they adopt American lifestyles.

Every wave of immigration that fully assimilates and acculturates tends to view the next wave with suspicion. The earlier arrivals regard themselves as the "real Americans" and support immigration restrictions.

Bidimensional Acculturation

Current waves of Latino immigrants tend to have low educational and occupational aspirations and tend toward bidimensional acculturation with preservation of their language.

Tamar Jacoby, a Senior Fellow at the Manhattan Institute, sees maintaining a shared sense of American identity as a formidable contemporary challenge.[15] Some minority groups have not assimilated in mainstream society for generations. Though parts of our national identity are optional, most of it is not. Multiculturalism and diversity can obscure our American cultural identity that emphasizes tolerance, democracy and meritocracy. Contemporary Latino immigrants show a tendency to develop separate economies and social structures that hinder their assimilation and acculturation.

The social mobility that immigrants enjoyed over much of the twentieth century may not continue in the future.[16] Employment opportunities for immigrants are unlikely to provide the same advancement as did the rapidly expanding manufacturing sector a century ago.

A COMPARISON OF IMMIGRANT ASSIMILATION

More than sixty million people—about 22% of the total U.S. population—are foreign-born or of foreign parentage.[17] Twenty percent of children in the U.S. now live with at least one foreign-born parent; 80% of these children are American citizens, and nearly 50% speak English and another language at home.

In gateway cities such as New York and Los Angeles, immigrants and their children make up a majority of the population.

Comparative Social Mobility in New York City

Immigrants living in New York City and its environs from the Dominican Republic, Colombia, Ecuador, Peru, the West Indies, China, Taiwan, Hong Kong and Russia were compared with native-born Puerto Ricans, Whites and Blacks.[18] Adolescents from better-educated families typically went to college. Chinese adolescents were particularly upwardly mobile. They received support from more adults and had fewer siblings. They concentrated on education and forgoing childbearing. Asian-American families tended to be intact and influenced by filial piety and a reverence for education consistent with Confucianism. Forty-six percent of Chinese youngsters whose parents had only a high school degree or less went to college. The percentages for the other groups were under 19%.

Native Puerto Ricans with both poorly and even better-educated parents had especially low rates of upward mobility. Native Blacks showed downward mobility. They received less support from their parents, had children earlier and had less education.

The housing market funneled Puerto Rican and Black families into neighborhoods with declining schools where early parenthood was common. Of those working and not attending school, only 7% of the Chinese young adults had children while 62% of native Blacks had children followed closely by West Indians, Dominicans and Puerto Ricans. Childbirth clearly reduced educational attainment and hampered entry into jobs.

Native Blacks and Puerto Ricans had the highest one-parent homes, drug-infested neighborhoods, grade retentions and arrests with West Indians and Dominicans not far behind. Chinese and Russian adolescents had far less exposure to these risks.

Comparative High School Graduation Rates

Because high school graduation rates are not uniformly reported, significant discrepancies occur between analyses of them.[19]

According to the Manhattan Institute, the high school graduation rate for all students in 2003-2004 was 70%.[20] Graduation rates ranged from 22% in Detroit to 83% in Fairfax County, Virginia. Thirty-nine states increased their graduation rates from 2001 to 2003 while most southern states, Alaska, the District of Columbia and New York, showed declines.

Ethnic graduation gaps have been closing for four decades but remain substantial. For subgroups the graduation percentages were: Whites—78%, Asians/Pacific Islanders—72%, Blacks—55%, Latinos—53%, American Indians—51%, girls—72% (59% Black; 58% Latino) and boys—64% (48% Black; 49% Latino).

According to the Economic Policy Institute, the high school graduation rate during the same time was 82% when the retention of students in the ninth grade was taken into account.[21]

In 2005, Asian-Americans averaged a combined math-verbal SAT score of 1091, compared with 1068 for Whites, 982 for American Indians, 922 for Latinos and 864 for Blacks. Forty-four percent of Asian-American students took calculus compared to 28% of all students.[22]

CONTEMPORARY ADOLESCENT PARENTHOOD
CULTURAL PATTERNS

Throughout much of the world, girls still achieve social status largely through marriage and motherhood in the middle (15-17) to late (18-19) adolescent years.[23] In these cultures, adolescent parenthood usually occurs in the context of marriage, often arranged. Brides are expected to be virgins. Pregnancy is expected within the first two years of marriage, since children have economic value. In rural areas of Latin America, the pattern is similar except that young persons have more freedom to choose their partners.

Although marriage ages are increasing in most regions of the developing world, more than one-third of all women from 20 to 24 were married before 18. If present patterns continue, over 100 million girls will be married as minors in the next ten years. The practice of child marriage is perpetuated by a number of factors, such as gender discrimination; parental concerns surrounding premarital sex and pregnancy; dowry pressures; the perception that marriage protects from sexually transmitted diseases; and the desire to secure social, economic or political alliances. A poor family may calculate that marrying into another family will be to their advantage.[24] In most tribal societies, reproductive rituals cloaked by cultural symbolism are attempts by families to gain material advantage rather than to satisfy the needs of individuals. As a result, international human rights declarations advocate protections against child marriage by:[25]

- requiring that parties exercise "free and full consent" in the marriage decision and
- setting the minimum age of marriage at 18.

In Maylasia up to 25% of adolescents engage in premarital sexual activity. Many Philipino adolescents see virginity as important, but premarital sex is permissible when there is love and intention to marry. Filipino-Americans, the United States' second-largest Asian and Pacific Islander group, have more adolescent pregnancy and HIV infections than other Asian and Pacific Islanders.[26] One-tenth of Japanese adolescents are sexually active.

In rural Rajasthan, India, the mean age at which couples start living together is 15 for girls and 16 for boys.[27] Many couples go through a marriage ceremony arranged by their families much earlier, but they do not enter married life until later.

In Northern Bali, many couples engage in premarital sex to see if a female is fertile.[28] If she becomes pregnant, the male is likely to marry her. If she fails to become pregnant, he is likely to desert her, leaving her with a damaged reputation. Females must negotiate the treacherous path of attracting a mate and holding a reputation for chastity.

In many Asian societies, the sexual freedom that accompanies modernization has resulted in increasing numbers of young people turning to prostitution to generate money required to live in cities. As a result an increasing number contract HIV/AIDS.[29]

Prior to the 1970s, adolescent childbirth in the United States was handled in a variety of ways including marriage to an adult husband, adoption or child abandonment. These culturally defined arrangements did not include creating a family headed by either an adolescent mother or by adolescent parents as is currently the case.[30]

Under favorable economic conditions, immigrants who move from high-fertility to low-fertility regions ultimately adopt the reduced fertility patterns of their new country.[31] The challenge for immigrant parents in the United States is to bring up their children consistent with their cultural traditions and with successful assimilation into their new society. To do so, they must deal with our pop culture.

POP CULTURE IN THE UNITED STATES

Abetted by our pop culture, adolescent sexual intercourse is regarded as a part of growing up in many segments of American society.

Strong elements in our society encourage immediate gratification, impulsive actions and indulging fantasies.[32] Technological innovations supposedly designed to make our lives easier have fostered longer working hours and a sense of urgency. This social context discourages short-term restraint and long-term planning. It also makes it difficult for people to deal with problems outside their own lives, such as poverty, racism and adolescent parenthood.

The pop culture has drifted free from reality and tends to make adolescents more like participant-observers in their own lives, as if they are actors playing themselves.[33] They buy new clothing made to look old. They use drugs and alcohol to keep their authentic feelings at bay. They use steroids and body piercing to alter athletic abilities and appearances. The idea has taken root that we need not heed anxiety as a warning signal in our lives.

The actor Tom Cruise epitomizes contemporary celebrity life. Married twice with a son and a daughter and having a third child with his fiancée, Cruise said: "I can create who I am." He used Oprah Winfrey's sofa as a trampoline while shouting his love for his current fiancée.[34]

Rap/Hip-Hop

The original rap/hip-hops appeared in the 1950s initiating the "Hip-Hop Generation" and have united young people since.[35] Rapping, breakdancing, "call and response" singing and rapper expressions, such as "scratching" (making instruments "talk") come from African culture. Jamaican Blacks fused soul music, funk and disco as the Soul or Ska/Reggae Generation.

Hip-hop reflects an evolving strain of Black sentiment as did the emergence of the Blues during the days of Jim Crow.[36] It began in South Bronx as an expression of the hopes and nightmares of a generation afflicted by unemployment and spread throughout the nation providing a new definition of what it means to be "cool."

The negative influences of hip-hop on adolescent sexual behavior appear to be based less on sexual content and more on degrading misogyny.[37] Futures of fame, wealth, cars and exploiting women are envisioned. Exhibitionism is encouraged by seductive clothing and sexual, violent lyrics. Both "use-or-be-used" and "get-it-while-you-can" attitudes enhanced by alcohol and drugs create one's identity and confer personal power. Profane, violent language conveys the image that being Black is about music, sex, guns, drugs and living on "the street." In videos, females are pets to be walked on leashes and given profane names in pimping and prostitution:[38]

> In a New York City middle school stairwell, a 12-year old girl performed oral sex on a 12-year-old boy arranged by a 13-year-old girl, who was pimping for her 12-year-old girl friend.

Rap music has evolved into a medium of misogyny, materialism and murder. A rivalry between two rappers culminated in a shoot-out at a New York radio station, Hot 97, in 2005. The growth of this lethal genre of pop art testifies to an industry's greed and lack of self-control. As Orlando Davis, a Tampa rap personality, put it:[39]

> (It's) like a cancer, or like crack going though neighborhoods. . . Gangsta rap has been as destructive as the Klan (to Black culture).

Fueled by hip-hop music promoted by major corporations, what was once a code of silence among criminals, is now being marketed as "Stop snitchin"—a catchy hip-hop slogan that encourages not cooperating with the police.[40]

There is a trend toward more positive hip-hop.[41] The playright-musician Will Power wants to reverse the sense held by many young Blacks that they are destined to repeat the mistakes of their fathers and mothers. Byron Hurt's documentary *Hip Hop Beyond Beats and Rhymes* questions the degradation of women and homophobia seen in rap videos.

Media

American adolescents are exposed to self-defeating messages about sex through our unrestrained media.[42] Sexual intercourse often is depicted as a goal in itself with little reference to its risks and responsibilities. The intimate, affectionate aspects of sexual expression are dehumanized and depersonalized. Adolescents receive little information about the consequences of sexual activity and about the realities of marriage.

The media has been shown to affect a broad range of adolescent health-related attitudes and behaviors including violence, eating disorders and tobacco and alcohol use.[43] Research shows that television and film violence contribute to both a short-term and a long-term increase in aggression and violence in young viewers. Television news violence also contributes to imitative suicides and homicides. Video games are associated with increased aggression and violence.

Television plays a central role in the lives of adolescents, who watch an average of three hours a day. Many studies have shown that exposure to sexual content in music, movies, television and magazines accelerates adolescents' sexual activity.[44] An Associated Press poll found that most Americans think rude behavior is on the rise and blame parents for not teaching civility, the media for displaying rudeness and celebrities for being poor role models.[45] Common sense and research leads policymakers and parents to advocate regulating television content.

"Celebrity-moms" play a subtle but important role in encouraging adolescent motherhood. They suggest that anyone can "make it" if they just work harder, laugh more and buy the right products. Under the veneer of celebrity maternal joy and love lurks narcissism that trivializes the struggles and hopes of authentic women.

The Internet

While internet use among youth is widespread, differences in access across socio-economic lines exist. Eighty percent of Whites have internet access from home, compared to 66% of Blacks and 55% of Latinos. A study found that 59% of 15 to 24-year-olds believed internet pornography encouraged young people to have sex before they are ready; 49% thought it implies that unprotected sex is okay.[46] Forty-nine percent thought that it promotes oppressive attitudes toward women. Still, some women believe that criticizing pornography is reactionary.

Pop Culture Support of Adolescent Parenthood

In 2007 an Orlando, Florida, hip-hop radio station *102 Jamz* named a *Baby Mama* of the week. The winner received clothes and lunch with a celebrity, Fantasia Barrino, who, as a high school dropout pregnant at sixteen, inspired the song *Baby Mama*.[47]

Krishawa

On days when motherhood seems overwhelming, 17-year-old Krishawa Bostick, who attends Marchman Technical Education Center for high school parents in New Port Richey, Florida, said: "I can listen to *Baby Moma*[48] that says it's like a badge of honor to be a baby moma and it's like, okay, well, I'm not the only one."

In Krishawa's neighborhood, children were called "seeds." Her 8-month-old son's father was "My baby daddy." In the eight months after his birth, he saw his child two or three times. Krishawa did not know where he lived.

Jordan

Sixteen-year-old "baby momma" Jordan said:

> I think there's two different messages in Baby Mama. One, it's supporting those girls who are going through a hard time. But the other message is letting girls say, "Wow, it's okay." I would hate to see another girl go through what I'm going through. It's a scary thing. I don't know how to be a parent. I've never done it before.

ADOLESCENT PARENTHOOD IN OUR SEXUALLY ACTIVE SOCIETY

The National Center for Health Statistics notes that the contraceptive revolution in our society disconnected sex from pregnancy.[49] The sexual revolution disconnected sex from marriage. The legalization of pregnancy termination disconnected pregnancy from childbirth so that the birth rate went down as the pregnancy rate went up. These trends disconnected childbearing from childrearing marriage. As a result, Americans are less likely to marry, more likely to divorce and more likely to be single parents. Advertising directed at young girls encourages them to be sexually attractive. And many adolescents are sexually active.

Open acceptance of adolescent and adult sexual activity in our society leads to the belief that adolescent parenthood must be supported because little can be done to prevent it.

PREJUDICE AND DISCRIMINATION IN ADOLESCENT PARENTHOOD

Prejudice and discrimination play important roles in adolescent parenthood. Adolescent girls can be victims of sexism and ageism. If they are in a minority, they can be victims of racism as well. When adolescent girls of minority groups are encouraged to become, and are supported as, parents, sexism and ageism can be combined with racism.

Sexism

Until recent decades, early motherhood was the career of choice for White working class families, in part because of stereotyped roles for women.[50] Early marriages strengthened girls' identifications with their mothers and provided boys with socially sanctioned sexual gratification. The inroads made by feminists on sexism altered this pattern. Still, the sexist exploitation of females remains a powerful force as is apparent in the rape of adolescents by older men and dating abuse among adolescents. Boys maul and molest girls in video games.

A bias placing responsibility for the control of sexual activity solely on females was suggested when a judge in Panama City, Florida, told a woman to "close her legs and stop having babies."[51]

Ageism

Prejudice and discrimination based on age usually is thought of as neglect of the needs of the dependent elderly. But ageism also is expressed through neglect of the needs of children and adolescents. An adolescent requires a legal guardian and is not an independent person. When adolescent girls and boys are treated as adults and supported as parents, their own developmental needs are compromised. They are deprived of the opportunity to fully experience a vital stage in their physical, emotional, social and educational development. Treating their babies as their possessions reflects ageist prejudice and discrimination against the babies as well.

Racism

A latent bias against Blacks, Latinos and poor people having too many babies can lead to punitive actions against them.[52] Consequently, minority groups with the greatest exposure to racism may regard efforts to reduce adolescent pregnancy and parenthood as racist genocide.

Sensitivity to racial eugenics is crucial, but the claim that reducing minority adolescent childbirth constitutes genocide lacks credibility. Political agendas underlie the genocide argument. Increasing their numbers can be seen as the best way for a group to rise from minority status. Fear that a child adopted by persons of another race might experience discrimination and be unable to develop self-respect also can lead to opposition to trans-racial adoption.

However, accepting adolescent childbirth as an appropriate expression of any minority in contemporary society in the United States — "that's just the way they are" — reflects prejudice when it means continuing the disadvantaged status of minorities resulting from the cycle of adolescent childbirth. It also expresses the racist attitude that minority adolescents do not have the same aspirations as do White adolescents. It implies that minority adolescents and their families are incapable of using counseling that might lead them to make adoption plans.

Racism is evident when well-meaning persons and charitable organizations presume that early childbearing is inherent in Black and Latino cultures. It is racist to presume that they do not need to fully experience adolescent development as do White adolescents.

CONCLUSION

Adolescence is the proving ground for the core functions of any civilization–socialization and reproduction. From indigenous to modern societies, sexual and aggressive behavior is socialized by cultural values and practices.

The developmental goals of adolescence are the same in all cultures: to prepare young people for responsible roles in the society in which they live. Throughout much of the world, girls still achieve social status through arranged marriages and motherhood in the middle to late adolescent years.

Over one fifth of the population in the United States is foreign-born or of foreign-born parentage. High school graduation rates are related to the degree to which immigrants successfully assimilate and acculturate in mainstream society. The social mobility enjoyed by immigrants in the past may not continue in the future. Recent immigrants are tending to develop separate economies and social structures that hinder their assimilation and acculturation.

Some initially disadvantaged groups can achieve high rates of upward mobility. The parents of these adolescents have fewer children to support, hold high expectations for educational achievement and seek access to good schools.

As it now stands, some biological, societal and cultural pressures encourage adolescent parenthood: the earlier onset of puberty, the earlier initiation of sexual intercourse and the social and peer pressures for sexual activity abetted by commercial exploitation of sexuality. Overlooked is the likelihood that girls are the victims of sexism and ageism when they are impregnated. Minorities can be victims of racism as well. When minority girls are encouraged to become, and are supported as, parents, sexism and ageism combine with racism.

America's prosperity depends on the continued assimilation of new waves of immigrants who enrich our culture. We need to find common ground across cultures to encourage nurturing parents, education and productive citizenship.

Chapter 23

Black Adolescent Parenthood

Our elders saved us from action paralysis and self-pity by putting our present problems in spiritual and historical perspective. They shared lessons of the mighty oppression of slavery, of the great dashed promises of the Reconstruction, and of the violent Klan lynchings aided and abetted by powerful economic interests and a silent citizenry. They made us see that our individual struggles were part of an ongoing struggle for freedom and justice that had to be won over and over again and that never can be taken for granted. They also made us see that we did not have to fight these battles alone—that God was on the side of truth and righteousness, which would eventually prevail.

Marian Wright Edelman
Guide My Feet 19951

Black adolescent parents supported by their extended families today are reminiscent of the West African tribal structure cultivated during American slavery.[2] But during the first half of the twentieth century, Black nuclear families predominated. In 1965, the Moynihan Report reported the transition of Black and White families from nuclear to single-parent families.[3] This chapter reviews the historical, social and cultural context of contemporary Black families.

THE IMPACT OF SLAVERY

Both Whites and Blacks came to America as indentured servants in the 17th century. But only Blacks subsequently came as slaves, who were dehumanized in a pitiless racial hierarchy.

Dorothy Roberts, professor of law at Northwestern University, believes that Black women's reproductive decisions are rooted in slavery that valued fertility because it benefited the slave owner economically.[4] Slave women were given incentives to bear children and often were punished for failing to procreate. Their children were the property of their owners. Fertility determined slave women's auction prices. Roberts notes that by taking away the rights of motherhood, slave masters took away part of Black women's humanity and worth.

According to Roberts, slavery gave way to the icons of "Jezebel"—a sexually insatiable character—and "Mammy"—loyal to her master and his family. These historical images persist today in the current icons of "welfare queen" and "matriarch." In slavery, a Black man could not be a father or a husband and offer security or identity to a mother or a child.[5] This tradition in which mothers could not rely on the presence of fathers has resurfaced in today's ghettos.

THE EMERGENCE OF BLACK FAMILY LIFE AFTER SLAVERY

Hortense Powdermaker, professor of anthropology at Queens College, described an underclass of single mothers, peripatetic men and an undertow of crime and violence in the South following the Civil War.[6] Most sharecroppers lived in unstable common-law arrangements, except for a small Black elite. Non-marital births prevailed.

The century of segregation that followed slavery's abolition did little to end Black social isolation. Adolescent's children were raised in poor multigenerational families. The book *Cotton Field of DREAMS* depicts the lives of families in the Arkansas delta.[7] It memorializes James and Ethel Kearney who taught their seventeen children that nothing was out of reach if they put their minds and hearts into it. The Kearnys exemplified the faith and dreams of poor Black families.

The Black Nuclear Family

From the 1890s to the 1970s unwed parenthood was not a Black tradition in the United States. U.S. Bureau of the Census data reveals that before 1950 young Black women were more likely to be married than were young White women. In every census from 1890 to 1960 the percentage of Black households with two parents remained essentially unchanged at about 80%.[8] As the mechanical cotton picker created massive unemployment in the South from 1940 to 1970, five million Black southerners moved to Northern cities. They gave rise to the Black middle class, one of the great success stories of the 20th Century, but they also created urban ghettos.

The percentage of Black households with two parents dropped from 64% in 1970 to less than 40% in 1992, contradicting the assumption that unwed parenthood is a cultural tradition for American Blacks.[9] One survey reported that 77% of Black adults from 19 to 35 said they wanted to marry. A 2006 Gallup Poll found that Blacks were more likely than Whites to say that marriage is important.[10] Yet, young Blacks are losing hope that a good marriage is attainable.

Since the Great Depression of the 1930s, Blacks who moved out of urban ghettos to suburbs have shown a decrease in unwed births and female-headed households.[11] A significant number have created an elite Black upper class.

From slavery onward most Black families have prevailed over adversity.[12] Now most girls do not become pregnant. Most boys do not end up on the path of drugs, crime, incarceration and death. Enrollment of Black freshmen at the nation's highly ranked universities and liberal arts colleges has increased by nearly 10% since 1994.

A memoir: Marian Wright Edelman

Marian Wright Edelman, Executive Director of the Children's Defense Fund, was a child in the 1940s and 1950s in a small, segregated South Carolina town.[13] The internal world of her family and Black elders felt safe, nurturing and spiritually enriching. The external world of legal apartheid felt like a prison constraining and controling her mind, movements and dreams:

> White people and black people lived both totally separate yet totally intermingled lives. Most of the parents of my playmates and the members of my church cleaned and cooked in white folks' homes, raised white folks' children, and were the hidden, undereducated and underpaid labor cogs which kept Southern town life going. However, everybody knew the white and black families in our community who shared a common granddaddy or father.
>
> Much has changed in the South since my childhood years: some good and some bad. When I go home today, I can sit and sleep and eat in whatever public hotels and restaurants I can afford. But too many people still cannot find enough jobs to escape poverty and too many college-educated young people of both races can't wait to leave.
>
> The critical sense of community and spirituality that immunized my generation of children against external challenges appears weaker. 50 years ago many black adults refused to let external barriers become internal ones by wrapping children in a cocoon of caring and activity. They knew that the care of the mind and the body needed to be grounded in the care of the spirit, which was the glue that held our families and our community together.

COMPARISON OF CONTEMPORARY BLACKS AND WHITES

During the second half of the 20th century legalized and culturally sanctioned overt segregation and discrimination were effectively undermined. But during that same period economic inequality grew more rapidly than at any other time in our nation's history.[14]

The 2006 Urban League's Equality Index revealed that despite significant progress, the overall status of Black Americans was assessed at 73% of their White counterparts:[15]

- *Economic*—Black economic status 56% of White; unemployment 10% vs 4.4%.
- *Health*—Black health 76% of Whites, and life expectancy 6 years shorter.
- *Education*—Black educational status 78% of Whites
- *Social Justice*—Equality in sentencing and victimization 74% of Whites.
- *Civic Engagement*—Voter registration, volunteering and government service 104%.

The number of Black unwed mothers has increased because of jobless Black males.[16] As long as there are limited employment opportunities, remedial education, training, wage subsidies or other benefits will not enable members of the underclass to sustain stable family lives.

White girls are inclined to terminate pregnancies or make adoption plans. Black girls disapprove of these options for a variety of reasons.[17] A boyfriend may conceive a baby to demonstrate his masculinity and expect the girl's mother or grandmother to care for the baby.

Blacks are six times as likely as Whites to have been in prison at some time in their lives. At this rate, one in three Black males will be in prison at some time.[18] More needs to be done to end incarceration for non-violent crimes and to rehabilitate released prisoners.

Public Schools

There is no undisputed evidence for the genetic superiority of either race, but environmental factors contribute to the IQ gap between Blacks and Whites.[19] The cultural and psychological dynamics of Black academic underachievement are related to social inequality.

The disparity in wealth between school districts results in corresponding differences in the quality of teachers, courses, materials, equipment and facilities as reflected in the following 2005 survey of high school students by the U.S. Department of Education [20] (See Figure 23.1).

Ashley

The experience of being a successful Black student in a White environment is illustrated by Ashley, a 16-year-old 11th grade student at East High School in Madison, Wisconsin. She described being the only Black student in an Advanced Placement class:[21]

> I feel the need to prove to my teachers and classmates that I belong. I am expected to fail because some of my Black peers do. My presence allows white students and teachers to see many of us work to break down barriers.

Marriage

The lack of successful Black marriages grows out of a scarcity of marriageable men.[22] Blacks are less likely to cohabit around the time of a baby's birth; less likely to marry;

Category	White	Black
Teaching is good at my school.	82%	76%
I get along well with my teachers.	78%	61%
I like school a great deal.	21%	29%
I do not feel safe at my school.	9%	17%
Something was stolen from me at school.	38%	46%
I had a physical fight at school.	12%	20%
Grades are very important to me.	47%	62%
Education is very important in later life.	96%	98%
Subjects are interesting and challenging.	52%	63%

Figure 23.1.

and marry later than Latinos, who in turn are less likely to marry than Whites. Black divorce rates are higher than for Whites. Black women appear to benefit less from marriage than White women.

Married Blacks earn more, have higher levels of occupational prestige and are more likely to own their own homes compared to unmarried peers.[23] They report more happiness and fewer emotional problems. They are less likely to be involved in crime.

Compared with those in single-parent families, Black children living with their married parents are less delinquent, have higher self-esteem, are more likely to delay sexual activity, have lower rates of adolescent pregnancy and have better educational outcomes.[24] Married Black mothers' babies are healthier. Parental marriage is especially important for Black boys.

Black cultural values can be uniquely supportive of marriage as articulated in Martin Luther King's vision for a "beloved community."[25]

RACISM IN BIRTH CONTROL

Poor Black mothers have been blamed for perpetuating social problems by transmitting deviant lifestyles to their children. A *Philadelphia Inquirer* editorial noted:[26] The main reason more Black children are living in poverty is that the people having the most children are the ones least capable of supporting them.

In contrast, Dorothy Roberts says that reproductive liberty includes the right to bear a child even in the context of wealth and power inequities.[27] She points out that Black women were denied reproductive liberty in slavery, by sterilization during the 1960s and 1970s and by Norplant and Depro-Provera use in the 1990s. She sees reproductive control as perpetuating the view that racial inequality is caused by Black people themselves not by an unjust society.

In 1990, the ACLU's Reproductive Freedom Project found that 70% of pregnant women prosecuted for drug use were Black. Roberts points out that other substances are harmful to a fetus.[28] Although alcohol abuse far exceeds crack abuse, crack-addicted women are prosecuted more than alcohol-addicted mothers. This inequity led appellate courts to invalidate prosecution for drug use during pregnancy. The American Medical Association expressed concern about reporting drug use in pregnant women when it leads to their incarceration rather than treatment.[29]

RESPONSIBILITIES OF THE BLACK MIDDLE CLASS

Above all, the better classes of the Negroes should recognize their duty toward the masses. They should not forget that the spirit of the twentieth century is to be the turning of the high toward the lowly, the bending of Humanity to all that is human, the recognition that in the slums of modern society lie the answers to most of our puzzling problems of organization and life, and that only as we solve those problems is our culture assured and our progress certain . . .

W.E.B. Du Bois, 1899[30]

A large Black middle class is committed to education, civic involvement and responsible parenthood. Many who moved out of poverty want to help others do the same. On the other hand, fear of being dragged back into the ghetto life deters some from helping the less fortunate.

A Pew Research Center survey found that Blacks see a widening gulf between the values of middle class and poor Blacks. Nearly 40% say that Blacks no longer constitute a single race.[31] Sydney Duncan, noted social worker in Detroit, Michigan, sees three classes of Black families:[32]

- *Middle class*—It includes professionals and entertainers who see adolescent pregnancy as interrupting advancement and either use the extended family or agencies for informal and formal adoptions.
- *Working class*—It has two levels: one barely a pay check away from poverty and one a notch above with jobs in the service economy. When their adolescents become pregnant, they are likely to incorporate the child in the extended family.
- *Poor class*—They comprise 25% of the Black population but produce 50% of the children. Many are dysfunctional, often because of crack cocaine.

In 2004, Bill Cosby spoke to a National Association for the Advancement of Colored People meeting and criticized poor Blacks for not assuming more responsibility for raising their children. He brought out one side of a controversy shared by Juan Williams, journalist and commentator, that emphasizes the lack of personal responsibility as a greater cause of Black crime and educational shortcomings than racism.[33] That side implies that racism is used as a crutch. It reflects a desire for people to be seen as Americans without reference to race.

Michael Dyson, Black radio host and author, expresses the other side of the controversy.[34] He does not deny poor Black parents' problems, but he emphasizes the colossal barriers they face just getting up in the morning and making ends meet. He advocates a relentless effort to lift the poor through the hard work for which they often are given little credit.

Tavis Smiley, Black radio host and author, successfully surmounted abuse as an adolescent and became an advocate for resolving the political, economic and medical problems confronting Black society.[35] He edited *The Covenant with Black America* as a manual for action.

Juan Williams calls for a new generation of Black leadership to fill the vacuum left by those who abandoned the tradition of hard won pride and self-determination.[36] *Fortune* magazine writer, Cora Daniels, points out that Black business persons see the business world as the nexus of power rather than government.[37] Instead of seeking change through governments or churches, they are opening doors in the corporate world or building businesses themselves. Rather than fighting the power structure, they seek to take power to uplift the entire race. They embrace a Black world of shared culture and experience. The National Center for Black Philanthropy, Inc., was established in 1999 to promote Black participation in all aspects of philanthropy.[38]

Traditionally, Black women have been moral anchors and driving forces in supporting roles. Now they are rising to positions of leadership.[39] Daniels believes that women will dominate the next Black generation. She estimates that 24% of all Black women will be in the professional-managerial class compared with 17% of Black men.

The sobering reality is that if middle and upper-class Blacks are in the wrong place at the wrong time, or if they get into trouble with the law, or if they do something their White superiors do not like, they still may encounter prejudice and discrimination.[40]

Darice Jones

Darice Jones, a journalist, offered three steps for achieving Black unity:[41]

1) to really begin to reunite with our collective African power by understanding ourselves not just as survivors, but as innovators, creators, artists, storytellers, healers and educators;
2) to become better risk-takers by realizing ourselves as one big family and pulling our little sons and daughters out of foster care and youth facilities into our homes, whether we know the children or not; and
3) to become reacquainted with our history before and after the enslavement. As we honor and understand our legacy, it will be easier for us to live together without longing to live apart to feel important.

BLACK SOCIALIZATION

As with all ethnic groups, Black socialization is influenced both pro- and anti-socially by families, peers, neighborhoods, communities, the media and socio-economic status.[42]

Black Community Support

Arline Geronimus, a professor of public health at the University of Michigan, calls attention to the social support in Black communities for Black adolescent mothers:[43]

> Relatives actively contribute to the nurture of the young. This provides a form of "social insurance" against unemployment, loss of welfare benefits, homelessness, disability, imprisonment and premature death. Early childbearing makes it less likely that grandparents will have to compete with their own grandchildren for support from their adult children. It provides a larger set of descendants to support them as their risk of disability increases.

Parenting Styles

Overall, a mother's beliefs in her ability to influence her child and her environment are strong predictors of her child's academic success.[44] Adolescents whose parents provide consistent discipline are more successful than those who do not, especially in dangerous environments.

Preparation for racial bias is an important feature of parenting in ethnic minority groups. In one study, ethnic culture, history and pride appeared to be more prevalent among Black than Dominican or Puerto Rican parents.[45]

Black families prepare girls for menarche better than White families when they celebrate it as an important milestone without shame.[46] Black girls who have positive family relationships during puberty may successfully adapt to bodily changes in forming their identities.

"Acting White"

Philip Cook and Jens Ludwig, professors of economics at Duke University, followed 25,000 public and private students from the 8th grade through high school in North Carolina. They concluded that Black students were as eager to learn as White students although they dropped out of school slightly more than White students.[47]

Black young people are beset on all sides by myths about race.[48] The most poisonous one defines middle-class normalcy and achievement as "White," while embracing violence, illiteracy and drug dealing as authentically "Black."

Richard Sennett, a sociologist who grew up in Cabrini Green in Chicago, described the plight of the boys there:[49]

> You survive in a poor community not by being the best or indeed the toughest but by avoiding eye contact on the street, which can be taken as a challenge; in school if you are gifted you try to render yourself invisible, so that you will not be beaten up for getting better marks than others.

High achieving Black boys and girls may be accused of "acting White" by their peers. They become isolated when they also are not accepted by Whites. Even not having a baby can be seen as "acting White" by Black peers.[50]

Bob Herbert, a New York Times columnist, called attention to the pressures Black and Latino adolescents face when they try to advance themselves academically and socially. He quoted David Blocker and Ms. Jhingory:[51]

David Blocker

When 15-year-old David took a summer math course at a private prep school, he got an A-minus. When he came back to his regular school, he failed math. He said:

> The pressure was mostly to chill and, like, do what you want to do. People were not doing their work, just coming to school for fun, coming to school high, just playing sports, not really knowing what school was for. To be like everyone else, my sister turned into this wild child, this ponytail honey who was out there cursing and being bad and just didn't care.

Ms. Jhingory

Twenty-year-old Ms. Jhingory came face-to-face with the dilemma that many young Black adults encounter as they try to improve their lives by studying and going to college.

> When I went off to college, I eventually woke up from la-la land and realized that I would have to get an education and a job, something a little more concrete than fantasies about the hip-hop underground.

She noticed that when home on visits, some of her friends treated her differently.

I don't know if it was from jealousy or resentment or whatever, but they would say to me, "You're acting white now."

Threatened Group Cohesion

Signithia Fordham, professor of anthropology at the University of Rochester, and John Ogbu, former professor anthropology at the University of California-Berkeley, proposed that Black youths sabotage themselves academically by deprecating school achievement.[52] Ogbu suggested that Blacks from other countries come to the United States expecting to improve their lives. In contrast, Black Americans already in our society may not have this expectation.

Anthropologists note that social groups seek to preserve their identity when their internal cohesion is threatened. The more successful members enhance the power and cohesion of a group as long as they are loyal to it. But if a group risks losing them, the group tries to prevent the outflow. Amish communities are examples of threatened cohesive groups. They limit their children's education, fearing that contact with the outside world risks their survival.

Avoiding "acting White" also can be a way to cover up skill and knowledge deficiencies or the self-defeating feeling that White racists are correct about Black capabilities. But the economists Donald Austen-Smith and Roland Fryer affirm that the best strategy to preserve a minority group in school is to 1) signal loyalty to the group by reducing educational effort and 2) condition group acceptance on continued low educational effort.[53] They suggest this strategy can be broken by: increasing immediate benefits, such as cash rewards for good grades, and increasing immediate costs by meaningful penalties for disruptive behavior. Suspensions do not work. Conspicuous community service does.

The Social Context

In order to place "acting White" in the general social context, Duke University political scientists studied Black and White students in North Carolina and found:[54]

- There is a general sentiment against high academic achievement among adolescents in North Carolina regardless of race.
- There is no evidence of racial opposition to achievement in elementary school, suggesting "acting White" is not widely believed in the Black community.
- There is evidence of racial peer pressure against achievement in high school classes where Black students are underrepresented. In schools with 40% to 60% Black students, those in honors classes are likely seen as "acting White."

Roland G. Fryer, a fellow of the National Bureau of Economic Research, reviewed the literature and concluded that "acting White" is more prevalent in schools with more interethnic contact.[55] The pressure to behave in self-defeating ways was described by a father:[56]

"Dad, if I show them how smart I am, they say I'm trying to be white." My teenage son tried to explain why he was failing every class, despite having an IQ well above average. My Black son is failing because his peers will deny him both his identity and their friendship if he dares to succeed.

To gain friendship, even to be defined as a Black man, my son must hide his brain with the bigoted implication that all things "white" are to be avoided. He'll also hear he can't use his brain because white people victimize him.

"Cool-Pose" Culture

Psychologist Richard Majors and sociologist Janet Mancini Billson vividly described the behavior of some Black males in the United States in their book *Cool Pose*.[57] They point out that the unflinching self-assuredness of "cool" behavior has its origins in African tribal expressions of masculinity reinforced in the United States by slavery.

The "cool-pose culture" of young Black men consists of hanging out on the street, dressing sharply, sexual conquests, party drugs and hip-hop music.[58] This can lead Black boys and young men to believe that academic excellence is not "cool."

From his observations in Brazil and the Netherlands, anthropologist Livio Sansone sees the Black subculture as a mixture of protest and conformity.[59] He notes that following their tradition of musicality, sensuality and physical strength is the best way for Black males to gain status and make it in the White world. Not only is living in their subculture fulfilling, it brings respect from Whites as advertisements purvey hip-hop, professional basketball and "homeboy" fashions. The "cool-pose" feeds Black pride and affirms their disconnection from the mainstream and their unrealistic aspirations. Boys want to be street hustlers so they can someday cash in on grandiose fantasies of becoming celebrities as "gangsta" rap stars.

Howard Stevenson, professor of psychology at the University of Pennsylvania, sees "hypervulnerability"—a sense of vulnerability resulting from feelings of annihilation and dehumanization by others and society—as underlying the "cool pose".[60] Internalizing negative images of Black maleness promulgated by the media result in abusive relationships, dangerous behavior and hurting others to avoid rejection. The angst of this identity leaves many Black boys feeling "missed, dissed and pissed."

James Comer and Alvin Poussaint, professors of psychiatry at Yale and Harvard Universities, point out that racism continues to deny Blacks the secure feeling of being part of mainstream society.[61] They need encouragement to enter all fields. They need to know that only 1% of college athletes become professional rookies. Less become professional entertainers.

Rejection of Black Feminism

T. Denean Sharpley-Whiting, professor at Vanderbilt University, writes that Black feminism is not widely understood as a movement to end sexism, racism and male privilege, but as White and as a move to unseat aspiring Black men:[62]

> For many Black women feminism is the equivalent of kicking a Black man while he is down, kneeing him in the groin to make him holler, "Uncle" when we know full well that

groin will more likely be consumed by prostate cancer because of unequal access to health care.

Sharpley-Whiting adds that too much of our culture—both hip-hop and mainstream— gives men and boys every reason to continue gender violence.[63]

Hip hop culture offers sexual liberation and expressivity to young Black women, but the "new Niggaz" pose of sex and beauty really perverts freedom.

David Ikard, professor of English at the University of Tennessee, points out that many Black men have become oppressors, venting and displacing their anxieties, frustrations and rage on to Black women. In turn, Black women compound their victimization by becoming enabling agents, openly embracing self-sacrificial models of Black womanhood that reify patriarchy.[64]

Joan Morgan, journalist and author, crticized negative Black female relationships:[65]

Ain't a Black woman alive who hasn't experienced the jealousy, duplicity, backstabbing, and competitiveness sistas are capable of. What are you waiting for girl? You got the job, the house—when are you going to have a baby?

"White Guilt"

In *White Guilt*, Shelby Steele, Hoover Institution fellow at Stanford University, said that since the 1960s some Black leaders stimulate "White guilt" unlike Martin Luther King, Jr., who appealed to moral character.[66] For them racism is the core of Black life. Steele sees the absence of actual prejudice and discrimination as irrelevant to claims of victimhood:

"White guilt" is an incentive to exhibit racial woundedness. The result is a political identity that manipulates white guilt. We got remedies pitched at us for injustices rather than academic excellence—school busing, black role models as teachers, black history courses, "diverse" reading lists, "Ebonics," multiculturalism, culturally "inclusive" classes, standardized tests corrected for racial bias, and so on. Reading, writing and arithmetic? Later. Maybe.

The linguist John McWhorter sees separatism and "victimology" as obstacles to advancement.[67] Victim status is a source of sometimes lucrative leverage over a White guilt-ridden society. Bill Cosby and Alvin Poussaint, professor of psychiatry at Harvard University, wrote *Come on People* to inspire Blacks to shift from being "victims" to being "victors."[68]

BLACK FATHERS

Low levels of education and income are not in themselves insurmountable obstacles to fathers' involvement in their families.[69] Many Black fathers who live separately from their children and mothers are highly involved with their children.

At the same time, the lack of jobs or the inability or unwillingness to sustain employment contribute to the lack of involvement of fathers in the lives of their children. In inner cities, more than half of all Black men do not finish high school.[70] The share of young Black men without jobs has climbed relentlessly. In 2000, 65% of Black male high school dropouts in their twenties were unable to find work, not seeking work or incarcerated. By 2004, this had grown to 72%, compared with 34% of White and 19% of Latino dropouts. Even when high school graduates were included, 50% of Black men in their twenties were jobless in 2004, up from 46% in 2000—more than double the rates for White and Latino men.

Total incarceration rates reached historic highs in recent years.[71] In 1995, 16% of Black men in their twenties who did not attend college were in jail or prison; by 2004, 21% were incarcerated. By their mid-thirties, 60% of Black male school dropouts spent time in prison.

Two reasons have been advanced for the plight of young Black men.[72] First is the high rate of incarceration and subsequent flood of former offenders into neighborhoods who are shunned by employers. Second, the stricter enforcement of child support leaves young men overwhelmed with debt and deterred from seeking work where their earnings could be seized.

Curtis Brannon

Curtis Brannon, 28, told a typical story at the Center for Fathers, Families and Workforce Development in New York City.[73] He quit the 10th grade to sell drugs, fathered four children with three mothers and had been in jail for drug possession, parole violations and other crimes.

> I was with the street life, but now I feel like I've got to get myself together. I live in a flat with my girlfriend and four children. I get tired of incarceration. I plan to look for work, and I have not been locked up in six months.

The health of Black men is worse than for women.[74] Two-thirds of men in urban ghettos are likely to die before completing their productive years, not just from homicide or drug abuse. The principal killers are heart disease, cancer and chronic iilnesses that Whites face at later ages.

A Black mother's unresolved feelings about an absent father may be projected on to one of her sons who assumes the role of father surrogate.[75] These sons are seen as being like their fathers, who haunt their relationships. They show a precocious interest in sex. They may be unable to distinguish themselves from their fathers as unique persons in their mothers' eyes.

The positive influence of Black fathers in the lives of their children was illustrated by Oronde Miller, Executive Director of the Institute for Family and Child Well-Being:[76]

Oronde Miller to his father

> I remember when you sat me down in the family room and shared with me some of your observations of the American political and criminal justice systems, especially as they re-

late to African American families. Your message was neither exclusively about "personal responsibility" nor exclusively about "blaming the system." Instead it was about critical observation, study, and reflection, as well as our responsibility to be socially and politically engaged.

Mark Anthony Neal, professor of women's studies at Duke University, describes the New Black Man as strong in new ways: commitment to diversity in his community, support for women and feminism, faith in love and aware of the value of listening.[77]

THE BLACK GHETTO

The Black ghetto did not appear until Blacks migrated from the South after World War I. Several Black ghettos, especially Harlem, prospered until manufacturing declined in the 1970s.[78]

William Julius Wilson, former professor of Afro-American studies at Harvard University, vividly described the impact of de-industrialization on Black communities that became ghettos as their living conditions deteriorated.[79] The contemporary Black ghetto is a self-sustaining world with a set of contradictions and dilemmas, especially in attitudes toward adolescent parenthood.

The journalist Leon Dash interviewed Black boys and girls in Washington, DC.[80] He found they knew about sex and birth control as young as eleven. But their poor academic preparation, poverty and isolation from mainstream society all contributed to their becoming parents. Dash concluded, as did the Black child psychiatrist James Comer,[81] that successful students strove for high school diplomas, and unsuccessful students achieved recognition by having babies.

A 2004 Motivational Educational Entertainment Productions, Inc., survey revealed the attitudes and behavior of 2,000 Black adolescents.[82]

Most reported growing up in environments where sex is commonplace, marriage is rare, and teen parenthood is prevalent. They agreed that teen parenthood carries little stigma and can confer immediate "adult" status. They said that Black girls who choose not to have sex can feel unpopular, but those who give in to sex are often seen as good only for one-night stands.

Willingness to have unprotected sex with a steady partner may be seen as proof of fidelity. Many girls worried that "if I don't sleep with him, someone else will." Girls said they don't turn to each other for support, accusing each other of gossiping and "stealing" men. Some saw no point in marriage because "everybody cheats."

Girls reported they had little support from the adults in their lives. Some of their parents tried to act "young" and engaged in risky sexual behavior. Some tacitly or overtly approved becoming an adolescent parent.

Boys showed unspoken respect for girls who were virgins. Many sexually active boys and girls said they wished they had waited longer to have sex. They wanted to hear more about the emotional consequences of sex.

Despite the fact that over 60% had been sexually active in the last three months, most felt that pregnancy, STD's or other possible consequences of sex couldn't happen to them.

BLACK GANGS

Fights between White and Black gangs became commonplace following World War I.[83] In Chicago, White social athletic clubs—that city's version of New York City's political gangs—fiercely resisted penetration of their neighborhods by Blacks. The 1919 race riots were among the most serious eruptions of violence in the United States and were instigated by White gangs.

In major U.S. cities, the ideologies of groups such as the Black Panther Party, the Brown Berets and the Young Lords Organization attracted many adolescents away from gangs. They initiated community service agencies, started local businesses and obtained federal grants for education and job training. For example, the Conservative Vice Lord Nation, a Chicago gang that organized in the 1950s, began many social programs and businesses in the 1960s.

But the 1960s ended in a flurry of violence. Revolutionary organizations such as the Black Panther Party were broken up. Social programs run by gangs lost funding. Thousands of gang members and political activists were incarcerated. While the political groups disintegrated, gangs persisted and maintained ties to prisons. In the 1970s, James Jacobs, a sociologist and legal scholar, carried out a seminal study of Stateville, a maximum-security prison in Illinois, and demonstrated how prison life was linked back to the community through gangs.[84]

Gangs joined with revolutionary and Black Muslim groups in demanding better prison conditions. Some gangs adopted religious doctrines and rituals. But in the 1970s and 1980s, when many gang leaders were released from prison, the neighborhoods were even more rundown than when they left them. Since legitimate work was disappearing, gangs embraced the underground economy. The advent of crack cocaine allowed for profitable business plans. Violence soared in the late 1980s and early 1990s as gangs competed for crack markets.

Ironically, gang clothing, language and music have been commercially exploited worldwide. Black gang members adopt certain colors; blue for the "Crips" and red for the "Bloods." Some gang sets have special names, such as British Knights, where BK stands for Blood Killer, and Colonial Knights, where CK stands for Cop Killer.

THE NATION OF ISLAM

The Nation of Islam in the United States was founded by Wallace Fard Muhammad in 1930 as a social movement committed to changing the existing political and economic structure.[85] It was reorganized by Warith Deen Muhammad as the largest group of Black Muslims in the United States. When his father, Elijah Muhammad, died in 1975, he changed its name to the World Community of al-Islam in the West. He abolished the Fruit of Islam, the Nation's paramilitary organization, and eliminated dress codes for men and women. Ministers became imams and temples mosques. His focus no longer is solely on Blacks. He pursues inter-faith, inter-denominational alliances, including the Focolare Movement.

Louis Farrakhan is the current controversial leader of a reconstituted Nation of Islam whose national center is in Chicago. He warns that Black adolescents are being demonized by hip-hop's gangsta posturing. His advocacy of a drug-free, moral society with Blacks sharing their material and moral gains with fellow Blacks may make him a positive role model.

The Nation of Islam is seen by some as incompatible with mainstream Islam and by others as exploiting its adherents. But, according to James Baldwin, Elijah Muhammad was able to do what generations of welfare workers, committees, resolutions, reports, housing projects and playgrounds failed to do:[86]

> to heal and redeem drunkards and junkies; to convert people who have come out of prison and to keep them out; to make men chaste and women virtuous; and to invest both the male and the female with pride and a serenity that hangs about them like an unfailing light.

CONCLUSION

Many contemporary Black families have extended families reminiscent of the West African tribal structure cultivated during American slavery rather than the nuclear family that prevailed in Black families in the first half of the 20th century.

In today's inner cities profoundly affected by the lack of jobs, the re-entry of ex-convicts and the enforcement of child support deter young men from marriage and from employment where their earnings could be seized.

The prevalence of avoiding "acting White" in racially mixed schools suggests that social pressures play a role in the ethnic gaps in SAT scores; the underperformance of Blacks in schools; and the lack of representation of Blacks in elite colleges and universities.

Underlying the Black "cool pose" attitude, grandiose fantasies of becoming celebrities vie with awareness that hard work and education are essential for success.

The last forty years have created a large Black middle class, in which many persons feel a need to help others gain economic and political security. In contrast, the advent of crack cocaine led to the development of profitable business plans for gangs that persist to this day.

Motivations for adolescent parenthood arise from limited life goals. Successful students strive for high school diplomas, and unsuccessful students achieve recognition by having babies. There is social support in Black communities for Black adolescent mothers and fathers.

Chapter 24

Latino Adolescent Parenthood

A quinceañera celebrates a girl's fifteenth birthday. Originally signifying eligibility for marriage, it now signifies that a girl is ready for dating.

Roberto Suro, 1994
Strangers Among Us[1]

The original explorers and settlers in America were Spanish. The first permanent settlement in the United States was Spanish at St. Augustine, Florida, in 1565. As late as 1783, Spain laid claim to roughly half of the continental United States.[2] Its discoveries spurred the English to colonize North America.

Latinos now come to the United States as immigrants and as temporary workers who return to their homes. They come from countries with unique traditions and perspectives. Puerto Ricans in New York are different from Cubans in Miami and Mexicans in Los Angeles. Most Latinos are Mexican, but Puerto Ricans comprise a significant group that holds U.S citizenship.[3]

There are three patterns of Latino acculturation.[4] The first is assimilation and acculturation embracing American traditions and life styles over one or more generations. The second is assimilation while retaining Latino identities and language. The third is neither assimilation nor acculturation and isolation from mainstream society.

DEMOGRAPHICS

The number of Latinos in the United States has grown from 500,000 in 1900 to 40 million in 2005. They now comprise the largest minority in the United States, making up over 15% of the total population and 17% of the adolescent population.[5] The Latino adolescent population will grow by an estimated 60% over the next 20 years.

Sixty-five percent of Latinos in the United States are Mexican.[6] The next largest group is Puerto Rican at 10%. Latinos comprise 20% of the population in Texas, 32% in New Mexico and 21% in California. These figures are projected to increase by 25%

in 2020. One third of the Latino population is under 18. One third of Latino immigrant families live in poverty.[7]

The Mexican-born population in the United States has increased dramatically over the last 30 years. Until the 1980s, they migrated to the United States at modest rates—50,000 a year.[8] When the Mexican economy collapsed in the 1990s, the rate began to exceed 500,000 a year.

Mexicans currently constitute 30% of all of the foreign born in the United States. In 2003, more than 20% of all Latinos were living below the poverty level compared to 25% of Blacks and 8% of Whites.[9] In 2001, two-thirds of Latinos under 18 lived in two-parent homes.

LATINO ACCULTURATION

While past waves of European immigration generally had a beginning and an end, Mexican immigration has been virtually continuous for the last century.[10] Mexican Americans include unassimilated newcomers who have been regarded as foreigners longer than other ethnic groups. Mexican immigrants remit back to Mexico over $20 billion a year.[11] These remittances improve living conditions, but they also leave towns bereft of men and fuel inflation. Some Mexicans immigrants are not as attached to their families as those who do not emigrate.[12]

According to Lionel Sosa, an advertising and marketing executive, some Mexican Americans and other Latinos have attitudes that obstruct moving into the main-stream:[13]

- *Resignation of the poor:* "It's good to suffer in this life because in the next you will find eternal reward."
- *Low priority of education:* "The girls don't really need it. They will get married any-way. And the boys? It's better they go to work to help the family."
- *Fatalism:* "We must not challenge the will of God. The virtues so essential to suc-cess in American business are sinful."

In addition to these traditions, the American Dream for Latinos can be frustrated by racism and economic exploitation.[14]

Herman Badillo, the nation's first Puerto Rican-born Congressman, urges Latino parents to stress education with their children.[15] He hopes that this may stem the "five-hundred year siesta" Spain induced in Latin America, which is now "exporting its poor to the United States."

The longer Latinos live in the United States, the better their jobs and the higher their incomes. But the continuing influx of unskilled newcomers depresses the overall sta-tus of Latinos.[16] From 1994 to 2006, median Latino household income rose 20% to $37,800 a year. During that time, the percentage of 18- to 24-year-old Latinos who graduated from high school or obtained a general equivalency diploma rose from 56% to 66%. Twenty-five percent were enrolled in college, up from 19% in 1994.

The Importance of Language

Latino adolescents live in two societies:[17] one at home where they adhere to the traditional values of Latino culture and speak Spanish and the other in school and the community at large. Schools are ill-equipped to compensate for their accumulated disadvantages.

The more Latinos speak Spanish, the more conservative they tend to be on social issues and the more fatalistic they tend to be about their own lives. The more English-speaking they are, the more they hold mainstream views.[18] In one survey, nearly 60% of Spanish speakers compared to 15% of Whites were so fatalistic they saw no point in planning for the future. In contrast, 75% of second-generation English speaking Latinos felt that they were in charge of their lives.

Eighty percent of third-generation Mexican-Americans cannot speak Spanish.[19] Rapid assimilation can have negative effects for Latino adolescents as they become less subject to parental control. They are more likely to adopt the attitudes and cultural styles of U.S.-born disaffected adolescents. An extensive literature indicates that a higher assimilation rate for Latinos is associated with younger age at first intercourse, adolescent pregnancy, premature birth, low birth weight and neonatal mortality as well as undesirable maternal behaviors, such as smoking and drug use during pregnancy and decreased breast feeding.[20]

Latinidad

Puerto Ricans and Mexicans in Chicago articulated the idea of Latinidad, a political project that questions the American national identity and privilege in the United States.[21] It aims to educate others about Latino cultures and needs and to promulgate their arts.

Commercial marketing and contemporary multiculturalism promote Latinos as comprising a nation within the United States with a distinct culture and language. It appeals to contrasting images of the moral, spiritual Latino and the materialistic Anglo.

Chicanoism

Chicanoism merges Mexican and U.S. cultural elements in an effort to establish a unique identity. The melting-pot model is seen as unachievable and undesirable.[22] Chicanoism bridges difficult choices for adolescents between traditional virginity and family ties and mainstream sexual activity and competition. Family networks are highly valued and are critical to maintaining a Chicano code of honor. Chicano families take pride in helping each other in emergencies and periods of unemployment and through childcare.

LATINO SEXUALITY

Growing up Latino often is growing up Catholic with the belief that God blesses those who get married and have large families. The Virgin Mother is one of the most important religious symbols for Latino Catholics, symbolizing the sexual purity of women.

The Patriarchal Tradition

Gender roles are prominent in traditional Latino families. For a male virility, prowess, honor and providing for his family are strong values. In this "machismo" context, males may be encouraged to be sexually active from adolescence onward. In contrast, Latinas are expected to show the patience and forbearance of "marianismo."[23] The role of an honorable woman is self-sacrificing and subservient to her husband.

The strong patriarchal orientation of Latinos places the control of sexual relations largely with males. The honor of a man is besmirched if his daughter is not a virgin at the time of marriage. The husband-wife bond may be based more on procreation than on companionship. Since an unrelated man and a woman may become sexually involved when together, only male relatives can be trusted with women. This creates a dilemma for Latino parents. Freedom risks a daughter's loss of her virginity, but close supervision risks alienating her.[24]

The *Quinceañera*

A *quinceañera* celebrates a girl's 15th birthday.[25] Originally signifying eligibility for marriage, it now signifies readiness for dating. In this context, although her sexual behavior may be considered shameful, after the initial shock and anger her family often supports a pregnant adolescent and looks forward to the birth. The girl often marries or lives with the father. Leaving school is more acceptable for Latinas than non-Latinos.

> Eighteen-year-old Lorene Rodriguez in New York City was six months pregnant when she said: "I think it was just the influence of seeing all my friends getting pregnant and having kids that made me want one too."[26] Lorene is unemployed, has no high-school diploma and lives with her parents. The baby's father, an older Dominican immigrant, who has fathered three other children, does not make enough money to support them. As one 16-year-old girl put it: "When you are pregnant, you are a queen."

Parent-adolescent Communication

A National Campaign to Prevent Teen Pregnancy Survey of Latino adolescents found:[27]

- Almost half said they have never had a helpful conversation with their parents about sex, yet 82% of their parents said they had such a conversation. Parents consistently underestimate their adolescents' sexual involvement.
- 68% said they do not share their parents' values about sex, even though an equal percentage of parents think their offspring do.
- Almost three-quarters of the girls regretted having sex too soon.

- Over half of the girls said it is acceptable to date older boys and men.
- Over half of the girls said they receive the message that looking sexy is important.
- Only 38% said being an adolescent parent will keep them from reaching their goals.
- Two-thirds agreed that boys often receive the message they are expected to have sex.
- 40% of the boys agreed that adolescent pregnancy is "no big deal."
- Three-quarters of the adolescents and parents agreed that parents give inconsistent messages to their sons and daughters.

Latino parents apparently are less likely than White and Black parents to know their adolescent's friends.[28] Most Latino adolescents are close to their parents and feel a strong sense of responsibility to them but do not think they can offer useful advice. Their parents may need their help with business affairs. Some adolescents drop out of school to help support their families.

Robert Suro, director of the Pew Hispanic Research Center, described his experience with a Latino family at the time of a *quinceañera*:[29]

> I interviewed a girl just turned 15 in a very solid family with four children and strong Mexican family values. They organized a *quincenera*, spending a lot of money and invited all their friends. The next day she announced at breakfast that she a) was pregnant, b) was dropping out of school, and c) was going to move in with her Mexican-American boyfriend, who didn't speak Spanish and whose family lived on welfare. The father and mother had absolutely no idea that she had been living an entirely different life.

Latino parents need assistance in talking with their adolescents about sexuality and pregnancy prevention, especially fathers and sons. The Latino concept of *personalismo* places great importance on exchanging sensitive information privately.[30] Group discussions about adolescent pregnancy are likely to be more awkward than one-to-one conversations for them.

Machismo is harmful when *macho* boys think they are invincible and do not need condoms. But *machismo* in the form of male responsibility for family support can be used to promote greater male responsibility for sexual relationships as well.

MARRIAGE

There are significant differences in the ways in which Mexican-Americans approach marriage compared to Blacks and Puerto Ricans who live in the same socioeconomic circumstances.[31] Although extramarital affairs for men are tolerated, there often is anguish when an unmarried woman becomes pregnant. Mexican Americans are more likely to marry after the birth of the first child than Puerto Ricans, who are more severely affected than Mexican Americans and Blacks by family breakups and poverty.

The traditional, religion-based cultural pattern of Mexican-American families took for granted that all men and women would marry and have children, and many did so as adolescents. Childbearing was considered the ultimate fulfillment of a woman's life.[32]

The good woman is a wife and a mother. She is non-erotic and saintly. She tolerates her husband's sexual needs and does not develop her own sexuality.

In Mexico, husbands sometimes are more sons of their mothers than they are husbands.[33]

RISKS OF ADOLESCENT PARENTHOOD

The children of undocumented immigrants born in the United States are U.S. citizens. This can provide an incentive for immigrant females of all ages to give birth in the United States.

A survey of Latino and Black adolescent males in Houston, Texas, revealed that 90% had high-risk behaviors, such as failing subjects in school, sexually transmitted diseases, drug and alcohol use, smoking, delinquency and conceiving pregnancies.[34]

More than 50% of Latino boys and about 40% of Latina girls have had sex, similar to the general population.[35] However, fewer Latina than White and Black adolescents report using contraception the first time they have sex. Despite Catholic opposition to birth control, Latinos usually use contraception for birth spacing or to limit family size.

Over one-third of Latinas reported their first male partner was four or more years older. Latina adolescent mothers are more likely than White or Black mothers to say that their pregnancy was intended. Latino boys are more likely than White or Black boys to report they would be pleased if they got a partner pregnant. One boy said:

Once I became a parent all of a sudden I got a lot more attention from my family. Before I only got attention when I did things wrong.

When there is unemployment, inadequate education and low social status, motherhood can be attractive to Latino adolescents who live in a cultural context in which motherhood has high social value.[36] This attitude often does not prevail when opportunities for self-development for both boys and girls are available.

Rates of Latina adolescent pregnancy and birth have not declined as much as for other groups. Between 1990 and 2000 White adolescent pregnancy rates declined by 28%, Black by 32% and Latino by 15%. Because of the increased number of adolescent Latinas, the number of births actually increased.[37] Twenty-three percent of all adolescent pregnancies and 30% of all adolescent births in the U.S. are to Latinos. Fifty-one percent of Latino girls are pregnant at least once before the age of twenty— 20% higher than the national average.

Adolescent mothers in largely Latino neighborhoods are more likely to be married than other adolescent mothers.[38] However, negative or ambivalent views on birth control and pregnancy termination and socioeconomic disadvantage combine to create an environment conducive to unwed adolescent childbearing without marriage. Consequently, 80% of Latina adolescent mothers live at home one year after giving birth.

LATINO GANGS

Latino gangs differ from their Black and Asian counterparts.[39] Homicides among Latino gangs often are displays of manhood. Black gangs typically fight over drug trade issues. Asian gangs' usual crimes are extortion and home invasion.

Many females in gangs adhere to a mixture of traditional as well as gang values. Many are not treated well, yet they remain with abusive males.

Latino gangs play an important role in adolescent pregnancy and parenthood. In Chicano gangs studied by Joan Moore, professor of sociology at the University of Wisconsin-Milwaukee, one third of the members were girls.[40] Forty-three percent of the females but only 19% of the males regarded parenthood as a turning point in their lives. When gang girls become pregnant, they may leave the gang or leave their children with relatives and continue to tag along with their male companions. They also may marry gang members with resulting unstable marriages.

Cholo

The term "Cholo" refers to a fashion style and to families in which members engage in illicit activity and fail to control their children.[41] "Cholo" families teach their children to lie to social workers, law enforcement officers and teachers to cover for their wayward parents.

MS-13

A violent civil war began in El Salvador in the 1980s and lasted more than twelve years. Some 100,000 people were killed, and more than one million fled to the United States.[42] Some had ties with La Mara, a violent El Salvador gang. Others had been members of paramilitary groups like the Farabundo Marti National Liberation Front (FMNL). Many had been guerilla fighters.

Most of the Salvadorian refugees settled in Latino neighborhoods in Los Angeles. They were not accepted by the communities and were frequently targeted by local gangs. In response in the late 1980s, members of La Mara and FMNL formed the Mara Salvatrucha (MS-13) gang. MS-13 quickly became violent and continues to be fed by refugees from El Salvador. It has an estimated 10,000 members in the United States and 50,000 in Central America. Together with the Los Angeles 18th Street gang, the combined membership may be closer to 25,000 in 30 states.

In general, MS-13 members show no fear of law enforcement. They have executed federal agents and shot and booby-trapped law enforcement officers.

LATINO/BLACK RELATIONS

Families are important to both Blacks and Latinos. Latinos who are proud of their own ethnicity tend to rate Blacks more positively than those who are not. Promoting Latino pride tends to increase positive attitudes toward Blacks.[43]

The Latino belief that government programs favor Blacks probably is related to Latinos encountering Black employees in public service settings, where they may see them as cold and distant if not hostile. Blacks in turn may see Latinos as foreigners.

The more Black and Latino leaders impress on their followers that the two groups have common interests, the greater the chances for unifying them around common causes.

CONCLUSION

Latinos come to the United States from over twenty countries, each with their own culture and motivation for emigrating. Most are Mexican.

Mexican immigration has been virtually continuous for the last century, increasing dramatically over the last 30 years. Second and third generation Mexican Americans usually assimilate and move up the economic ladder.

Religion has a strong effect on Latino sexuality and reproductive behavior. Growing up Catholic is a part of growing up Latino. God blesses those who get married and have large families. Still, most Latino adolescents do not think their parents can offer useful advice.

Puerto Ricans and Mexicans in Chicago articulated the idea of Latinidad, a political and commercial project that questions American national identity and privilege in the United States. Chicanoism merges Mexican and American cultures in an effort to establish a unique identity.

When there is unemployment, inadequate education and low social status, motherhood can be attractive to Latino adolescents who live in a cultural context in which the role of mother has high social value. The children of undocumented immigrants born in the United States are U.S. citizens, providing an incentive to give birth in the United States.

Having their own children leads many of the girls in gangs to rethink their lives at least temporarily. The MS-13 gang fanned out across the United States from ethnic enclaves in California. Together with the 18th Street gang, also based in Los Angeles, the combined membership may be close to 25,000 in over 30 states.

Promoting Latino ethnic pride tends to increase positive attitudes toward Blacks. Family ties are important to both Blacks and Latinos.

Latino culture's warmth, love of children, respect for the elderly and parenthood and exuberance for life are strengths. All of these can be preserved without adolescent parenthood.

Chapter 25

American Indian Adolescent Parenthood

> I was never allowed to go out alone after I was that way the first time (menarche). That was the custom. And that's why in the old days no girl had a baby until she was married; now every little girl has one. All that has changed since the Whites have come.
>
> Red Lake Chippewa grandmother[1]

There are 562 federally recognized tribal governments in the United States. Although the federal designation is American Indian/Alaska Native, many people prefer their own tribal name or another name, such as Indigenous Peoples or First Nations. Nearly 70%—2.8 million—live in or near cities.[2] Generalizations about American Indians are fraught with exceptions.

Because of treaties, federal statutes, executive orders and court decisions, the federal government has trust responsibilities for American Indians. Those residing on reservations have a unique political status subject to federal but generally not to state control.[3]

The American Indian population is young and growing faster than the national average with 60% under the age of 25.[4] A few tribes have dramatically bolstered their economies through casino gaming. Improved living conditions tend to reactivate tribal traditions.

PUBERTAL INITIATION RITES

In the past, American Indian societies had widely varying traditions regulating sexual practices.[5] Although pubertal rites of passage have largely disappeared, two examples in Navajo and the Ojibway tribes are worth noting.

The Navajo Ha Mah Tee pubertal ceremony for a boy when his voice changes and the Kinaaldá ceremony for a girl at the onset of menstruation are the first steps on the path to adulthood, which takes several years to complete.[6] Young people receive guidance from elders in the responsibilities of men and women and in sexual matters.

The onset of menstruation is announced to the community in a four-night Kinaaldá ceremony with special rituals. Until the 1960s, Navaho maintained the tradition that menstruation indicates readiness for marriage.[7] Helen Williams, a Navajo Culture teacher at Ganado Middle School, sees girls behaving less respectfully of others and encourages them to participate in the Kinaaldá ceremony.[8]

In the Ojibway tradition, when a young male was deemed to have reached the age of understanding by the elders and was ready to be inducted as a full member of the tribe, his parents were given notice of his initiation through the performance of the Hah-Mah-Tsa ceremony.[9] In the four-day ceremony of fasting and meditation, the initiate chooses between selfishness and selflessness. If he chooses the latter, he will be admitted to the community.

Yurok Indian women in California traditionally viewed menstruation as spiritually potent and as a potential route to knowledge and wealth.[10]

MARRIAGE

In early American Indian Societies, as soon as a girl reached menarche and adult status, she and her parents began making plans for her marriage. In the Papago tradition, marriages of girls were arranged by parents.[11] When she left home, she became part of her husband's family and was expected to obey her mother-in-law. She would have no contact with her family unless arranged by her husband. These practices persisted until the mid 20th century. Contemporary remnants are seen when extended families expect young marriages.

Most tribes traditionally viewed woman as the natural complement to man.[12] Premarital chastity often was a cultural ideal, but young people were allowed a certain amount of dalliance. As examples, Natchez girls did not attempt to conceal their sexual exploits. When an unmarried Huron girl discovered her pregnancy, her lovers came to her, each saying the child was his. She picked the man she liked best to be her husband.

ADOLESCENT PREGNANCY AND PARENTHOOD

The American Indian adolescent childbearing rate generally is higher than the national rate except in Kansas.[13] Almost 2% of American Indian births are to mothers less than 15 years old—seven times the national average.

Christianity successfully penetrated Indian cultures, bringing shame and guilt regarding sexuality, which previously was largely regarded as a natural human expression. Still adolescent pregnancy usually is not seen as shameful today in some tribes. Pregnancy termination is uncommon when adolescents' babies are seen as gifts from the Creator.[14]

HEALTH

The general health status of American Indians is lower compared to other Americans, including sexually transmitted diseases.[15] Life expectancy is lower, and infant mortality is higher. The death rates from alcoholism, tuberculosis, diabetes, accidents and suicide are higher. Approaching these problems requires an understanding of their life circumstances, including substandard education, poverty, limited access to health services and cultural differences.

Unhealthy behaviors are substantially greater among American Indians compared to other populations.[16] Eighth, 10th and 12th grade students report higher uses of cigarettes (32%), alcohol (47% tied with Latinos) and marijuana (22%) compared to other ethnic groups. Poor diet and lack of exercise contribute to adverse health outcomes. The rates of injury, mortality, morbidity and suicide for American Indian adolescents are almost double the national rate. Alcohol-related deaths are 17 times the national average. A survey of the Red Lake Indian Reserve in Minnesota revealed that 81% of 9th grade girls and 43% of boys had considered suicide.[17] Nearly half of the girls and 20% of the boys said they had attempted suicide. A despondent 16-year-old, Jeff Weise, shot eight students and himself. One was a 15-year-old father.

All of these health problems occur in the context of a loss of strong cultural identities, limited opportunities and contemporary discrimination stemming from a history of oppression.[18]

POVERTY

The average unemployment rate in most Indian reservations is 45%, although in some it can be as high as 90%.[19] Thirty percent of those who are employed live below the poverty level. Even when American Indians move to urban areas from reservations, their participation in the labor force is low. Comparative median earnings in 2005 for males were: Asian $48,693; White $46,807; Black $34,433; American Indian $33,433; Latino $27,380.

Forty-three percent of American Indian children below the age of 5 live below the poverty level. They are less likely to reside with two parents than the national average.

EDUCATION

For over a century, many American Indian children and youth were educated in institutions away from their reservations. In Indian boarding schools, many children were victims of sexual and physical abuse. Off-reservation schools resulted in inter-tribal marriages, the blending of traditions and mixed tribal children.

In tribal schools now, American Indians have the lowest educational attainment of all groups in the United States. Fifty-one percent complete high school or its equivalent, and less than 15% obtain a college degree.[20]

CRIME AND TRIBAL LAW ENFORCEMENT

In 2004, the property crime arrest rate for 10- to 17-year-old American Indians was less than half and the arrest rate for violent crime was 9% higher than the general population.[21]

Tribal Healing to Wellness Courts are components of tribal justice systems that offer opportunities for communities to address alcohol and drug abuse through supervision, drug testing, treatment services, immediate sanctions and incentives, team-based case management and community support.[22] This non-adversarial system reflects traditional American Indian problem-solving methods that restore persons as contributing members of their communities.

GANGS

In 2000, 23% of tribal communities reported adolescent gangs, which are expanding across the nation.[23] The extent of the gang problem varied considerably among communities. On average, 80% of gang members were male, and 20% were female. Although some gang members were involved in crime, their activities most often were limited to graffiti and vandalism.

NATIONAL AMERICAN INDIAN ORGANIZATIONS

The Bureau of Indian Affairs administers and manages 56 million acres of land held in trust for American Indians and Alaska Natives.[24] Developing forestlands, leasing assets on these lands, directing agricultural programs, protecting water and land rights, developing and maintaining infrastructure and economic development are all Bureau responsibilities. It also provides educational services to approximately 48,000 Indian students.

Because of the diversity of American Indian tribes, national organizations have been formed for clearinghouse and advocacy purposes.

National Congress of American Indians

The National Congress of American Indians (NCAI) was founded in 1944 in response to the policies forced upon tribal governments that contradicted their treaty rights and status as sovereigns.[25] It stresses cooperation among some 250 tribes and serves as the major national tribal government advocacy organization.

Current issues and activities of the NCAI include: protecting programs and services to benefit Indian families; promoting Indian Head Start, elementary, secondary and adult education; enhancing Indian health care; preventing substance abuse, HIV-AIDS and other diseases; supporting environmental protection and natural resource management; protecting Indian cultural resources and religious freedom rights; promoting Indian economic opportunities on and off reservations; and protecting the rights of all Indian people to safe and affordable housing.

National Indian Child Welfare Association

The National Indian Child Welfare Association (NICWA) is a nonprofit organization dedicated to the well-being of American Indian children and families.[26] The NICWA was founded in 1987 to: promote safe, healthy and culturally strong environments for children; promote the spirituality of children and a positive cultural identity; and provide technical assistance and a clearinghouse for children's programs.

The NICWA has a model of practice and technical assistance called the "Relational Worldview," which provides a culturally based theory of change and community development. NICWA provides assistance in planning, developing and operating systems of care, especially where the social challenges are serious.

National Indian Education Association

The National Indian Education Association (NIEA) is a membership based organization committed to increasing educational opportunities and resources for American Indian, Alaska Native and Native Hawaiian students while protecting their cultural and linguistic traditions.[27]

Founded in 1969, NIEA is the largest and oldest Indian education organization. It provides a forum for Indian educators to discuss current issues and long-range strategies.

National Indian Gaming Association

The National Indian Gaming Association (NIGA), established in 1985, is a non-profit organization of 184 Indian Nations.[28] It operates as a clearinghouse and educational, legislative and public policy resource for tribes, policymakers and the public on Indian gaming issues and tribal community development.

According to Mark Van Norman, executive director of NIGA, gaming's most important achievement is the ripple effect gaming revenues provide for Indian entrepreneurs.[29] Tribal governments use gaming proceeds to fund services and basic infrastructures. These revenues have helped to reduce adolescent behavior and addiction problems on some reservations.

INDIAN CULTURAL REVIVAL

American Indians exemplify how assimilation can occur in American society without complete acculturation. There is interest in reviving the traditional role of Indian elders.[30] Traditional American Indian song and dance groups and rituals can help vulnerable adolescents regain important cultural traditions and values.

CONCLUSION

Generalizations about American Indians are fraught with exceptions. Tribes vary in their levels of affluence related to the prominence of revenues from gaming.

Each American Indian society had rites of passage for its members. In the past, as soon as an Indian girl reached menarche and adult status, she and her parents began making plans for her marriage.

American Indian adolescent childbearing generally is higher than the national rate and usually is accepted by extended families. American Indians experience lower health status compared to other Americans. The average unemployment rate on most reservations is high. Many who are employed live below the poverty level.

Tribal Healing to Wellness Courts are components of tribal justice systems that address alcohol and drug abuse by establishing structure and accountability for those affected.

The National Congress of American Indians now serves as the major national tribal government organization positioned to monitor federal policy and coordinate efforts to inform federal decisions that affect tribal government interests.

If at-risk Indian adolescents can be reached by connecting them with their tribal culture through traditions, tribal elders may once again function as role models.

Chapter 26

Muslim Adolescent Parenthood

A healthy, intimate relationship can only exist in the context of marriage.

Muslim Women's League[1]

Muslim children learn about the Qur'an (from God) and about the Hadith (from Muhammad). They are expected to work hard in school under strict discipline and to spend time with their families. At about 13, they are expected to carry out their religious duties as adults. Muslim adolescents are both attracted by and critical of the ideas, products and practices of Western societies.

In the Muslim tradition, boys often are circumcised at the head shaving ceremony on the seventh day of life. A boy may be deemed to reach adulthood when one of the following occurs: seminal emission, pubic hair or the age of 15. For girls, it is the onset of menarche.[2]

The Muslim transition to adulthood traditionally was accompanied by marriage. Economic and social pressures have lessened the relevance of that marker as adolescence has come to be recognized as a stage of life with its own characteristics and challenges.[3]

MUSLIM SEXUALITY

The Muslim Womens' League offers details about sexuality, which is only supposed to be expressed in the context of marriage.[4]

Historical Perspective

Leila Ahmed, professor of divinity at Cambridge University, calls attention to the misogynistic Jewish and Christian beliefs that preceded Islam during the 6th and 7th centuries in the Mediterranean area.[5] These beliefs were part of a broader ethos that sexuality was legitimate only for procreation. They were adopted by Muslims.

Sense of Shame ('ayb)

Although shame regarding one's body has no scriptural basis in Islam, Muslim parents may fear that if they do not discourage their children from touching their genitals, they will encourage them to explore sexuality. The sense of shame ('ayb) can be taken to extremes. Girls might be afraid to cleanse their genitals properly because to touch themselves is 'ayb. Muslim parents are being encouraged to accept their children's interest in their genitals to avoid preoccupation with them and to enhance the development of a positive sexual identity.

Menstruation

Muhammad's view of menstruation differed significantly from the Jewish attitude during his time, which restricted women while they were menstruating. Muhammad said, "Associate with them and do everything except sexual intercourse." His wives affirmed his tolerant attitude.

Although most Muslim women do not view menstruation negatively today, many Muslims believe that menstruating women should not enter a mosque or touch the Qur'an. Some Muslim women apparently suppress menstruation medically during Hajj, a once in a lifetime event not to be disturbed by menstruation.

Virginity

While many of the cultural traditions involving proof of a woman's virginity are less prevalent than in the past, an intact hymen is regarded as a marker of virginity in many parts of the Muslim world. As a result, activities that might damage the hymen may be forbidden, such as bicycle and horseback riding and gymnastics. These prohibitions are not in the Qur'an or Hadith and, unfortunately, may not be accompanied by explanations, leading girls to feel arbitrarily barred from activities enjoyed by other girls.

Sex Outside of Marriage

In Islam, both males and females are expected to be chaste and to seek fulfilling relationships in marriage. Pre- and extra-marital relations are prohibited. Each individual is responsible and accountable to God for a state of purity prior to marriage. The Qur'an and Hadith texts describe adultery as *zina*, which is considered a sex crime (*hadd*) to be punished by 100 lashes or stoning to death. The requirements for proof of guilt are so strict that the chances of actually being convicted through the contemporary Islamic legal system are remote.

Masturbation

An often quoted Hadith text advises fasting to quell the sexual appetite. Frustrated urges do not justify sexual behavior outside of the marital relationship. Masturbation prevents illicit sexual contact and is permitted by Hanbali jurists.

Contraception

While the value of family and raising children is undisputed among most Muslims, contraception is practiced at the discretion of a couple. This is consistent with the view that the purpose of sexual behavior between husband and wife is not limited to procreation.

Pregnancy Termination

Like the other monotheistic religions, Islam prohibits taking the life of another human being without just cause. The Qur'an describes the stages of embryonic development with the fetus acquiring a soul at a certain point. According to interpretations of the Hadith, ensoulment occurs somewhere between 40 and 120 days of gestation. Medieval Islamic jurists' documents suggest that pregnancy termination was used as a form of birth control.

In spite of the positions of major jurists, many Muslims today believe that pregnancy termination should be avoided under any circumstances unless a woman's life is endangered.

Female Genital Mutilation

Female genital mutilation is a custom in a few Muslim countries, particularly in Africa, that pre-dates Islam. It is not based on Islam and is used to limit the sexual activity of women. It involves varying degrees of mutilation from removing the clitoris to all labia and sewing the vagina to an extent that only a small opening exists to allow passage of menstrual blood. It is expected to make girls less likely to "misbehave" before or during marriage.

Sex Education

The strong position in the Qur'an and Hadith against unlawful sex contributes to a negative attitude toward sex in general. Fear of retribution is often used to discourage young people from engaging in premarital sexual behavior and contributes to repression and guilt that can interfere with healthy sexuality in marriage.

At the same time, Muhammad frankly discussed sex and sexual development. According to the Muslim Women's League, Muslims can follow the his example to use "wisdom and beautiful preaching" to talk about sexuality from an Islamic perspective, especially with Muslim young people growing up in societies that foster sexual activity.

Muslims may disagree about the age at which sex education begins, but it is acceptable in the United States.[6] Unexplained rules only stimulate young persons' curiosity and interest in risky behavior depicted by the media and practiced by peers.

MARRIAGE

Islamic marriage is a civil contract not a sacrament.[7] It requires free and unfettered consent of the parties. Marriage is prohibited between genetic relatives and during pilgrimages. Under Muslim Law, a husband is entitled to have as many as four wives. All of the wives are entitled to exercise marital rights. *Mahr* is a husband's cash or in-kind obligation at the time of marriage as a sign of respect for his wife.

Divorce is only allowed in extreme situations. If she is divorced, a woman usually becomes the responsibility of the men in her family. According to many Muslim schol-ars, after divorce a mother is entitled to the custody of her male child until he has com-pleted the age of seven years. She is entitled to the custody of a daughter until puberty and is married. In the United States, Muslims usually abide by state laws in which the interests of the children are foremost. *Iddat* is the period of chastity a Muslim woman is expected to observe for three months after divorce and four months and ten days af-ter the death of her husband.

A Muslim wife's first responsibility is to look after her home and family. Tradi-tionally she does not work away from home, although in the United States many do. She helps teach her children about Islam.

In the United States, Muslim spouses' expectations for their marriage can be writ-ten in a prenuptial contract in a way enforceable by the U.S. courts.[8] This can be an effective approach for certain rights, particularly payment of dower, a wife's right to work or not to work and the rights of the spouses to maintain separate property.

For some Muslims, adolescent marriage is based on the belief that the younger the bride the more likely she is to be submissive to her husband, dependent on his family and unaware of the outside world.[9] Girls in Iran now are required to wait until 13 to legally marry. For boys the legal age was raised from 14 to 15, unless court permis-sion is granted for a younger age. The adoption of this law was seen as a victory for women's rights activists.

ISLAM IN AMERICA

Islam has a long history of interacting with other cultures. At the same time, authori-tarian Muslim regimes portray the West as hostile to Islam to deflect attention from their domestic problems.[10] In this context, *jihad* can be seen as a protest against glob-alization, change and opportunity inequalities.

A Pew survey of Muslim Americans found them to be largely assimilated, happy with their lives and tolerant of many of the issues that have divided Muslims and Westerners around the world.[11]

American Muslims usually choose as a matter of conscience to follow specific doc-trines of Islam.[12] For them *jihad* refers to the "*inner jihad*" persons wage against their selfish desires and whims. Growing numbers of Muslim women interpret the Qur'an in non-patriarchal ways. The single most important idea is the equality of human be-ings in the sight of God.

Dar al Islam is an American, non-profit, educational organization devoted to living Islam in North America.[13] Muslims in the United States reflect a conservative-liberal spectrum. As an illustration of the latter, 60,000 Muslims in the U.S. and Canada elected ex-Catholic Ingrid Mattson president of the Islamic Society of North America.

CONCLUSION

Muslim children are expected to work hard in school and to spend time with their families. At about 13 they are expected to carry out their religious duties as adults.

Jewish and Christian thinking during the 6th and 7th centuries influenced the Muslim view that sexuality was legitimate only for procreation. This belief contributed to maintaining women in positions of subservience to men.

The concept of shame regarding one's body has no scriptural basis in Islam. Muslim women today can view menstruation as a fact of life without a negative bearing on their value as human beings.

In Islam, both males and females are expected to be chaste and to seek fulfilling relationships in marriage. Contraception is practiced at the discretion of a couple.

Teaching about sexuality from an Islamic perspective is necessary for Muslim young people who are growing up in societies that foster sexual activity. Muslim parents need to be encouraged to discuss sexual issues openly with their children.

Marriage under Islam is a civil contract and not a sacrament. Under Muslim Law, a husband is entitled to have as many as four wives. For some Muslims, adolescent marriage is based on the belief that the younger the bride the more likely she is to be submissive to her husband, dependent on his family and unaware of the broader world.

American Muslims often choose to follow certain doctrines of Islam. Growing numbers of Muslim women interpret the Qur'an in non-patriarchal ways. Islam teaches morality, personal decorum, modesty, mutual respect and discipline in dress and comportment.

Chapter 27

Hmong Adolescent Parenthood

In Laos, we helped you fight the war. If the Americans came to our house, whatever we ate we treated the Americans equally. If we found an injured soldier, we carried the American to the base. We considered Americans as our own brothers. Now we have lost our own country.

Tim Pfaff
Hmong in America[1]

The Hmong culture has a history of resistance, accommodation and transformation as an ethnic minority—in China, in Laos and now in the United States. For many Hmong who have grown up in the United States, the story of their diaspora offers a unique sense of their identity.[2]

Significant class and status differences shaped the Hmong diaspora. The first Vietnam War Hmong refugees from Laos consisted of the political and military elite who were able to draw upon pre-war connections with politicians and educators in France or to join a CIA-sponsored airlift from the U.S. military base at Long Tieng. These refugees were initially selected from a refugee camp in Thailand for resettlement in the United States in the mid 1970s. They were the most educated and had held high positions within General Vang Pao's army. Recent arrivals from Thailand speak different languages and have had different experiences.

The Hmong in the United States are from Laos, where some 315,000 still reside.[3] Several million live in southwestern China, 500,000 in Vietnam, and 120,000 in Thailand. There are two groups of Hmong with a long history of intermarriage and harmonious relations: the *Hmong der* (White Hmong) and the *Hmong Leng* (Blue Hmong).

By 2006, there were at least 275,000 Hmong refugees and their descendents residing in the United States.[4] The major Hmong centers are in the mid-west and in California. The largest urban concentration of Hmong in the world is in St. Paul, Minnesota.

HMONG ACCULTURATION

The Hmong culture in the United States is in the process of change. Many Hmong-Americans converted to Christianity during their time in Thailand refugee camps.

Hmong immigrants have achieved significant progress since their arrival in the United States.[5] Most have achieved educational and material success, but almost one-third receive some form of public assistance and are struggling economically. The 1990 median Hmong family income was $14,300 compared to $32,076 in 2000; 67% received public assistance in 1990 and 30% in 2000; and 13% owned their own homes in 1990 and 40% in 2000. Hmong students are graduating from high school and attending college in increasing numbers.

Hmong families must cope with the inherent inequalities in our society's social, economic and political structures. Kinship networks have been important factors in the ability of Hmong immigrants to overcome adversity before and after arriving in the United States. Hmong marriages tend to be more stable than others in part because of a Hmong tradition of kin counseling for marital problems.[6] This concept of mutual assistance is evident in the more than 100 Hmong-run community-based organizations.

Hmong adolescents are actively reworking, negotiating and contesting their cultural traditions.[7] Their behavior is influenced by their parents' traditions and their own acculturation. Some Hmong adolescents are involved in criminal gangs and drug abuse. The Hmong Women's Action Team is working to support the Hmong culture and to educate communities about the destructiveness of sexist beliefs as well as of customs, such as polygamy and early marriage.

HMONG FAMILY LIFE

Although the Hmong culture is patriarchal, traditional Hmong society does not have a caste system. It acknowledges that children have much to learn from those who came before them and that being an adult requires caring for and preserving the larger community and society. Their leaders earn their status and authority.

Southeast Asian fathers in general have difficulty understanding and parenting adolescents in the United States because of the differences in Hmong and American approaches to adolescence.[8] Past experience of these fathers with obedient, polite children does not equip them to parent their adolescents in American society, which prolongs adolescence, encourages independence and self-expression and emphasizes gender equality. Most Hmong parents try to monitor their adolescents' activities that can bring pride or shame to a family.

When parents do not speak English, their offspring communicate with teachers and other professionals. This can give adolescents inappropriate power at home.

HMONG WOMEN

The experiences of Hmong and Cambodian women and girls are far more complex and heart-wrenching than those of most immigrants. Beaten down by war, flight, confinement in prison-like refugee camps and the challenges of moving from peasant societies to a technologically advanced country, they are survivors in every sense of the word.[9]

Refugee Hmong women traditionally have been the nurturers and caregivers in their families. They were conditioned to be diligent, obedient and respectful of the men in their lives. Hmong women obtained value and respect through their roles as wives to their husbands, mothers to their sons and daughters-in-law to their husbands' family. The patriarchal Hmong culture has dictated that Hmong women be quiet, patient and obedient persons, who meet the needs of their men and family members. These cultural dictates tend to limit Hmong women's opportunities in education and career development in the United States.[10] Hmong daughters were considered respectable if they could accommodate daily family demands and display proper etiquette to their future family-in-law. Thus, young girls seldom obtained an education in Laos and Thailand.

In the United States, Hmong women are redefining these traditional roles as the necessity of education and employment become essential for economic survival.[11] They are faced with the difficult task of being American enough to succeed in America and Hmong enough to fulfill their roles in the Hmong culture. Successful women are challenging the Hmong's patriarchal social structures and are acculturating and assimilating into mainstream American society.

A study of three generations of Hmong women in California revealed that traditional culture was maintained by adults through garden plots, needlework, Hmong New Year celebrations and living close to relatives.[12] They also were assimilating through interacting with health care providers, social service agencies and public schools. Their adolescents were learning to shift between the American world at school and the Hmong world at home.

MARRIAGE

Marriage in the Hmong culture offers a context for procreation and continuing family lineages. Young Hmong often were not considered mature until they were married and had children. When arrangements were completed between a groom's and a bride's families, a girl became a member of her husband's family under the control of her husband and his parents.

In Laos, the pattern of Hmong marriage was between 18 and 20 for males and 14 and 16 for females.[13] In Australia, a Hmong girl may feel that if she is too old no one will want to marry her. If a girl wants to hold on to a boy, she needs to marry before another girl comes and takes him away from her.

A 1994 study revealed that 53% of Hmong females were married while in high school.[14] Seventy-five percent of them graduated from high school. Compared to nonmarried Hmong adolescents, early marriage did not appear to have a significant impact on school performance or personal well-being. Recent anecdotal evidence from 2- and 4-year colleges in the St. Paul area indicates that substantial numbers of Hmong students continue their educations, even though the majority of the female students at this level are married and have children. The primary child-care responsibilities are borne by parents, siblings or the extended family.

A 2000 study focused on the perception of early marriage and future educational goals of Hmong female adolescents living in Minnesota and Wisconsin.[15] Sixty percent of the respondents were born in the United States. Thirty-five percent of the respondents were in high school, and 40% were married. When there was a positive perception of early marriage, there were lower educational goals for Hmong girls. Eighty-five percent of single college Hmong students ages 19 to 26 agreed that the most important reasons for early Hmong marriage was that their friends married early, and they did not want to feel left out. Married Hmong girls without children have higher educational goals than married Hmong girls with children.

Education is an important value in most Hmong families, because before coming to the United States it was only available to the relatively wealthy. The greatest obstacles for Hmong girls' pursuit of higher education are early marriage, childbearing and lack of financial resources.

Early marriage, low academic achievement and dropping out of school in Hmong communities in the United States cannot be attributed solely to tradition.[16] Early marriage may be a form of opposition to family and schooling. For some girls, marriage allows them to leave their parents' homes. Ironically, girls who marry to escape their parents' control find themselves under a mother-in-law's control. Some parents-in-law may prohibit their daughters-in-law from pursuing higher education, even if they and their parents wish her to continue. Divorce is an infrequently chosen option in Hmong society.

Hmong organizations are addressing the challenges to improving the status of Hmong women.[17] Along with the negotiations between men's and women's work contributions in their families, Hmong women also have gained new footing in marriage decisions. Some Hmong American women choose to postpone marriage until their personal aspirations are fulfilled.

For many Hmong, the being Hmong is far from central to their lives. At the same time, one young, unmarried Hmong woman described her dilemma:[18]

Many of the issues I have faced as a single Hmong woman in her mid-twenties come to mind. Should I discuss the functional reasons why marriage is so important in the Hmong culture, especially for women? Or do I talk about the lack of eligible, older Hmong men? Better yet, should I complain about the attempts by my relatives to find me a good husband as if it were an unfortunate circumstance that I was single instead of a conscious choice? Thinking it over, though, I decided that all those questions boiled down to one fundamental truth – the Hmong community is still trying to learn how to treat the increasing number of Hmong women who, like me, are making the choice to stay single in their mid-20s.

Interviews with Hmong families from two different generations in the Minneapo-lis-St. Paul area suggest that there will be few changes in the near future in Hmong kinship and marriage practices, except for bridal dowery, brother marriage of a widow and polygyny, but that adherence to them will be inconsistent.[19]

HMONG GANGS

Hmong gangs are similar to other gangs in their propensity for antisocial behavior. Fif-teen percent of male and 8% of female 8th and 10th grade Hmong students identified themselves as belonging to gangs in Eau Claire, Wisconsin, in 1999. Twenty percent of males and 13% of females had been victims of gang violence.[20]

A study of Hmong adolescents found that strong parental attachment and monitor-ing prevented delinquent behavior while harsh and inconsistent discipline practices promoted delinquent behavior as in other cultures.[21]

A survey of Hmong adolescents in Dane County, Wisconsin, found higher rates of cigarette, alcohol and drug abuse than for other adolescents.[22] They were twice as likely as White adolescents to have had a physical fight with weapons in the past year and to feel pressure to join a gang. Hmong males also were more likely to skip school and to report being treated unfairly by other students and teachers than any other ethnic group.

CONCLUSION

The Hmong culture has a history of resistance, accommodation and transformation as an ethnic minority in China, in Laos and now in the United States. The story of their diaspora provides a sense of continuity in the face of disruption and trauma.

Hmong immigrants have achieved significant progress since their arrival in the United States over 30 years ago. Welfare rates have dropped, employment rates have risen and Hmong students have been graduating from high school and attending col-lege in increasing numbers. The Hmong spirit of mutual assistance is evident in Hmong-run community-based organizations.

Although the Hmong culture is patriarchal, traditional Hmong society does not have a caste system; their leaders earn their status and authority. Traditional Hmong expec-tations of wives and mothers are no longer appropriate in America as the necessity of education and employment become primary factors for economic survival.

Early marriage, low academic achievement and school dropouts in Hmong com-munities in the United States cannot be attributed solely to tradition when girls marry to escape their parents' control. Ironically, they then find themselves under the control of their mothers-in-law.

Substantial numbers of Hmong students continue their educations beyond high school, even though the majority of female students are married and have one or more children. The students' primary child-care responsibilities are borne by parents or siblings. At the same time some Hmong boys and girls have become involved in antisocial gang activities.

The beliefs and practices of the Hmong marriage system are not likely to change, except for bridal dowery, brother marriage of a widow and polygamy. The emerging nuclear family system probably will overtake the traditional Hmong family system.

Part 8

SOCIETY

These states are the amplest poem,
Here is not merely a nation, but a teeming nation of nations.

Walt Whitman
Chants Democratic and Native American[1]

Society plays a central role in amplifying or dampening the outcomes of adolescent parenthood.

Public policies in the United States treat parenthood as an acceptable choice for adolescent girls. These policies are influenced in part by those who see efforts to reduce the birth rates of the poor as reflecting covert eugenics or genocide.

Programs intended to promote the aspirations and maturity of adolescent parents have disappointing results because adolescent parents often are multiply disadvantaged. In addition, the services they need are not effectively coordinated, are of low quality or have requirements that adolescents do not meet.

A striking aspect of most welfare-to-work programs is their inattention to the children of adolescent mothers. They often include sanctions that make it difficult for mothers of all ages to meet the requirements of child welfare services.

Recent positive trends reveal a shift in the attitude of adolescents toward serving their own self-interests rather than following their impulses and fantasies. As a result, adolescent sexual behavior, pregnancy and childbirth are decreasing, although formidable barriers to a realistic approach to adolescent parenthood remain.

Chapter 28

Impact of
Adolescent Parenthood on Society

We Americans don't know what we want to be when we grow up, so we never do. We languish in the semi-dependent, semi-virile, semi-conscious, semi-irrelevant self-destructiveness of perpetual adolescence.

Lee Thayer
The Functions of Incompetence, 1976[1]

Most adults agree that adolescents are too young to enter parenthood. However, we give them financial, educational and emotional support when they do. Most of us feel compassion toward adolescent mothers, particularly when they are in distress. The impulse to support an adolescent mother and her baby overrides considering other alternatives for both of them. This is understandable because adolescent mothers do include successful students as well as school dropouts; conscientious family planners as well as those with repeated childbirths; the socially skilled as well as the unskilled; and competent workers as well as the unemployable.

Still, most girls and boys who become parents have significant behavior, emotional, cognitive and social problems. The short and long-term consequences of adolescent parenthood are straining our educational, health care, social service and correctional systems.[2]

HISTORY OF PUBLIC SUPPORT FOR ADOLESCENT PARENTHOOD

When adolescent pregnancy was identified as an "epidemic" in the 1960s, the focus was on preventing it through the Title X Family Planning Services Program and Research Act of 1970. It funded family planning clinics to dispense contraceptives to sexually active adolescents.[3] A parallel movement to provide special educational facilities for adolescent mothers was reinforced in 1972 by Title IX of the Higher Education Amendments, which prohibited the expulsion of pregnant students from schools.

The legalization of pregnancy termination by the Supreme Court in 1973 underlay much of the concern about adolescent pregnancy and childbearing at that time. Congressional impetus for supporting adolescent mothers came from "pro-life" legislators who saw these programs as alternatives to termination.[4] The Reagan Administration emphasized postponing sexual activity and helping young mothers raise their children in the Title XX Adolescent Family Life Program.

The Family Support Act of 1988 required adolescent recipients of Aid to the Families of Dependent Children to continue their schooling or enroll in job training programs.[5] The Personal Responsibility and Work Opportunity Reconciliation Act of 1996 added the requirement that they live with parents, other adults or in supervised facilities. The Temporary Assistance for Needy Families (TANF) block grant aims to help adolescent parents "end dependency, reduce out-of-wedlock pregnancies, and form and maintain two-parent families."

PUBLIC ASSISTANCE FOR ADOLESCENT PARENTS

Contemporary public policies in the United States treat parenthood as an acceptable choice for adolescent girls. When they give birth, they are supported with the expectation that they will become competent parents.

Even though intended as crisis-oriented interventions, public financial assistance and publicly supported education are obvious signs that our society supports adolescent parenthood. Without clear statements of this intent and of society's expectation that the children of adolescent parents should have competent parents, both public assistance and parent education programs condone adolescent childrearing.

In spite of welfare reform, there still are financial incentives for adolescents to enter parenthood. In some states, adolescent girls with babies are eligible for public benefits that initially seem substantial to them. If girls make an adoption plan, they lose these benefits and their babies in addition to possibly being criticized by their peers and families. Consequently, adoption is an unpopular option for most childbearing adolescents.

The public and private support of adolescent parenthood is costly for society in direct educational, welfare and health care expenditures and in the later social and health problems of the adolescents and their offspring.

THE IMPACT OF ADOLESCENT PARENTHOOD ON WELFARE

Respected studies reveal differing pictures of the welfare impacts of adolescent motherhood with welfare recipient rates of between 55% and 70% and "doing reasonably well" rates of between 18% and 33%.

The Furstenberg, et al, Review

A review of the literature in 1987 and in 1997 revealed that the life trajectories of adolescent mothers are highly variable, with about 33% doing reasonably well as young adults.[6] About 25% do not become economically self-sufficient, and many more move on and off public assistance. About 55% of all mothers on welfare were adolescents at first childbirth.

The Baltimore Study

A Baltimore follow-up in the early 1990s of adolescents who became mothers at 18 or younger, found that two-thirds were on Aid to the Families of Dependent Children at some point during the 20 years following their first births.[7] By the end of the study, 71% of Black adolescent mothers had entered welfare and were grouped in three categories.

Almost one-half were *early-exit* recipients who had more favorable family and personal resources. They were more likely to graduate from high school, successfully limit further births and enter stable marriages. Many left welfare after one or two years. They found jobs or married and never returned to welfare again.

Almost one-half were *cycling* recipients who were in and out of welfare use because of erratic and changing life circumstances. Lacking in educational and job skills and burdened by larger numbers of children than the early-exit recipients, they were continually vulnerable to events, particularly marital and job instability, that undermined their attempts at self-sufficiency.

The remainder were *persistent* recipients who came from families with few social supports and resources. They were youngest at first pregnancy and were likely to drop out of school and have more pregnancies. They eventually left welfare through the slow process of combining work and welfare or when they entered marriage.

Of adolescents who were younger than 16 at their first pregnancies, 51% entered welfare within two years of the first birth, compared to 32% of older adolescents.[8] Girls whose mothers received welfare continue to be more likely to receive welfare themselves than girls whose mothers never received it.

The Robin Hood Foundation Study

The Robin Hood Foundation commissioned seven coordinated teams of leading scholars to study the connection between adolescent parents and social problems.[9] The teams compared adolescents who had their first babies at the age of 17 or younger with mothers who delayed their first births until the ages of 20 or 21. The studies separated the differences between these two groups attributable to age and to background factors such as race, ethnicity, socioeconomic class and parental education. They also took into account motivation, self-esteem, peer-group influence and community impact.

The teams found that mothers 17 and younger spent four times more of their young adult years as single parents. Half of the difference was due to adolescent childbearing and half to background factors. They also had 50% higher rates of welfare dependency.

The Notre Dame Study

Fifty-five percent of the original Notre Dame sample that did not include the most at-risk mothers were evaluated after three years.[10] Although none of the mothers in the study said they regretted having their children, a common theme was that they wished they had waited longer. When their children were three and five years old, these adolescent mothers tended to be undereducated, underemployed and to have additional children. After five years, 50% were employed; 76% were single; 76% had two or more children; and 70% were receiving public support. Only 18% of the adolescent mothers could be regarded as living successful lives in all areas by meeting the needs of their children, continuing to pursue their own educational and career development and establishing constructive social relationships.

IMPACT ON ECONOMY AND GOVERNMENT REVENUES

Joseph Hotz, professor of economics at the University of California at Los Angeles, and his colleagues compared just the earnings and taxes paid by adolescent girls who miscarried and did not become parents and those who became parents.[11] They found no significant differences in their earnings over time. Extending this analysis to the probability that these mothers would require public aid, the authors cast doubt on substantial savings in government costs from delaying childbearing. They theorized that from the ages of 17 to 34 delaying childbearing for 2 to 2.5 years would make using public assistance more rather than less likely.

This hypothetical calculation did not take into account our society's total costs of adolescent childbearing. It focused only on earnings and taxes paid. If the total financial impact of adolescent parenthood is taken into account, another conclusion is evident.

National Campaign to Prevent Teen Pregnancy estimates are based on a very conservative approach that only include costs that can be confidently attributed to adolescent childbearing rather than to other accompanying traits or social disadvantages, such as poverty. When the costs of educating adolescent mothers is included, that cost to society estimate is $20 billion a year.[12] The 422,043 annual births in 2004 to adolescents 19 and younger cost taxpayers at least $9.1 billion. Between 1991 and 2004 there were 6,776,230 births to this age group. The estimated cumulative public costs of adolescent childbearing during that time is $161 billion dollars. The reduction in adolescent childbearing between 1991 and 2004 saved taxpayers an estimated $6.7 billion in 2004 alone. Because not all costs can be measured, and because the estimates themselves are conservative, the full public sector costs of adolescent childbearing are larger than those noted in this analysis.

The extent to which adolescent parenthood reduces education has a financial impact on our economy.[13] Education clearly increases productivity and wages. According to the U.S. Census Bureau in 2005, workers 18 and over with bachelor degrees earned an average of $51,206 a year, while those with a high school diploma averaged $27,915. Those with advanced degrees averaged $74,602, and those without a high school diploma averaged $18,734. Adolescent fathers, who were one third as likely to become active parents as girls, earned $4,732 less annually than those who delayed fatherhood until the age of 20 or more. A 1% increase in the high school completion rate of all men from 20 to 60, including the fathers of children born to adolescent mothers, would save as much as $1.4 billion a year in reduced costs from crime. Voting also is strongly affected by education.

The public costs of adolescent parenthood include paying the salaries of professionals in adolescent pregnancy and parenting educational and supportive programs. These professionals are understandably reluctant to turn their backs on adolescent mothers who wish to care for their children and pursue their educations. These professionals need reassurance that reducing the numbers of adolescent parents need not threaten their employment. Their expertise and resources will still be needed to help adult parents.

PRIORITIZING RISKS TO OUR SOCIETY

When we want to prevent diseases and environmental pollution, we focus on risk reduction. As we detect risks to the quality of our lives, we prioritize them in terms of their probability of occurring and their costs. For example, the range of risks is from 1 in 10,000 for federally regulated drugs to 3 in 100 for factory-work injuries to 1 in 10 for lung cancer for smokers.[14] *The risk of serious harm to children from adolescent parenthood is at least 1 in 3.* The risk for children created by adolescent parenthood is the greatest hazard of all in frequency and cost. Yet it is not managed as are other risks and is supported by public and private funding.

Our approach to adolescent parenthood needs incentives that have meaning to adolescents and their families. In 1742, David Hume wrote:[15]

> every man ought to be supposed to be a knave and to have no other end, in all his actions, than private interest. By this interest we must govern him, and, by means of it, make him, notwithstanding his insatiable avarice and ambition, cooperate to public good.

Contemporary sociological research suggests a modification of Hume's maxim:[16]

> Good policies support socially valued ends not only by harnessing selfish preferences, but also by evoking, cultivating and empowering public-spirited motives.

CONCLUSION

Contemporary public policies in the United States treat parenthood as an acceptable choice for adolescent girls. When they give birth, adolescent girls usually are supported as parents without consideration of the costs to society in direct educational, welfare and health care expenditures and in the later social and health repercussions of their children's problems.

Adolescent parenthood costs our society over $20 billion annually. The long-term welfare usage rates of adolescent parents range between 55% and 70% with self-sufficiency rates between 18% and 33%.

Adolescent parenthood is a greater risk factor for children than diseases and environmental pollution. As a social problem to be addressed, it warrants the highest priority because solutions are within our reach.

Chapter 29

Programs for Adolescent Parents

Human beings are governed more by passion and prejudice than by an enlightened sense of their interest. A degree of illusion mixes itself in all the affairs of society.

Alexander Hamilton[1]

This chapter illustrates the extent to which public and private resources are mobilized when babies have adolescent parents. An extensive array of programs presume that adolescents can assume the responsibilities of parenthood with help. Most are for mothers in schools and include services, such as counseling, childcare, transportation, residential care, financial benefits, job training, parenting and life skill education, family planning, child support, agency coordination and follow-up care.[2]

CHALLENGES POSED BY ADOLESCENT MOTHERS

Most adolescent parents live in poverty, often in dangerous neighborhoods, with few role models to guide them toward social and economic independence. Over two-thirds have been physically or sexually abused.[3] These disadvantages inspire private and public agencies to support them. The challenges faced by these programs are illustrated by Alecia's experience:[4]

Alecia

Alecia, the oldest of six children, was 14 when her father and primary caregiver died. She was placed in a foster home. Because of her defiance, she was transferred to a second foster home. When 17 she became pregnant. Her boyfriend promised her he would "be there" for her and the child. After Bryan's birth, he ended all contact with them after two visits.

Complications with the pregnancy led to two months of bed rest for Alecia. Three weeks before childbirth, she was hospitalized with anemia. Bryan was delivered by cesarean section and placed in neonatal intensive care.

After two weeks in the hospital, they returned to Alecia's previous foster home. In a few months, Alecia began violating curfew. She and Bryan were transferred to a group home for adolescent mothers.

Alecia and Bryan received intensive counseling from a parent educator for two years in the group home. Three months after Bryan's second birthday administrative changes resulted in Alecia and Bryan being transferred to a foster home where they both had difficulty adjusting. Alecia lost interest in school and work and cancelled counseling appointments. Her counselor arranged for Bryan to receive preschool special education with a support group. Alecia used the group as a way of not having to take care of Bryan.

Over the course of the next two years, many service providers worked with Alecia and Bryan, each using a different approach.

As Alecia's story reveals, adolescent parent programs must address multiple issues. At another level, adolescents receive various messages in programs. For example, a study of the *Chicago Pilot Program for Teen Mothers* revealed less emphasis on forming a worker-to-be identity for the mothers and more on ways they could become responsible welfare users.[5] Four years later, 10 of the 17 participants in the pilot program were located. Four had finished their GEDs, 3 had at least one more child within two years, 2 were in jail, and the young mother who was the most promising was working part-time at a minimum wage job.

THE REWARDS OF ADOLESCENT MOTHER PROGRAMS

The *Ounce of Prevention Fund* in Illinois found that adolescents described becoming a parent as a transforming experience. Parenthood gave them a sense of purpose and direction. Although becoming a parent so young may have been a mistake, they were clear that being a young parent had made them better people. One girl put it this way:[6]

> They helped me with, well I was going through some emotional changes. . . They stayed on me about finishing school. . . I could have been out on the streets, young girl pregnant you know, just at home on welfare you know, but they showed me I could be more than that . . . I see I can be anything I want to be and still take care of my baby. . . They showed me I'm a person.

ADOLESCENT MOTHER SUPPORT STRATEGIES

Adolescent parent support strategies can be described as *deficit-based* or *strength-based*. *Deficit-based* strategies, which are currently dominant, focus on identifying risks and weaknesses and treating them. *Strength-based* strategies focus on building competencies, promoting healthy development and strengthening social environments.

An optimal *strength-based* strategy addresses the following considerations:[7]

- *Adult Supervised Settings.* In families or facilities.
- *School Attendance.* Homebound instruction and school programs for mothers.
- *Supportive Services.* Both crisis intervention and long-term services.
- *Parenting Education.* Learning parenting skills and about nutrition and health care.
- *Family Planning.* Adolescent parents need effective birth control.
- *Childcare.* With screening and preventive health services.
- *Transportation.* For school, job training or work, childcare and health care.
- *Father Involvement.* Paternity establishment, child support and services for fathers.
- *Service Collaboration.* Multiple systems require collaboration.

The Harvard Family Research Project has a Guide to Online Resources on Family Involvement,[8] and the National Youth Development Information Center maintains information on programs for adolescents.[9]

The rest of this chapter is devoted to examples of programs for adolescent parents. They target mothers through: 1) home visitation, 2) childcare and early childhood education, 3) education, 4) alternative living arrangements, 5) community programs and 6) public financial services. Comparable systematic evaluations of most of these programs are not available.

HOME VISITATION

The dominant form of prevention and intervention assistance for adolescent mothers is home visitation by private and public professional and paraprofessional personnel. Since these programs are voluntary, they do not reach or retain mothers who need help the most.

Healthy Families America

Healthy Families America draws upon research and the experiences of the original *Hawaii Healthy Start* program.[10] It offers intensive services for expectant and new parents at least once a week over three to five years in 440 communities in the United States and Canada. Half of families remain in the program for at least one year. Trained home visitors see themselves as coaches rather than as teachers. They try to create an individually tailored, nurturing family environment that allows time for reflection. Three-quarters of the family support workers have at least two and 30% have three or more years of experience.

Three *Hawaii Healthy Start* programs were successful after two years in linking families with medical care, improving maternal parenting efficacy, decreasing maternal stress, promoting nonviolent discipline and decreasing injuries from partner violence.[11]

In 2002, the Centers for Disease Control and Prevention Task Force on Community Preventive Services reviewed twenty-five studies and found an overall 39% reduction of child maltreatment in high-risk families with parents of all ages.[12]

The Nurse-Family Partnership

The *Nurse-Family Partnership* serves some 20,000 low-income families.[13] It focuses on first-time mothers and encourages fathers and grandmothers to participate. Visits begin during pregnancy and continue for two years. They include continuing the parents' education, personal and environmental health, parenting education, maternal support and linkage to needed services.

In the *Louisiana Nurse-Family Partnership*, 36% of 1,000 mothers of all ages finished the program. When turned two, almost 60% of the mothers over 20 were employed, and 41% who started the program without a high school diploma or equivalency obtained one.[14] Alexis, an adolescent mother in rural Louisiana, exemplifies the challenges of voluntary home visitation:

> Alexis initially responded favorably to home visits. Her baby was overweight and lethargic because she found that he slept when she fed him. She ultimately moved into an apartment with her baby's father who left her. Alexis miscarried a new boyfriend's baby. He was eager to try again. Alexis said, "And next I want a little girl." She left the home visitation program.

Randomized trials of the *Nurse-Family Partnership* were conducted in three cities beginning in Elmira, New York, in 1977; in Memphis in 1987; and in Denver in 1994.[15] All three trials targeted first-time, low-income mothers who were mostly adolescents. The mothers from the 15-year follow-up of the Elmira trial of *Nurse-Family Partnership* had 61% fewer arrests. The children at the age of 15 had a 48% reduction in abuse and neglect; 59% reduction in juvenile arrests; and a 90% reduction in adjudications of incorrigible behavior.

The rate of participant attrition in the national *Nurse-Family Partnership* program sites is about 60%. In the Denver program, 38% of the mothers dropped out within two years.[16]

Parents as Teachers

Parents as Teachers (PAT) offers the *Born to Learn* model of services worldwide to families with parents of all ages.[17] These services include home visits, parent group meetings, child screenings and referrals to community resources. Certified professionals bring customized child development information to parents from pregnancy until their child enters kindergarten.

PAT expanded from four Missouri pilot sites in 1981 to more than 3,000 sites in 2006. A number of studies have found favorable results. One follow-up revealed that only 3% of PAT children compared to 25% of a control group performed unsatisfactorily in the third grade.[18]

Colorado's Bright Beginnings

Colorado's *Bright Beginnings* is a public-private partnership that offers home visitation programs for parents of all ages of newborns and childrearing materials for the parents of toddlers. 11,500 families were visited in 2005. Of this number, 527 were under 18.

An evaluation completed by 36% of the families of which 70% had high school diplomas revealed that 76% used *My First Picture Book* with their child; 88% of children tested in the normal range of development; and 83% of the children were up to date on their immunizations.[19]

Rosalie Manor

The *Supporting Today's Teen Parents Program* was created by Rosalie Manor in Milwaukee to offer parenting and child development support to first-time parents. It includes a Teen Parent Unit that served 1,014 adolescent mothers and a father's outreach component that served 99 fathers from 2000 to 2005.[20] Over 65% of the adolescent mothers met a minimum of one of their personal goals as a result of participating in this program. Over 90% had a primary care doctor. The repeat pregnancy rate was 7-13% compared to 20% for the city.

Welcome Home and Early Start in Cuyahoga County, Ohio

A University of Chicago Chapin Hall study documented the characteristics and experiences of 325 new mothers of all ages who received an initial *Welcome Home* visit and were referred on to the Early Start nurse home visitation program and 193 pregnant women or new mothers referred to Early Start by their Ohio Works First caseworker.[21] Interviews were conducted at the time of referral and 3 and 11-month post-enrollment between 1999 and 2002.

One third of *Welcome Home* referrals did not want to participate in the Early Start program. Sixty-nine percent of those visited received the number of visits necessary to achieve positive change in parents' levels of depression, stress and competence.

Teenage Parent Home Visitor Services Demonstration Program

Three-year demonstrations between 1995 and 1997 of the *Teenage Parent Home Visitor Services Demonstration Program* in Chicago, Dayton and Portland, Oregon, were compared to control groups.[22] The program aimed to reduce welfare dependence of adolescent parents by completing their educations and delaying additional pregnancies.

The average number of home visits with each adolescent was 28 of 84 potential visits. The months the mothers were in school, job training or employment were not increased. Financial sanctions were imposed on 45%. High school diplomas or GEDs were obtained by 58% in the program and 56% of the controls. Over 90% of the program and control mothers were sexually active. Twenty-five percent of the program versus 19% of the control group reported using condoms. The program did not lead to lower pregnancy or repeat births rates.

Reasons for the program's limited success included the chaotic lives of the mothers, their unwillingness to meet home visitors, the multiple resources needed and the inertia of agencies.

Infant Health and Development Program

An 18-year follow-up of *Infant Health and Development Program* pre-term babies at eight birthing centers found that program adolescents had higher achievement scores in math and reading and fewer risky behaviors than controls.[23] The 3-year intervention consisted of weekly home visits for the first year of a child's life and every other week in the second and third year, along with daily center-based education beginning at 12 months and a support group for parents.

Parent-Child Home Program

The *Parent-Child Home Program,* which began in 1965, serves more than 5,000 families in 150 replications world-wide. It is for parents of all ages and their 2- and 3-year-olds to help them achieve academic success through intensive home visiting. This program emphasizes parent-child interaction around books and toys to promote cognitive and socio-emotional development through twice-weekly, half-hour visits over two years by paraprofessionals.[24]

At-risk preschoolers in the *Pittsfield Parent-Child Home Program* evaluated 16 to 20 years later were less likely than randomized controls to drop out of school (16% vs. 40%) and more likely to have graduated (84% vs. 54%).[25]

Maternal Infant Health Outreach Worker

The *Maternal Infant Health Outreach Worker* program, a partnership between Vanderbilt University Center for Health Services and community based organizations in Nashville is dedicated to parent-to-parent interventions to improve health and child development for low-income families across the Southern United States using peer home visitors. They visit pregnant girls and women and families with children up to three to promote health and self-sufficiency.[26] Compared to state rates more of the participants had prenatal care in the first trimester, less had low-birth-weight babies, more had well-child visits and more had health insurance.

The Chicago Doula Project

The *Chicago Doula Project* was started in 1996 by the Irving Harris Foundation. Doulas counsel pregnant girls and women on the birthing process, breast-feeding, developing the mother-child relationship and baby development. Of high-risk participants with an average age of 17, 80% initiated breastfeeding at birth and 22% were still breastfeeding at 6 months compared with 45% and 12% of other adolescents.

Eight percent had Cesarean sections compared with 13% for other adolescents.[27] The *Project* is being replicated across the country. There are 24 Projects in Illinois, serving 750 mothers a year at an annual cost of $2 million.

Baby FAST

Baby FAST is a multi-family group process developed by Lynn McDonald, professor of education at the University of Wisconsin. It usually supplements home visitation programs. It brings together families of new mothers, especially adolescents, in 8 weekly meetings to enhance relationships with their babies and peers who do and do not have babies and community agency professionals.[28] The activities fit the needs of the babies, mothers, fathers and grandmothers.

Baby FAST described its outcomes as: 1) increased healthy child development; 2) improved parent-adolescent relationships; 3) improved peer and inter-generational social capital; and 4) reduced child neglect and abuse.

Community-Based Family Administered Neonatal Activities

Community-Based Family Administered Neonatal Activities is a program home visitors can use to promote emotional engagement between adolescent parents and their unborn babies and newborns.[29] The program spans six prenatal visits and four weeks after birth.

Parenting Support and Literacy

Some programs increase the literacy and childrearing skills of young mothers.

National Center for Family Literacy

The *National Center for Family Literacy* was established in 1989. It has pioneered educational initiatives that open pathways for life improvement for the nation's most at-risk children and families. More than one million families have made positive educational and economic gains as a result of NCFL's work, which includes training more than 150,000 teachers and thousands of volunteers.[30]

Home Instruction for Parents of Preschool Youngsters

Home Instruction for Parents of Preschool Youngsters is a parent-centered, school readiness program that helps parents prepare their 3-, 4- and 5-year-old children for success in school. Home visitors role play activities with parents at home and in group meetings. A model HIPPY site serves up to 180 children with one coordinator and 12 to 18 part-time home visitors. The 160 sites in the U.S. serve over 16,000 children.[31]

Home-based Mentoring Program

A home-based intervention by college-educated, Black, single mother mentors ("big sisters") that targeted adolescent development and interpersonal negotiation skills was found to be effective in preventing repeat births within two years among low-income, Black adolescent mothers.[32] The curriculum extended biweekly until a baby's first birthday.

EARLY CHILDHOOD EDUCATION AND CHILDCARE

A popular strategy is to increase access to high-quality, center-based early childhood education programs that include home visits for low income 3- and 4-year-olds.[33]

Early Head Start

Early Head Start (EHS) is a federally funded community-based program created in 1995 for low-income mothers of all ages to enhance the development of young children and to promote healthy family functioning from pregnancy to age three.[34] EHS *Center-based programs* provide childcare and early education services with at least two home visits a year. *Home-based programs* consist of weekly home visits with families attending group activities at least once a month. *Mixed-delivery programs* combine the center-based and home-based approach.

Adolescents under 18 comprised 20% of mothers participating in EHS in 2006.[35] Although EHS participation is linked to positive outcomes, the impact on child development and parenting was greater for parents over 19 and those who were in the program longer.

Evaluation of participants two years after completing Early Head Start showed favorable impacts on children's socio-emotional development, behavior problems and approaches to learning—the greatest with Black children.[36] There were no improvements in aggressive behavior, in behavior during play with parents or in attention, letter-word identification or problem-solving. There were improvements in parental depression, but adolescent parents were no more likely than a control group to obtain a high school degree or GED.

School-based Childcare

School-based childcare programs encourage young mothers to return to or stay in school.[37] One study found that adolescent mothers were more likely to complete their educations and less likely to become dependent on welfare when they utilized childcare in their schools.[38]

ADOLESCENT MOTHER PROGRAMS IN SCHOOLS

Public schools have a variety of programs for school-age parents. In Wisconsin, school districts are required to accommodate school-age mothers and fathers.[39] Public schools cannot deny participation in any school activity because of pregnancy, marital or parental status. State aid is available to help offset the costs of serving school-age parents.

Two organizations have established guidelines for school-based programs: the Center for Assessment and Policy Development and the Adolescent Parent Network of the Minnesota Organization on Adolescent Pregnancy, Prevention and Parenting.[40]

School-Age Parent Program

The Metropolitan School District School-Age Parent Program (SAPAR) in Madison, Wisconsin, is a full-day program that serves students through the age of twenty. Course work is offered in English, social studies, math, computer technology, consumer education and family education. Childcare and other supportive services are provided. Students generally enroll for one to four quarters.

In Madison, 37% of school-age parents graduate from high school, compared with 85% of other students. 46% of the school-age mothers who enroll in SAPAR graduate from high school.[41] SAPAR serves 40 mothers a year at an estimated cost of $12,000 each above the regular education cost, including childcare. The state subsidizes $500 of the cost for each student.

New York City Programs for Pregnant Students

New York City's four Programs for Pregnant Students served 1,500 students in the late 1960s and 323 in 2006—a small portion of the 7,000 girls in public schools who became pregnant each year.[42] They have had low test scores, poor attendance and inadequate facilities even at the cost of $33,670 a year for each student. Less than 50% returned to high school. The decision to close the schools in 2007 came after the Education Department concluded that the girls were in second-class schools and treated more like mothers-to-be than students.

ALTERNATIVE LIVING ARRANGEMENTS FOR ADOLESCENT MOTHERS

Minor mothers who are unable to live with their families are likely to be homeless or in foster care. The Personal Responsibility and Work Opportunity Reconciliation Act of 1996 stipulated that they must live with family members or other responsible adults in order to receive cash assistance. If they cannot, states are expected to provide alternative living arrangements.

Maternity Homes

After the death of his 4-year-old daughter Florence, Charles Crittenton, a New York businessman, established the first *Florence Crittenton Center* in Los Angeles County in 1892. In the 1960s, the shame of unwed pregnancy abated, and girls no longer sought the confidentiality of maternity homes. Some, like the *Florence Crittenton*

Home in San Francisco, now serve an indigent population of adolescent mothers, who receive support services, supervision and sometimes residence.[43] There now are about 30 *Centers* in the United States.

Most maternity homes, such as the *Gladney Center for Adoption* in Fort Worth, TX, are for pregnant girls oriented toward adoption.[44] The girls usually pay no fee and may be court wards. Some maternity homes offer longer stays for mothers and babies while helping them find another place to live. Some assist fathers with parenting and preparation for employment.

Private Homeless Parent Programs

A number of privately financed shelters for homeless adolescent mothers and their children provide counseling, mentoring and assistance in obtaining educational and financial support. An example is the *Interfaith Hospitality* program in Madison, Wisconsin.[45] It adds the component of moving families into monitored independent living.

Waunita

18-year-old Waunita dropped out of high school in Chicago when she had her first child at 16. She had been an honor student and athlete. The father of the first child abandoned her after the second child was born, and her own family was unable to provide a home for her. She came to Madison, WI, and entered the *Interfaith Hospitality* program, which houses families in churches.

Waunita finished high school and moved into the program's Apartment Project where she continued with her caseworker and mentor family. She now is employed and attending college.

Second Chance Homes

Second Chance Homes refer to group homes, a cluster of apartments or a network of homes that include services for mothers under 19 and their children.[46] In 2005, there were 105 in the United States. Mothers are required to learn parenting, budgeting, health and nutrition skills to promote their long-term economic independence and the well-being of their children.

Second Chance Homes can be transitional or long-term. The two largest sources of federal funds for states come from the Departments of Health and Human Services and of Housing and Urban Development through Temporary Assistance for Needy Families Block Grants and Social Services Block Grants. Other federal funding sources are Child Welfare and Foster Care, the Independent Living Program and the Transitional Living Grant Program.

A Mathematica study of maternity group home programs in seven states found that many residents stayed for a year or more, but just as many left within a month or so of entry.[47] In 2005, the cost of 43 homes with 355 residents was over $18 million or $51,000 for each girl and baby.

The Massachusetts Alliance for Young Families estimates that 16,000 girls and boys in Massachusetts have 13,000 children.[48] Massachusetts operates a statewide network of 21 homes for over 180 mothers from 13 to 19 called *Teen Living Programs* under the Department of Social Services and the Department of Transitional Assistance. The average annual cost is about $60,000 for each family in addition to public school special education costs. Virtually all of the children have access to health care. Over 90% have their immunizations. Parents are connected to Early Intervention, Food Stamp and Women Infant and Children services. Eighty-five percent contacted several years later were in stable living situations—50% in their own apartments.

A *Hull House Teen Pregnancy and Parenting Program* evaluation in Chicago in 1991 found that parents' knowledge of contraception, child development and parenting increased.[49] There were no improvements in education, employment or repeat pregnancies. In 2001, 46% of the participants completed high school, 64% were employed and 22% lived in their own homes.

COMMUNITY PROGRAMS FOR ADOLESCENT MOTHERS

Adolescent mothers who live at home can be assisted by community-based programs.

Teen Parent Services

The Illinois Department of Human Services *Teen Parent Services* helps adolescent parents receive education, transportation and childcare and to delay subsequent pregnancies with the help of case managers.[50] Participants are expected to obtain a high school diploma or GED. To receive TANF benefits, they must help contact the child's father or mother. If they receive TANF cash, they also receive up to $50 of the child support collected by the state each month. When they no longer receive TANF payments, they receive the full amount of child support.

Parents Too Soon

Since 1982, the Ounce of Prevention Fund's network of *Parents Too Soon* programs has supported a statewide network of community based programs, including Doulas, long-term home visiting and parent resources.[51] It operates in 42 communities in Illinois and serves nearly 4,000 persons. It presumes that about one half of adolescent mothers can respond to support:

> The challenge is not to arrange handholds and direct routes into the mainstream for the one or two in a dozen with exceptional talent, exceptional intelligence. It is to help six or seven of that dozen into the mainstream.

Evidence-based program models are used to achieve positive outcomes for pregnant and parenting adolescents and their children from birth to three years of age.

Teen Parent-Infant Project

The *Chances for Children: Teen Parent-Infant Project* is a program for school-age mothers sponsored by a psychoanalytic institute and a public school in New York City.[52] It relies on "mothering the mother" to foster adolescent development and to improve parenting skills.

Treatment sessions include play therapy with the children and psychotherapy with the mother-baby dyad in a school setting in addition to informal contacts. The therapists believe that on-site school programs for adolescent mothers and their babies can create a "transitional space" in which the mother-baby pair learn how to play together.

New Chance

New Chance was a national welfare demonstration program in the 1990s designed to provide services six hours a day five days a week for mothers ages 16 to 22 without high school degrees or GEDs. The program addressed the mothers' reproductive behaviors and educational, vocational and parenting skills in addition to the children's development and education.

An evaluation found that program participants experienced some positive, but many negative, effects.[53] At a 42-month follow-up at 16 sites, program mothers were more likely to be depressed, to report behavior problems with their children, to have difficulty finding a place to live, to have a second child sooner and to experience parenting stress than the control group. One third had reading skills below the 6th grade. The cost of childcare, recruitment and case management was about $9,000 a year for each participant.

Adolescent Family Life Demonstration and Research Program

The *Adolescent Family Life Demonstration and Research Program* (AFL), created in 1981 as Title XX of the Public Health Service Act, gives grants to develop, implement and evaluate interventions to promote abstinence from sexual activity among adolescents and to provide health care, education and social services to pregnant and parenting adolescents.

In 2006, there were 42 AFL care programs entering their 1st, 4th and 5th years as partnerships between community organizations and the federal government. Most projects reach out to fathers as well as adolescent mothers, encouraging them be involved in their children's lives and aiming to prevent risky behaviors and sexually transmitted diseases in addition to enhancing parenting skills and reducing child neglect and abuse. The Office of Adolescent Pregnancy Programs administers the program funded at $30.3 million in 2007.[54]

PUBLIC BENEFITS FOR ADOLESCENT MOTHERS

The first national welfare legislation was in the Social Security Act of 1935 for widows of men covered under the law's insurance provisions. Assistance also was provided through Aid to Dependent Children (AID) to children in poor families where the mother was widowed, separated, divorced or unwed. In 1962, AID was changed to Aid to Families with Dependent Children (AFDC), which was expanded in 1964 and 1965 to include Food Stamps and Medicaid.

In 1967, the Supplemental Security Income Work Incentive Program (WIN) was enacted to encourage employment of welfare mothers by permitting them to keep some of the earnings while receiving AFDC. In 1988, the Family Support Act included the Job Opportunities and Basic Skills Training (JOBS) program. It provided for a range of services, including education, training, job search and placement, childcare, transitional childcare and Medicaid.

Subsequent legislation reflects a national concern that policies should not foster, and should discourage, adolescent and non-marital childbearing.[55]

Personal Responsibility and Work Opportunity Reconciliation Act

The Personal Responsibility and Work Opportunity Reconciliation Act of 1996 (PRWORA) replaced AFDC and aims to strengthen families and to assist mothers of all ages to become gainfully employed. Its goals include preventing non-marital births, encouraging marriage and strengthening two-parent families.

PRWORA represents a departure from the earlier emphasis on education as a means of enhancing employability. The requirement that most TANF recipients work after 24 months of receiving cash assistance combined with time limits on the receipt of cash assistance and rules about caseload participation levels exert strong pressure for rapid entry into the work force. States may terminate assistance for failure to comply with work requirements.

PRWORA requires work for parents with babies and toddlers, although states may exempt those with babies under 12 months. It mandates that states establish paternity for 90% of all births to unwed mothers. States also are required to strengthen enforcement techniques to increase child support collections. Adolescent mothers may be required to establish their children's paternity, a problem when they are in abusive situations:

> An adolescent mother left the state to get away from an abusive partner. She reluctantly gave paternity information to TANF workers in her new location and dropped out of sight. Her partner may have found where she was living through the paternity process and harmed her or caused her to flee again.

Temporary Assistance to Needy Families

PRWORA replaced previous welfare programs with a block grant called Temporary Assistance for Needy Families (TANF). It allows states flexibility in implementing new programs except that states cannot use TANF funds for a family that includes an adult who has received TANF for over 60 months. Recipients must be working within 24 months after commencing receipt of assistance. A state may allow exceptions for up to 20% of its cases. States can provide extensions with their own funds for families that reach the time limit. In addition to payments the annual cash equivalent for recipients can be: food stamps—$2,500; Women, Infants and Children—$1,800; housing aid—$6,000; and Supplementary Social Security Income—$6,500.

Adolescent parents constitute 17% of the total TANF caseload and 13% of adolescents who live in TANF families.[56] States vary in the eligibility of minor parents to receive cash benefits. TANF generally prohibits an unwed, minor parent from receiving federal benefits unless she is living with a relative, legal guardian or in a supervised facility.

Child support collections are withheld from families who receive or have received TANF assistance. States pay between 50% and 76% of retained support to the federal government. State policy options under the Deficit Reduction Act of 2006 range from passing on child support payments only to former TANF recipients or to them and current TANF recipients as well.[57]

The Wisconsin welfare-to-work program Wisconsin Works (W-2) recognizes that although minor parents carry the responsibility of caring for a child, they are still children and need the guidance of a parent or adult. It holds that under the supervision of an adult "a minor parent can obtain the life skills necessary to become a productive, independent adult and reduce the need for continuing support from government programs."[58] The presumption appears to be that they would be successful in school and later in life if they were not parents.

Regardless of their living arrangements or eligibility for TANF, minor parents may be eligible for Medicaid, food stamps and child care. Any minor parent is eligible to meet with a W-2 Financial and Employment Planner (FEP). The FEP provides information regarding eligibility for childcare, education, financial planning, family planning services, community resources, employment, Medicaid, food stamps and other nutrition programs. Adolescent parents also can be covered by kinship care payments when living with their parents.

Many public assistance programs are under-utilized by adolescent mothers. In one city, 31% of those eligible who never applied for benefits thought that TANF was "too much hassle."[59]

The TANF and Child Welfare Systems

The TANF and child welfare systems share overlapping histories, populations and philosophies.[60] The two systems impose competing—often conflicting—demands on families that make it difficult to comply with both TANF and child welfare requirements. Neither system has sufficient resources to help parents keep jobs and rear their children. They are not equipped to deal with the causes of poverty and child maltreatment.

REWARDS & SANCTIONS IN PUBLIC FINANCIAL PROGRAMS

Both positive reinforcement and negative sanctions have been used to try to improve the lives of adolescent parents who receive public financial benefits.

Ohio Learning, Earning, and Parenting Program

Ohio's *Learning, Earning, and Parenting Program* (LEAP) sought to promote school attendance through financial incentives and penalties for pregnant and parenting adolescents on welfare. Adolescents who complied with LEAP rules had bonuses added to their monthly welfare payment—$62 for school enrollment and $62 for regular school attendance—whereas those who failed to comply without an acceptable reason had $62 deducted from their payments.

Manpower Development Research Center's controlled study of LEAP began when the program was launched in 1989 and continued until 1997.[61] This study revealed that three years after involvement in the program General Educational Development (GED) rates increased among adolescents who were enrolled in school when they entered LEAP, but not for adolescents who were not enrolled in school when they entered LEAP. Two-thirds of the adolescents did not receive a high school diploma or a GED within the three-year follow-up period. However, one-sixth of the adolescents were still in school at the end of that period and could have graduated or received a GED subsequently. Sixty-one percent of LEAP and 60% of the control group were employed four years later.

Cal-Learn

The *Cal-Learn* program was designed to reduce adolescent pregnancy rates and long-term welfare dependency of adolescent parents receiving CalWORKs cash aid and services.[62] It serves 15,000 girls monthly and consists of coordinated services to help them become self-sufficient adults and responsible parents. Bonuses and sanctions encourage school attendance and good grades. Four $100 bonuses/sanctions per year may be earned or deducted based on report card results, plus a $500 bonus for graduating or attaining a GED.

An evaluation of the Cal-Learn demonstration project revealed that 32% of the participants graduated from high school or earned GEDs compared to 24% in the control group. The program had no effect on subsequent childbearing or employment and earnings.[63]

Wisconsin Learnfare

The *Learnfare* program under the Department of Workforce Development required participants to attend school or receive sanctions. A study by the Wisconsin Legislative Fiscal Bureau found that sanctions had no effect on school attendance.[64]

PROGRAMS FOR ADOLESCENT FATHERS

Programs for adolescent fathers who have emotional ties with their children aim to help them handle their responsibilities for their children and decrease subsequent pregnancies.[65] They include parenting classes and support groups involving both parents.

Teen Father Collaboration

The *Teen Father Collaboration*, a two-year national demonstration project started in 1983, was designed to determine the most effective ways to help adolescent fathers.[66] Eight social service agencies provided nearly 400 young fathers and prospective fathers—most 17 or 18—with a variety of services, including counseling, educational assistance and job training. Many fathers wanted to contribute financially to their children's upbringing but could not because they were unemployed. By the end of the project, of the 400 participants only 23% had full-time and 14% part-time employment. Only half of the participants who were not enrolled in school when they entered the program had returned to school or obtained their GEDs. Ambivalence on the part of cooperating agencies may have been a factor in diminishing the effects of the program.

A Program for Young Black Fathers

Inner city young fathers in a Southwestern city were offered an array of health, social and community services to help them function as responsible fathers.[67] In a follow-up of 181 participants, only 17% could be located and reported gains in self-improvement; 13% reported gains in family relationships. The program highlighted the young fathers' struggle to meet their own needs and provide for their families.

Center for Urban Families

The *Center for Urban Development* (CFUF) founded in 1999 as the *Center for Fathers, Families and Workforce Development* is committed to assisting fathers in regaining personal power to benefit their families and communities.[68] Based in Baltimore, CFUF includes 1,700 low-income men and women each year. Ninety-eight percent are Black, 61% are males, 47% have been convicted of a felony or misdemeanor, 32% have a history of substance abuse and nearly all live in poverty. Program evaluation was underway in 2007.

META-ANALYSES OF ADOLESCENT PARENT PROGRAMS

Over half of 19 studies reviewed by Lorraine Klerman, professor of maternal and child health at Brandeis University, reported that some adolescent mothers in these programs had postponed additional pregnancies.[69] With the exception of those in which adolescents used contraceptive implants, few carefully evaluated programs reduced additional births in the two years after the first birth to less than 25%—a rate close to that without any intervention.

An analysis of why programs for adolescent fathers have been ineffective was carried out in Austin, Texas.[70] Non-custodial fatherhood is not high on the public policy agenda. As a result, these fathers do not receive needed health, mental health, welfare, workforce development and legal services. Many have been involved with the criminal justice system. When they are unable to find jobs they become discouraged and turn to gangs and the illegal drug industry.

NEED FOR RIGOROUS PROGRAM EVALUATION

The disappointing results of programs designed to help adolescent parents reveal the limits of voluntary educational and job training programs.[71] Participants with higher education or skills generally benefit from them. But they are unable to help most adolescent mothers and fathers overcome their dysfunctional situations.

Even "evidence-based" programs intended to promote the aspirations and maturity of adolescent parents have had disappointing results.[72] Policy makers confronted with evaluating "evidence-based" social programs need to know that applying the methods of physical science research to the social sciences is not straightforward. They need help in evaluating what "evidence" means. Statistical significance can mean a 5% change without practical significance. Identifying markers for biological processes also is far easier than for social processes. This means that evidence for the causes of changes must be compelling and obvious.

Researchers need to develop and evaluate approaches to adolescent pregnancy prevention that target all pertinent systems and employ designs that are sensitive to system interactions over time. The linkages between systems may be more important than the individual systems.[73]

Social science research must be evaluated with the following caveats:

- Some outcomes, such as parenting skills and self-esteem, are difficult to measure. *What Do Children Need to Flourish? Conceptualizing and Measuring Indicators of Positive Development* offers guidance for markers to measure changes.[74]
- Many key outcomes can only be measured after long time lapses.
- Outcomes must be robust and far exceed statistical significance.
- Upward and downward trends may reflect periodic cycles unrelated to programs.
- Successful programs are likely to involve the most favorable subjects.
- Small samples conducive to service delivery make statistical evaluations difficult.
- Methodology must include control groups. Where there is more demand than capacity to serve, applicants can be randomly selected into programs as space allows.[75] Those not selected can be controls.

In effect, cultural values are distillations of what works over time in a particular society. In this sense, cultural values are "evidence-based" guidelines for social programs that have stood the test of time. Policy makers need to balance "evidence-based" considerations with cultural values. If "evidence-based" programs conflict with cultural values, their long-range integrity may well be compromised. By the same token if "evidence-based" programs have robust research support, they likely reflect underlying cultural values. For example, if a program for adolescent mothers results in 75% high school graduation compared to 33% for comparable controls, it probably is because it builds upon the cultural value of personal responsibility.

Strong evaluation findings on programs generate interest from communities and funders.[76] But to successfully duplicate results of model programs, new sites need to replicate models with fidelity and include performance measurements.

The National Science Foundation is encouraging the development of a hybrid field in universities called "services science" that would use technological and management expertise to improve the performance of services that now employ more than 75% of American workers.[77] High-speed internet, wireless networks and specialized software can improve service delivery.

CONCLUSION

A wide variety of programs intended to promote the aspirations and maturity of adolescent mothers have had disappointing results at costs that can exceed $60,000 a year. These results expose the limitations of voluntary programs that help older more than adolescent mothers and do not reach the most needy. Programs for adolescent fathers have had even more disappointing results.

There are two dominant explanations for these disappointing results. First, the personal, social and economic circumstances of adolescent parents pose formidable obstacles. In addition to being young and living in poverty with few social and family supports, they lack basic educational skills and are beset by personal problems ranging from clinical depression to alcohol and drug abuse often related to neglect and abuse earlier and currently in their lives. Many have difficulty conforming to the schedules and routines of education and employment.

Second, the multitude of resources adolescent parents need are not effectively coordinated and are overburdened. Federal legislation culminating in the Personal Responsibility and Work Opportunity Reconciliation Act of 1996 requires far more resources than are currently available to meet its objectives. Existing programs can include sanctions that make it difficult for mothers to meet the requirements of child welfare services

All of this points to adolescent parenthood as a symptom of core dysfunctions in our society rather than a situation that can be remedied in isolation from these dysfunctions.

If adolescent parenthood was in the best interests of the adolescents themselves, their babies, their families and our society, the high costs of its support could be justified. However, this support clearly is a damage-control measure that does not reach the most vulnerable parents and their babies. At the least, it betrays adolescents' trust in our society to protect them from making decisions that compromise their development and their futures. At the most, it permits babies to be used in efforts to stimulate adolescent maturation and to further ideological agendas.

Chapter 30

Dampening and Amplifying Trends

The process of making human beings human is breaking down in American society.

James S. Coleman, 1982
The Asymmetric Society[1]

Attitudes toward adolescent parenthood vary across societies. In Scandinavian countries, adolescent childbearing is unacceptable. Sexually active adolescents are encouraged to use contraceptives or pregnancy termination to prevent it.[2] In the United States, the ambiguous message to adolescents is: "Try not to get pregnant, but, if you do, we will support you."

The positive and negative trends that dampen and amplify adolescent and dependent adult pregnancy and childbearing in the United States merit consideration.

DAMPENING TRENDS REDUCING ADOLESCENT PARENTHOOD

Kristin Moore of Child Trends sees incompatibility with modern society—as the most compelling explanation for the decline in adolescent pregnancy and childbirth.[3]

Greater Emphasis on Family Life

Parents are spending more time actively engaged with their children.[4] Even while involved in the workforce, mothers are spending at least as much or more time with their children as they did forty years ago. Fathers' participation in childrearing has increased as well.

A variety of programs strengthen families, such as family resource centers, home visitation for the parents of newborns and fatherhood initiatives. Community development efforts, such as *Making Connections*, are creating safer neighborhoods.[5]

Improving Quality of Education

More children are enrolled in high-quality early childhood and after-school programs. Elementary math scores in 2007 were the highest ever for 4th and 8th graders.[6]

Progress has been made in comprehensive sex and HIV education programs.[7] Twenty years ago none of them resulted in significant changes in behavior; currently about two-thirds do.

Decreasing Violence

Many indicators of social breakdown, which shot upward in the late 1960s and 1970s and leveled off at high levels in the 1980s, have been declining since the early 1990s. Family violence has dropped by more than half since 1993. Violent crime overall is down by 55% since 1993.[8]

Crime began to fall roughly 18 years after pregnancy termination was legalized in 1973, accounting for as much as 50% of the decrease.[9] States with higher pregnancy termination rates in the 1970s and 1980s had greater crime reductions in the 1990s.

Declining Drug Abuse

Drug abuse by adolescents has been declining since 2001.[10] Drug abuse treatment is being used by courts instead of incarceration that breaks up families.

Taxpayer Resistance to Supporting Adolescent Parents

The consequences of adolescent parenthood for taxpayers are focusing their attention on public financial support of adolescent parents. Businesses also recognize the adverse impact of parenthood on the education and work skill development of adolescents.

The following comments were made on a blog about contemporary families:

- Almost any careless 14-year-old can get pregnant and give birth. Therefore, we should not be subsidizing it. With the availability of birth control, adoption and pregnancy termination there is no excuse for having children you cannot afford.
- Parents already use more resources than the childfree, and they already pay less in taxes—they don't call children "little deductions" for nothing. To provide an even bigger free ride to those who breed irresponsibly is to encourage even more of the same kind of irresponsibility in the next generation.

Increasing Reluctance of Relatives to Parent Adolescent's Children

The parents and extended families of adolescent parents are becoming increasingly reluctant to sacrifice their own goals in life to accommodate the children of their offspring. Many want them to avoid repeating the cycle of adolescent parenthood they experienced.

Increased Access to Adoption

The dramatic shift in recent decades from adoptions in the United States to foreign countries is beginning to reverse. The large number of potential adoptive parents has made it possible to find adoptive homes for minority babies in the United States.

Feminist Emphasis on Career Development

The feminist movement has empowered girls to pursue careers in the workforce and has fostered awareness of male exploitation of girls and women. Role models offering hope for achievements other than by motherhood are appearing in disadvantaged communities.

Welfare Reform

More stringent welfare and child support policies have reduced non-marital childbearing and single motherhood to some extent.[11]

Welfare innovations in Minnesota and Connecticut and non-welfare experiments, such as Wisconsin's "New Hope" and Canada's "Self Sufficiency Program," that raise the incomes of single mothers have reduced divorce and increased marriage somewhat.[12]

Programs to improve communication and relationship skills for new mothers and fathers may help genetic fathers play a greater role in the lives of their children.[13] These programs also try to obtain needed services, such as for mental health treatment and employment.

Child Support Enforcement

The National Directory of New Hires, the Federal Case Registry, the passport denial program and the Financial Institution Data Match have enhanced child support collection.

The Personal Responsibility and Work Opportunity Reconciliation Act of 1996 streamlined paternity determination. More than 17 million children and their families received $24 billion in child support in 2006 through the Child Support Enforcement Program.[14] This federal-state partnership now collects $4.58 for every dollar spent.

AMPLIFYING TRENDS—BARRIERS TO REDUCING ADOLESCENT PARENTHOOD

There are barriers to realistically approaching adolescent parenthood in addition to the earlier onset of puberty, the earlier initiation of intercourse and peer pressure for sexual activity.

Mixed Messages

Our adolescents are exposed to the most self-defeating of all possible messages about sex through media that convey the impression that non-marital sex is exciting and present a romanticized view of marriage and parenthood.[15] Few sources of information they take seriously inform adolescents about the consequences of sexual activity and the realities of marriage.

Adolescents see their own parents or their parents' friends involved in multiple sexual relationships. Early childbearing is acceptable and even adulated in some settings.

Public assistance policies and parent education programs clearly condone adolescent childrearing. Girls learn that with babies they become eligible for public benefits that seem substantial and independence awarding. If they make adoption plans, they lose these benefits and possibly face criticism by peers and families.

For many adults, the compassionate impulse to support a vulnerable adolescent mother and her baby overrides considering other alternatives for her and for her child.

Lack of Parental and Institutional Accountability

Our society's reluctance to require accountability for individual and institutional behaviors underlies many of the barriers to dealing effectively with adolescent parenthood. This lack of accountability results in irresponsible parents. It also results in institutions and policies that tend to perpetuate rather than solve these problems.[16]

The "my personal life is none of your business" attitude is an outgrowth of individualism. It brushes aside parents' responsibility to society to raise responsible citizens. It obscures the fact that preparation for responsible citizenship begins with being a responsible family member.

A Sense of Helplessness

Efforts to reduce adolescent pregnancy encounter resistant beliefs that contribute to a sense of helplessness and to damage control rather than preventive policies. One is the belief that public attitudes toward sexual behavior cannot be changed. When pregnancy occurs, the focus is either on termination or on supporting the adolescent mother. Heated arguments revolve around notifying parents. The competence of adolescents to make life-course-altering decisions and their competence to rear their children are seldom considered.

Another belief is that stress and despair resulting from intractable racial, socioeconomic, psychological and abusive factors lead many adolescents to turn to drugs, alcohol and sex for relief. The resulting pregnancies and births involve issues that are too complicated to resolve.

Nonjudgmental Ethos

Contemporary professionals are strongly inclined toward nonjudgmental approaches to human behavior. Human relationships go much more smoothly without stereotypical prejudices.

On a nonjudgmental-judgmental continuum, health professionals are at one end and law enforcement professionals are at the other end. Mental health professionals especially must be nonjudgmental in order to establish rapport with patients.

But no one can avoid making judgments. Our innate tendency is to be judgmental. Being nonjudgmental means suppressing or consciously dealing with our instinctive negative reactions to people who differ from us in appearances, attitudes or behavior. Stranger anxiety is a biological wariness of unfamiliar individuals that can be measured physiologically.[17]

We all are guided by values that are inherently judgmental. The question is where to draw the line in expecting one's own values to apply to others. Behavior that offends others is generally regarded as uncivil. But an offended person may either be reacting to the unreasonable judgments of others or be unreasonably sensitive. Because this distinction may be difficult to make, we tend to avoid saying or doing anything that might offend others. Two undesirable consequences can result. First, resentment can build up if we restrain ourselves from expressing our feelings. Second, persons who need it are deprived of our constructive criticism.

Being nonjudgmental can be carried to a counterproductive extreme. Our society has evolved from being predominantly judgmental to being predominantly non-judgmental. The days are gone in which blatant public prejudice and discrimination generally prevail. The pendulum has swung to the opposite extreme. Now avoiding offending people has led to extreme non-judgmentalism. Misbehavior is defined by laws rather than values. Public disapproval of behavior that is not illegal is discouraged. The acceptance of overtly sexual behavior has shifted such adjectives as "promiscuous" to "sexually active," "adultery" to "affair" and "illegitimate" to "unwed." Just as judgmental approaches can foster prejudice and discrimination against the innocent, nonjudgmental approaches can condone uncivil and self-defeating behavior.

We need a balanced view of the nonjudgmental principle. Certainly judgments based on stereotypes, especially reflecting racism, sexism or ageism, must be avoided in public policy making. But judgments that reflect cultural values, especially as encoded in statutes, are necessary to preserve the integrity of our society. Avoiding making these judgments is a disservice to those who need feedback about their attitudes and behavior.

Misapplication of Cultural Competence

Cultural competence is an essential concept for professionals and organizations that deal with people with backgrounds and traditions differing from their own. The National Center for Cultural Competence suggests the following principles for effective cross-cultural work:[18] institutionalizing cultural knowledge; involving consumers, stakeholders and communities; adapting to the diversity of communities; and self-assessments of cultural sensitivity.

But cultural competence can be construed to mean that behavior and values of cultural origin should be accepted on that basis alone. This misunderstanding can result in withholding advice that could prevent individuals from engaging in behaviors contrary to their own self-interests. Misunderstanding cultural competence can impede the process of assimilation that enables people of diverse backgrounds to live together harmoniously. For example, accepting adolescent parenthood as a valid expression of a cultural tradition perpetuates maladaptive life styles in modern society and actually can reflect prejudice against minorities—"That's just the way they are."

Minimizing the Hazards of Sexual Behavior

The freedom to engage in aggressive behavior is limited by numerous laws because of its obviously damaging effect on other people. In contrast, sexual behavior is relatively unregulated because it is regarded as a private activity. This obscures the fact that sexual behavior often has more serious and lasting consequences than aggressive behavior, such as the emotional damage of sexual abuse, the physical damage and lethality of sexually transmitted diseases (especially AIDS) and pregnancy. Regarding diseases and pregnancy as the only undesirable consequences of sexual behavior leads to overlooking guilt and loss of self-respect. Because sex is regarded as a private activity, we fail to openly recognize two epidemics: 1) the sexual abuse of one in five girls and women and 2) the one in four adolescent girls with sexually transmitted diseases.

The assumption that adolescents can be induced to handle their sexual impulses wisely through education and the use of contraceptives ignores the fact that the risk of pregnancy is not realistically managed by the most vulnerable, even with sex education and contraception.

Parenthood Undermining Factors

Social, attitudinal and psychological factors undermine parenthood in the United States.

Self-Assertive Individualism

The freedom to act without restraints is a treasured principle in the United States. One facet of individual freedom is the privacy of one's personal life, home and family. On the positive side, this privacy relieves individuals of pressures to conform and the prying eyes of others. On the negative side, it diminishes the accountability of parents to society and conceals child neglect and abuse. The emphasis on individual freedom has led to a lack of commitment in personal relationships, cohabitation, divorce and avoidance of child support.

Self-assertive individualism is expressed in the following images:

- "Yankee know how and can do"—"I will be a winner;"
- "macho" independence with an audacious defiance of authority;
- prizing excellence and acquiring more things through "doing it all;"
- doing "my own thing" and being "cool;"
- being strong willed and seeking outrageous thrills; and
- "fighting for what I believe is right."

Self-assertive individualism grants us freedom to do as we wish and gives us license to ignore our responsibilities to others. It drowns out our ethic of caring. It underlies the belief that anyone can overcome the constraints of disadvantage through ambition and hard work. Herbert Gans, professor of sociology at Columbia University, and Lawrence Mitchell, professor of law at George Washington University, point out how this emphasis affects our society's values:[19]

- reluctance to postpone gratification and make unpleasant long-range decisions;
- obscured awareness that sexual can be more harmful than aggressive behavior;
- exploitation of sexual and aggressive behaviors for commercial purposes;
- failure to help disadvantaged and self-defeating persons lead effective lives; and
- minimizing the societal and economic sources of our social problems.

Self-assertive, individualistic American values prize material success.[20] In this ethos, voluntary organizations are expected to solve social problems that require governmental action. Politics is dominated by competing elites. Winners, notably athletes and corporation executives, are admired. There is no public recognition of self-sacrificing, successful parents.

Excessive Dependency on Experts in Childrearing

Dependence on childrearing experts can be an expression of self-assertive individualism when based on a desire for perfection. Much recent expert advice has stressed non-punitive approaches to misbehavior. As a result, parents avoid frustrating their children because they want them to be happy and fear stifling their creativity. They fear their children's anger or rejection. Their frustration as they attempt to win their demanding children's love heightens their dilemma because they do not know how to handle their anger toward their children. They feel guilty because they are told not to react in anger or physically limit their children. Their children's resulting misbehavior severely strain two-parent relationships and can overwhelm single parents.

Psychological Factors

The psychological factors that undermine parenthood are related to absent or insecure early child-parent attachment bonding that interferes with developing the capacity for empathy, forming committed relationships and acquiring self-discipline.

Insecure Attachment Bonding

A child's psychological self is formed from internalizing models of self-regulation from parents. The internalized image of a dependable parent provides continuity of the self. Trust in a parental, at first literal, "holding environment" leads to trust of the world (reality). The mistrust of a parent (insecurity regarding love and limits) leads to difficulty dealing with reality.

The continuity of society depends upon stable relationships between persons based upon reciprocal attachment bonding developed in early child-parent relationships. In contrast, personal insecurity from insecure attachment bonding results in a lack of commitment in adult relationships. This is seen in a lack of empathy for others, which leads to a lack of respect for others, for oneself and for cultural values.

The future of our society depends on the ability of individuals to learn from the past, live comfortably in the present and plan for the future. Respect for the past comes from respect for parents. Respect for others and the capacity to plan for the future flow from secure relationships with parents who model self-control and set limits. When attachment bonding between children and parents is absent or insecure, family life is unstable with adverse impacts on society.

The Lack of Shame and Guilt

The threshold for disapproving behavior has moved from informal social cues to breaking a law. Behavior is not limited unless it violates a law or unless it does not meet an age-grading or competency test. This means that speech is unlimited unless it poses an immediate danger to others or is libelous. The result is a gradual disappearance of external disapproval of behavior in the form of shame. The ability to feel shame depends upon the capacity for empathy with others and sensitivity to the feelings and attitudes of others. Guilt limits behavior through disapproval in one's own eyes. The ability to feel guilt depends upon having a conscience. A significant segment of our population lacks conscious shame and guilt as internal controls of their behavior.

Psychological Defense Mechanisms

The denial of powerful emotional states can lead to untoward behaviors and events in families. For example, a depressed person can engage in angry, impulsive behavior or can seek relief through drugs, overeating or childbearing. Hatred, envy, jealousy and greed can lead family members to project their problems on others and avoid assuming responsibility for their own behavior. All of these defensive feelings distort and disrupt family relationships.

Waiving Adolescents into Adult Courts

In the mid-1990s in the midst of a spike in violent juvenile crime and an ethos of punishing offenders, many states made it easier to waive adolescents into adult court.[21] Wisconsin allows 10-year-olds to be tried as an adult for certain crimes and 15-year-olds for any crime. Transferring juveniles to adult prisons avoids the higher costs of juvenile institutions.

Adolescents incarcerated in adult facilities are more prone to recidivism from more serious crimes than those treated in juvenile facilities.[22] This "hardening" process for adolescent offenders makes them less likely to ever be able to function as competent parents.

The "Family Values" Controversy

There is bipartisan political endorsement of "family values." For the far right "family values" may mean that mothers should stay at home.[23] For the far left "family values" may mean that childcare should be provided or subsidized by government. The former wants government out of the family, except on "right to life" issues. The latter wants government out of the family, except on parent support issues. Both equate parents' wishes with what is best for children. Neither takes into account the children's interests.

The far right, devoted to family privacy, advocates that disadvantaged parents take care of themselves. The antidote to contemporary irresponsibility is moral regeneration. An embryo's right to life is not followed by a child's right to competent parenting after birth.

The far left, devoted to individual freedom, advocates caring for disadvantaged families through governmental programs. It believes that the disadvantaged are victims who cannot be held responsible for their behavior. The ills of society are to be cured by eliminating injustice.

The emphasis on the privacy of the family and on individual freedom stymies the prevention of child neglect and abuse. For example, the far right may oppose home visitation programs because they invade the privacy of families. The far left may not support them because they compete with childcare for public funds. Opposition to governmental involvement in family life by both extremes hinders public debate about adolescent parenthood.

Emphasizing the Heroism of Adolescent Mothers

Efforts to reduce adolescent parenthood have been thwarted by an emphasis on the heroic mastery of adversity by some adolescent parents who manage to thrive with support. There is an understandable desire to avoid offending women who mastered the challenges of adolescent parenthood and became successful parents and outstanding career women. This laudable intent can be counterproductive when their examples justify supporting all adolescent mothers. Even for the successful, the question always remains: How much better would their lives have been without the burdens of adolescent parenthood?

The following adolescent mothers became successful adults:

Mary Childers

Mary Childers wrote about her own life as an adolescent mother in *Welfare Brat*. Her ambivalence about the parenthood of her niece illustrates how adolescent parents who succeed in the face of adversity can be seen as heroines:[24]

> One of my nieces, Lisa, is pregnant again. She already has two kids she cannot support, emotionally or financially. She's repeating the mistakes of her mother (my sister Jackie) and her grandmother (my mother). I fear she'll end up begging for welfare and put herself and her kids through the same humiliation that soured my childhood and my mother's life.

Why do some poor women replicate mistakes they surely hear others operatically lament? How could my niece do this to the two children she already has? How could she do this to herself? Although she loves her children, she has often regretted the loss of her youth to them. Just when she could taste freedom, she may have slipped into believing the myth that you can keep a man by hatching him a baby. He fled, of course.

I question my niece's behavior, but I also empathize with her. What a heroine you have to be to drag yourself out of bed day after day into minimum-wage jobs, aware that you'll never get ahead and fearful that everything will collapse. No wonder she may have hoped again that love would subsidize her life. Now, with abortion out of the question because of her religious beliefs, she will of course give birth to another cherished obstacle. The child is an excuse, an accident, a gift and a burden.

Jolly

The novel *Make Lemonade* by Virginia Euwer Wolff is recommended by some professionals for adolescent mothers.[25] The message of the book is that young people can accomplish much if they work together. It describes the struggle of 17-year-old Jolly, a mother of two who hires LaVaughn, a 14-year-old, as a babysitter.

> LaVaughn babysits everyday after school while Jolly goes to work. LaVaughn plants lemon seeds and waters them. The lemon seeds do not sprout. Before long, LaVaughn is spending a lot of time at Jolly's home. She sleeps over because of Jolly's late shifts.
>
> One day Jolly comes homes crying. She tells LaVaughn that her boss got a little "touchy-feely" with her and that she quit. Her rent is due; she has no way to pay LaVaughn, who agrees to babysit without pay while Jolly searches for a job. With LaVaughn's encouragement, Jolly finally decides to go back to school and earn her high school diploma, and the children begin daycare. LaVaughn babysits one hour a day while Jolly does her homework.
>
> Shortly after the children begin daycare, the lemon seeds sprout.

Nicole

Melinda Robertson, a former adolescent parent, wrote a book that presents the complexities of adolescent parenthood in an effort to reduce adolescent pregnancy. At the same time she hopes to inspire adolescent parents by Nicole's example.[26]

> Nicole is a 15-year-old girl from an upper middle class family who gets pregnant the first time she had sexual intercourse. She initially tries to hide her pregnancy but decides to take responsibility for her actions and have the baby. Juggling the demands of motherhood and school is more than she imagined. But she succeeds with the help of her family and supportive services.

Prejudices

Three subtle, but powerful, prejudices underlie our society's failure to deal effectively with adolescent parenthood:

- sexism against females ("good girls say no"; no such expectation for boys),
- ageism against adolescents (ignoring adolescence as a developmental stage), and
- racism against minority groups (they are destined to early and single parenthood).

The combined force of these prejudices is seen most poignantly with the Black adolescent girl who is impregnated to prove a male's fecundity (sexism), treated as an adult and deprived of the opportunity to complete her adolescent development (ageism) and seen as destined to adolescent motherhood by her cultural heritage (racism).

Other examples of sexism and ageism are evident in societies that encourage early marriages. For example, Muslim and Hindu parents may arrange a daughter's marriage before her first menstruation and thereby avoid out-of-wedlock pregnancies but perpetuate a subservient role for women.[27] The developmental aspects of adolescence are ignored.

CONCLUSION

The timing appears to be propitious for developing social policies that discourage adolescent and vulnerable adult pregnancy and parenthood. Recent trends reveal a shift in adolescent attitudes toward serving their own self-interests rather than following their impulses and fantasies. Adolescent sexual behavior, pregnancy and childbirth rates are decreasing.

Our society's reluctance to require accountability for individual and institutional behaviors and a nonjudgmental ethos underly many of the barriers to dealing effectively with adolescent parenthood. We are rapidly reaching the point at which limits must be set on the freedom of individuals to do as they wish when other people are affected by their sexual behavior, particularly when those other people are children. We can no longer presume that childbearing and childrearing are private matters without consequences for society.

Adolescent parenthood exposes a variety of anti-parenthood attitudes in the United States. Childless adults may believe that parents already have unfair advantages. The far right opposes governmental involvement in parenthood because it invades the privacy of families. The far left does the same because it infringes on personal freedoms.

Support for adolescent parenthood is a default position that lacks holistic thinking about adolescent pregnancy prevention and planning. In an effort to help adolescent parents, we honor and publicize the achievements of the few who are successful without recognizing how even more successful their lives might have been without the responsibilities of parenthood.

The combination of three prejudices is seen when a minority adolescent girl is impregnated to prove a male's fecundity (sexism), treated as an adult and deprived of the opportunity to complete her adolescent development (ageism) and seen as destined to adolescent motherhood by her cultural heritage (racism).

We need to capitalize on the adolescent trend away from irresponsible sexual behavior. If we shift to a paradigm in which parenthood is seen as a valued career, we can create a tipping point that aligns social values with our integrative cultural values and reduces the likelihood of adolescents becoming parents.

Part 9

SOLUTIONS

In politics there is no agreed-upon solution reached by sheer brainpower and logic, but rather an ongoing and never-ending struggle between contested versions of the truth.

Joseph J. Ellis, 2007
American Creation[i]

Fortunately, the initial conditions and subsequent amplifying influences of adolescent parenthood can be averted by preventing adolescent pregnancy in the first place and by fostering a social and cultural context in which adolescent parenthood is not encouraged. An extensive array of programs aims to prevent adolescent pregnancy in the United States.

The inescapable fact is that too many children are growing up in the United States under circumstances that prevent them from becoming responsible, productive citizens. These obstacles could be mitigated if our society strengthened our struggling families. We need to value sacrificial parenthood as a life-long career vital to the future of our society. We need to make it possible for parents to compete economically with adults without children. We need to set minimum standards for parenthood.

Adolescent and dependent adult childbirth should be recognized as a serious public health crisis. Parenthood Planning Teams composed of existing family planning, prenatal care, child welfare services, home visitation and legal professionals can be organized in the same way crisis intervention teams are formed in other health and child welfare matters. When adolescents and dependent adults choose parenthood, a legal procedure is needed to ensure that their babies have competent custodial guardians.

When an adolescent's baby is born, there are three reasonable outcomes after all parties have carefully considered the available options with the assistance of a Parenthood Planning Team: 1) relatives continue custodial guardianship of the adolescent mother and assume temporary custodial guardianship of the baby; 2) a voluntary adoption plan is made for the baby; and 3) an involuntary adoption plan is arranged for the baby when relatives cannot effectively function as custodial guardians of the adolescent and her baby.

Chapter 31

Preventing Adolescent Pregnancy and Parenthood

Does anyone understand that the jobless father often destroys himself, his family, and his community? Does anyone understand the frustration of the mother who knows that her children will need the best education possible, but she can't afford it and the national community won't help pay for it? Does anyone understand that the young men who make city streets dangerous and destroy themselves with drugs could have been proud, productive citizens. Does anyone understand that these problems can destroy this country?

Richard Gordon Hatcher
Mayor, Gary, Indiana, 1971[1]

We are a second-chance society. We believe everyone can succeed in life if they try. We spend enormous amounts of money on rehabilitating adolescents and adults involved in addictions, crime and welfare dependency. But James Heckman, a University of Chicago economist, points out that the track records of all of these efforts are disappointing.[2] We overinvest in adults with a low return and underinvest in early life where the return is high.

The evidence is clear that interventions with disadvantaged children early in life have much higher economic returns than "deep end" interventions later in life. Public policies designed to create the "good society" usually stress improving education, employment and wages.[3] *None of these policies will make a significant difference unless we ensure that all children have competent parents.*

The RAND Corporation found that the returns from early childhood preventive interventions are up to $17 for each dollar invested.[4] The best returns are from home visitation for the parents of newborns and home visitation combined with early childhood education. Preventing adolescent and dependent adult pregnancy and parenthood is even more cost effective.

We do need effective "deep end" interventions, but we need to do much more at little cost to prevent these problems from developing in the first place. Just as prevention is the key to personal health, prevention is essential for our society's health as well.

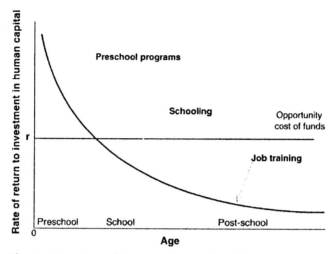

Figure 31.1. Rates of Return to Human Capital Investment.

The theme of this book is extending efforts to prevent social problems to before babies are born in order to reap the greatest humanitarian and economic benefits. Supporting adolescent parenthood flies in the face of this aim. It overlooks the obvious fact that adolescent pregnancy prevention really is intended to prevent adolescent parenthood.

A MODEL FOR ADOLESCENT PREGNANCY AND PARENTHOOD PREVENTION

Joseph Allen, a professor of psychology at the University of Virginia, suggests a nutritional model for preventing adolescent pregnancy and parenthood.[5] Some adolescents are psychosocially "poorly nourished" in a way that leaves them susceptible to a wide array of maladaptive behaviors. This "nutritional-risk" model focuses on nurturing an adolescent's development into a productive citizen. It focuses on managing risky behaviors that result from the lack of nurturance. It focuses on building their human capital through self-respect and self-confidence. It focuses on their families and where they live. It focuses on their *social capital*.

Whereas *physical capital* refers to material things and *human capital* refers to characteristics of individuals, *social capital* refers to connections between individuals—social networks based on reciprocity, good will and trustworthiness. Nourishing adolescents' human capital means fostering their social capital by improving the quality of their family lives, neighborhoods and communities rather than just by fixing individual problems.[6]

Social capital binds families and communities together and makes cooperative action possible.[7] It is based on trust that acts like a lubricant that makes any group run more efficiently and effectively. Communities with higher social capital have lower crime rates, better health, higher educational achievement and better economic growth. There can be a downside. Groups with high social capital can isolate themselves from *Them* who are not *Us*.

When the focus is on fixing problems rather than on building social capital, the emphasis is on managing, housing, educating and employing adolescent mothers and fathers.[8] We need to focus on building adolescents' human and social capital before they become mothers and fathers. They need safe places for conversations about responsible decision-making based on accurate information. They need positive role modeling and opportunities that motivate them to pursue education and training. The key to preventing adolescent parenthood is nourishing adolescent development and thereby preventing adolescent pregnancy.

ADOLESCENT PREGNANCY PREVENTION

Efforts to prevent adolescent pregnancy must recognize the fact that significant numbers of adolescents are not inclined to avoid and may actually seek pregnancy. In one study, one-fifth of the girls described their pregnancies as planned, and over one-half desired to give birth once they found they were pregnant.[9] Furthermore, the predatory behavior of men and boys is encouraged by the prevalent sexist attitude that responsibility for contraception lies with girls.

Capitalizing on their decline, the *National Campaign to Prevent Teen Pregnancy* challenges our nation to reduce adolescent pregnancy rates by one-third by 2015.[10] The *Campaign* advocates ten steps for building adolescents' social capital:

- Recognize the problem is not solved. The United States still has the highest rates of adolescent pregnancy and births among comparable nations.
- Parents must do more. Parents need to model loving relationships and offer guidance about sexual behavior.
- Stop fighting about abstinence versus contraception. The best choice is to delay sexual activity, but adolescents also need accurate information about the benefits and limitations of contraception.
- Intensify efforts in communities with high rates of adolescent pregnancy, especially Latino.
- Make the connection between adolescent pregnancy and poverty.
- Help fathers fulfill their roles in adolescent development.
- Start early. The conversation parents, faith leaders and other key adults must have with children about sex begins during early childhood.
- Involve the powerful. Sustained change requires that the entertainment media, elected officials, corporate executives, press leaders, foundation heads, faith leaders and educators be involved.
- States and communities should set goals for reducing adolescent pregnancy.
- Stay on the cutting edge of ever-changing technologies.

These objectives can be attained by applying the principles of social marketing in the context of education and law enforcement to developing adolescents' human and social capital.

SOCIAL MARKETING TO DEVELOP HUMAN CAPITAL

Social marketing aims to develop human capital by showing the benefits of healthy behavior through persuasion and education in the context of law enforcement.

Michael Rothschild, a professor of business at the University of Wisconsin, describes social marketing as tool for changing maladaptive behavior.[11] It can be used to change adolescents' behavior by identifying and nurturing their self-interests as opposed to their desires and impulses; by creating and delivering benefits that promote those self-interests; and by reducing barriers to achieving those self-interests.

The decisions people make often are determined by emotions, incomplete information and a host of other factors.[12] Future goals often are discounted in making difficult decisions. Human beings tend to overspend and undersave resources in the short-term, which leads to long-term debt. Adolescent parenthood is an example of a long-term debt that results from short-term decisions that lead to pregnancy, childbirth and parenthood.

Adolescents can be placed on a continuum from "prone to behave as we wish them to" to "resistant to behave as we wish them to." Those who are prone to behave as we wish them to are likely to be optimistic about the future and to see the value of delayed gratification. They are likely to live in affluent, educated families. They are not the targets of social marketing.

Those who are resistant to behave as we wish them to are likely to be pessimistic about their futures and to choose short-term benefits. Members of this group are more likely to live in poor, less educated families with little social capital. Many are only likely to change their behaviors through law enforcement. They are not the targets of social marketing.

Those in the middle of the continuum are neither prone nor resistant to behave as we wish them to. They are open to opportunities and inducements. Social marketing applies to them. They usually try to make the best decisions they can, but peer and family factors push them toward short-term thinking. They can be influenced by opportunities and by rewards for appropriate behaviors. The video *Tanisha's Choice*, which depicts an adolescent mother's choice of making an adoption plan, is an example of marketing to this group.[13]

Adolescents tend to be wishful thinkers who lack a future orientation because of their sense of invulnerability and their attraction to risks. They can be swayed by the belief "it can't happen to me." This omniscient and omnipotent flavoring of adolescence underlies the attitude "I don't care about that now" in spite of knowledge that smoking, drugs, noise and steroids produce disease, addiction, deafness and a shortened life span. Similarly, an adolescent can fail to take into account the realities of childrearing. These immaturities are inherent in adolescence, but they can be modified by thoughtful decision-making and self-restraint.

A social marketing strategy to help adolescents overcome the slide into the debt of parenthood is to add short-term benefits to choices that pay out in the long-term. The most effective rewards for making wise short-term decisions are *self-respect* and *self-confidence*—good feelings about oneself and about one's abilities.

The National Campaign to Prevent Teen Pregnancy maintains *Putting What Works to Work*, a project that applies research on adolescent pregnancy prevention and related issues in user-friendly materials for practitioners, policymakers and advocates.[14] Programs that aim to develop human capital by increasing self-respect and self-confidence can be classified as *curriculum-based*, *mental health screening*, *mentoring*, *service-based* and *comprehensive*. They aim to help participants plan for their futures in accord with their self-interests. For those who do not respond, the authority of the legal system is required to achieve this end.

Curriculum-based Education

The general quality of education plays a vital role in determining whether or not adolescents are absorbed in schoolwork and activities rather than creating pregnancies. Athletics offer girls and boys opportunities for non-sexual physical activities and to acquire identities unrelated to sexuality. Athletic training helps develop self-discipline.[15]

In a survey of high school students, 82% said they had a place where they could discuss sexual issues.[16] 86% knew where a provider of contraception to prevent pregnancy and sexually transmitted diseases (STD) was located. Only 62% had been shown the correct use of contraception and had at least one teacher in school who taught them to avoid risky behavior. They felt the emotional consequences of risky sexual behavior including heartbreak, depression and suicide were not discussed sufficiently. They turned to friends to discuss sexual choices. They felt their parents were too "uptight."

Sex Education Classes

Kristin Luker carried out an extensive review of sex education in the United States.[17] She attributes present-day hostilities toward sex education to the sexual revolution of the 1960s. She found that "sexual liberals" hold that sex is a healthy, quasi-recreational activity. For them, sex education helps young people manage sex risks by giving them facts. "Sexual conservatives" consider sex sacred in marriage but destructive outside it. For them, conventional sex education teaches adolescents to be irresponsible and drains sex of its mystery and power. Luker plausibly believes that this disagreement about sex underlies the political polarization of our nation.

Traditional sex education classes teach biology and safe sex. Abstinence education promotes delaying sex until marriage. Comprehensive sex education aims to convince adolescents that not having sex or using contraception if they do are in their self-interests and will enhance their self-respect. Older adolescent mothers who want to discourage girls from becoming sexually active have an important role to play in sex education programs.[18]

Sex education programs that focus on both abstinence and contraception generally have a positive effect by delaying the initiation of sex and improving contraceptive use or both.[19] The most effective classes have well trained leaders and focus on personalizing information, peer pressure and communication skills. Still, an Indiana survey revealed a disconnect between curricula that educators think is most effective and what they are actually using.[20] Most did not feel that their principals, parents and communities supported what they do.

The Personal Responsibility and Work Opportunity Reconciliation Act of 1996 significantly increased funding for abstinence education that is not supported by a majority of the public nor the scientific community.[21] A Mathematica study found that youth in four abstinence-only programs were no more likely than a control group to have abstained from sex. A National Survey of Family Growth survey found that teaching about contraception did not increase the risk of adolescent sexual activity or STD. The survey also found that adolescents who received comprehensive had a lower risk of pregnancy than adolescents who received abstinence-only sex education or none.

One quarter of school-based health clinics provide some type of contraception, according to the National Assembly on School Based Health Care.[22] Portland, Maine, high school clinics decided to extend contraception to middle school after learning that 17 middle school students had become pregnant in the preceding four years.

Although adolescents need to know facts about sex and contraception, this is not enough to curtail adolescent pregnancies.[23] In the absence of social capital and in the presence of media and peer encouragement to be sexually active, adolescents cannot be expected to establish control over their emerging reproductive capacities through school-based education alone.

Baby Think It Over

Baby Think It Over can be an effective pregnancy prevention program for both girls and boys. An artificial baby is cared for at home by students and brings out the realities of parenthood, although the experience may make motherhood appealing to some girls:[24]

> When asked to recount their "parenting" experiences, most of the students found it filled with "constant headaches," and "hardly any fun." Another said, "Me and my girl, neither one of us have time for a baby. We don't have any money. We're just kids ourselves. What do we look like having a baby now?"

Draw the Line/Respect the Line

Draw the Line/Respect the Line is a STD and pregnancy prevention program, consisting of five lessons for 6th graders and seven each for 7th and 8th graders. In a controlled study, it delayed sexual initiation among boys, who had more positive attitudes toward not having sex.[25] The benefits for girls were limited.

Wise Guys

Wise Guys is a North Carolina-based adolescent pregnancy and STD curriculum designed to promote sexual responsibility in boys.[26] Over 2,300 professionals nationwide have been trained to implement this program with a variety of ethnicities. *Wise Guys Male Responsibility Curriculum* and the Latino version, *Jóvenes Sabios,* is being used by community, school-based and faith-based organizations in over 40 states.

Aban Aya Youth Project

The *Aban Aya Youth Project* targets Blacks in 5th through 8th grade classrooms with the aim of instilling self-empowerment and pride. For grades 9 and 10, it adds five all-day Saturday workshops each year in addition to parental involvement, peer mentoring and school staff training coordinated by a Local School Health Promotion Task Force. An evaluation of the Project showed significant effects for high-risk but not for medium- or low-risk adolescents.[27]

Mental Health Screening

The chance that an adolescent will have a treatable psychiatric illness is over 20%.[28] The National Comorbidity Survey revealed that 50% of all serious adult psychiatric illnesses start by 14 and 75% by 25. Yet most mental illnesses in young people are unrecognized and untreated. In 2005, according to the Centers for Disease Control and Prevention, 17% of high school students seriously considered suicide, and 8% had attempted suicide at least once during the preceding year. The vast majority gave no warning to parents, siblings or friends.

These statistics provide a rationale for mental health screening of adolescents. *TeenScreen*, a voluntary, school-based questionnaire-interview program was developed under the direction of David Shaffer, professor of psychiatry at Columbia University.[29] In 2005, 55,000 young people in 42 states were screened. About one-third were identified as needing a clinical interview by the questionnaire. One-half of those were referred for further evaluation after the interview. In a follow-up survey of the parents of participants, 72% reported that their adolescent had significantly improved and was seeing a mental health professional.

The potential consequences of false identification are far less dire than failing to identify an adolescent with a mental illness, as seen in high school and college shootings.

Mentoring

Ideally, adolescents should be able to turn to their parents or relatives for advice. Professional counseling may well be needed for both families and individual adolescents but often is in limited supply. Mentoring through school counselors or community volunteers can offer support and referrals to available services.

The *MENTOR/National Mentoring Partnership* estimates that, although over 17 million young Americans need or want mentoring, only 3 million are in high-quality mentoring relationships.[30] In one study, 46% of adolescents with a mentor reported a high sense of self-respect and self-confidence compared to 25% who did not have a mentor.

Big Brothers Big Sisters

Big Brothers Big Sisters has been the leader in professionally supervised mentoring for young persons from 6 through 18 for more than a century and has had lasting impact on the lives of many.[31] Participants are more confident in their schoolwork performance; able to get along better with their families; 46% less likely to begin using illegal drugs; 27% less likely to begin using alcohol; and 52% less likely to skip school than controls.

Beating the Odds Foundation

Beating the Odds Foundation provides motivational demonstrations and mentoring programs through schools for at-risk students.[32] They help school districts establish and expand mentoring programs to help young people learn to take control of their lives and gain self-respect. The program has documented positive effects on students' grades and classroom behavior in the William P. Kimmel Alternative School in Altoona, Pennsylvania.

Alpha Phi Alpha Fraternity

Alpha Phi Alpha Fraternity offers Black adolescents mentoring.[33] Since 1922, it has sponsored the *Go-to-High-School, Go-to-College* program that emphasizes completing high school and college by providing information and strategies to facilitate success. Together with the March of Dimes Birth Defects Foundation, the Fraternity initiated *Project Alpha* in 1980. The program promotes motivation, self-confidence and skill-building in personal responsibility and relationships for boys ages 12 through 15. It taps boys with leadership potential to help them become forces for change through workshops conducted by fraternity brothers.

Service-Based Youth Development Programs

Youth development service-learning programs combine community service with curriculum-based learning and improve academic achievement more effectively than lecture-style classes.[34] According to the *National Survey on Service-Learning and Transitioning to Adulthood,* adults who engaged in service-learning during their school years were more likely than their peers to be politically and socially connected to their communities; to serve as role models; to understand the importance of lifelong learning; to obtain advanced education; and to engage in service activities. Service learning programs offer a promising strategy for influencing sexual behavior as participants build self-respect and self-confidence.

Reach for Health Community Youth Service

Compared to other adolescents, middle school urban Black and Latino economically disadvantaged youth enrolled in *Reach for Health Community Youth Service* were more likely to delay first sex and less likely to have had sex recently.[35] The program includes three hours of weekly community service; a two-year, 40-lesson health promotion curriculum; and reflection to help students learn from their community experiences.

Teen Outreach Program

The nine-month *Teen Outreach Program* for high-risk minority high school boys and girls aims to reduce the likelihood of pregnancy.[36] Programs include volunteer service and discussions related to key social and developmental tasks in more than 400 sites involving over 12,000 adolescents throughout the United States. A University of Virginia study found that it reduced adolescent pregnancy and school failure rates by 40% compared to controls.

4-H Youth Development Program

The *4-H Youth Development Program* began in 1902. Community service has always been an important component of 4-H with adults and adolescents working together with community organizations. 45% of the participants are in rural, and 55% are in urban areas. A 2001 survey found that 4-H helped young people gain self-respect and empowered them to try new activities, work as a team and become leaders.[37]

Comprehensive Programs

Comprehensive programs combine academic assistance, sex education, participation in the arts and sports, health care, employment assistance and some degree of parent involvement.

The Carrera Program

In 1984, Michael Carrera and the Children's Aid Society developed a model that incorporates parent participation with educational support, career awareness and job club, lifetime sports, creative expression, comprehensive medical and dental services, mental health services and family life and sex education.[38]

The program offers a supportive environment in which young people can learn about sexual responsibility while developing life goals. There are 21 replications and 30 similar programs in 20 states. A follow-up survey in the New York Program in 2004 revealed that 86% of the participants graduated from high school compared to 66% of controls.[39] The program reduced pregnancy and births and increased high school graduation and college enrollment.

Boys and Girls Club of America

The mission of *Boys and Girls Clubs of America* is to inspire and enable young people, especially from disadvantaged circumstances, to realize their full potentials.[40] A Club offers a safe place to learn and grow, ongoing relationships with professionals, life-enhancing and character development experiences and hope. More than 4.4 million boys and girls participate in 3,700 Clubs served by 44,000 staff persons.

Challenge Academies

The *Wisconsin National Guard Challenge Academy* is one of 30 similar programs in 27 states.[41] It is a 17-month program for high school drop-outs, habitual truants, expelled students or students deficient in credits from 16 through 18. Academy cadets complete a 22-week residential phase during which they can earn their General Equivalency Diplomas and work on character development. A 12-month post-residential phase follows in which they go on to jobs, post-secondary education or military service. 25% of the cadets drop out during the first two weeks. Of those who remain, 85% earn GEDs, and 75% complete the post-residential phase.

BUILDING ADOLESCENTS' SOCIAL CAPITAL

Building social capital involves strengthening families, neighborhoods, schools, communities and society. The Center for Law and Social Policy outlines a plan for building social capital through a *Community-Wide Continuum of Support*.[42]

Family-oriented Change

The developmental characteristics of adolescence and family influences are more important causes of adolescent pregnancy than socioeconomic disadvantage and can be treated through home-based therapies.[43] Antipoverty measures alone do not address family relationships.

Doris Entwisle and Karl Alexander, professors of sociology at Johns Hopkins University, collected data on Baltimore school children who began the first grade in 1982. They found that it was difficult for schools to compensate for family disadvantage.[44] Richard Rothstein, a research associate of the Economic Policy Institute, also found that educational reforms are inadequate unless there are changes in economic and social circumstances that adversely affect children at home.[45] At their best, schools are partners with parents.

Childrearing Practices

Contemporary childrearing practices tend toward overindulgence abetted by the commercial exploitation of the tastes and wishes of the young. This attitude can lead poor families to desire and obtain unaffordable material items for their adolescents. They also can fail to challenge an adolescent's wish to become a parent.

Parents who permit a high degree of freedom in choosing friends, staying out at night, dating and other unsupervised activities encourage risky socializing.[46] Parents who are highly intrusive and excessively limit their adolescents' freedom invite rebellion. When the relationship between parents and adolescents is one of mutual respect and authoritative limit setting, adolescents are less likely to become involved in risky behaviors.

Parental Advisory Role

Many parents need support in their advisory roles with their daughters and sons, especially in decisions regarding continuing a pregnancy and making an adoption plan.

A nationally representative survey of adults and adolescents in 2006 revealed that the proportion of adolescents who said parents most influence their decisions about sex increased since 2004 (47% vs. 37%).[47] More said that they have had a helpful conversation with their parents about sex (71% vs. 63%).

Parent-Child Connectedness Intervention Activities are designed to help community-based organizations improve parent-adolescent relationships.[48] *Terms of Engagement* offers practical advice on how to involve parents in programs to prevent adolescent pregnancy.

An editor of the magazine *Seventeen* provided the following advice to adolescents:[49]

> When life is moving fast with scenarios you haven't yet rehearsed, your first instinct might be to pull away from your parents. When you've lost yourself, it's uncomfortable to be around people who can tell you are in a mess. But that's when you need them the most. Plus, they're the only ones who are willing to do the hard work necessary to help you find yourself again. Self-medicating with alcohol, drugs, and the fake friends will just push you deeper into the hole. The real medicine is love and honesty. It doesn't taste good, but it's the only thing that will work. If you find yourself in a black hole, run to the ones who love you.

Strengthening Families Program: For Parents and Youth 10-14

The Strengthening Families Program: For Parents and Youth 10-14 aims to reduce adolescent substance abuse and behavior problems by improving parents' nurturing and management skills and improving adolescents' interpersonal competencies. Parents and adolescents attend seven separate skill-building and family activities. Four booster sessions six months to one year later reinforce the skills gained in the original sessions. Randomized evaluations have indicated favorable outcomes.[50]

Families and Schools Together

Families and Schools Together (FAST) is a peer and multifamily intervention for 10- to 14-year-olds.[51] A FAST Club is a 14 session peer group designed by participants, a FAST team's youth representative and an adult advocate. The program is shaped by participants' interests and needs to help them develop leadership skills. A multifamily group meets for 10 sessions in which parent-adolescent communication is rehearsed. Monthly multifamily meetings are held for two years following the program to keep families connected in support networks.

Health Care

Many adolescents in a Motivational Educational Entertainment survey said that health care facilities were not "youth-friendly" and that they had been "disrespected" and "shamed" during visits to them.[52] These incidents discouraged them from seeking additional services.

Programs to improve family relationships should be incorporated in public health services and health insurance programs and family-centered medical clinics because they prevent more expensive health services.[53]

Neighborhood Oriented Change

The Commission on Children at Risk advocates that service organizations, governments, employers, faith and civic leaders, philanthropists, foundations, scholars, families and individuals build social capital in "authoritative communities."[54] When adolescent and community development are seen as two sides of the same coin, the creativity and energy of young people can change their own lives and their neighborhoods and communities.

Harlem Children's Zone

Founded in 1970, *Harlem Children's Zone* is an integrated network of educational, social service and recreational resources that builds the fabric of community life in some of New York City's most devastated neighborhoods. Formerly known as Rheedlen Centers for Children and Families, its 15 centers serve more than 12,600 children and adults, including over 7,500 at-risk children. The organization employs over 650 people in more than 20 programs. It reports that evaluations of its program components have shown positive results.[55]

Time Banks USA

Time Banks USA seeks to build social capital by rewarding decency, caring and justice with a new medium of exchange called Time Dollars.[56] One hour helping others yields one Time Dollar that can be spent to have someone do something for you.

The services people share in a Time Bank depend on what people need, such as childcare, caring for the elderly and helping with homework. Tested in communities and organizations throughout the world, Time Banks allow those formerly labeled as "problems" to become partners in solutions. Youth Courts can use Time Bank hours as fines and to compensate jurors.

School Oriented Change

Although the United States spends more money per student on education than any other nation, numerous experiments are underway to restructure our schools. When students enter high school with inadequate reading and math skills, their prospects for success are limited.[57]

The Teaching Commission and the Alliance for Excellent Education point out that our nation is at a crossroads in education.[58] Over the next decade, two million new teachers will be needed in our public schools. Filling these openings will be difficult, especially in inner-city schools where turnover is high. A new compact is called for with teachers built around raising teacher salaries, teacher mentoring and compensation based on student progress.

When their parents are supportive, adolescents attend school more regularly, are better behaved and are more likely to continue their education beyond high school.[59] The Center on School, Family and Community Partnerships conducts and disseminates research on policies and practices that help families, schools and communities work together. In some large cities, the alignment of schools with city government has proved to be helpful. The American Youth Policy Forum reconnects out-of-school adolescents to the social and economic mainstream.

The Evolution of High Schools

In 1961 in *The Adolescent Society: The Social Life of the Teenager and Its Impact on Education*, James Coleman pointed out that peers were superceding adults in shaping behavior in high schools.[60] Standard-setting young people were those with athletic prowess, good looks and winsome personalities not those who were doing well academically. Course and program selection shifted from guidance counselors and educators to students. Schools came to resemble educational shopping malls with students searching for easy courses that satisfied graduation requirements. In some ways, the 1970s marked the low point of high school education. Many adolescents continue to drift through high school unchallenged and uninspired.

High School Reform

Chester Finn, Professor of Education and Public Policy at Vanderbilt University, concluded that high-schools present multiple problems that need multiple solutions.[61]

A new wave of high school reform efforts led by the Gates Foundation is based on the belief that smaller high schools can develop a shared sense of mission and relationships between faculty and students.[62] There is much to commend reducing the anonymity and alienation many students experience in large high schools. But sociologists Douglas Ready and Valerie Lee found that schools within schools have the same the courses and expectations as in large high schools.[63]

Another strategy, also promoted by the Gates Foundation, is to make high schools more like colleges with open campuses and electives that employ college faculty. The hope is that greater autonomy and more challenging material will help keep students engaged in school.

Four years after it was enacted, vast numbers of students were not getting the tutoring the No Child Left Behind law offers.[64] In New York City, fewer than half of the 215,000 eligible students sought free tutoring in the 2004-2005 school year; 34,055 children did not successfully complete the terms of their tutoring contracts.

Orienting education to adolescent physiology and brain development is gaining attention.[65] Adapting school hours to sleep requirements of adolescents and to the working hours of their parents deserves serious consideration. One-fourth to one-half of adolescents report having insomnia for periods of one to four years.

Without radical change in our educational system, large numbers of minority adolescents will continue to leave high school without the skills and knowledge needed to do well in life.[66]

KIPP Schools

Knowledge Is Power Program is a network of free, open-enrollment, college-preparatory public schools in under-resourced communities throughout the United States.[67]

There currently are 52 locally-run KIPP schools in 16 states and Washington, DC, serving over 12,000 students. Students, parents and teachers create and reinforce a culture of achievement and support through a range of formal and informal rewards and consequences for academic performance and behavior. With an extended school day, week and year, students have more time to acquire academic knowledge and skills, as well as for extracurricular activities.

School Busing

The Metropolitan Council for Educational Opportunity (METCO), Boston's 40-year voluntary school desegregation program, was founded by Black parents and activists to bus Black children from inner city neighborhoods to White suburban schools.[68] Students prepare for college by learning how to build bridges to our predominantly White society. Although shifting between Black and White worlds can make Black students feel they do not belong in either one, the vast majority are grateful for METCO.

School Development Program

Over the past four decades, James Comer, a child psychiatrist at Yale University's School of Medicine, has been expanding the *School Development Program*.[69] It builds on the principle that strong relationships are the only way to help children become successful in life as well as in school. It centers around three teams with the goal of cultivating a nurturing, democratic school community: 1) teachers, administrators and nonprofessional staff; 2) parents; and 3) support professionals, such as social workers, psychologists and nurses. It now exists in schools in 20 states and has shown dramatic improvements in schools, often within five years.

Alternative Schools

A growing number of communities have programs for school dropouts operated by entrepreneurial citizens working through community organizations.[70] Charter school legislation with public funding is especially important for these alternative programs.

The all-male *Eagle Academy for Young Men* opened in 2004 in New York City. Its curriculum is based on how boys learn and on boys' competitive nature. The school day lasts until 5:30 P.M. and includes study groups, tutoring and dinner. Saturday mornings are devoted to intramural sports, as well as classes on topics, such as managing finances and leadership.[71]

The *Technical Assistance & Leadership Center* in Milwaukee is committed to personalized learning environments; different school governance structures; and permitting families to choose options that best fit their needs.[72] Milwaukee's experience since the 1980s demonstrates that charter schools can provide at-risk students pathways to successful lives. In 2003-2004, Shalom High School and NOVA High School had 100% graduation rates.

After School Programs

After school programs were evaluated in two studies.[73] An evaluation by Policy Studies Associates resulted in a model that emphasizes an array of enrichment opportunities: dance, music, art and organized sports; opportunities for skill-building and mastery; relationship-building; a staff with diverse backgrounds and skills; an experienced site coordinator with strong ties to the community; the administrative and fiscal support of a committed sponsoring organization; and ongoing communication and relationship-building with schools and families.

A meta-analysis of after-school programs by the Collaborative for Academic, Social, and Emotional Learning found that improvement occurred in self-respect, positive social behaviors and levels of academic achievement. Significant reductions occurred in problem behaviors and drug use. Programs that used evidence-based approaches to achieve objectives and active forms of learning had better results than those that did not.

An evaluation of 21st Century Community Learning Centers revealed that participants were more likely to have classroom discipline problems.[74] They may have been tired of being in school, discipline may have been lax or the programs may have been poorly implemented.

Community Oriented Change

Hundreds of community development organizations, human service agencies and state and local governments have initiated projects based on community building strategies. Documentation of the opportunities and challenges of a community building approach to neighborhood transformation is available on the *Community Builders* web site.[75]

Industrial Areas Foundation

The *Industrial Areas Foundation* builds a political base of religious congregations and orders, labor locals, homeowner groups, recovery groups, parent associations, settlement houses, immigrant societies, schools and seminaries.[76] The Foundation has 56 organizations that directly benefit adolescents and their families. It focuses on recruiting and training community leaders.

Communities Organized for Public Service is composed of 50 predominantly low-income Latino parishes in San Antonio. Founded in 1974, it is the oldest of the Interfaith Area Foundation organizations in the Industrial Areas Foundation network.[77] It has brought over a billion dollars worth of new streets, drainage, sidewalks, libraries, parks, streetlights and affordable housing to poor neighborhoods. It emphasizes leadership development.

YouthBuild USA

Founded in 1990, *YouthBuild USA* helps low-income young people rebuild their communities and their lives in 200 programs.[78] Unemployed and undereducated young people from 16 to 24 obtain their high school diploma or GED while learning job skills by building housing for homeless and low-income people. Emphasis is placed on leadership development, community service and creating a community of adults and adolescents committed to success.

YouthBuild USA's outcome data affirms its value in transforming low-income youths' lives. More than 6,500 adolescents are enrolled in *YouthBuild USA* each year.

Since 1993, they have helped create more than 10,000 units of affordable housing in their communities.

Homelessness and Housing

Some adolescents face the choice of staying in an abusive situation or being homeless. They need emergency housing and, as do those who age-out of foster-care, safe long-term living arrangements.[79] Many exchange sex with intravenous drug users and multiple partners for the necessities of life. Their STD rates range from 23% to 46%.

Moving to Opportunity for Fair Housing is a 10-year demonstration program that offers poor families Housing and Urban Development vouchers to move out of high poverty to lower poverty neighborhoods.[80] Evaluations found that four and seven years after moving to lower poverty neighborhoods there were improvements in personal safety; housing quality; mental health and obesity among adults; and mental health, staying in school, delinquency, and risky behavior among adolescent girls. However, there were no improvements in school performance.

Community Coalition Partnership Programs for the Prevention of Teen Pregnancy

Community Coalition Partnership Programs for the Prevention of Teen Pregnancy was a demonstration program from 1995 to 2002 conducted in 13 cities to demonstrate whether communities could mobilize and organize resources to support programs for preventing initial and subsequent pregnancies.[81] The evaluation identified barriers to implementation, including problems in obtaining funding, high rates of staff turnover and low levels of community concern about adolescent pregnancy. It suggested approaches to address these problems.

Society-Oriented Change

A thriving economy is essential to providing young, poor and undereducated people with tools and advocacy to navigate out of poverty.[82] Focusing only on schools diverts attention from state and federal policies that affect work productivity and our nation's global competitiveness. Creating investment incentives, dealing with trade deficits, funding technology research and supporting job-retraining all are policies that improve our economic competitiveness. Most of these policies have long-range goals, but many have goals within our reach now.

Media

Targeted media education in minority communities is needed to encourage successful passage through adolescence to self-fulfillment in modern society.

Since 1997, the Kaiser Family Foundation and MTV have partnered on a campaign to inform young people about STD and related issues.[83] The partnership includes advertisements, documentaries, entertainment, news, *It's Your (Sex) Life: Your Guide to Safe and Responsible Sex* and an extensive website.

MEE Productions, Inc., offers strategies to reach and influence urban populations.[84] It uses insights gained through years of focus group research, media production experience and industry-proven marketing and advertising expertise. MEE has a Website for the *Be On The Safe Side Campaign*—Washington DC's adolescent pregnancy prevention campaign.

Public Policies

Taxpayers need to understand that supporting adolescent parents now and the later costs of unemployability, welfare dependency and crime are major factors in the level of state and county taxes. Public policy should not be guided by the fact that some minors are capable of handling parenthood with support. It should be guided by the fact that the majority are not.

Male Employment. The focus needs to extend beyond girls to boys and men. As long as boys fail to postpone fatherhood until they have steady employment and as long as men do not support their children, mothers and children will remain trapped in poor neighborhoods where social problems incubate.

Since the 1970s, the loss of jobs is the most important factor in the decline of urban neighborhoods.[85] Increasing employment opportunities improve the social organization of ghetto neighborhoods. Expanding eligibility for earned-income tax credit for fathers would raise incentives to accept low wage jobs, as it has for single mothers.

The 2006 *State of Black America* report by the Urban Institute recommends specific policies and actions:[86]

- The minimum wage must be a living, not a poverty, wage.
- Strengthen the Community Reinvestment Act that helps banks make mortgages available and affordable.
- Increase Business Development and Entrepreneurship in urban communities by doubling the size of the New Markets Tax Credit Program.
- Strengthen and improve the Community Development Block Grant program and other urban economic opportunity and job training programs.
- Expand job training and career counseling efforts for young urban males.
- Develop a comprehensive re-entry program for ex-felons.
- The Black middle class should increase their commitment to supporting Black colleges and universities, churches and civil rights organizations.

These policies would benefit couples who wish to marry and not pressure women to enter or remain in relationships they would not otherwise choose.

Welfare Reform. After peaking in 1994, the welfare caseload fell by 60% over the next decade from 5 to 2 million families.[87] Welfare roles started to decrease before the 1990s boom and the 1996 welfare reform act, perhaps because of growing recognition of welfare as an undesirable life style. Wisconsin took a "work first" approach to welfare reform (W-2), which many states copied. The goal was to put people to work as rapidly as possible without assessing barriers to employability.

W-2 mothers' employment rate increased from 44% in 1993 to 66% in 2000, and the poverty rate dropped from 15% to 11%. Sixty percent who left welfare were working, and 70% held at least one job after leaving welfare. However, increasing numbers lose their jobs and move back into W-2. Low paying jobs convert the welfare poor into the working poor.

Because of time-limited benefits, 10-15% of America's former welfare recipients are neither working nor on welfare and appear to be worse off now than before welfare reform. They include people with mental or physical disabilities or other severe limitations. Mark Courtney, professor of social service administration at the University of Chicago, found that many of the parents coming into welfare offices today are too poorly educated and too service-needy to work.[88] They have limited capacities to raise their children. Courtney's study of 1,100 Milwaukee W-2 families revealed that Wisconsin's work-first approach did not help a number of parents:

- At the beginning of W-2 more than 20% of all parents reported at least one potential barrier to employment—disability; disabled family member; poor or fair health; no high school or general equivalency diploma; mental illness; alcohol or drug addiction; or involvement in a physically abusive relationship. Of this 20%, more than 50% had two or more barriers to employment, and 30% reported three or more.
- Four years later, 75% of the parents remaining in W-2 still had at least one barrier. More than 50% still lacked a diploma or GED; 20% had mental health problems; and 20% had a disability.
- More than 50% of the parents had been previously investigated for child maltreatment. When they applied for welfare in the next five years, 20% were investigated, and 17% had a child placed in foster care.

It is time for welfare to focus on helping parents in the work of childrearing by: [89]

- Treating developmentally disabled, mentally ill and addicted parents.
- Raising the incomes of the working poor through education and training.
- Employing men so they can pay child support.
- Expanding maternity leaves to six months to permit breast feeding.
- Enabling their adolescents to stay in school and delay pregnancy.

The irony of welfare reform is that for the foreseeable future millions of poorly educated and unwed young mothers face living in poverty on welfare or while employed.

Correctional Systems—Incarcerated Parents. Over the last thirty years, the prison population in the United States has increased more than sevenfold to over 2 million people. The growth in incarceration is taking its toll on the social and economic fabric of many American communities. Almost 60% of Black male high school drop-outs have spent time in prison by their early thirties.[90]

In 2004, there were 2,010,814 males and 190,309 females in U.S. prisons and jails. 60% of the males and 70% of the females were parents.[91] Women made up 7% of inmates in state and federal prisons in 2004, up 4% from 2003. There were an estimated 2,473,300 children of male prisoners and 319,718 children of female prisoners. Incarcerating parents for non-violent offences exacts high economic and humanitarian costs because of its adverse effects on children.

Because of their incarceration, young Black men did not benefit from the economic boom of the 1990s.[92] Mass incarceration left 10% of Black children with a father in prison by 2000, perpetuating the cycle of broken families, poverty and crime.

Incarceration places extreme burdens on relationships between parents and children.[93] Incarcerated mothers and fathers must learn to cope with the loss of contact with their children, infrequent visits in inhospitable surroundings and lost opportunities to contribute to their children's development. The children must come to terms with absent parents, the stigma of parental imprisonment and living with relatives or foster parents. One study found that over 33% of all genetic mothers of children in foster care had criminal convictions at some point in their lives.[94] Some incarcerated mothers may never be fit to resume parenting responsibilities, but the evidence is compelling that underlying substance abuse is treatable through drug courts.

Maintaining family ties during incarceration benefits both children and their parents. The *Living Interactive Family Education* program in Missouri brings children and adolescents to monthly meetings with their fathers in prison in a comfortable atmosphere conducive to positive interactions.[95] They work together on arts and crafts projects. All fathers in the program attend monthly classes to help them become positive influences in their children's lives.

An evaluation of the program disclosed that the most significant gains for the young persons were in social skills and academic performance. They became friends with other children in the same situation. The fathers developed better relationships with their children as well.

Juvenile and Family Law Enforcement. Juvenile and family justice reformers have avoided incarceration by creating specialty courts. Drug Courts have been created because 65% of all arrested persons test positive for illegal drugs, as do over half of those returning to prison.[96] The best strategy to reduce drug-related incarcerations is to hold individuals responsible for their actions through drug courts that provide community treatment.[97] A drug court handles drug-using offenders through supervision, drug testing, treatment and incentives. There were 1,621 drug court operations in the United States in 2004; 357 were juvenile drug courts. "Meth prisons" are examples of treatment facilities that replace prisons.

In one study, more than 80% of juvenile drug court participants returned to, or remained in, school full-time.[98] Adults who had court-ordered treatment for alcohol and drug problems had the same rates of abstinence, employment and re-arrest as peers who sought help on their own. In 2001, there were 2,100 drug-free babies born to mothers in drug court programs.[99]

According to the National Association of Youth Courts there are 1,255 youth court programs in 49 states and the District of Columbia.[100] They are run by adolescents, usually in schools. They use peer pressure to help adolescents avoid re-offending. Adolescents who admit commiting minor offenses, such as petty theft, alcohol use or disorderly conduct, receive consequences from a "jury" of their peers whom they are more likely to respect than adults. The juries hand down "sentences" ranging from community service to apologies, essays and educational workshops. Successful completion of the program usually means avoiding a juvenile court record and school suspension or expulsion.

Probation departments in California have shifted from punishing youthful offenders to focusing on strengthening families with a decrease over the last decade in juvenile arrests and incarcerations; adolescent pregnancies; the number of adolescents living below the poverty level; and high school drop-outs.[101] These declines have been greater in California than in other states, suggesting that this initiative has positive effects beyond an improved economy.

Protective Law Enforcement. While law enforcement has improved its understanding of adult domestic abuse, this has not reached adolescents. An adolescent girl may have difficulty obtaining a "protection from abuse" order. Police officers also may be slow to respond to her calls because they have difficulty evaluating their validity.

Community Policing. In the 1990s, the New York City Police Department delegated operational decisions to precinct commanders. Community policing led to training and deploying 5,000 new officers; integrating housing and transit police into the Police Department; clearing a backlog of 50,000 unserved warrants; a robust "zero tolerance" campaign against petty crime and anti-social behavior; removal of graffiti; moving over 500,000 people into jobs from welfare; and housing vouchers that enabled poor families to move to better neighborhoods.[102] As a result, crime turned downward more than any time in the past.

Restorative Justice. Restorative justice practices focus on repairing the harm done to people and relationships rather than on punishing offenders, although it does not preclude incarceration of offenders or other sanctions.[103] Originating in the 1970s as mediation between victims and offenders, in the 1990s it broadened to include victims' and offenders' families and friends participating in collaborative processes called "conferences" and "circles."

The International Institute for Restorative Practices in Bethlehem, Pennsylvania, is a graduate degree-granting institution for training in this practice.

Multisystemic Therapy. *Multisystemic Therapy* is intensive family therapy designed to prevent juvenile crime.[104] It encompasses family, peer, school and neighborhood systems as the "client." Using the strengths of each system to facilitate positive change, it strives to build social capital and promote behavioral change in adolescents' natural environments. It has reduced delinquency.

THE ADOPTION OPTION

Once an adolescent decides to carry a pregnancy to term, the only way to prevent adolescent parenthood is to make an adoption plan. Most importantly, pregnant adolescent girls and the fathers need to understand that the sacrifice of making an adoption plan is in the spirit of personal sacrifice for offspring required of all parents.[105]

Infant Adoption Awareness Training

Growing out of legislation by Congress in 2000, the primary purpose of the Infant Adoption Awareness Training Program (IAATP) is to train pregnancy and health counselors to present adoption as an option to persons with unplanned pregnancies.[106] IAATP has trained more than 16,000 individuals from all 50 states, 94% of whom rated the training "excellent." The curriculum is designed to train professionals to help pregnant persons understand the legal, emotional, psychological and social processes of adoption and make fully informed, realistic choices. It helps pregnancy counselors become aware of, and sensitive to, family, cultural, religious and social influences that affect pregnancy decision-making.

Benefits of Adoption

The benefits of an adoption plan for an adolescent parent and for her baby need to be emphasized through the media, education and counseling. One study compared adolescents who made an adoption plan for their babies with those who did not.[107] In both instances, 84% described the option of pregnancy termination as morally unacceptable and contrary to their religion. Those who decided to make adoption plans for their babies cited realistic reasons: 75% said they were not ready for parenthood; 56% said adoption would be better for their baby; and 37% said they would have a better education through adoption. In contrast, those who decided to enter parenthood cited emotional reasons: 52% said they could not handle the thought of adoption; 42% said it would be better for them to raise a child than make an adoption plan; 37% said they could not bear to make an adoption plan for a baby they had carried through pregnancy.

CONCLUSION

Public policies designed to create the "good society" usually stress improving education, employment and wages. None of these efforts will make a significant difference unless we ensure that all children have competent parents. Inexpensive interventions with struggling families during early life have much higher economic and humanitarian returns than costly "deep end" interventions. The most cost-effective intervention is preventing adolescent pregnancy, which really is preventing adolescent parenthood. The prevention of our social problems should begin before childbirth.

Our usual approach to preventing adolescent pregnancy is with the adolescents themselves through sex education, contraceptives and expanded health care. None of these measures makes an impact on the premature foreclosures of personal, educational, occupational and developmental opportunities that occur when adolescents deliberately choose to become parents.

Some adolescents are psychosocially "poorly nourished" and are susceptible to a wide array of maladaptive outcomes. A "nutritional-risk" model focuses on managing risky, sensation-seeking behaviors that result from the lack of nurturance. It focuses on nourishing adolescent development in their families and the places in which they live.

The aim of social marketing is to develop human capital by showing that the value of healthy behaviors exceeds that of other options. The most effective rewards for making wise short-term decisions are self-respect and self-confidence—the elements of strong character and identity.

The development of adolescents' human capital is directly related to the quality of their social capital—their families, neighborhoods, schools, communities and society. Numerous efforts to improve schooling are underway, but students who lack supportive families will continue to fall behind. Legislation is required for those who do not respond to social marketing. Criminal justice and child support reforms are needed to encourage involvement of fathers with their children.

Once an adolescent decides to carry a pregnancy to term, the only way to prevent adolescent parenthood is to make an adoption plan. The benefits of adoption for an adolescent parent and for her baby need to be emphasized by the media, education and counseling.

Public policy should not be based on the fact that some minors are capable of handling parenthood with support. It should be guided by the fact that most are not. We need to confront the fact that our society does not value parenthood enough to place a high priority on ensuring that all of our children have competent parents.

Chapter 32

Valuing Parenthood

The only way women can achieve equal citizenship is for the entire society to contribute to the provision of public good that everyone desires: well-raised children
who will mature into productive, law-abiding citizens. And that means that all free
riders—from employers to governments to husbands to communities—have to pitch
in and help make the most important job in the world a top national priority and a
very good job.

Ann Crittenden
The Price of Motherhood.[1]

Thirty years ago we were assured that technology would give us more leisure time for
our families. The opposite has occurred. The more we can do, the more we want to do.
The more money we have, the more money we want. Still, most of us yearn for deeper
fulfillment in life.

One way to find fulfillment is to share the wonders of life by growing with children.
But too many parents and other adults miss this opportunity by doing things for, rather
than with, children. Too many parents have little time to be with their children. Even
worse, too many families are dysfunctional.

Why does our society seem to adulate children but fail to recognize parenthood as
essential to our prosperity? Emulating the audacious behavior of celebrities and acquiring wealth often eclipse family relationships. "Having children" can seem to be
more important than raising them. Acting like adolescents can seem to be more important than parenting them.[2] All of this reflects uncommitted relationships that result
in cohabitation, divorce and adolescent childbirth.

Most importantly, the fact that childrearing families subsidize our society is not
fully appreciated.[3] Governments and businesses are "free-riders" that depend upon the
labor of parents, who care for the young now, and on the productive citizens their children become. Our society owes parenthood a social and financial debt, as is recognized to a degree in tax benefits.

We all pay an enormous price for neglecting parenthood. In Wisconsin, 26% of
state and 45% of county expenditures are related to failing to strengthen struggling

families. A neglected and abused child who becomes a habitual criminal or welfare dependent costs our economy $2.4 million.[4] Thriving childrearing families contribute $1.2 million to our economy for each child they raise to become a productive citizen. Even those of us without children gain from having more children who become workers that contribute to our economy and to our old-age benefits.

We need a vision for America in which parenthood is valued as much as a paid career.

WHY WE NEED TO VALUE PARENTHOOD IN AMERICA

As we enter the 21st century, we have a clear vision of the pleasures we seek from material things. We are only beginning to envision the kind of citizens we need in our society.

The vitality of our science, technology and economy made the United States the world leader at the end of the 20th century. We benefited from a high standard of living and unprecedented freedom of action. But in a world where knowledge is widespread and low-cost labor is readily available, our advantages are eroding.

The National Academies, our most prestigious scientific voice, calls for a comprehensive federal effort to bolster our competitiveness so that we will gain, rather than lose, from globalization.[5] In 2005, our 12th-graders were below 21 countries in mathematics and science.

Without a major push to strengthen the foundations of America's competitiveness, we will lose our privileged position. Our economic progress has come from new industries created by the ideas of exceptional scientists and engineers. Continuing to improve this human capital depends upon a well-educated citizenry as we move into an information/cognitive skill era.

The well-being of our society has been traditionally measured by the goods and services produced and consumed in the Gross Domestic Product (GDP). But the GDP does not measure the actual well-being of our society. Persons with long, expensive illnesses have more economic value than when they are healthy.[6] Expenditures for social services and prisons increase the GDP.

The National Academies point out that working more to spend more on goods and services contributes to the disconnection of many persons from their communities and society.[7] Alexis De Tocqueville, the 19th century French observer of America, predicted this outcome when he highlighted individualism in the United States:[8]

> The prospect really does frighten me that they will become so engrossed in the cowardly love of immediate pleasures that their interest in their own futures and in that of their descendents may vanish, and that they will prefer to tamely follow the course of their destiny rather than make a sudden energetic effort necessary to set things right.

According to Richard Florida, professor of public policy at George Mason University, the key to the global economy no longer is competition for goods, services or capital. It is competition for creative people—for human capital.[9] Creativity is a common good, like liberty and security. It must be nourished, or it will slip away.

The United States ranks 11th in developed nations in population percentage considered to be creative and competitive.[10] We rank 9th on the Global Talent Index based on the percentage holding college degrees and the number of research scientists and engineers.

Compared to other developed nations, our society does not place a high value on parenthood. We have the highest child poverty rates and the lowest childrearing benefits. We should not be surprised that we have the highest incarceration rates as well.

The causes of crime and welfare dependency are hotly debated. Are they environmental—unemployment, poverty, and racial discrimination—or are they personal—dysfunctional families, poorly educated mothers and derelict fathers? Of course, they are both.

Crime and welfare dependency abound where there are extreme differences between the "haves" and the "have nots." One of the most important differences between "have nots" who are habitual criminals or welfare dependent and the majority of "have nots" who are not is the latter's ability to empathize with others learned through attachment bonding with their parents.

We no longer can afford to focus only on economic factors that contribute to our social problems. Inadequate, strained and disrupted parent-child relationships are more important. At the core of the lonely, unhappy undercurrent in our society lies an inability to form and sustain intimate relationships. Competent parents foster their children's capacities for commitments to others through secure attachment bonding with them during the early years of childhood. Competent parents prevent our social problems. Incompetent parents contribute to them.

We must confront the prevalent belief that little can be done to strengthen families, therefore, institutions must assume responsibility for rearing our children. This belief leads to turning to childcare, schools and professionals to fill in when parents fail—thus contributing to the GDP. Consequently, parents are not held as responsible for their actions with their own children as they are for their actions with persons outside of their families.

On the positive side, many women and men choose to give their careers as parents as much or more priority as their paid work. Many struggling parents are receiving education and support. Family-friendly neighborhoods and communities are being created. Parents have increasing access to private and public resources.[11]

These trends reflect our cultural expectation that all children should grow up to be responsible citizens. This expectation depends upon children forming and sustaining intimate relationships in early life with competent parents who temper individualism with cooperation.

We no longer have the leisure of drifting with the illusion that our GDP measures our society's well-being while our human capital erodes. The prominence of self-centered, impulsive and exploitative persons endangers our nation's future. Valuing parenthood requires a paradigm shift from self-assertive social values to integrative cultural values.

A PARADIGM SHIFT FROM SELF-ASSERTIVE TO INTEGRATIVE VALUES

The family is the most fragile of all human institutions. Yet, it is the bedrock of civilization. Its strength lies in the cohesion and loyalty of the parent-child relationship around which the larger world of kin, community and nation revolve. Parenthood is the source of our moral stature and our social organization.[12] It is the source of the "work ethic" and our human capital. It is the crucible in which self-assertive social and integrative cultural values are blended.

Families produce future generations. They help protect members against ill health, old age, unemployment and other hazards throughout life. In the United States especially, family relationships are strained by tension between self-assertive social values and integrative cultural values as reflected in the view of the parent-child relationship. Is a child a parent's private property (self-assertive)? Or is a parent a child's temporary custodial guardian (integrative)?

Both the extreme political left and right espouse self-assertive values that regard children as the private property of their parents. The far left advocates the right of parents to do as they wish. The far right advocates the privacy of the family. Both political extremes reflect the belief that parenthood is outside of the public domain. Both avoid holding parents responsible for the behavior of their offspring. To do so is "parent blaming." These extreme self-assertive views need to be balanced by integrative values.

In our society, balancing self-assertion and integration leads to social progress. Edward Chambers, executive director of the Industrial Areas Foundation, sees competitive self-assertion that produces winners and losers as dominating the way the *world is* and cooperative integration as moving us toward the *world that ought to be*.[13] George Lakoff, professor of linguistics at the University of California-Berkeley, reminds us that devotion to the common good has been the strength of our nation. But balancing self-assertive and integrative values requires actions that create friction between competing interests and the heat of controversy.

CHALLENGES FOR OUR SOCIETY

We live in two worlds. The *world that is* and the *world that ought to be*. Like the encircling polarities of the Chinese yin/yang symbol, the two worlds interact. Philosophers refer to the back-and-forth tension between the opposing poles as dialectical.[14] Goethe described the successful life "as the intensification of inborn talents through judicious surrender to the natural rhythm of opposing tendencies."[15]

Edward Chambers points out that self-assertive capitalism regards the family as a unit for generating money to be spent on goods and services.[16] This consumerism characterizes the *world as it is*. Lester Thurow, an economics professor at the Massachusetts Institute of Technology, points to the inherent unfairness of self-assertive capitalism.[17] For example, no individual can invest in the stock market with the same sophistication as Wall Street firms. Stephen Marglin, professor of economics at Harvard, points out that market relationships undermine reciprocity, altruism, and mutual obligation—vital ingredients of a sense of the common good.[18]

At the same time, commercial marketing uses *world as it ought to be* symbols. Slogans such as "be all that you can be," "reach out and touch someone" and "own a piece of the rock" appeal to cultural values of the *world as it ought to be* and aim to turn wants into needs.

Our mediating institutions—families, congregations, service clubs, athletic groups, parent-teacher associations and social organizations—counterbalance self-assertive capitalism. They are the glue that holds our society together.[19]

Our mediating institutions are under pressure. Families have become money machines that generate income to pay off debts. Work schedules are more important than family schedules. Neighborhoods corrode families through drug abuse and violence. Television pumps out images that oppose cultural integrative values. All of these pressures weaken our civil society without which the marketplace itself cannot survive. Some of the resources poured into capitalistic endeavors need to be used to strengthen families in order to preserve our marketplace system.[20]

Children's social, economic, health and educational problems require integrative community and societal efforts that are sensitive to racial and cultural diversity. But our service systems tend to view children apart from their family and community contexts. Competing programs for different categories of problems treat children as freestanding units and focus on school, peer, social class, racial, neighborhood and societal factors rather than on their homes.

All of these problems could be minimized if our society recognized parenthood as a career with economic and social value and as the essential foundation of our society.

CHALLENGES FOR PARENTS

Genetic and peer influences play important roles in children's temperaments, fashions and interests that can override parental influences. However, overemphasizing these factors overlooks parents who shape character—empathy, self-discipline, perseverance and morality.

Childrearing is a stressful economic burden. Our society expects parents to rear our children without providing adequate resources for many.[21] Not having access to childcare, health care or quality education saps the rewards of parenthood and is detrimental to our society.

Parents are confronted with the following detractors from the fulfillment of parenthood:

- the decline of committed, sacrificial relationships that weakens family bonds;
- pleasing children rather than expecting them to contribute to family well-being;
- viewing children as extensions of themselves rather than as life companions;
- guilt for being imperfect parents; and
- stress making employment away from home attractive and straining marriages.

Parental efforts to integrate childrearing and employment expose the dilemma over how many parenting functions can be delegated without undesirable consequences. After sixty years, the Israeli kibbutzim discontinued childcare for babies because of its long-term negative effects on parent-child relationships and adult outcomes.[22] Virtually all kibbutz babies now receive maternal care at home as mothers gradually increase their workloads during the rest of the first year. As it did in Israel, it will take years to assess the long-term effects of current practices of delegated childcare in the United States on child development and adult outcomes.

CULTURAL EXPECTATIONS OF PARENTHOOD

Because adult interests overshadow children's interests, our society has not clearly articulated its cultural expectations of parenthood. The general assumption is that parents will raise their children as they wish, although it is expected that children will be educated. The lack of articulated cultural values for childrearing does not mean that they do not exist.

The United States is a creedal nation based on the cultural presumption that all human beings are created equal and endowed with certain rights. These values inspired the Declaration of Independence, the Constitution and the Bill of Rights. They evolved from ideas about freedom and justice that accommodate diverse ethnic origins and creeds. They are generally shared by the variety of subcultures in the United States.

American cultural values support raising children to become responsible citizens capable of committed attachments to other people and of contributing to the common good. The cultural expectation of parenthood is developing *both* children's and parents' potentials to function as responsible citizens. Family relationships are as important for adults as for children. The family still is the only institution that provides unconditional acceptance for both. Childhood and parenthood are vital stages in life for developing competence and personal responsibility.

We Expect Competence

Our cultural expectation of competence is reflected in laws and regulations based on personal responsibility that curb the exploitation of individuals by others and the marketplace.

We expect that telephones will work, that checks will be honored, that prices will be honestly displayed, that the contents of foods will be labeled, that contracts will be honored, that manufactured goods will be warranted, that schedules will be dependable and that laws and regulations will be enforced. Travel through foreign countries makes one realize how much we take fulfillment of these expectations for granted. The stark exception is that we do not expect the genetic parents of children to be competent, as we do the parents of adopted children.

Because we hold no articulated expectations for parents who conceive and give birth to children, child neglect and abuse have reached epidemic proportions in the United States, exceeding that in all other developed nations. At a substantiated rate of over 900,000 annually, over 11 million children have been neglected or abused.[23] Many will become violent, habitual criminals or welfare dependent.

If we wish to preserve the quality of our lives, we must reverse the deterioration of parenthood in our nation. We only intervene after child neglect and abuse have occurred, often ineffectively. Enormous public expenditures on treatment, rehabilitation and incarceration result.

All of this would dramatically change if our vision for America was that all of our children will be raised by competent parents.

We Expect Children to Become Responsible Adults

We can expect competence and responsibility in business and professional transactions in the United States because of our laws and regulations. But compliance with these expectations depends upon persons having internalized values that support competence and responsibility. Persons who have not internalized these values exploit others on grand scales as white-collar criminals and on small scales as underclass criminals.

Children become responsible adults when they internalize the values of responsible parents.[24] These parents set limits for their children who learn to respect them. Children learn to be responsible for their behavior when they see their parents acknowledge their mistakes.

When parents do not model prosocial values, their children may overtly or covertly rebel against them or adopt their parents' antisocial values, both with self-defeating consequences for the children. In extreme instances, parents misuse their power and abuse or abdicate their responsibilities and neglect their children. More commonly, parents do not use their culturally supported authority to set limits for their children.

THE EROSION OF CULTURAL CHILDREARING VALUES

Families originated out of clans where fathers had absolute power over their wives and children. In medieval times, parents coped with excess heirs or unwanted children by selling them, giving them to the church as oblates or abandoning them.

The Jewish tradition introduced marriage as a sacred bond between a husband and a wife with procreation as its goal. Fathers remained heads of their households but no longer had absolute power over their children. In the context of individual rights, Christianity introduced the idea that wives and husbands should respect each other and that children were autonomous beings whose primary loyalties were to God.

Still in the eighteenth century, many European mothers either abandoned babies or sent them to wet-nurses.[25] Some desperately poor mothers apparently were infanticidal.

The Industrial Revolution stripped away many of the functions of the family, which was the dominant social institution during the Agricultural Age. Production moved out of homes and education shifted to schools. More recently, the trend in developed countries has been to sidestep the nuclear family as the preferred unit for childbearing and childrearing. The results are fatherless families, uncommitted parents and unprecedented levels of child neglect and abuse, necessitating more governmental involvement in childrearing.

Relying on science and technology instead of on our culture for childrearing guidance contributes to the present ambiguity regarding parenting styles. Research is being conducted on whether or not mothers and fathers matter to children. In her book *The Revolution in Parenthood: The Emerging Global Clash Between Adult Rights and Children's Needs*, Elizabeth Marquardt asks: Are children commodities to be produced by the marketplace?[26] What role should the state have in defining parenthood? When adult rights clash with children's needs, how should the conflict be resolved? She says that our society will either answer these questions through serious reflection and public debate, or they will be answered for us by the marketplace. The choice is ours. At stake are the most elemental features of children's well-being—their social and physical health and their moral and spiritual wholeness.

Fortunately, our pluralistic American cultural values are a rich source of principles for rearing children. All but a few antisocial subcultures in the United States agree that children need a dependable, nurturing environment in early life with a few competent adults with whom young children can form enduring attachment bonds. They agree that the family is the primary agent for child development, especially for developing self-discipline. They agree that the objective of childrearing is developing the ability to function competently and responsibly within our society.

Our cultural values define clear boundaries between childhood and parenthood. When those boundaries are blurred, the rights of children and parents are not balanced by their responsibilities. Those rights surface when divorce or child abuse or neglect occur. But they also occur in family life where the question of whose way will prevail frequently arises.

One of the reasons for blurred boundaries in families is that parents do not clearly define children's responsibilities. When parents are not in charge, the natural exploitative tendencies of children can make parenthood especially stressful. When stressed parents have a choice, delegating parenting functions to childcare workers and to teachers can be appealing.

Unfortunately, our cultural childrearing values are not enforced until after children have been neglected or abused. Even then, conflicting social values often trump cultural values.

THE TENSION BETWEEN SOCIAL AND CULTURAL VALUES

When a social and a cultural value conflict, the integrity of a society depends upon the cultural value prevailing in the long-range. History demonstrates that self-assertive social values dominate the public arena until the excesses they create provoke an ultimately prevailing counter-reaction based on cultural integrative values.

We currently are in a phase in which our social values have become detached from our cultural values in critical ways. The most obvious example is in our underclass. The historian, Carl Nightingale, spent six years with Black young people in a Philadelphia ghetto and saw how they were saturated with self-assertive social values.[27]

> From designer sportswear to gold jewelry, they turned to expensive material goods to bolster self-respect and resorted to violence to obtain money to buy them. Many of them aspired to move to better neighborhoods and to improve their lives. To compensate for the humiliation and frustration of poverty and racism, they turned to our society's self-assertive consumerism.

Nightingale found that these young people were detached from our integrative cultural values of personal and collective responsibility because of their lack of experience with those values.

Major political issues often involve conflicting social and cultural values. They revolve around social values associated with individual liberty that conflict with cultural values that affirm the common good. Nowhere is this more evident than in the dilemma posed by adolescent parenthood where the following conflicting social and cultural values dominate debates as illustrated in figure 32.1. Contemporary dominance of these social values over cultural values in the United States undermines family life. These social values devalue parenthood by supporting adolescent parenthood. We need to align our social values with our integrative cultural values.

ALIGNING SOCIAL VALUES WITH CULTURAL VALUES

There is a palpable yearning for fulfilling careers and for fulfilling family lives in the United States. Aligning our social and cultural values that affect families would relieve the conflicts between these goals.

Aligning a social value with a cultural value goes through a process of identifying an issue; discussing it in organizations; and the media and persuasion through editorials, essays and political activities.[28] Legislation ultimately crystallizes the cultural value in law.

Self-Assertive Social Values	Integrative Cultural Values
parental rights	parental responsibilities
passion (follow emotions)	wisdom (follow thoughtful reasoning)
gratification now	postponing gratification
impulsiveness	tolerating frustration
freedom to make decisions	capacity to make decisions
reproductive liberty	capacity to enter parenthood
baby as a parent's property	baby's right to a competent parent

Figure 32.1.

For example, racism was expressed though slavery at one time. A cultural value contradicted slavery, but that value did not penetrate American society. A long process evolved with identification of slavery as racism, discussion of the issue, education about its harmful effects and ultimately the Civil War that crystallized the 13th Amendment outlawing slavery. Since then a series of laws addressed racism so that social values ultimately were aligned with integrative cultural values that disapproved of prejudice and discrimination.

More recently, the cultural value of protecting children from harm was identified, discussed, educationally disseminated and ultimately crystallized as a social value in state laws protecting children from neglect, abuse, labor and accidents with car seats. Mandatory education and immunization laws protect the developmental interests of children.

Legislation ultimately is necessary in a democratic republic in order to align a social value with a cultural value because an individual's freedom to act requires constraints so that others are not harmed. Although persuasion and education are enough to gain the compliance of most people with a cultural value, there is a segment of the population that does not respond to those measures and requires the constraint of laws. In fact, the success of our society has been based on the rule of law—the tangible repository of our cultural values. We are able to transact business with checks and credit cards rather than cash because of the trust we all have in the enforcement of our laws. But we still are reluctant to legislate standards for competent parenthood. The prime example is our failure to deal with the crisis of adolescent childbirth.

THE PERSONAL AND SOCIAL CRISIS OF ADOLESCENT PARENTHOOD

The possibility of influencing conflicting public attitudes toward adolescent parenthood is greater than might be expected. All that is needed is to mobilize cultural values that support children's and adolescents' rights to competent parents. Then society's interest in each pregnant adolescent is apparent. That interest is not primarily in educating and funding adolescent parents. It is primarily in insuring that adolescent parents and their babies have competent parents.

The Self-interests of Adolescents

The most important question for each pregnant girl and conceiving male is what is in my self-interest?

- Should I be free to pursue my own development, education and career or should I assume the responsibilities of parenthood and compromise my own self-interests?
- Should short-term emotions, fantasies and unrealistic attitudes determine my life course or should my long-term self-interests prevail?
- Should my baby's developmental needs be compromised to suit my short-term desires or should my baby's long-term interests prevail?

- Should society bear the costs of supporting me as a parent and the likely costs of crime and welfare dependency later?

The Interests of Society

Looking at adolescence from society's point of view, should the chaos engendered by the crisis of adolescent childbirth be approached reactively with "damage control" that can amplify its effects or thoughtfully with holistic planning that can dampen its effects? We have sufficient knowledge and capabilities to prevent damage in the first place if we connect adolescent parenthood with its consequent social problems. We do not need to feel helpless when an adolescent girl gives birth. We can apply the knowledge and problem-solving skills we have.

Adolescent pregnancy does not stop being a social and personal crisis when a baby is born. Adolescent parenthood is an even greater crisis with health, child welfare and legal elements. The legal system has statutes that use the age-grading concept to protect minors from activities beyond their capabilities and to protect society from their inappropriate actions.

Articulating cultural values that discourage premature coitus can dramatically change adolescent behavior, as was shown in this country in the early 20th century and is evident in other countries today. This can be done through a public health campaign highlighting the disadvantages of adolescent coitus and pregnancy, as has been mounted against smoking, drug abuse and driving while drinking. Civic groups, churches and celebrities can articulate standards for sexual behavior and parenthood, as has been done to promote the importance of education.

In 1983, Marie Winn called attention to many children who were growing up then without childhoods.[29] This is even more evident today. One symptom of our society's denigration of childhood and parenthood is supporting adolescent parenthood, which ignores adolescence as an essential preparation for adulthood, especially in our increasingly complicated world.

If we recognize adolescence as a developmental stage, and if we define parenthood as an adult responsibility, we can restore childhood for children of coming generations. Our society must realize that it cannot afford to shorten the period of nurture and protection of its young by allowing them to assume adult responsibilities prematurely.

If we truly wish to prevent adolescent pregnancies and childbirth, we need to understand that the developmental characteristics of adolescence and the influences, or the lack thereof, of parents are more important causes of adolescent parenthood than ignorance and socioeconomic disadvantage. Antipoverty measures alone do not address parent–child relationships. Ronald Mincy and Susan Weiner of the Urban Institute found that poverty is less important than the behavior of her own parents in influencing an adolescent girl's chances of becoming pregnant.[30]

Most importantly, we need to recognize that our charitable impulse to support adolescent parents can have unintended consequences. We need to shift from a damage-control attitude to offering hope and empowerment to adolescents and their families.

Valuing parenthood enough to set minimum standards for it could be a tipping point for our society by shifting from self-assertive social to integrative cultural values. The most important issue facing our society today is whether or not we value children and the future of our nation enough to value parenthood as a career.

HOW OUR SOCIETY CAN VALUE PARENTHOOD AS A CAREER

As it now stands, the link between incompetent parents and our social problems is obscured by other issues. But parents can be held accountable to society, as attested by the progressive enactment of child labor, mandatory education and child abuse and neglect laws. Because it is vital to the future of our society, parenthood should be recognized as a privileged career supported by our society.

The logic for societal support of parenthood is compelling.[31] All of us depend upon the quantity and quality of other peoples' children. Our cultural values expect that adults who are not parents have a responsibility to support rearing the next generation. Support in return for service is an American rationale that combines respect for both individual freedom and an obligation to the common good. Social Security and the post-World War II GI Bill are prime examples.

In the 1970s, most industrialized nations began to publicly support parenthood. They refused to accept the risks to healthy development posed by inadequate care for babies and toddlers.[32] These governments now protect them through paid parental leaves for childbirth and sick children care, regulated and subsidized childcare services and flexible work hours. President Nixon vetoed the Comprehensive Child Development Act in 1971. Passed with bipartisan Congressional support, the Act would have provided our families the support being instituted then by other nations. As one consequence, all states fell far short of meeting basic requirements for childcare in 2005. Out of 150 possible points, the average state score was only 70 points.[33]

Although Americans work much longer and irregular hours than Europeans, we provide far less childcare and family leaves. We would profit from learning from the experience of other developed countries in supporting parenthood.

The focus also needs to extend to men. As long as boys fail to postpone fatherhood until they are employed and men do not support their children, mothers and children will remain trapped in poor neighborhoods. The 1988 Family Support Act and the Personal Responsibility and Work Opportunity Reconciliation Act of 1996 widened the gaps in advantages females have over males by helping mothers prepare for jobs without provisions for fathers.

Increasing the number of fathers who are involved in the care of their children means improving their employment prospects and adopting workplace policies that include paternity leaves, flexible scheduling, employment-based childcare and reasonable work loads.[34] It means parent counseling to help couples manage their disagreements and keep fathers involved with children. It means mentoring and other community programs to model responsible fatherhood. For example, the Chicago Black Star Project focuses on low-income Black, Latino and American Indian boys in low-achieving schools. It organizes a Million Father March that urges fathers to take their children back to school.[35] Non-custodial fathers also could be sent report cards and invited to parent-teacher conferences, school assemblies and graduations of their children.

Social policies that support parenthood would go a long way toward removing the need to choose between raising children and a paid career.[36] If women were assured of childcare and economic assistance while pursuing higher education and career development during their optimal childbearing years, fewer would delay childbearing until late in their reproductive years.

Although individual parents have little power, local, state and national organizations could unite and work toward recognizing the service that parents provide to society through the personal sacrifices they make in rearing our nation's children.

THE NEED FOR GOVERNMENTAL INTERVENTIONS

We would not need law enforcement if every citizen considered the rights of others. We would not need welfare if every individual was capable of, and had the opportunity to lead, an economically productive life. Unfortunately, everyone does not have these qualities and opportunities. We always will need law enforcement and some form of welfare. We always will face the repercussions of incompetent parents if we do not set standards for parenthood.

Parents are in the best position to represent the interests of their children, but they are accountable to society, as attested by the progressive enactment of child labor, mandatory education and child neglect and abuse laws; the licensing of foster parents and childcaring facilities; standards for adoptive parents; and divorce custody and visitation laws. Standards also are set for childcare, pre-schools, schools and others who are responsible for children's lives.

Now all parents are assumed to be competent until they damage their children by neglect or abuse. A more accurate assumption is that the vast majority of parents are competent, but children need protection from the millions who are not.

We cannot assume competence in parenting any more than we can assume competence in any other activity that affects others. Irresponsible people conceive and bear children. Children and society need protection from having incompetent parents through the prevention provisions of child neglect and abuse statutes. When parents are unable or unwilling to become competent, these statutes require that parental rights be terminated and that their children be adopted.

Parents' abdication of their responsibilities has necessitated laws that mandate parental participation in school conferences, the liability of grandparents for the children of their children, the liability of parents for their children's actions and the liability of non-custodial parents for the financial support of their children. However, because of the subtle, but powerful, presumption that children are the property of their genetic parents cloaked by family privacy and individual freedom, we intervene in families only after children have been damaged by neglect or abuse.

If all parents were competent, there would be no need for governmental involvement in family life. Because the neglect, abuse and exploitation of children damage the next generation, government has a clear-cut role in preventing child neglect and abuse by articulating standards for parenthood. All of us are paying an ever larger share of the cost of rearing, educating and treating children and have a financial stake in preventing child neglect and abuse.

Around the world, governments are defining and regulating parenthood because of conflicts between adult rights and children's needs.[37] Underlying these conflicts is the erosion of the nuclear family. Children also are being increasingly viewed as commodities to be traded in the artificial fertilization and adoption marketplaces.

We have come to the point at which a new paradigm for parenthood is needed. Now anyone who conceives and gives birth has custodial guardianship of the child until that child is damaged by neglect or abuse. We need to implement our cultural expectation that parents will be competent.

We have standards for responsible adulthood. They are supporting oneself legally and abiding by our laws and regulations. We need the minimum standards for parenthood outlined in Chapter 33 to protect children from neglect and abuse and all of us from the consequences.

CONCLUSION

The National Academies call for a comprehensive federal effort to improve our nation's human capital so that we can benefit from globalization. Although the smallest and seemingly most fragile of all social institutions, parenthood produces our human capital.

The inescapable fact is that too many of our children are growing up under family circumstances that prevent them from learning essential social and work-related skills and becoming responsible, productive citizens.

Compared to other developed nations, our society does not place a high value on parenthood. We have the highest child poverty and incarceration rates and the lowest childrearing benefits. The cycle of adolescent parenthood and resulting child abuse and neglect is the most preventable source of our society's habitual crime and welfare dependency.

Our society needs a paradigm shift from our dominant self-assertive social values toward our integrative cultural values that can protect the future of our nation by ensuring that all children have competent parents. We would then value parenthood as a career with economic and social value as much as remunerated employment. We would make it possible for parents to compete economically with adults without children.

Competent parents are essential for the survival of our society. Because it is vital to the future of our society, minimum legal standards should be set for parenthood. Legislation is needed to make parenthood planning counseling available to pregnant adolescents and dependent adults and their families and to ensure that their babies have legal custodial guardians.

Chapter 33

Parenthood Planning Teams and Certification of Parenthood

Politics is not a game. It exists to resolve the largest questions of the society—the agreed-upon terms by which everyone can live peaceably with one another. At its best politics creates and sustains social relationships—the human conversation and engagement that draw people together and allow them to discover their mutuality.

William Greider
Who Will Tell the People[1]

The adolescent parenthood dilemma seems unsolvable. Few politicians want to take on an issue that raises controversies over poverty, race, families, childrearing and individual rights. Even one of these controversies is enough to derail political action. It seems that all we can do is make the best of an undesirable situation.

It seems this way not because we lack knowledge. We know that adolescent childbirth creates initial conditions that adversely affect the lives of adolescents, their babies and their families. These initial conditions are amplified or dampened by interacting circumstances that can lead to crime and welfare dependency. We know that taxpayers pay for the consequences.

If we know that everyone is burdened by adolescent parenthood, why do we support it with public and private funds?

There are many reasons. The most important is our emotional response to childbirth. Even though they are still girls and boys, adolescent parents are mothers and fathers. Their babies belong to them. How can anyone separate a mother or a father from their baby?

The next is the belief that being a parent will cause an adolescent to mature rapidly. The Horatio Alger theme is deeply embedded in our culture. Adolescent parents have successfully raised their children and become productive citizens. Many have overcome adversity to become celebrities and leaders. They can "make it" through diligent effort. Parenthood gives meaning and purpose to life for adolescents who have little else going for them in modern society.[2]

Another deeply felt reason is that when a girl and a boy make a mistake, they must take the consequences. The honorable response to adolescent childbirth is marriage or for the unmarried mother and father to rear the baby. Many families step forward and assist their minor parents or assume responsibility for rearing their babies.

Finally, we recognize that poverty is a major factor in adolescent parenthood. Our charitable impulse is to help the less fortunate. We feel obliged to minimize adversity for adolescents and their babies. We can try to improve their babies' lives by providing parenting education and childcare so adolescent parents can attend school.

All of these reasons make supporting adolescent parents seem to be the most practical solution to adolescent childbirth. But none of them should deter us from trying to find better solutions to the adolescent parenthood dilemma. None of them change the following facts:

- Adolescents are not adults.
- Adolescents require parents or other adults as custodial guardians.
- The first weeks, months and years are critical in child development. Babies do not benefit from temporary living arrangements while their adolescent parents mature.
- Parenthood adversely affects adolescents, their babies and their families.

We need to remember why we so strongly advocate preventing adolescent pregnancy—adolescent parenthood is an *undesirable life style* in modern society. The objective of preventing adolescent pregnancy really is preventing adolescent parenthood. Ironically, the American Humane Society requires that one be an adult to adopt an animal, but a minor traditionally is accorded parental rights and presumed to be capable of entering parenthood.

In our society, the principle that *undesirable life styles* should be prevented is generally accepted. We devote considerable effort to preventing child neglect and abuse, drug abuse, alcoholism, smoking, obesity, sexually transmitted diseases and adolescent pregnancy. In spite of these interventions, individuals persist in behaviors that contribute to these undesirable conditions. Our health care and human service systems care for them. However, when their behavior harms others, public health and law enforcement systems intervene. Parenthood has repercussions far beyond individual adolescent parents. It is an *undesirable life style* that has harmful short- and long-term effects on others—their babies, their families and society.

The shift from prevention to support when an adolescent becomes a parent is based upon a perceived lack of alternatives and an effort to minimize adverse outcomes for the baby. However, when the focus is only on the baby, the interests of the adolescent parent can be overlooked. When the focus is only on the adolescent parent, the interests of the baby can be overlooked. In both situations, the interests of the families and society can be overlooked. The birth of babies to minors should invoke considering the interests of the babies first, of the adolescent parents second, of the relatives third and of society fourth.

Because we have not carefully thought through the issues and options surrounding adolescent childbirth, our responses are reactive rather than proactive. Paul Trad, a child psychiatrist, noted that adolescent childbirth is a "high-risk" event that warrants sensitive, realistic intervention.[3] We need a paradigm that proactively protects the interests of everyone affected by adolescent childbirth. That paradigm is recognizing *adolescent childbirth as a public health crisis.* It can be resolved by combining the resources of the health care, social welfare and legal systems. We need to do this with cultural competence and without harming adolescent parents. The high-risk status of adolescents' babies can be recognized by designating giving birth under the age of 18 as a public health crisis. This principle also can be applied to dependent adults with legal guardians and adults who have been adjudicated to be unfit parents.

ACTING ON THE PUBLIC HEALTH CRISIS OF ADOLESCENT PARENTHOOD

Any *undesirable life style* harmful to individuals and to others falls within the scope of public health. Violence, sexually transmitted diseases, drugs and incarceration are public health issues because their prevention involves behavioral changes. Adolescent pregnancy already is a public health crisis. Adolescent childbirth is an even more serious public health crisis.

The public health system is firmly grounded in law.[4] It is devoted to preventing physical, mental and social disorders. It promotes education, advocacy, services and enforcement guided by legislation. The Child Abuse Prevention and Treatment Act of 1974 placed the moral weight of the federal government behind professional interventions with struggling families.[5]

As knowledge emerges about preventable conditions, new legislation is enacted, such as protecting the health of children during early life by testing for phenylketonuria and by requiring immunizations. The Keeping Children and Families Safe Act of 2003 requires states to ensure that health care providers report babies affected by prenatal drug exposure to child protective services. Physicians in New Jersey are required to educate expectant mothers and their families about the signs and symptoms of postpartum depression and screen new mothers for the disorder.[6] Routine HIV testing of pregnant women has been introduced in some states because the rights of the unborn child are violated if a mother refuses HIV testing. All of these measures are precedents for legislation to deal with the crisis of adolescent and dependent adult childbirth.

The adolescent childbirth crisis now draws attention to supporting the girl as a mother rather than to her own and to her baby's developmental needs. As a result, the fact that there are two young persons with developmental needs is ignored. Also overlooked is the likelihood that adolescent mothers are vulnerable girls with pre-existing problems. Some see pregnancy as more appealing than finishing school. Some advocates regard openly dealing with these facts as intruding on an adolescent's privacy or as on a slippery slope to undesirable paternalism. As a result, the idea of "soft paternalism" has been advanced.

Soft Paternalism (*Parentalism*)

Soft paternalism has been suggested as a way to help people who are likely to make self-defeating decisions avoid self-defeating behavior.[7] Missouri makes it illegal for compulsive gamblers to enter casinos in order to help them break their addiction to gambling. Rebecca Maynard, professor of education and social policy at the University of Pennsylvania, suggests that soft paternalism be applied to adolescent pregnancy and parenthood as well.

But paternalism has a sexist flavor. It also evokes images of a slippery slope to governmental control of our private lives and abuse of disadvantaged persons. However, soft paternalism really means protecting individuals through regulations that serve their interests.

We all need protection from the acts of others and from our own impulses. We need speed limits and traffic lights. We need protection from unethical businesses and professionals. The philosopher Harry Frankfurt submits that we only really act freely when we thoughtfully act on a desire since we can be slaves to our impulses.[8] Long-term goals can be easily sacrificed to uncontrolled short-term desires. Our lower brain centers seek immediate gratification. They become subservient to the reasoning part of our brain in the cerebral cortex only through our learning how to restrain our impulses and to tolerate frustration during childhood and adolescence by having externally imposed limits. This neurological fact necessitates externally imposed laws in order to maintain freedom in our society by restraining undesirable actions.

The "slippery slope" argument is valid when a public policy can have unintended consequences that override its benefits to society. This can happen when policies are based on preferences, such as that all cohabiting couples should be married. However, this argument is not plausible when policies are based on scientific evidence and when possible adverse effects are enormously overridden by demonstrated benefits. This is the case with adolescent parenthood.

A less controversial term for soft paternalism might be *parentalism*. Parentalism means protecting and nurturing. Government already applies parentalism in its *in loco parentis* role under the *parens patriae* doctrine by supporting parental authority and by limiting the privileges of minors to prevent them from making decisions that permanently alter their lives and that they will regret later, especially when the stakes for society are high.

Primary, Secondary, and Tertiary Prevention

The public health concepts of primary, secondary and tertiary prevention of health and social problems help place adolescent childbirth in perspective. Preventing adolescent pregnancy where the risk is to the girl is primary prevention. Managing adolescent pregnancy where the risk is to the girl and a fetus is secondary prevention. Managing adolescent childbirth where the risk is to the girl, baby, father, relatives and society is tertiary prevention.

The public health, child welfare and legal systems can collaborate in focusing attention on the secondary and tertiary prevention of adolescent parenthood in the same way that we prevent handicaps from physical illnesses and disabilities. The most important strategy is to create opportunities for thoughtful dialog with pregnant adolescents and their families. This would permit working through conflicting motives and perceptions using problem-solving techniques based on realistic goals. This can be done by including *Parenthood Planning Counseling* in the clinical management of each pregnant adolescent and dependent adult.

PARENTHOOD PLANNING COUNSELING

Health care professionals are in a key position to provide Parenthood Planning Counseling for pregnant girls, dependent women, fathers and families.

Title XX of the Public Health Service Act already specifies that Adolescent Family Life Demonstration Projects include Parenthood Planning Counseling in the form of adoption counseling and referral services; education on the responsibilities of sexuality and parenting; and counseling for the immediate and extended family members of the eligible adolescent.[9] The following programs can play key roles in offering or arranging for Parenthood Planning Counseling as is required for Adolescent Family Life Demonstration Projects:

- Family planning and health care clinics that provide pregnancy diagnosis.
- Medicaid Prenatal Care Coordination services.
- Prenatal care clinics.
- Prenatal home visitation programs.

Professionals can contribute to positive counseling outcomes by engaging individuals and families in respectful ways. Their ethical obligation is to enter every clinical situation with an open mind and develop a shared understanding of concerns, priorities, strengths and challenges with sensitivity to cultural factors. To this end, materials have been prepared to assist counseling with Black, Latino, American Indian and southeastern Asian families.[10]

Pregnancy usually is the first time an adolescent is confronted with a life-course altering decision. She and the father can be expected to vacillate in decision-making. Most adolescents have little or no information about pregnancy or its termination. Their fears, fantasies and anxieties need to be explored along with offering facts and reassurance. Guilt on the part of the adolescent and her family is common. Parents' guilt may be projected in the form of anger at a daughter or her boyfriend. They need to explore their feelings to prevent untoward reactions.

Pregnancy may be a way of avoiding loneliness and isolation. An adolescent may be too fearful to face her own emptiness and inadequate resources. This is accentuated by abandonment by the putative father. The resulting feelings of despair and unworthiness create a precarious time for decision-making.[11]

Timing of Parenthood Planning Counseling

The best time for decision-making regarding the course of a pregnancy is when it first becomes known. It is a time when the interests of everyone can be considered: the mother, father, fetus and their families.

Although the discovery of pregnancy is an emotional event for all concerned, the physical and emotional changes of advanced pregnancy and childbirth have not yet occurred. It is the time when the potential mother and father and their families are in the best position to weigh the pros and cons of each possible course. If the decision is to continue the pregnancy, the interests of the unborn baby should be foremost in the minds of everyone. There is time—usually five to seven months—to work through guilt, shame and fantasies about childbirth for all concerned.

Late in pregnancy, hormonal and physical effects produce mental and emotional states that cloud objective thinking. After childbirth, prolactin and oxytocin activate neural codes that motivate mothers to become attached more strongly to their babies, who have been parts of their bodies. Pitressin produces similar responses in fathers. This is the time of least capacity for objective decision-making.

Consummating the decision-making process during pregnancy also is critical because the first weeks and months in the lives of babies have profound developmental consequences, especially for the bonding process. The interests of the unborn baby should take precedence over the traditional view that mothers need time after birth to decide to make an adoption plan.[12]

Shifting from Short-term Desires to Long-Term Interests

Our pop culture glorifies self-indulgence and self-defeating actions.[13] Most people believe that they should eat reasonably, live within their means, avoid addictions, be sexually responsible, keep promises and hold undesirable impulses in check. Yet most of us violate some of these tenets, not because we want to harm ourselves but because we cannot control our urges.

In this ambivalent social context, pregnant girls, conceiving boys and dependent adults and their families need Parenthood Planning Counseling to help them make decisions that truly are in the interests of the unborn baby first and then in the self-interests of the adolescents or dependent adults, their families and society.

Parenthood Planning Counseling should not simply be based on supporting the status quo or satisfying the desires of the individuals involved. It should be based on the goals of productive citizenship for the adolescents and dependent adults and for their children. It should be based on placing long-term interests ahead of short-term desires.

Adolescents and dependent adults who become pregnant have difficulty envisioning alternatives and reasoning about the consequences of childbirth. They need counseling about which alternative would be best for themselves and for their babies. They need help in identifying and acting upon their own self-interests. They need to understand the burdens of parenthood. They need to realize that a baby is not a personal possession but is a human being entitled to competent parenting. They need to appreciate the impact of imposing the burdens of childrearing on their own parents and relatives. They need help to see adoption realistically.[14]

Young people need to have accurate information about the choices they face. They need to know that adolescence is an important stage of life that is truncated by the physical, emotional and psychological consequences of parenthood. A girl needs to know that her decision to enter parenthood exposes her and her child to elevated risks of poverty, poor education, depression, welfare dependency and prison. Parenthood does not remove disadvantaged circumstances.

We need to create opportunities and a language for sharing our knowledge with young people and helping them make life-altering decisions.

THE MOTHER-BABY BOND

The deepest human bond is between mother and child. It has a sacred aura. Our instinctive response to the image of a mother and a newborn baby is one of awe and empathy. The baby is her own flesh and blood. This natural response underlies our legal framework that protects the privacy of the family and of parental rights. It creates a climate in which the image of a baby as the possession of the mother overrides consideration of a newborn as a separate human being. As a result, the question of "true mother love" is seldom raised today, as it was in the proverbial wisdom of Solomon:[15]

> Two women claimed the same child as their own. Solomon offered to cut the baby in half to settle the dispute. One woman replied she would rather forfeit the child than see him killed. Solomon judged her to be the true child's mother and awarded her the child.

At the core of assessing mother love is whether it is self or baby oriented. Is a baby viewed as a mother's possession or as a mother's responsibility? Is a mother an owner or a guardian of a baby? Is a mother seeking what the baby can do for her or what she can do for her baby? Is a baby's purpose to fulfill a mother's desires or to develop as an autonomous person?

These questions need to be raised with adolescents and dependent adults as they consider the options of entering parenthood or making an adoption plan. Are her or his motives egocentric or are they centered on the interests of her unborn baby?

Enhancing Adolescent Development

Approaching adolescent pregnancy with a problem-solving attitude can enhance personal growth rather than create obstacles to achieving personal goals. It can help adolescents learn how to question their egocentric desires and thereby gain self-respect and self-confidence.

Adolescence is a critical time for learning how to resolve personal dilemmas in ways that lead to discovering and serving one's own true self-interests. Without efforts to grow in awareness, knowledge, wisdom and planning one's life self-fulfillment cannot occur. The experience of deferring one's own wishes and urges for the benefit of others is character building for adolescent mothers and fathers. When they acknowledge they made a mistake in conceiving a child, they can make decisions for themselves and their babies to avoid further mistakes with grave consequences for both of them. When caught up in a cycle of failure in their academic and social lives, they can be helped to reverse this cycle by building their self-respect and self-confidence through realistic achievements other than parenthood.[16] They can be empowered to face and master the challenges of adolescence without the responsibilities of parenthood.

Involving Families

An adolescent's or a dependent adult's family is crucial in determining the course of a pregnancy and its aftermath. A family can choose to assume responsibility for assisting a dependent parent in childrearing. However, because most adolescent parents have significant mental and emotional vulnerabilities in addition to immaturity, family members should not assume responsibilities for caring for their adolescents' babies without having commensurate authority to make decisions for the babies through custodial guardianship. Still, the parents of minor parents cannot be presumed to be competent parents themselves. In situations involving incest, abuse, alcoholism or drug abuse, parental involvement may not be desirable. Intervention may be needed to obtain a custodial guardian for the adolescent and her baby.

Minors and their parents can disagree about a course of action. Parents might pressure a couple to marry against their wishes or withhold permission when minors desire marriage. Given the vulnerability of many young mothers and fathers, counseling is needed to help them choose the most appropriate route for establishing paternity, including the choice not to do so in cases of rape, incest or domestic violence. Law enforcement referral may be appropriate.

Child welfare workers can be helpful in assessing whether or not relatives are capable of assuming childrearing responsibilities for an adolescent or dependent adult mother and baby.

THE CHILD WELFARE SYSTEM

Child welfare interventions should be shifted from the secondary goals of preventing subsequent births and securing the safety of babies to the primary goal of preventing adolescent parenthood in the first place. Child neglect and abuse statutes already provide for terminating parental rights at childbirth when circumstances warrant.[17] These statutes could be expanded to include the unavailability of a qualified custodial guardian.

Child welfare workers can draw upon the research on adolescent pregnancy and parenthood and knowledge of adolescence as a critical developmental stage in which adult physical capacities can lead to actions that are regretted later in life. They have access to training in counseling pregnant adolescents and in making adoption plans, including transracial adoption. They also are in a position to participate in the education of public and policy makers.

In order to function effectively and expeditiously, child welfare workers need the support of the legal system.

THE LEGAL SYSTEM

Because it can be abused, the power of government to intervene in private lives is restricted to circumstances in which serious harm to others or to society is likely to occur. These interventions are intended to benefit and protect individuals, especially children. They also protect taxpayers from the costs of dependency and crime.

We are free to lead our own lives without governmental intervention as long as we do not harm others and, under certain circumstances, ourselves. Yet people frequently abuse their freedom to act as they wish. The challenge is to distinguish between irritating abuses of our freedom to act and those that warrant legal limitations.

The freedom to procreate and to be a parent is one of the most cherished human freedoms. Limiting the rights of parents is highly controversial, but child neglect and abuse laws clearly state that parents are not free to neglect or abuse their children.

In *Carey v. Population Services International*, the U.S. Supreme Court noted "the incidence of sexual activity among minors is high, and the consequences of such activity are frequently devastating. . ."[18] This recognition opens the door to a role for the state when a minor gives birth, especially since minors already have limited legal privileges.

Legal Limitations of Adolescent Behavior

Childhood is regarded as a legal "disability." The gradual maturation of young persons' abilities to act independently is legally regarded as growing out of the "disability of infancy." Our age-grading laws recognize that adolescents are not capable of making life-course altering decisions. Progressively awarding adult privileges protects the healthy development and safety of adolescents. Driver training and graduated licensing programs reduce the fatal accidents of 16-year-old drivers.[19] This age-grading principle can be applied to parenthood as well.

In spite of the age-grading principle, courts tend to follow antiquated common law that does not recognize adolescence as a developmental stage of life. Adolescence also is seen as a temporary status that will be outgrown. Legal traditions that treat adolescent parents as legally qualified custodial guardians of their babies and ignore their immaturity as expressed in the age-grading principle need to be challenged. These traditions also ignore the fact that weeks and months are long times with significant developmental consequences for adolescents' babies.

Adolescent parents need double protection from the incompetence of their own parents and from being incompetent parents themselves. Their children may well need protection from them and their relatives as well. We need a realistic way to think about the legal status of adolescent parenthood if we are to ensure that they and their babies receive competent parenting. This brings us to the legal status of minors' babies.

Custodial Guardianship of the Babies of Minor Parents

The evolving legal trend is to place the interests of children above the rights of parents when they conflict. This means that the interests of the babies of adolescent parents should take precedence over the wishes of adolescent parents and their families.

In fact, the babies of minors do not automatically have custodial guardians to:

* Ensure that they receive nurturance and the material necessities of life.
* Make decisions affecting their welfare and well-being.
* Arrange for and authorize their medical care.
* Advocate their interests.

Although some states regard childbirth as emancipating minors from parental authority, minors cannot be custodial guardians of their babies, as is recognized now when a guardian *ad litem* (an officer of the court representing the minor's interests) is appointed to represent a minor parent in adoption proceedings.

Minors cannot exercise custodial guardianship of their own children (and be competent parents) because they require custodial guardians themselves and the age-grading principle prevents them from assuming responsibility for the life of another person. They are not competent to exercise parental custodial guardianship rights because their brain development and emotional and social maturity have not progressed to the point where they can make decisions that permanently affect their own lives, the lives of their babies, their families and society.

Grandparents may have statutory financial liability for the support of their grandchildren, but they do not have custodial guardianship. They and other relatives need relief from feeling obliged to sacrifice their own interests in order to parent the children of their adolescents without the authority of custodial guardianship. Some states now permit *defacto* guardianship when the defaults of minor parents force relatives to care for their children.[20]

We must see adolescent childbirth from the baby's point of view. We need a vision in which the birth of every baby in the United States is a cause for celebration. When it is clear that this will not be the case, we need a way to bring a baby's birth as close as we can to this vision. Because adolescent childbirth is a public health crisis masked by powerful emotional reactions, we need to pull together existing health, social welfare and legal resources when pregnancy is identified and establish best practices to ensure that the unborn baby's interests are served first.

We need to emphasize prevention in our child neglect and abuse statutes. The present stance of intervening only after children are damaged is inhumane and costly. We need to craft legal and clinical procedures to deal with the fact that the babies of adolescent parents need protection, as do the adolescent parents themselves. This can be done by mandating Parenthood Planning Counseling for pregnant minors and dependent adults and their families when they choose to become parents during the five to seven months prior to childbirth.

Our failure to resolve critical parenthood issues before a baby is born is the single most important preventable cause of crime and welfare dependency. As it now stands, the adolescent childbirth crisis evokes a number of interventions ranging from paternity determination to finding a home for the mother and baby that may take months to years to resolve. During that time, the baby's interests usually are submerged with resulting adverse effects for the baby. *Parenthood Planning Teams* are needed to provide Parenthood Planning Counseling.

PARENTHOOD PLANNING TEAMS

A public health approach to the adolescent parenthood crisis would involve case re-porting (a standard public health procedure), counseling (now available at clinical lev-els) and law enforcement (now available for suspected child neglect or abuse). Child welfare and legal procedures can be based on augmented prevention provisions in child neglect and abuse statutes and legislation mandating Parenthood Planning Coun-seling by *Parenthood Planning Teams*.

The composition of a Parenthood Planning Team would depend upon the circum-stances. It would consist of two or more of the following: a family planning counselor, prenatal care counselor or public health nurse; a child welfare worker; a juvenile or family court staff member who implements the guardianship petition process; a guardian *ad litem* when appropriate; and other professionals involved with the ado-lescent or her family. A Team can be established by connecting existing resources as is done through Coordinated Services and Wraparound Teams.[21]

A Parenthood Planning Team would be required for certain categories of dependent parents: 1) minors and 2) adults with developmental disabilities, previous terminations of parental rights, incarceration as violent felons or convictions as domestic abusers.

Dependent parents need to be considered on an individual case basis guided by the in-terests of each parent, baby, family and society. For example, most of the 84,000 women in federal and state prisons are serving a year or less for possession or trafficking in il-legal substances, shoplifting, bad checks and stolen credit cards. Of those in Illinois, most are in their thirties with three or four children; 63% are high school drop-outs; 60% have substance abuse problems; 85% are single mothers; and most are victims of do-mestic abuse.[22] We need to shift from incarceration to community management in sen-tencing and consider the life circumstances and abilities of each parent in order to iden-tify the most appropriate parenthood option. Because each parent's situation is unique and involves multiple issues, a Parenthood Planning Team is needed in order to facili-tate making appropriate choices. As is the case in evaluating adolescents' or adults' ca-pacities to give informed consent for health care, their decision-making capacities for entering parenthood or making adoption plans need to be evaluated.

Parenthood Planning Counseling through a Parenthood Planning Team can be man-dated since the *babies of adolescent parents do not have legal custodial guardians*. With relatively little cost or inconvenience, a Parenthood Planning Team can be acti-vated by family planning and prenatal care services through a legally mandated re-porting process beginning when an adolescent or dependent adult learns of her preg-nancy and decides to continue it to childbirth. We now have access to most pregnant adolescents and dependent adults through family planning clinics, Medical Assistance prenatal care, prenatal clinics and home visitation programs. Federal law requires in-hospital paternity acknowledgment programs to establish babies' paternity at birth. A Parenthood Planning Team would begin this process during pregnancy.

The first professional who becomes aware of a minor's or a dependent adult's de-cision to continue her pregnancy would connect the child welfare and legal systems with prenatal care by forming a Parenthood Planning Team and activating a *parent-hood certification* process.

PARENTHOOD CERTIFICATION

Parenthood is publicly supported now through tax benefits, public education and public assistance. In order to justify this public support, greater accountability of parents is needed. The benefits of parenthood need to be connected to the capacity to fulfill its responsibilities. Parents cannot expect public support if they are unable or unwilling to handle the responsibilities of parenthood.

The capacity to become a parent by conceiving and giving birth to a child says nothing about a parent's ability to rear that child. Still, there is a way to assess whether or not a genetic parent is capable of handling the responsibilities of parenthood. It is by setting minimum standards that translate our cultural expectations of parenthood into public policies by balancing self-assertive social with integrative cultural values.

Integrative cultural and social values are commonly articulated through rituals and celebrations. Patriotism is expressed through awards and holidays. Marriage is certified by a ceremony and vows as a legal contract and personal commitment between two people for the purposes of enhancing social stability, promoting standards for sexual relations and procreation, rearing offspring, transfering property and enhancing companionship. Although marriage may not result in parenthood, John Stuart Mill noted that the unborn child is the third party in marriage. Following this logic, the personal commitment of marriage should include a commitment to parenthood for unborn children of that union.

Standards for Marriage

We have a model for setting minimum standards for parenthood now—it is the marriage process that creates a social contract between a marital couple and traditionally has been regarded as a prelude to parenthood. Applying for a marriage license in itself demonstrates motivation for a committed relationship and a minimum level of social and intellectual competence. States usually have three requirements for a legally recognized marriage that reflect the Model Marriage and Divorce Act of the Uniform Law Commission:

1) *Affidavit:* a declaration under oath that information provided is true and that no legal impediment exists to entering marriage:
   - proof of age and residence eligibility,
   - information about previous marriages,
   - Social Security number, and
   - marriage is not between genetic relatives.
2) *License:* authorizes the marriage ceremony after a waiting period.
3) *Certificate of Marriage:* executed by a legally authorized person.

The vital importance of parenthood to our society justifies setting similar minimum standards to create a legal parent-child relationship both in and outside of marriage. This is more critical now than ever before because marriage no longer serves as a prelude to parenthood. Furthermore, the long-standing willingness of our society to assist childrearing families is being strained by the millions of contemporary incompetent parents. We need to align our social values with integrative cultural values that further the common good through committed relationships between people, especially between parents and their children.

Standards for Parenthood

In 2007, over one-third of all babies were born outside of marriage. Over one-half of the births to mothers under thirty were non-marital.[23] A growing number of babies are born to surrogate mothers. These trends have increasingly necessitated the legal determination and acceptance of both maternity and paternity. These trends have focused attention on ensuring that all children have parents who are capable of assuming responsibility for their custody and care.

Because of the public interest in ensuring that every child has a competent parent—a legal custodial guardian, we need a way to provide a legal basis for the social contract of parenthood as marriage does for the social contract between a marital couple. We now require fathers of non-marital children to assume financial support and, when appropriate, permit them to assume guardianship of their children. Parents who adopt through agencies or are involved in custody contests must meet minimum standards. Our society can no longer afford to presume that everyone who conceives and gives birth to a baby is qualified to assume the responsibilities of parenthood.

James Dwyer, professor of law at William and Mary University, proposes that certain categories of high-risk parents be required to apply for certification that they meet minimum standards in order to become the custodial guardians of their genetic or birth children.[24] Those minimum standards would be based on the principle that *a person who requires a guardian or who is legally unfit to parent cannot be the guardian of a child*. The most common category of persons who require guardians is legal minority, ordinarily in the form of their parents. Additional less common generic categories are: developmental disabilities, mental illness, adjudication of parental unfitness and incarceration.[25]

Legal standards for the need for guardianship vary across jurisdictions, but generally they embody limited capacities to understand relevant information and the consequences of actions, to reason about choices, to communicate choices and to control impulses.[26] Tools for assessing the need for guardianship of mentally ill and developmentally disabled parents are available.

Many jurisdictions require maternal and paternal grandparents of children born to minor mothers and fathers to be financially responsible for their grandchildren, as are the adult fathers of non-marital children. These maternal and paternal grandparents also should have custodial guardianship of the children of their children for whom they already have custodial guardianship.

Modifying the Birth Registration Process

A birth certificate actually is certification of a legally executed vital record submitted to a state agency by an authorized designee. It contains detailed information about the birth, baby, parents and family histories.[27] It could easily include informing parents of their parenthood responsibilities and their acknowledgement that they are committed to parenthood and meet minimum standards. This would affirm that our society places a high enough value on parenthood to certify that a newborn baby has a parent who meets minimum standards for parenthood.

Following Dwyer's reasoning, mothers who give birth or fathers who conceive would be presumed to be competent to assume the responsibilities of parenthood except when they require guardians themselves. Potential high-risk parents would be identified as soon as possible before childbirth. This could be done by combining the health, child welfare, correctional and birth registration systems to make the birth registration process more than reporting a birth. This process could be initiated at three points in order of desirability: 1) when pregnancy is diagnosed; 2) when prenatal care begins; and 3) on admission to a hospital or birthing center. The age of the mother would be known, and child abuse and neglect and correctional databases could be accessed at the first point of contact. In the event the pregnancy is interrupted, at least the fact of a pregnancy would be known for health statistical purposes. Some states already require reporting of pregnancy terminations and fetal deaths.

The birth certificate could be modified to become a certificate of parenthood—in legal terms, it would affirm a mother's and father's custodial guardianship of their newborn. Because the babies of minor parents do not have custodial guardians, a statutory requirement would be created requiring that babies born before the mothers attain the age of 17? be assigned custodial guardians who would meet parenthood certification requirements.

The model in figure 33.1 offers an outline for a feasible procedure for modifying the birth certificate to certify that a newborn baby has a custodial guardian who meets minimum standards for parenthood. This model would be implemented through the following steps:

Automatic Certification	*Certification by Application and Court Approval*
Legal adults	Minors with or without Parents (Custodial Guardians) Developmentally Disabled Adults Adjudication as Unfit Parent Current Incarceration
Procedure	*Procedure*
The adult attests that she or he understands and accepts the responsibilities of parenthood in the birth registration application.	1) Parenthood Planning Team is formed to provide Parenthood Planning Counseling at diagnosis of pregnancy. 2) Qualified and willing relative is appointed custodial guardian of the baby. 3) Formulation of a voluntary adoption plan is considered. 4) If there is no relative qualified to be the custodial guardian of the parent and newborn, a guardian ad litem is appointed to institute an involuntary termination of parental rights with an adoption plan.

Figure 33.1.   Model for a Parenthood Certification Process.

1) Identify dependent parents requiring custodial guardians at the earliest possible time. Pregnancy diagnosis, initiation of prenatal care or admission to a hospital or birthing center are points to establish parental age and consult child abuse and neglect and correctional registries.

2) Modify the birth registration process to include informing parents of their parenthood responsibilities to this baby consistent with existing statutory criteria for child custody, such as: 1) to provide shelter, clothing and food; 2) to nurture this child's development; and 3) to arrange for health care.

3) Automatic certification of parenthood would take place with parents who are legal adults informed of the statutory responsibilities of parenthood and who attest that they understand and accept these responsibilities.

4) An application for the court appointment of a custodial guardian for the baby would be required under the following circumstances:
   a) Legal minor status: a mother or father under 17? when a birth is expected.
   b) Developmental disability or mental illness with guardian.
   c) Adjudication as an unfit parent.
   d) Incarcerated mother or father who is under the custodial guardianship of a state.

5) Process for obtaining certification:
   a) When a pregnancy is diagnosed, those eligible for automatic certification would be informed about the requirement of attesting to an understanding and acceptance of the responsibilities of parenthood. They would affirm this by signing the birth registration form.
   b) When a pregnancy is diagnosed, those who are not eligible for automatic certification would be contacted by a child welfare worker, and a Parenthood Planning Team would be formed to provide Parenthood Planning Counseling for the parents and their families.
      i) The counseling process would include identifying adults who are qualified to assume custodial guardianship of the baby and information about making an adoption plan.
      ii) Adults desiring to become custodial guardians under i) would be assisted in applying to the court of jurisdiction for custodial guardianship until the court determines that the dependent parent is capable of assuming custodial guardianship and in applying for Kinship Care status if indicated. This would be a summary legal procedure with uncontested applications. The custodial guardians would attest that they understand and accept the responsibilities of parenthood.
      iii) When an application for certification is required under 4) and there is no qualified adult under ii), a guardian *ad litem* would be appointed as a member of the Parenthood Planning Team to represent the unborn baby, seek termination of parental rights and make an adoption plan. A state agency would be recorded as the guardian on the birth certificate until the adoption is finalized.
      iv) If an adolescent or dependent adult gives birth without prenatal care, a referral by the hospital to child welfare services would occur. This medical neglect of the baby would be rebuttable presumptive grounds for a

termination of parental rights action and making an adoption plan. The state would be recorded as the legal guardian on the birth certificate until an adoption is finalized.

Resistance to Parenthood Certification

This proposal for parenthood certification will encounter resistance because it appears to add burdens on legal and social service systems that already are strained by child neglect and abuse cases. It also invokes images of government restricting individual liberties, invading the privacy of families and stigmatizing dependent parents in addition to allegations of discriminating against persons living in poverty. It might appear to "presume guilt unless proven innocent." Placing professionals in the position of reporting pregnancies also raises potential conflicts with their codes of ethics and might increase distrust of professional systems.[28] In fact, this proposal affirms existing societal expectations and would reduce existing burdens on professionals and courts.

These resistances can be overcome by involving relevant professionals, advocates and policy makers in a process to devise a collaborative health, social welfare and legal procedure to ensure that all children have competent parents. The costs of planning and implementing this system are miniscule compared to the resulting economic and humanitarian benefits.

We need clear thinking about our priorities and the consequences of continued helplessness in the face of babies being born with one, two and even three strikes against them. We must link the enormous public financial and humanitarian costs of crime and dependency to their roots in adolescent and dependent-adult childbirth. This can be done by establishing Parenthood Planning Teams as a "best practice" for managing adolescent and dependent-adult pregnancies. Such a Team can dampen initial adverse conditions in a baby's life before birth.

Qualification for parenthood certified by a birth certificate would signify that our society places a high value on ensuring that all of our children have competent parents and that we recognize parenthood as a life-time commitment—indeed, as a valued career for which we have minimum standards.

CONCLUSION

We know that adolescents gradually become ready to assume adult responsibilities and set ages for awarding them. Because of the great impact adolescent parenthood has on our society and because the onset of menarche is occurring earlier, we need to establish an age at which custodial guardianship (parenthood) for a child can be assumed.

We need to overcome our sense of helplessness and squarely face the adolescent parenthood dilemma by clearly thinking through the options available to adolescents and their families and to us as citizens and as a society. Paralyzing political and ideological agendas and emotions need to be replaced by objectivity.

In modern society, parenthood is an undesirable life style for girls and boys. In spite of this fact, we provide financial, educational and supervised living support for adolescent mothers in an effort to help them function as parents. We do this presumably to help their babies.

The most striking aspect of adolescent parenthood is that the child of a minor parent does not have a legal custodial guardian. This is particularly significant because having an adolescent parent places babies at risk for morbidity, developmental problems and abuse and neglect.

The most sensible and realistic approach is to recognize dependent parent childbirth as a serious public health crisis. Parenthood Planning Teams composed of existing family planning, prenatal care, child welfare, home visitation and legal professionals could be organized in the same way crisis intervention teams are formed in other health and child welfare matters. These teams could guide adolescents and dependent adults and their families in making the most appropriate decision for all concerned, as required for federal Adolescent Family Life Demonstration Projects.

Setting minimum standards for parenthood through modifying birth registration to become a parenthood certification process would signify that our society places a high value on ensuring that all of our children have competent parents.

When an adolescent's baby is born, there are three reasonable outcomes after all parties have carefully considered the available options and their consequences: 1) relatives continue guardianship of the adolescent mother and assume temporary custodial guardianship of the baby; 2) a voluntary adoption plan is made for the baby; and 3) an involuntary adoption plan is made for the baby when relatives cannot be custodial guardians of the adolescent and her baby.

Adoption offers the most practical and available access to competent parents for many babies.

Chapter 34

Adoption

The Way I See It

I wish couples who desperately take every means to conceive a child would realize that adoption is a wonderful alternative. A child who becomes your child though adoption completes a family. Just as when you commit to your spouse or partner there are no biological ties, yet a family is formed, this child enters a family in the same way. It is not blood and flesh that form a family, but the heart.

Michele Johnson, Wamego, Kansas[1]

Prior to the 1970s, adoption was the most frequent sequel to adolescent childbirth in the United States. Now it seldom occurs.

The word "adoption" can evoke a variety of emotions—*sadness* for separating children from their genetic parents; *fear* of the consequences of placing children in strange families; *shame* and *guilt* for resorting to adoption; *anxiety* in an adopted child; and *anger* at professionals who might seem to treat children as commodities. Adoption also can evoke feelings of *gratitude* and *affection* by parents who have adopted children; by children who have been adopted; and by genetic parents who have seen their children thrive in adoptive homes. A mixture of these feelings is common in persons involved in adoption.

The desire to adopt children conceived by other persons reveals that the human need to nurture children is stronger than the human need to procreate.[2] The existence of adoption affirms that parenthood transcends bloodline.

Parents who adopt through an agency are prime examples of competent parenthood. They voluntarily choose parenthood, and they meet rigorous childrearing standards.

This chapter puts human faces on the process and consequences of adoption.

THE CONCEPT OF ADOPTION

Denis Donovan, a child and adolescent psychiatrist, calls for a shift from an adult-centered to a child-centered model of adoption.[3] The commonly held adult-centered model is *providing children for parents who want them*. This model runs the risk of making children means to adult ends. In contrast, a child-centered model views adoption as *a process that provides competent parents for children who need them.*

A child-centered model of adoption focuses on the needs of children, not just on the needs of adults. Children's needs for parents are more fundamental than adults' needs for children. Adults can thrive without children. Children cannot thrive without competent parents.

Babies adopted at birth have the genes of their conceiving parents and prenatal and postnatal interactions with their genetic mothers. They do not have reciprocal attachment bonds with anyone and do not have a family identity. They do not have formed

ADULT CENTERED		CHILD CENTERED
PROVIDES CHILD FOR ADULTS	VS	PROVIDES PARENTS FOR CHILD
CHILD MEETS ADULT'S NEEDS	VS	ADULT MEETS CHILD'S NEEDS
CHILD STRANGER IN ADULT'S HOME	VS	ADULT'S HOME IS CHILD'S HOME
CHILD REMINDER OF ADULT INFERTILITY	VS	CHILD IS JUST A CHILD
MUTUALITY OF DIFFERENCES AND LOSS	VS	FAMILY MUTUALITY OF BELONGING
CHILD'S IDENTITY DEVELOPS IN RELATION TO IMAGINED OTHERS	VS	CHILD'S IDENTITY DEVELOPS IN RELATION TO PARENTS
IDENTITY BUILT ON DISCONTINUITY UNCERTAINTY AND LOSS	VS	IDENTITY BUILT ON CONTINUITY CERTAINTY AND CONNNECTION
SEARCH NECESSSARY TO DISCOVER TRUE IDENTITY	VS	SEARCH UNNECESSARY TO DISCOVER TRUE IDENTITY

Figure 34.1.   Adoption.

personalities. Their first reciprocal attachment bonds are with the parents who adopt them—their "real" parents. They are the real children of their real parents. They do not have a lost identity with unresolved emotions.

The persons most likely to have unresolved emotions are genetic and adoptive parents. Genetic parents need to work through their feelings about adoption without burdening adoptive parents and their children. Parents who adopt need to work through their own reasons for adoption *before adopting* so that the children they adopt are not seen as filling a lost space or function for them. The later-life identity problems and "rootlessness" attributed to being adopted actually are due to inferences and professional practices that interfere with children's natural attachment bonding with their real parents. There is no need to search outside the adoptive home for a child's "true identity."

THE MYSTIQUE OF BLOOD RELATIONSHIPS

The popular assumption is that blood ties are the deepest and most enduring human relationships. Parents and children love each other because they share the same genes. Adopted children seem to seek genetic parents because of a genetically determined attraction to them.

In fact, "blood ties" have genetic proclivities but are determined by life experience. The strongest human bond is between genetic mother and child because of its genetic, neurological, hormonal, emotional and experiential basis. Babies are programmed to send cues (coos, gurgles, cries, smiles and frowns) to which mothers and fathers are genetically predisposed to respond. Babies also appear to be predisposed to distinguish maternal from paternal responses to them.[4]

But the mutual affection shared by genetically related persons is based on human interactions not on their genes. Some adopted persons and stepchildren have gone through life believing they were the genetic offspring of their parents without ever knowing they were not.

Without DNA testing, fathers have no way of knowing about their parentage other than what they believe to be true. The perception of being blood relatives defines the relationship, not the actual sharing of genes. Babies do not bond to their genetic fathers unless interaction occurs creating father-child reciprocal bonding. A father's reaction to discovering that a child is or is not his is based on his perceptions not on his genes.

Babies and children form reciprocal attachment bonds with parents who interact with them. Children who discover they were adopted have reactions to that information, but they do not shift their bonding relationships from their adoptive parents to their genetic parents. Their reactions are determined by their perceptions and their emotional bonds not their genes.

Genes actually are designed to take their cues from nurture. The more we lift the lid on the human genome, the more we see how strongly genes are influenced by experience.[5] Life experience is the basis for parenthood, not genes.

Seeking Genetic Kin

The idea of genetic kinship still deeply influences human perceptions and behavior. This is illustrated by the interest people have in establishing genetic ties.

The Donor Sibling Registry is a web site where children conceived by donor insemination can be registered for possible matching with half siblings or the donor himself.[6] The importance of perception in genetic ties is illustrated by the growing number of persons who are the products of *in vitro* fertilization and discover genetic relationships through the Registry:

- Sixteen-year-old Danielle and 15-year-old JoEllen were excited to become sisters when they found they came from the same father's sperm and two different mothers. They enjoy a relationship based on the perception they are genetically related through records that could be erroneous.
- An 18-year-old girl discovered that her father's sperm had contributed to the pregnancy of a surrogate mother. Excited by this discovery, she tracked down the implantation and found a genetic half sister. Her feelings were determined by her perception of that connection. Her newly discovered half sister did not share her excitement.

The voices of donor-conceived children reveal how important knowing one's genetic father can be. They have an instinctual hunger for the presence of a father:[7]

- A 23-year-old woman conceived through confidential donor insemination said: "I had to grieve. It wasn't until I was 17 or 18 that I felt very angry. How dare someone take my choice to know my father away from me?"
- A 15-year-old boy submitted his own DNA to an on-line DNA-testing service. He matched it to a family surname and found his genetic father.

Artificial Insemination

Some single women choose to conceive through artificial insemination in order to give birth to a baby with their own genes. One third of the patrons of the California Cryobank are single women.[8] Their desire to have a genetically related baby enables them to undergo costly hormone treatments, hospitalizations, miscarriages and the risks of frozen sperm.

HISTORY OF ADOPTION

Adoption in the United States has changed over the years.[9] Massachusetts was the first state to regulate adoption in 1851. In the late 1880s, orphan trains sought homes for children in Western farming communities. As a result of the exploitation of children delivered by these trains, adoption agencies with confidential legal procedures were established in the early 1900s.

Adoption within the United States

The stigma attached to unwed pregnancy throughout most of the 20th century led to the creation of maternity homes where girls could give birth, nurse their babies and make adoption plans.[10] As bottle feeding increased, these mothers could choose adoption immediately after birth.

The existence of adoption agencies and statutes affirms that parenthood is a public responsibility, not simply an informal arrangement between individuals.[11] Agencies accept responsibility for the welfare of the children they serve. While maintaining confidential adoption records, most states have procedures through which information can be obtained from them.

In 1973, *Roe vs. Wade* sharply reduced the number of babies available for adoption by creating a legal right to pregnancy termination.[12] The normalization of single parenthood through welfare support for unwed women and girls as well as increased job opportunities removed the stigma of "illegitimate birth." Two Supreme Court decisions increased the legal rights of genetic fathers in adoption. As a result, young parents infrequently make adoption plans for babies now.

In the 1980s, most domestic adoptions came from foster care. Because some children were not free for adoption and others required unavailable subsidies, more children entered foster care than permanent homes. Young persons who "aged out" of foster-care in the Casey Family Programs between 1988 and 1998 illustrate the unfavorable outcomes of foster care.[13] Sixty-five percent had seven or more school changes; 22% were homeless after 18; 17% received public assistance; 33% had incomes at or below the poverty level; and 33% had no health insurance.

An emphasis on permanency planning and the timely adoption of foster children gradually evolved. When there is no reasonable prospect of parental reunification, federal legislation allows courts to accelerate the termination of parental rights for babies and preschool children. Under the Adoption and Safe Families Act of 1997, states must terminate the rights of parents whose children have been in foster care for 15 of the past 22 months.[14] The Act created a state "bonus" of $4,000 to $8,000 for each foster care adoption above the previous year.

The Adoption Assistance and Child Welfare Act of 1980 provided federal funds for state-subsidized adoption payments. The Adoption and Safe Families Act of 1999 and the Promoting Safe and Stable Families Amendments of 2001 increased the number of older child adoptions.[15] The InterEthnic Placement Act of 1996 prohibits considering race or ethnicity in adoptive or foster placements except in the "best interest of the child" under exceptional circumstances.

International Adoptions

After World War II, many families adopted orphans from war-torn European countries, setting the stage for contemporary international adoptions.

Since 1995, international adoptions by Americans have increased by more than 140%.[16] Couples often cite the lack of American babies as the reason for adopting from abroad. Many want children who resemble them and seek adoptions from Eastern European countries.

Fees for international adoptions are usually about $30,000 with a waiting period of nine to eighteen months. Because of laws in the countries of origin, most foreign children adopted by Americans are more than one year old when they arrive in the United States.

ADOPTION DEMOGRAPHICS

In 2000, over 6 million persons of all ages in the United States were adopted.[17] Over 2% of American children—1.5 million—have been adopted. One third live with relatives or stepparents. In 1996, 45% of adoptions took place through public agencies; 31% through private agencies; and 24% through attorneys without agency involvement.[18]

The National Adoption Information Clearinghouse prepared the following statistics:[19]

- 2% of unwed women at any age make adoption plans for their children.
- About 120,000 children are adopted annually.
- In 1972, 20% of White and 2% of Black unwed mothers made adoption plans. In 1995, the figures were less than 3% for White and 2% for Black unwed mothers.
- In a 1995 survey, 51% of pregnant adolescents gave birth.
- Women who make adoption plans are likely to have greater educational and vocational goals than those who do not.

NEGATIVE ATTITUDES TOWARD ADOPTION

Because of its complexity and of the adjustment challenges for all parties involved, adoption continues to be stigmatized in spite of decades of education and experience that affirm its benefits for children, genetic parents, parents who adopt and society. As the stigma of unwed pregnancy and single parenthood diminished, young mothers became reluctant to make adoption plans, especially if their families were willing to help with childcare and financial support.

Taking Responsibility for the Baby

The negative aura of adoption may be fueled by the belief that a genetic mother and father must take responsibility for making a mistake by entering parenthood. This belief justifies compromising a genetic parent's own education, social life, career and financial independence and adding the burden of childrearing to their families. It makes an adoption plan a shameful choice for a girl and possibly for a boy, especially when it is shared by their families and peers.

Adoption as Abandonment

Making an adoption plan may be seen as child abandonment and be criticized by families and peers. In later life, the baby might feel betrayed by the genetic mother.

A Feeling that Irreparable Wounds Are Caused by Adoption

The depth of feeling evoked by adoption is poignantly revealed in this blog:[20]

> I am one of the millions of Mothers and children of adoption wounds. Many of us are sick or dying young from the grief of having our children taken from us by adoption brokers. Only in America will a community tell a Mother and adopted person that have lost each other to coercion to be grateful. Adopted persons and Mothers have committed suicide due to the trauma of adoption. Many adopted teens are in treatment centers. These are truths you will seldom hear because adoption is politically correct now.

A radical feminist view of prevalent adolescent baby adoption prior to recent decades is expressed in the following excerpts:

> In the past, experts recommended that the girl and her family must arrange her disappearance from the community.[21] Then the unwed mother must undergo intensive psychological treatment; and most important, she must agree to relinquish her illegitimate child to a married couple, for without a husband, the young woman was not a mother, according to the ideology of the era. Having cooperated, the unwed mother could ostensibly deny the entire episode and resume development toward middle-class womanhood.
>
> Maternity homes were considered a reform over the days when "fallen women" were stigmatized.[22] The new, professionalized staff rarely imagined the devastating, lifelong consequences many unwed mothers of that era suffered for having been shamed and coerced into relinquishing their babies. At first they were places of refuge and spiritual development for women who had been seduced and abandoned. After World War II, they became places to sequester girls until they could give birth and surrender their children for adoption. These mothers did not have a chance to fully grieve their losses.

As the experience of the vast majority of persons who make an adoption plan attests, the separation involved in adoption in itself does not cause mental illnesses. It can become the displaced focus of emotional and psychological problems generated by other factors.

THE ADOPTION PROCESS

Adoption is complicated by the lack of uniformity and application of state adoption laws. There also are federal statutes and constitutional principles that pertain to adoption. For example, the Indian Child Welfare Act governs the adoption of American Indian children.

Adoption makes an adult the legal parent of a child equivalent to a genetic parent.[23] A petition for adoption is not granted unless a court determines that the genetic parents have executed voluntary, informed consents or that their parental rights have been legally terminated and that the "best interests" of the child will be served by qualified adoptive parents.

Intra-family adoptions are the least regulated. They legally recognize a *de facto* custodial family, thereby allowing children to preserve ties to members of their original families. Still they can generate bitterly contested proceedings, especially when a non-custodial parent objects; when grandparents seek a relationship with a child and custodial parents object; and when maternal and paternal relatives compete to adopt a child of deceased or legally unfit parents.

Open Adoptions

Open adoption was conceived as a remedy for the closed system in which genetic parents felt stigmatized and adopted persons felt deprived of their genetic heritage. It has become the dominant form for babies because it is attractive to genetic parents. However, since it is a relatively recent practice, little is known about the long-term outcomes for all parties involved.[24]

Attorney-arranged open adoptions that permit genetic and adoptive parents to select each other are increasingly prevalent. Agency waiting periods and standards are avoided. Ann Powers described her experience with an agency-mediated open adoption:[25]

> A counselor from Open Adoption and Family Services called to say that a 16-year-old high schooler had selected us from a pool of 60 families. Mallory was seven months pregnant and wanted to meet us. Her mother was convinced that open adoption would provide her family with the best possible outcome. She called us when she went into labor and invited us to come. We stayed in the room next to them and left the hospital the next day walking with Mallory as she parted with Rebecca. Mallory visited us every several months. Now a college student, Mallory has a picture of Rebecca in her room. We all have gained from staying connected.

The process of choosing an adoptive family in Georgia is illustrated by the following information provided by AAA Partners in Adoption, Inc.:[26]

How do I choose a family for my child? When you contact us you will be given a number of families' picture books from which to choose. You will have the option of speaking with the families on the phone or meeting them in person before you make your final decision.

What information do I have to provide to the adoptive family? A detailed medical history, including any illnesses that run in your families, is important information to pass on.

How much contact will I have with my baby and the adoptive family after the adoption? You can choose to have no contact with the adoptive family and have the agency select the adoptive family for you. You can choose to receive letters and pictures of your child, or you can have face-to-face or telephone contact with the adoptive family and your child.

If I am under the age of 18 do my parents have to sign for me to be able to place my baby for adoption? No, your parents do not have to sign for your adoption regardless of your age. They can neither force nor prevent the adoption.

Once I sign the adoption papers, can I change my mind? State laws vary on the amount of time, if any, that you have to change your mind after you have signed adoption consent documents. In Georgia, genetic parents cannot sign the consent for adoption until the baby is at least 24-hours-old. Thereafter, genetic parents have 10 days to change their mind.

AAA Partners in Adoption, Inc., offers free Parenthood Planning Counseling and emotional support during the pregnancy, delivery and after birth. Waiting families are approved by the agency. Genetic parents can receive assistance with medical care and living expenses.

A counselor meets with the genetic mother who signs documents relinquishing rights to the child to enable adoption. The baby usually goes home from the hospital with the adopting family. In Georgia, the genetic father receives notice of the adoption plan. If his cooperation cannot be secured, a termination of his parental rights is obtained at no cost to the mother.

The Bethany Christian Service of Waukesha, Wisconsin, found that 25% of genetic mothers changed their minds after birth. Of those who did not, 50% had open adoption with visits; 50% had open adoption with letters and photos; 20% of the placements were biracial. Another study found that contacts between genetic mothers and adoptive families continued for 44% of open adoptions.[27]

Genetic Parents' Perspectives

Adoption often is seen as only involving adoptive parents and children. But it includes a third set of persons—the genetic parents.[28] They and their extended families are present initially and later at least in the children's and adoptive parents' imaginations.[29]

Genetic Mothers

Making an adoption plan for a baby can have lasting effects for a genetic mother if she has not clearly thought through and emotionally accepted her reasons for choosing not to enter parenthood. One study found that 50% of the mothers experienced a sense of loss extending over 30 years.[30] Some had psychological repercussions related to adoption, preexisting conditions and their own personal problems. In the light of these findings, Kristin Luker believes that adoption deprecates maternal love, breaks family ties, values money more than love and does not guarantee that a stranger will love a child as much as a genetic parent does.[31]

In one study, genetic mothers in closed adoptions had less grief resolution than mothers who chose fully disclosed adoptions. The latter feel "less empty" because they can envision their children in another family.[32] Counseling can help work through grief over separation from a child when it is seen as the result of choosing not to enter parenthood. Dealing with feelings of shame and guilt is important for parents who make both voluntary and involuntary adoption plans.

Adoption is a wise choice for unwanted babies. Swedish and Czechoslovakian studies revealed that children raised by mothers who were denied pregnancy terminations showed long-term adverse psychological, emotional and social effects.[33] This does not imply support for pregnancy termination as a method of birth control. It highlights the importance of adoption when mothers are not motivated to raise babies.

Genetic Fathers

Once they acknowledge their parentage, many genetic fathers have a sense of connection even when they have never seen their offspring. They experience curiosity, a sense of responsibility, loss, guilt, love and regret in varying degrees of intensity.[34]

The U.S. Supreme Court affirmed the Constitutional protection of a putative father's parental rights when he has a genetic link and has participated in a child's rearing.[35] The Court did not address the fact that a putative father can have no more than a genetic link to a baby adopted at birth and what a putative father must do to protect his parental rights.

Genetic fathers are involved in about a quarter of adoptions.[36] A father's motivation may not be a desire to enter parenthood but the fear of losing the opportunity to know a child he has conceived. This need not happen since adoption registries allow children who were adopted and genetic fathers and mothers to contact each other by mutual consent.

The role of fathers in making pregnancy termination and adoption decisions has not been adequately explored. Putative fathers have used the Fourth and Fourteenth Amendments to challenge the termination of their rights when birth mothers make adoption plans.[37] Putative fathers generally are entitled to notice of proceedings to terminate their rights and adoption if they register in putative father registries or acknowledge paternity within a certain time. If he does not answer an adoption notice, his rights are involuntarily terminated for abandonment. In some states a previous termination of parental rights is a reason for involuntary termination of rights to a later child.

Perspectives of Persons Who Have Been Adopted

At one end of a continuum, the lives of children who were adopted early in life are the same as those of children raised by their genetic parents. At the other end, are those who suffered deprivations and disruptions in their lives prior to late adoption.

Adoption actually is an issue for all children. Most young children experience the "family romance" fantasy in which they imagine they have different, usually idealized, parents. For a child who was adopted this fantasy can idealize the genetic parents.[38] How much of a child's response to adoption is based on a "family romance" fantasy that also is experienced by children who were not adopted and how much is based on actual adoption may be difficult to separate.

Children who were adopted commonly raise the following questions:[39]

• Why was I not wanted by my genetic parents?
• How did my parents get me?
• Will my parents keep me, no matter what?

They may feel the stigma of adoption. But with the support of their parents most cope with these feelings. Some achieve a unique identity more fully than children who were not adopted.

Regardless of how satisfied they are with their families, children who were adopted have an interest in their genetic mothers and fathers.[40] Currently, 50% search for their genetic parents at some point in their lives. Feelings of self-doubt may intensify interest in finding genetic parents. There also is a growing interest on the part of many genetic parents in searching for their adult children. A number of organizations, such as OmniTrace Corporation, assist in searching for genetic relatives. One study found that over 90% of reunions were favorable experiences.[41] But they can be disappointing when genetic parents do not live up to expectations.

The Perspectives of Parents Who Adopt

Parents who adopt may be sensitive about their infertility and the genetic child conceived in their imaginations.[42] They may have idealized or deprecatory images of genetic parents.

The comfort of parents who adopt in discussing their feelings about adoption with their children is important.[43] They may be confused by expert advice that either encourages or discourages informing children of their adoption early in life. They need the latest information on this point, which essentially holds that the natural course of events will provide opportunities for discussing adoption without making a special effort to do so.

TRANSRACIAL ADOPTION

Adoption involves at least five parties: the child, the genetic parents, the parents who adopt, the agency or attorney arranging the adoption and the state. With minority children, additional cultural and political interests arise.[44]

History of Transracial Adoption

Transracial adoption began in order to accommodate children of color languishing in foster homes and institutions.[45] Almost half of the children in foster care are from minorities. Pregnancy termination, contraception and fertility rates reduced the number of White children available for adoption and made White couples more willing to adopt minority children. Adoption agencies were forced to reevaluate their tradition of matching races.

The first documented domestic transracial adoption occurred in Minneapolis in 1948.[46] Transracial adoption gained momentum in the mid-1950s and then declined in the early 1960s. The Civil Rights Movement in the mid-1960s led to another rise until the early 1970s when significant opposition caused a decline again.

By the mid-1990s, race matching policies led to excessive numbers of Black children in foster care because of the lack of adoptive families of the same race. As a result, transracial adoption was presented as "pro-family," "anti-racist" and "color blind."[47] In 1997, approximately 17% of all domestic adoptions were transracial— largely of Black children by White parents.[48] *Christian Homes* in Texas now reports that they can find homes for all their babies in the United States. *Adoption Associates* in Michigan reports that they have White families waiting to adopt Black babies. *Adoption-Link* in Chicago also has a waiting list of families for Black babies. Black parents seldom adopt White children but are foster parents for them.

The Adoption and Safe Families Act of 1997 aimed to clear the foster care logjam by accelerating terminating parental rights to permit adoption of foster children.[49] The Act implies that racial or ethnic characteristics are to be considered only when they directly affect a child's safety or permanent placement. The wishes of a child's genetic parents are not considered to be justifications for same-race placement in foster care or adoption. An exception is that American Indian children must be placed with America Indian families whenever possible.

The Promoting Safe and Stable Families Act Amendments of 2001 enables states to establish and expand community-based family preservation services, time-limited family reunification services, adoption promotion and supportive services for adoptive parents.

Opposition to Transracial Adoption

Transracial adoptions numbered 733 in 1968 and rose to 2,574 in 1971 as a result of the Civil Rights Movement. Organized opposition to transracial adoption began in the 1970s and caused a reversal in transracial placements by major adoption agencies.[50] Opposition was led by the National Association of Black Social Workers and leaders of Black political organizations, who feared that Black communities would be deprived of their most valuable resource: children. Transracial adoption constituted cultural genocide. Black children growing up in a White world would never take their rightful place among Blacks. As evidence of their loss of racial identity, one study found that 11% of transracially adopted Black children preferred to be called White.[51]

Opposition also came from some of the leaders of American Indian groups, who saw transracial adoption as genocide. The Indian Child Welfare Act of 1978 ended the practice of placing Indian children in White homes. The Act concluded that "there is no resource that is more vital to the continued existence and integrity of Indian tribes than their children."[52]

Both the Black and Native American groups who opposed transracial adoption agreed that White parents lack the skills, insights and experience needed for adopted children to grow up with awareness of their Black or Indian heritage.[53] The children belong in Black and Indian families where they can develop their racial and cultural identities.

However, Dorothy Roberts, professor at Northwestern University Law School, believes that transracial adoption will not decimate Black culture.[54] She views the transracial adoption issue as diverting attention from the harm child welfare practices inflict on minority families.

Support for Transracial Adoption

Those who have direct experience with transracial adoption tend to evaluate it more favorably than those who have had no experience with it.[55] In a Midwestern Black community, 57% were receptive to transracial adoption while only 7% were totally opposed. A 2003 survey of college students revealed overwhelmingly positive attitudes toward transracial adoption.

Research indicates that transracial adoptions fare well.[56] Over seventy-five percent of transracial adoptions are considered successful, a number comparable to same-race adoptions.

Social and cultural attitudes are learned, not inherited. Individuals develop self-awareness through social interaction. Sixty-eight percent of Black children who were transracially adopted said they did not feel any discomfort with their appearance.[57] Most experienced a positive sense of ethnic identity as well as a high comfort level living with White people.

Public opinion and experts are divided over race-matching in adoption. Some say that children should always be placed with families with at least one parent of the same race. Others say that if a family of the same race cannot be found, a child should be placed with any family that meets the child's needs. Others say that a loving family can meet the needs of any child.

The Psychology of Transracial Adoption

Although we may yearn for a "color blind" society, it is against human nature for individuals to be completely "color blind." Some degree of race-consciousness is necessary for making sense out of one's social environment. This is especially important for children, because their immaturity renders them vulnerable to absorbing racial stereotypes.[58] Even if White parents raise a Black child, society still sees the child as Black. The Black race is unique because it is the only group in the United States that was enslaved, and then, having been granted nominal freedom, was segregated, disenfranchised, brutalized and stigmatized.

The following anecdotes illustrate the psychological importance of racial background.

Julia Sudbury-Oparah[59]

When a white person says to me, "It doesn't matter if they're black, white, brown or green . . ." or "there's only one race, the human race," a shudder goes down my spine. As we grow into our teens, transracially-adopted children discover that being "human" is simply not enough.

Transracial adopted Black child[60]

I think whites adopting black kids should be made easier, but there should be some sort of education with new adoptive parents. Do you know what you are getting into? "Oh, I want to give love to some child!" Well, that's not enough.

Tara Wall[61]

Imagine yourself as a child without a family or anything to call your own. Think of the feelings of despair and not being wanted. Then one day a caring, loving couple comes along that wants to give you the home you never had and the opportunity for you to become all that you want to be. But that's all brought to a screeching halt when you're told "there was a family who wanted to take you home and make you a part of their family, but we can't allow it because of your skin color." This happens to black children every day.

Most of the kids waiting to be adopted in the U.S. are black. Most of the parents on adoption waiting lists are white, many of whom want to adopt black children but can't.

A group of black teens who spent their entire lives in foster homes said they'd rather be adopted by a loving white family than no family.

The last time I checked our primary "culture" is American culture. Considering the vast shortage of adoptive black parents for black children, I think it is a travesty to disregard the desires of loving, willing Caucasian, Hispanic and even Asian parents who are willing and able to bring these children into their homes. How can we teach children that racism is wrong and then tell them they can't be adopted because of their race?

More specifically, minority children's identity formation involves observing that members of their group are not in positions of power.[62] They may assume that they have the same limited rights, that they can only have limited accomplishments and that their minority group is not as good as those in power. They need encouragement to think critically about how racial categories influence their lives. Rejecting the assumption that children receive ready-made racial identities from their parents, genetic or adoptive, is one step in that direction.

Agencies should provide education and counseling for parents who adopt minority children in recognizing the meaning of racial differences; the importance of the children's culture; and how to raise them in the context of prejudice and discrimination.[63] At the same time, Gail Steinberg and Beth Hall, adoptive parents and advocates, point out that being a member of a transracial family can build character.[64] These children have more opportunities to learn how to deal with challenges and to value differences within families than other children.

Black Adoption

Historically, Black adoption has been informal. Because these children do not come to the attention of agencies, the misconception arose that Blacks do not adopt children. In 1998, 800,000 Black children lived in informal adoptive homes compared to 500,000 children of all ethnicities in foster care and 150,000 children waiting for adoption.[65] Black children often remain in foster care twice as long as do White children. Many potential Black adoptive parents cannot adopt because they do not meet the requirements of a middle-class income and lifestyle.

The National Association of Black Social Workers now recommends that when foster care or adoptive placement is necessary, children should be placed within the extended family first. If that is not possible, they should be placed with families in their own communities so that they can maintain connections and educational continuity. If that is not possible, they should be placed with families of the same race and culture. Lastly, transracial placements should be made with families who are aware of the impact of racism in America and who will assure that their children's experiences are racially and culturally inclusive.[66]

In one survey, traditional agencies placed minority children in minority homes 51% of the time with Black children and 30% of the time with Latino children.[67] Another survey disclosed that agencies specializing in placing minority children in minority homes placed 94% of their Black children and 66% of their Latino children in same-race homes. *Adoption by Shepherd Care* in Hollywood, Florida, places 90% of its Black babies in Canada, where most Blacks are middle-class and live in integrated neighborhoods. In the United States, Black families are waiting to adopt children through agencies that specialize in Black adoptions.

Adoption-Link specializes in the placement of Black babies and has a waiting list of families.[68] Pregnant mothers select parents who are given their background information. If prospective parents choose to proceed, a meeting is arranged with the genetic parent(s) if they live in the Chicago area or by telephone if out-of-state. The waiting period is 9 to 18 months. One-third of the children placed through *Adoption-Link* go to families in Europe.

American Indian Adoption

Although the structures of the Black extended family and the American Indian tribe are similar in many ways, there is a major difference in how the two groups fare legally. The United States has a trust responsibility for American Indian tribes that are quasi-sovereign nations subject to broad federal powers but generally not to state control. American Indians are granted preferences as members of sovereign tribal entities not as a racial group.[69]

Although tribes have different traditions and customs, the importance of community over the individual prevails in American Indian culture. Tribal governing bodies, rather than parents, are allowed to determine the circumstances in which American Indian children will be raised. An example of the extended family structure within the American Indian culture is the formation of a "kinship community" in the Potowatomie tribe, where the responsibility for the care of children falls to the grandparents, even when the parents are living and well.[70]

The extended family is the most widely applicable model for American Indian adoptions in the Indian Child Welfare Act of 1978 (ICWA).[71] The Act was a response to the "alarmingly high percentage of Indian families broken up by the removal, often unwarranted, of their children from them by non-tribal public and private agencies and the alarmingly high percentage of such children placed in non-Indian foster and adoptive homes and institutions."

The ICWA promotes the integrity of Indian tribes and families by establishing minimum standards for placing American Indian children in foster or adoptive homes and assisting family service programs. It does not to apply when a child is in the custody of a non-American Indian mother.[72] The New Jersey Supreme Court held that the

ICWA does not include an unwed, American Indian father who has not taken affirmative steps to establish paternity.

ADOPTION OUTCOMES

All research on intervention outcomes in human lives is fraught with methodological problems.[73] Adoption is not an event. It is a process with a past, present and future. It is difficult to separate out how much of a particular outcome can be attributed to the adoption process and how much is related to other factors in the individual, family and environment.

General Adoption Outcomes

Proponents emphasize the benefits of adoption over other options available to the children, such as institutional rearing, foster care or life with incompetent genetic parents. One study found that two-adoptive-parent are like two-genetic-parent families in investing resources in their children at higher levels than other types of families.[74] Other experts point out the problems associated with adoption. Both sides make important points.

A child's pre-placement experience, age at placement, family dynamics and demographic factors determine the outcomes of adoption placements. The following generalizations have been made about children who were adopted:[75]

- The vast majority do not have major adjustment problems.
- They have fewer behavioral and psychological problems, less adolescent pregnancy and higher educational attainment than those in similar circumstances at birth who were not adopted.
- They are at somewhat higher risk of having school-related, behavioral and psychological problems than children raised in two-parent genetic families, often attributable to genetic factors and adversity earlier in their lives.
- They may struggle to make sense of issues raised by their adoption especially during middle childhood when all children are trying to understand their lives.

A study of late-adopted children, all of whom had below-average IQ scores before adoption at the age of four found that as adolescents their IQ scores increased from 8 to 20 points.[76] A prospective study of children placed for adoption from foster care between the ages of 5 and 11 revealed that 23% of the placements were disrupted; 49% were continuing positively; and 28% were continuing with substantial difficulties.[77] Urban Systems Research estimated the national adoption disruption rate for special needs children to be between 6% and 20%.[78] A review of eight studies of baby placements found a disruption rate of 2%. Eleven special needs placement studies of older children found an overall disruption rate of 11%.[79]

A longitudinal Swedish study compared children who were adopted as babies with those whose mothers registered them for adoption and changed their minds and with children placed in long-term foster care.[80] These three groups were compared with controls matched for age and gender from the general population. The children who remained with their genetic mothers had two and one half times and those in foster care three times higher social maladjustment scores than the adopted children and controls. In another study in the United States, most internationally adopted children were well-adjusted although they received mental health services more often than those who were not adopted.[81] Older international children who were adopted were less often referred to mental health services than older domestic children who were adopted.

Financial support, social work coordination, legal services and support groups for parents and children involved in special needs adoptions are essential.[82]

Transracial Outcomes

Research suggests that transracial adoption produces children whose self-respect and adjustment are at least as satisfactory as that of children who have not been adopted.[83] One study found no difference in placement disruption between Black and White adoptions.

John Shireman and Penny Johnson found that most of the Black children who were adopted and reared in single parent, transracial and Black homes appeared to develop well, although racial development in transracial homes was of concern.[84]

Rita James Simon and Howard Altstein followed White families that adopted Black children over 20 years. They found no significant problems with the children apart from behavior attributable to other factors in 80% of the families.[85] In a review of the literature, transracial adoption was not detrimental for the children in terms of adjustment, self-respect, academic achievement, peer relationships and parental relationships.[86] Still, families with genetic siblings tended to be less successful with transracial adoption than those without them.

Racial issues sporadically occur in transracial families. However, pre-adoptive problems and delays in permanent placement account for more of the problems of children who have been adopted than does race itself.[87] For the most part, non-White children raised in White homes identify with both White and non-White communities. Though children who were adopted transracially have some degree of doubt and discomfort, there is strong evidence that most evaluate their non-White backgrounds and appearance positively.

As long as the number of minority children needing permanent homes exceeds the number of minority families able to accept them, transracial placement is an important resource.

SAFE HAVEN FOR NEWBORNS PROGRAMS

In Europe from classical and medieval times onward parents coped with excess or unwanted children by selling them, giving them to church oblates or abandoning them.[88]

Today states permit the mothers of newborns to give their babies to emergency services anonymously. An example is the Florida *A Safe Haven for Newborns* program[89] in which the police and the Department of Children and Families will not be called if an unharmed recently born baby is taken to a hospital, fire rescue station or emergency room. The receiving facility transports the baby to a hospital that provides medical services and contacts an adoption agency. The parent may claim the baby until a court terminates parental rights in 30 days.

Safe Havens are designed to avoid lethal abandonment of babies. At the same time, this approach means that parents who adopt have no information about the back-grounds of these babies and that these genetic mothers do not have Parenthood Planning Counseling.[90]

INCENTIVES FOR PARENTHOOD VS. MAKING AN ADOPTION PLAN

Neuroscience research suggests that when confronted with a choice between a risky and an uncertain outcome, the human tendency is to make the risky choice.[91] This is seen with adolescent parents who lack information and see adoption as having uncertain consequences.

For high-risk adolescents, the short-term incentives to become parents outweigh the long-term incentives of deciding not to enter parenthood. By becoming parents they gain financial benefits, counseling, educational accommodations, childcare and possibly status with their families and peers. The prospect of adoption is unappealing because it means they part with their babies and possibly evoke the disapproval of their families and peers.

The following chart compares the current incentives for adolescents to enter parenthood with those for deciding not to do so.

Elements	To Enter Parenthood	To Not Enter Parenthood
Family Planning	One of three options	One of three options
Prenatal Care	Medical Assistance	Medical Assistance
Financial	NOW: TANF, WICC & childcare benefits	LATER: Escape from poverty
Counseling	Welfare to Work Youth Assistance Adolescent Parenting	Adoption agency
School	NOW: Special programs & childcare	LATER: Higher education
Family	Encourages	Discourages
Peers	Model parenthood "Everyone is doing it."	Discourage
Media	Publicizes successes.	Does not connect parenthood to social problems.
Psychological	"Must keep a part of me." Gain status as a parent.	Sacrifice for well-being of self & baby.
Stress	Creates stress.	Relieves stress.
Adolescent Development	Interferes with	Allows for
Future Attitude	Regret	Satisfaction

Figure 34.2. Incentives to Enter vs. Not to Enter Parenthood.

ADOPTION AS A SACRIFICIAL CHOICE

Most people view childbirth as an awesome, even sacred, event. The birth of a child evokes compassion for the baby and mother. An image of inseparable oneness is conveyed by a mother holding her baby. Throughout pregnancy the mother has endured discomforts and inconveniences. Her baby literally has been attached to her body as she has to her baby.

The prospect of separating a mother and her family from a baby through adoption runs counter to the intent of nature that creates a symbiotic pair of human beings to become bonded to each other. Relatives of the mother and father also experience special feelings of pride and affection for the baby. They view this child as their possession that extends the family line.

In the light of all of these intense feelings, it is no wonder that mature judgment and courage are required for any mother to choose to not enter parenthood and make an adoption plan for her baby. This also is required for surrogate mothers who deliver a baby for others.

Education delays entry into marriage and parenthood and provides literate access to information that allow adolescents to consider their life choices.[92] For pregnant adolescents the choice is simple: *to or not to enter parenthood*. This shifts the focus from *the baby* to *the real-world obligations of parenthood*—from the idea of being a parent—to the personal obligations, responsibilities and sacrifices of parenthood. Accepting these sacrifices defines *motherhood and fatherhood*. The responsible fulfillment of parenthood creates the parent-child relationship.[93]

It is likely that mature adolescents with adequate financial and educational resources elect to terminate their pregnancies or make adoption plans for their babies as Laura did: [94]

Laura

It was a warm and sunny day in May that changed my life forever. The words "you're pregnant" ran through my head incessantly. How could this be? I was a 23-year-old college student who was getting ready to graduate in one month. As soon as I stopped feeling sorry for myself, my attention and energy turned to my unborn child, who was due in three months.

For me, adoption was the only real option. As much as I hated to admit it, I was not ready, or able to give my precious child the life he deserves. I wanted him to have a mother and a father, and all of the things that go along with being a real "family." I was not able to give him those things at that time.

So, I contacted several adoption agencies, and chose the one that I was most comfortable with. My social worker was my rock, the one who helped me get through it all. She worked tirelessly to find the perfect parents for my baby. She was there for me before, during, and after the birth, doing all she could to make me feel comfortable, happy and loved.

My son's parents and I have a semi-open adoption, and I love seeing our son grow up through pictures and updates. I thank God every day for my son's adoptive parents. They are the most wonderful people I have ever met. I am so grateful for their generosity in allowing me to see my baby grow up. We have developed a very special relationship: one that I hope will last for a long time.

For me, adoption was definitely the best option. There are still tough days emotionally, but you must believe in your heart that you are doing the right thing for your child. And I know that my child will grow up knowing that his birthmother loves him very much and only wanted what was best for him. It is my hope and prayer that one day I will again get to see the beautiful face of the child that I placed for adoption, so I can let him know how much I have always loved him and his parents.

Ironically, the mothers who would benefit the most from choosing not to enter parenthood and making an adoption plan for their babies are the least likely to do so. They are the immature, emotionally wounded and vulnerable adolescents. They are dominated by fantasies and short-term urges that undermine thoughtful decision making. When these urges are accompanied by uncertainty and misconceptions about adoption, girls understandably prefer to enter parenthood and try to raise their babies themselves, usually with the help of their relatives. For all of these reasons, Parenthood Planning Counseling is needed for each pregnant adolescent to ensure that a decision is made in the interests of all concerned.

The Decision-Making Process

In order to seriously consider whether or not to enter parenthood, a girl needs help in choosing the most advantageous course for herself and for her baby. She needs help to understand that her baby is not her possession but is a human being with a future life. She needs help to envision her future and the future of her baby. Then she can identify her self-interests and her baby's interests. She can see that entering parenthood would deprive her and her baby of vital opportunities in their lives. She can see that her responsibility to care for her baby can be fulfilled by ensuring that her baby has a family that can provide a better life than she can.

Choosing not to enter parenthood and making an adoption is a way for young persons to develop their identities as responsible, caring persons. It means they realize they are not ready to enter parenthood. It allows them to feel they can compensate for past mistakes by not making another mistake. It allows them to feel that they are doing the best they can for their babies, who are the innocent parties. It helps them mature by finding they can plan ahead and make painful decisions. They gain satisfaction from successfully mastering a confusing emotional crisis in their lives. They heal their own painful feelings by creating a better future for themselves and for their babies through adoption. Sixteen-year-old Stephanie chose to make an adoption plan:

I'm not a selfish person. . . A selfish person would have wanted to tough it out with her child and end up on welfare. . . The only thing I could give my child is love. I couldn't give her all that she needs. A mother who really loves her baby puts her up for adoption. I'm not going on welfare just to raise my child.

The sacrifice and altruism involved in adoption enables genetic mothers to see themselves as mature persons, who make decisions in their own and their babies' interests.

CONTESTED ADOPTIONS

When genetic parents arrange for adoption, they put the new parents on equal legal ground with them. Genetic parents can revoke their consent before an adoption is finalized if it is in the "best interests" of the child. They must show that they can provide a more stable and permanent family relationship for the child than the adopting parents can.

When genetic parents are pitted against adoptive parents over "possession" of a child, media and popular accounts usually invoke one of three narratives.[95] The first narrative depicts young morally suspect unwed people who have babies for whom they cannot care. Fortunately, there are hard-working, loving married couples, who are ready to live the American nuclear family dream if given a fair chance to raise children.

The second narrative forgives youth transgressions and looks favorably on young people who must struggle to make something of themselves as parents. Experts are portrayed as favoring couples who adopt and contributing to discrimination against the poor and minorities when they testify that a child will be irreparably harmed if returned to the genetic parents. Genetic mothers suffer when they are induced to "give up" their babies.

The third narrative characterizes adoption as a gift from genetic parents to parents who can provide a good home for a child.

These narratives obscure the fact that *adoption is a contract* in which the custodial guardianship of children is transferred by genetic parents who choose not to enter parenthood to parents who promise to rear the child and thereby relieve the genetic parents of their parental responsibilities.[96] This contract entailing responsibilities and privileges is made through the legal system and is subject to due process.

CONCLUSION

The word adoption evokes a mixture of negative and positive feelings about parents and children who do not share the same genes. But the mutual affection shared by both genetically and adoption-related persons are based on human experience not on genes.

Adoption involves adoptive parents, the children they adopt and a third set of people—the genetic parents and their families. It no longer needs to end one family and begin another. It can expand the families of all persons involved through open adoption that permits varying degrees of genetic and adoptive parent interactions.

Children who were adopted face different issues than those who were not. Parents who adopt children need to be aware of the emotions experienced by their children, who can feel alienated from their genetic parents in addition to feeling different from other children. This is especially true with transracial adoptions.

Some experts say that children should be placed with families with at least one parent of the same race so that the children can develop strong racial and cultural identities. Others say that if a family of the same race cannot be found, a child should be placed with any family who can meet the child's needs. Others say that any loving family can meet the needs of any child.

Age at placement, a child's pre-placement experience, dynamics within the genetic and adoptive families and demographic factors are important variables in determining adoption outcomes. The overall evidence suggests that children who have been adopted fare as well as other children.

By entering parenthood, adolescents gain financial benefits, counseling, educational accommodations, childcare and possible status with their families and peers. The prospect of adoption is unappealing because it means parting with their babies. Making an adoption plan also may evoke the disapproval of their families and peers.

The best time for decision making regarding whether or not to enter parenthood and make an adoption plan is when pregnancy first becomes known. The more mature adolescent parents are, the more likely they will choose not to enter parenthood and will make adoption plans for their babies.

Part 10

CONCLUSION

Just because we can reproduce doesn't mean that we should.

Sex education slogan

Contemporary adolescent parenthood is partly an aberration of nature. Nutrition and stress in modern civilization are causing the onset of puberty as early as the age of eight in girls. In dramatic contrast, in contemporary aboriginal societies relatively untouched by modern civilization the reproductive system still matures in harmony with the rest of the body.

Most importantly, the gap between the ability to conceive and the ability to raise children has widened. Adolescence has been extended by the earlier onset of puberty and the delayed transition into adulthood. Another gap—economic inequity—divides our nation. On one side are thriving families with well-paying jobs and safe neighborhoods. On the other side are struggling families with low-paying or no jobs in unsafe neighborhoods. This discrepancy in life circumstances can make motherhood seem to be a girl's best option and induce males to conceive without the ability to support their children. These factors and societal encouragement of sexual activity are powerful forces underlying adolescent pregnancies and parenthood.

At the same time, alarm over the "breakdown of the family" is a recurrent theme in our society. It usually triggers a focus on protecting children from "bad" parents.[1] But this "child saving" strategy has not worked. We now are overwhelmed by the prospect of "saving" millions of children. We must "save" families instead.

Thriving families produce the productive citizens our society requires for its prosperity. This gives government an essential role in ensuring that families thrive. High quality childcare and education can help competent parents, but they cannot replace them. Policies that strengthen families are more likely to offer every child an opportunity to become a productive citizen.

Government cannot rear children, but it can ensure that they have competent parents who have the resources needed to rear them. This is recognized reactively in welfare-to-work and child neglect and abuse statutes. It is recognized proactively in public education. It also needs to be recognized proactively by policies that fulfill children's rights to competent parents. The most feasible way of doing this is to ensure that every child has a legal custodial guardian (a competent parent) at birth. Then childrearing can remain a private responsibility of parenthood.

Our public policies seem to regard incompetent parents as an inevitable part of our society. So we support adolescent parents at great public cost. As a result, ingrained systems deal with the consequences of incompetent parents. All of this obscures the fact that ensuring competent parents for all of our children is within our reach at little cost if we have the will to align our public priorities with our knowledge about human development and our cultural values.

Adolescent parenthood is a dilemma not because we lack knowledge but because we lack the will to apply it. It is clear that adolescents are not adults. It is clear that childbirth adversely affects the lives of adolescents, their babies, their families and society. It is clear that choosing to become an adolescent parent seldom results from thoughtful planning. It is clear that our media, public policies and some professional practices encourage adolescent parenthood.

THE CONTEXT OF ADOLESCENT PARENTHOOD

Adolescent parenthood is a symptom of our society's inability to come to terms with parenthood as a life-long career and with adolescence as a vital developmental stage of life.

Our Adolescent Society

Some cultures venerate the elderly. We venerate the young. We are devoted to preserving youthful appearances and to displaying our vitality and strength. We are fascinated by sex and violence. We envy the enthusiasm, energy, risk-taking and audaciousness of adolescents. Our media encourage short-term gratification, impulsive actions and indulging fantasies. This social context discourages setting limits on behavior and promoting the long-term interests of individuals. It discourages recognizing and dealing with poverty, racism and the responsibilities of parenthood.

Adolescents hold up a mirror to us. They mirror our strengths and our weaknesses. The core issues of adolescence are those of our society—experimenting with new ideas and capacities and developing our identity as a global nation. Because our society is dealing with adolescent issues itself, celebrities rather than wise adults are role models, as they are for adolescents. They echo the Horatio Alger theme that anyone can fulfill their dreams.

Our False Beliefs

Our veneration of the young contributes to the belief that parenthood is a manageable challenge for adolescents. Public policies presume that harm to babies can be minimized by supporting adolescent parents. Their babies are expected to be resilient and to stimulate maturity in their parents. Their babies' developmental needs are secondary to the wishes of adolescent parents. Many public policies are based on the following beliefs:

- Parenting babies is simply childcare.
  Parenthood is more than childcare. It is forming attachment
  bonds and applying adult knowledge, skills and judgment.
- When parents struggle, providing parenting education and supplementary childcare is enough.
  Parenting education is not enough to change personalities and
  capabilities. Childcare cannot replace competent parenting.
  Neither ensures nurturing relationships with competent parents.
- Babies are not persons and are resilient. They do not remember neglect and abuse.
  Babies are persons and do remember. Traumatic experiences can
  have a more profound impact on them than on adults because
  their emotional memories are not susceptible to reason.

These facts are difficult for many of us to accept. Even though we know that everyone is burdened by adolescent parenthood, we support it with public and private funds for at least five reasons: 1) We respond emotionally to childbirth and the parent-baby image. 2) Parenthood will cause an adolescent to grow up quickly. 3) The honorable response to adolescent childbirth is for the mother and the father to rear the baby. 4) Our charitable impulse is to help the less fortunate without judging them. 5) Families will step forward and assist their adolescent parents or rear their adolescents' babies themselves.

All of these reasons make the support of adolescent parents seem to be the most practical response to adolescent childbirth. When our emphasis is on the resiliency of babies and adolescents and on supporting adolescent parenthood, we fail to see that adolescent parenthood is the most preventable cause of our nation's crime and welfare dependency.

Vulnerable Adolescents

Social class is the most important correlate of adolescent parenthood. Boys and girls who grow up in poverty are exposed to a number of risks. Their parents lack material resources. They have been exposed to a variety of toxic substances, ranging from drugs prenatally to high lead levels in their homes and schools. Many have experienced neglect and/or abuse and are likely to have attachment disorders. They are likely to lack self-discipline and self-respect because of inconsistent parenting and to have developmental disorders with consequent school failure.

Because they lack knowledge, judgment and coping skills, the most vulnerable boys and girls are the most likely to become adolescent parents. Sex provides immediate gratification and relief from stress and depression. For girls, sex can express fantasies of being loved by a partner who conceives a baby with her. For boys, sex provides immediate gratification and a sense of power from controlling girls and conceiving progeny. For both girls and boys, childbirth provides a sense of accomplishment and an identity as a mother and a father.

The developmental inability to fully anticipate the consequences of their actions often destines pregnant adolescents to repeat a family cycle of premature parenthood, educational failure, health problems, crime and welfare dependency. Their underlying lack of hope also may be concealed by fantasies that they can "have it all:"

> One Sunday afternoon at the St. John's County Juvenile Detention Center in St. Augustine, Florida, a group of Black, White, and Latino residents met with me and my wife. They all emphatically agreed that parents should be adults and that babies have a right to be well parented. However, when asked what they would do if they conceived a child, each one just as emphatically said that he or she would become a parent and would be able to raise the child. This was the right thing to do. One girl said, "When I spread my legs, I have to take the consequences."

These adolescents knew that they should not be parents, but as soon as they conceive a child, they believe they can be competent parents. Many high-risk adolescents today are primed to perpetuate the cycle of premature parenthood, welfare dependency and crime.

Prejudice

Three subtle, but powerful, prejudices contribute to our society's failure to deal effectively with adolescent parenthood:

- sexism against females (focusing more on female than male responsibilities),
- ageism against adolescents (minimizing the importance of adolescence as a developmental stage in life), and
- racism against minority groups. (Adolescent parenthood is in their culture.)

The combined force of these prejudices is seen most poignantly when a Black or Latino girl is impregnated to prove a male's fecundity (sexism), treated as an adult and deprived of the opportunity to complete her adolescent development (ageism) and regarded as destined to adolescent motherhood by her social class and cultural heritage (racism).

HOW WE ENCOURAGE ADOLESCENT PARENTHOOD

Values in high-risk populations, public policies, professional practices and religions can encourage adolescent parenthood. In spite of efforts to prevent adolescent pregnancy, these values lead to supporting a girl as a parent when she has a baby:

Family planning clinics usually present parenthood as an option for adolescents along with pregnancy termination and adoption. When pregnant adolescents receive information about becoming parents, it is no wonder that they see parenthood as an acceptable option for them. Our governments also support adolescent parents in welfare-to-work and poverty programs.

We say they should not become parents, but we support them when they do. They follow our actions not our words.

POSITIVE TRENDS

The decrease in adolescent pregnancy and childbirth rates reflects a number of trends in our society toward preventing and dealing with adolescent childbirth:

- Its high economic consequences are focusing attention on adolescent parenthood.
- The families of adolescent parents are becoming increasingly reluctant to sacrifice their own interests to accommodate the children of their offspring.
- Community development efforts are creating safer neighborhoods and are strengthening families.
- Drug abuse treatment is being used as an alternative to incarceration and consequent disruption of family life.
- Family resource centers and home visitation for the parents of newborns are increasingly available.
- Parenting education classes in schools are introducing adolescents to the responsibilities of parenting.
- An increasing number of role models are appearing in minority communities affirming that fulfillment can be achieved without becoming a mother or a father.
- The feminist movement has empowered girls to pursue goals in life other than motherhood and has exposed male exploitation of girls and women.
- Businesses recognize the adverse impact of parenthood on the education and work skill development of adolescents.
- Adoptive homes can be found for minority babies.

WHAT SHOULD WE DO?

In order to resolve the adolescent parenthood dilemma, we need to shift from an ambivalent attitude to one in which we offer realistic alternatives to adolescent parenthood.

Public Opinion

We admire anyone who overcomes adversity. We admire women who emerge from the adversity of adolescent parenthood to become national leaders. But this does not mean that we should accept and support adversity.

We have compassion for the less fortunate when we feel that we can help them, especially when their burdens are not self-imposed. However, adolescent parenthood is self-imposed. Pregnant adolescents have the options of termination or making an adoption plan.

Targeted education in minority communities is needed to stimulate a shift away from encouraging adolescent parenthood to encouraging successful passage through adolescence and self-fulfillment in our modern society.

Taxpayers need to understand that continuing the present policy of supporting adolescent parents with public funds and the later costs of crime and welfare dependency are major factors in the level of federal, state and county taxes.

We need to carefully think through how to discourage girls and boys from entering parenthood. We need to truly embrace a simple vision—every child in our nation needs and will have a competent parent. This vision can be achieved if we recognize two facts:

- parenthood is the most important career an adult can have and
- minors and adults requiring guardians themselves cannot be competent parents.

Individual Adolescents

Adolescent boys and girls need help in identifying and acting upon their own developmental interests. They need to understand the burdens of entering parenthood. They need to realize that babies are not personal property but are human beings with a right to competent parents. They need to be empowered to face and master the developmental challenges of adolescence without the responsibilities of parenthood. They need to appreciate the impact of imposing the burdens of childrearing on their own parents, relatives and society.

Pregnant adolescents need Parenthood Planning Counseling to help them and their families make wise decisions regarding their babies. Most importantly, they need to understand that the sacrifice of making an adoption plan for their babies is in the spirit of the personal sacrifices required of all parents for their offspring.

Adolescents' Families

The families of pregnant adolescents need to understand why cultural traditions that support the rearing of their adolescents' babies are inappropriate in modern America.

When grandparents and relatives do choose to help raise their own children's babies, they need legal custodial guardianship so that they can have the authority to act on these babies' behalf. Most of all, they need relief from traditions that oblige them to sacrifice their own interests to parenting the children of their children.

Professionals

The orientation of professionals needs to shift from the secondary goals of reducing repeated adolescent births and securing the safety of the babies to the primary goal of preventing adolescent parenthood itself.

Adolescent parents have given rise to millions of employees in the social problem industries, including law enforcement, special education, social services, corrections, courts, mental health, health and prevention. All of these professionals might constitute constituencies for maintaining the status quo. At the same time, they can be reassured by the fact that they are overburdened now and are not feeling rewarded by their frustrating work.

Immunization did not reduce the need for health care workers. Fluoridation did not reduce the need for dental professionals. If adolescent parenthood dramatically decreased, prisons could focus on rehabilitation rather than on controlling excessive numbers of inmates. Social workers could do their jobs more effectively, teachers could teach responsive students and prevention organizations could concentrate on refining effective prevention programs. All of these professionals would be able to work more effectively to strengthen struggling families.

Public Policies

Public policies should not be guided by the fact that with support some minors are capable of being parents. It should be guided by the fact that the vast majority are not.

Adolescent parenthood is one of our nation's greatest problems because of the burdens it imposes on present and future generations. Two strands of empirical research challenge the wisdom of voluntary programs intended to mitigate the consequences of adolescent parenthood: 1) Adolescent parenthood results from immaturity, personal problems, the lack of positive role models and the lack of opportunities for self-development. 2) Even with supportive services, adolescent parenthood has adverse outcomes for adolescents, their babies, their families and society.

Rebecca Maynard, professor of economics and education at the University of Pennsylvania, reviewed the evidence and found that:[2]

- Marginal changes in economic incentives have little or no effect on either adolescent pregnancy or birth rates.
- Advocating abstinence and providing universal access to contraceptives do not sufficiently lower adolescent pregnancy rates.
- Adolescent parents who need help the most are unlikely to seek it from voluntary programs.
- Comprehensive programs for adolescent parents do not significantly improve outcomes for them or their children.

Maynard suggests that future policies regarding adolescent parenthood should emphasize multi-pronged strategies that 1) emphasize prevention rather than support of adolescent parenthood; 2) establish behavioral expectations like those of adult parents; and 3) have clear consequences for not fulfilling these expectations.

We all have a compelling interest in ensuring that all of our children have competent parents. We should base our public policies on the fact that adolescent parenthood is contrary to the interests of an adolescent, of a baby, of their families and of society. Accepting and supporting adolescent parenthood denigrates the status of parenthood in our society. Instead, our public policies should support competent parenthood.

Statutes

The orientation of businesses and governments ordinarily is toward spending money to fix problems. At the same time, investing in research and development to avoid problems is the hallmark of successful businesses and governments.[3] The research and development aspect of public programs usually takes place in legislated model programs and outcome requirements. The legal status of adolescents can be used to guide our approach to adolescent parenthood.

Adolescence is regarded as a legal "disability" that precludes all adult privileges and duties, including marriage, but parenthood is not explicitly precluded. Common law tends to presume that minors have parental rights. Still our age-grading laws imply that adolescents are no more capable of decision making regarding their babies than they are in executing contracts, voting, entering the military service and other life-course influencing decisions. In fact, some states have specifically authorized minor parents to give informed consent for medical treatment of their children, tacitly recognizing that minors do not automatically have that privilege.

The values of our society are expressed in our laws. If our society is to take effective action, statutes must recognize that the babies of adolescent parents do not have custodial guardians (competent parents). Adolescents cannot be guardians of their offspring because they are minors and need custodial guardians themselves. Grandparents may have statutory financial liability for the support of their grandchildren, but they do not have custodial guardianship.

The *parens patriae* doctrine grants the state authority to protect adolescents, dependent adults and their babies from harm. We need statutory requirements that Parenthood Planning Counseling be provided for pregnant adolescents and dependent adults and that babies born to minors and adults with guardians be assigned legal custodial guardians. Relatives can assume this role when appropriate. This can be implemented by a process that expands birth certificates to become parenthood certificates. Most importantly, Parenthood Planning Teams could identify babies of adolescents without supportive families and trigger a Child in Need of Protective Services petition that enables their adoption before neglect and abuse occur.

Value Parenthood as a Career

Adolescent parenthood is the public health crisis on the edge of chaos that can stimulate us to articulate our integrative cultural values and reverse the relentless denigration of parenthood in our society. If we take effective action to manage this crisis, we can dampen the swirl of adverse humanitarian and economic consequences that follow. This action can be the tipping point in shifting from the paradigm that anyone who conceives a child can enter parenthood to a paradigm that values parenthood as a life-long career for competent parents.

The burden lies with those who advocate supporting adolescent parents to show how parenthood is in the "best interests" of adolescents, their babies, their families and society.

We need a positive approach to adolescent parenthood that converts a crisis into a healing growth experience that improves the lives of all concerned. For adolescents, the crisis can become a process of self-discovery that converts selfishness into self-respect and self-confidence by making decisions based on their own and their babies' true self-interests.

LAST WORD

We have come a long way through what might seem like digressions to conclude that there is a difference between being a parent and embracing parenthood as a career. We cannot expect adolescents to avoid entering parenthood until our society affirms our cultural value that parenthood is a rewarding, life-time, sacrificial calling for those who are capable of assuming its responsibilities. We betray their trust when we do not protect adolescents prior to childbirth from decisions that are contrary to their interests and that profoundly alter the courses of their lives.

Here is a vision. The prosperity of our nation depends upon all children and adolescents becoming productive citizens. All babies are entitled to the opportunity to become productive citizens. All adolescents deserve to be able to work through the joys and discomforts of adolescence without the premature distortion of their growing bodies, minds and personalities by the burdens of pregnancy and parenthood. All parents deserve to be able to raise their adolescents without assuming the responsibility of rearing another generation.

If all children had competent parents with the resources they need to grow up with skills and hope for the future, adolescent parenthood would no longer be a public issue. This vision is not "pie in the sky." We can move strongly toward its realization if we act upon the fact that minor and dependent adult parents require guardians themselves and cannot be the custodial guardians of other persons. They cannot be competent parents.

Notes

PREFACE

1. Kennedy, R. (2005) Finding a Proper Name to Call Black Americans. *The Journal of Blacks in Higher Education* 46: 72–83.
2. Tatum, B.D. (1997) *Why Are All the Black Kids Sitting Together in the Cafeteria?* New York: Basic Books.
3. Dávila, A. (2001) *Latinos, Inc.* Berkeley, CA: University of California Press, p. 2.

PROLOG

1. Degregory, Lane (2006) Good Intentions. *St. Petersburg Times* May 14. © *Copyright, St. Petersburg Times*. Reprinted with permission.

PART 1. THE PROBLEM

1. Children's Defense Fund (1991) *A Vision for America's Future*. Washington, DC: Author, p. xii.

CHAPTER 1. THE NEGLECT OF CHILDREN AND ADOLESCENTS IN THE UNITED STATES

1. Edelman, M. Wright (1995) Guide My Feet: *Prayers and Meditations on Loving and Working for Children*. Boston: Beacon Press, p. xxviii.
2. a) Kids Count (2006) Children in Poverty. Baltimore, MD: The Annie E. Casey Foundation. b) Cherlin, A.J. *(2005) Public and Private Families, 4th Ed.* Boston: McGraw-Hill.3. Louv, R. (2005) *Last Child in the Woods*. Chapel Hill, NC: Algonquin Books.
3. Louv, Richard (2005) *Last Child in the Woods: Saving Our Children from Nature Deficit Disorder*. Chapel Hill, NC: Algonquin Books.
4. Ibid.

5. a) Henderson, H. (1999) *Beyond Globalization*. Bloomfield, CT: Kumarian Press; b) Henderson, H. (2004) *Planetary Citizenship*. Santa Monica, CA: Middleway Press.

6. a) United Nations Development Programme (2006) *The 2006 Human Development Report*. New York: United Nations; b) Economics Discovers Its Feelings (2006) *The Economist* December 23, pp. 33–35.

7. a) Institute for Innovation in Social Policy (2007) *Index of Social Health*. Poughkeepsie, NY: Vassar College; b) Miringoff, M. & Opdycke, S. (2008) *America's Social Health*. Armonk, NY: M.E. Sharpe.

8. Quality Counts (2007) Connecting American Education from Birth to Adulthood. *Education Week* January 4.

9. Kids Count (2007) *Data Book 2007*. Baltimore, MD: The Annie E. Casey Foundation.

10. Land, K.C. (2007) Foundation for Child Development Child and Youth Well-Being Index, 1975–2005, with Projections for 2006. Durham, North Carolina: Duke University.

11. a) Bronfenbrenner, U., et al (1996) *The State of Americans*. New York: Free Press; b) Bronfenbrenner, Urie (2001) Growing Chaos in the Lives of Children. In Westman, J.C. (Ed.) *Parenthood in America*. Madison, WI: University of Wisconsin Press, pp. 197–199; c) Achenbach, T. & Howell, C. (1993) Are American Children's Problems Getting Worse? *Journal of American Academy of Child and Adolescent Psychiatry* 32: 1145–1154.)

12. Mansfield, H. & Winthrop, D. (Trans., Eds.) (2000) *Tocqueville, Democracy in America*. Chicago: University of Chicago Press.

13. Bronfenbrenner, U. (1986) Testimony before U.S. Senate Committee on Rules and Administration, *A Generation in Jeopardy*. Washington, DC, July 23.

14. Benson, P.L. (2006) *All Kids Are Our Kids, Second Edition*. Minneapolis, MN: Search Institute.

15. America's Promise (2006) *Every Child Every Promise*. Alexandria, VA: The Alliance for Youth.

16. Holzer, H.J. (2007) The Economic Costs of Child Poverty. Testimony Before the U.S. House Committee on Ways and Means. January 24.

17. Table C3 (2006) *Living Arrangements of Children under 18 Years*. Washington, DC: U.S. Census Bureau.

18. a) Federal Interagency Forum on Child and Family Statistics (2007) *America's Children in Brief*. Washington, DC: Office of Management and Budget. b) Bradbury, B. & Jäntti, M. (1999) Child Poverty across Industrialized Nations. *Innocenti Occasional Papers Economic and Social Policy Series no.71*. UNICEF International Child Development Centre, Florence & Social Policy Research Centre, UNSW, Sydney, Australia.

19. a) Kids Count (2006) Race and Child Well-Being. Baltimore, MD: The Annie E. Casey Foundation; b) Bureau of Justice Statistics (2006) *Key Crime & Justice Facts at a Glance*. Washington, DC: Office of Justice Programs. c) Bureau of Justice Statistics (2006) *Key Crime & Justice Facts at a Glance*. Washington, DC: Office of Justice Programs; d) Federal Bureau of Investigation (2006) *Arrest of Juveniles for Drug Abuse Violations from 1994 to 2003*. Washington, DC: Department of Justice; e) Federal Interagency Forum on Child and Family Statistics (2006) *America's Children in Brief*. Washington, DC: Office of Management and Budget.

20. a) Fingerhut, L.A. & Kleinman, J.C. (1990) International and Interstate Comparisons of Homicide Among Young Males. *Journal of the American Medical Association* 263 (24): 3292–3295; b) Schuetz, L. (2005) Juvenile Crime on the Rise. *Wisconsin State Journal*, November 22, p. 1; c) Garbarino, J. (2006) *Why Girls Are Growing More Violent and What Can Be Done About It*. New York: Penguin Group.

21. a) Uniform Crime Reports (2007) *Preliminary Annual Uniform Crime Report 2006.* Washington, DC: Federal Bureau of Investigation; b) Butts, J.A. & Snyder, H.N. (2006) *Too Soon to Tell.* Chicago, IL: Chapin Hall.

22. Zernike, K. (2006) Violent Crime Rising Sharply In Some Cities. *New York Times* February 12.

23. Herbert, B. (2007) Poor Kids Living in a War Zone. *New York Times* July 14, p. A25.

24. DeVoe, J.F., et al (2005) *Indicators of School Crime and Safety: 2005.* Washington, DC: Office of Justice Programs, Department of Justice.

25. a) U.S. Department of Education (2006) Threats to Teachers. *USA Today* December 28, p. 1A; b) Associated Press (2006) Parents, Teachers Divided on Education. *St. Petersburg Times* February 9, p. 8A; c) Bazar, E. (2005) A Busy Driver Acts as "Dad," Disciplinarian, Friend. *USA Today* November 27, p. 7A.

26. The National School Safety Center (2006) School Associated Violent Deaths. Westlake Village, CA: Author.

27. News and Notes. Child, 5, Shot Three Times by 7–year-old. *St. Petersburg Times*, February 8, B-1.

28. New Britain, CT (2006) Teens in Slay Case Said to Have Sought Fight. *Boston Globe* February 12, p. B-2.

29. Busack, M. (2006) Teen Accused of Making Pipe Bomb in Classroom. *Boston Globe* February 12, p. B-3.

30. Fries, J.H. (2006) In Teen's house, Police Find Guns, Hate. *St. Petersburg Times* February 18, p. A-1.

31. Associated Press (2006) Weapons and Bombs Found. *Wisconsin State Journal* September 1, p, B4.

32. Reddy, M., et al (2001) Evaluating Risk for Targeted Violence in Schools. *Psychology in the Schools* 38: 158.

33. No Child Left Behind (2004) *Unsafe School Choice Option.* Washington, DC: Department of Education.

34. a) National Commission on Excellence in Education (1983) *A Nation at Risk.* Washington, DC, U.S. Department of Education; b) Organization for Economic Cooperation and Development (2006) Education at a Glance 2004. Paris: Author; c) Greene, J.P. (2005) A "Comprehensive Problem". *Education Next*; Hoover Foundation; Stanford, California: Stanford University; d) College Board (2008) *Increase in Advanced Placement Student Success Achieved in All 50 States.* Washington, DC: Author.

35. Grigg, W., et al (2007) *The Nation's Report Card.* Washington, DC: National Center for Education Statistics.

36. a) Federal Interagency Forum on Child and Family Statistics (2006) *America's Children in Brief.* Washington, DC: Office of Management and Budget; b) American Institutes for Research (2006) *New Study of the Literacy of College Students Finds Some Are Graduating with Only Basic Skills.* Washington, DC: Author; c) Marcus, E.N. (2006) The Silent Epidemic. *New England Journal of Medicine* 355 (4): 339–341.

37. a) Kantrowitz, B. & Springen, K. (2005) *Newsweek* December 12, pp. 62–65: b) Demography (2006) College Prep in Elementary School. *The Futurist* 40 (2): 12; c) Finder, A. (2006) Debate Grows as Colleges Slip in Graduations. *New York Times* September 15, p. A-1.

38. Rimm-Kaufman, S.E., et al (2000) Teachers' Judgments of Problems in the Transition to Kindergarten. *Early Childhood Research Quarterly* 15: 147–66.

39. a) Bureau of the Census (2002) *Educational Attainment in the United States.* Washington, DC, Table 9; b) Diplomas Count. *Education Week* 25 (41S): 3 June 22, 2006; b) *Closing*

the Achievement Gap in American Schools. 109th Cong. 2005, September 29. Testimony of Margaret Spellings. Retrieved December 27, 2005.

40. Almeida, C., et al (2006) Making Good on a Promise. In *Double the Numbers*. Boston, MA: Jobs for the Future.

41. Cameron, S.V. & Heckman, J.J. (1993) The Nonequivalence of High School Equivalents. *Journal of Labor Economics* 11: 1–47.

42. Toppor, G. (2006) Dropouts Say Their Schools Expected Too Little of Them. *USA Today* March 2, p. 9D.

43. a) Federal Interagency Forum on Child and Family Statistics (2006) *America's Children in Brief.* Washington, DC: Author; b) Chartbook on Trends in the Health of Americans (2005) *Table 62. Suicidal Ideation, Suicide Attempts, and Injurious Suicide Attempts.* Hyattsville, MD: National Center for Health Statistics; c) National Adolescent Health Information Center (2006) *Fact Sheet on Suicide.* San Francisco, CA: University of California.

44. a) Westman, J.C. (1979) *Child Advocacy.* New York: Free Press, pp. 3–29; b) Achenbach, T.M. & Howell, C.T. (1993) Are American Children's Problems Getting Worse? *Journal of the Academy of Child and Adolescent Psychiatry* 32: 1145–1154; c) Shaffer, R.M., et al. (1996) The NIMH Diagnostic Interview Schedule for Children Version 2.3. *Journal of the Academy of Child and Adolescent Psychiatry* 35: 865–877; d) Keyes, C.L.M. (2006) Mental Health in Adolescence. *American Journal of Orthopsychiatry* 76 (3): 395–402.

45. Howe, N., Strauss, W. & Matson, R.J. (2000) *Millennials Rising.* New York: Vintage Books.

46. Federal Interagency Forum on Child and Family Statistics (2006) *America's Children in Brief.* Washington, DC.

47. a) Kantrowitz, B. & Springen, K.(2005) *Newsweek* December 12, pp. 62–65; b) Pollack, W. (1998) *Real Boys*. New York: Random House, p. 93; c) Pollack, W. (2001) *Real Boys Workbook*. New York: Random House/Villard.

48. Whitlock, J., et al (2006) Self-injurious Behaviors in a College Population. *Pediatrics* 117 (6): 1939–1948.

49. a) Fitzgerald, M.M., et al (2007) Youth Victimization. *The Prevention Researcher* 14 (1): 3–7; b) Hussey, J.M., et al (2006) Child Maltreatment in the United States *Pediatrics* 118 (3): 933–942.

50. a) Department of Health and Human Services, Administration on Children, Youth, and Families (2008) *Child Maltreatment 2006*. Washington (DC): Government Printing Office; b) Wang, C. & Holton, J. (2007) *Total Estimated Cost of Child Abuse and Neglect in the United States.* Chicago, IL: Prevent Child Abuse America.

51. Burns, B., et al (2004) Mental Health Need and Access to Mental Health Services by Youths Involved with Child Welfare. *Journal of the Academy of Child and Adolescent Psychiatry* 43 (8): 960–970.

52. a) Scannapieco, M. & Bolen, R.M. (1999) Prevalence of Child Sexual Abuse. *Social Service Review* 73 (3): 281–313; b) Freyd, J.J., et al (2005) The Science of Child Sexual Abuse *Science* 308 (22): 501; c) Leiderman, S. (2001) *Interpersonal Violence and Adolescent Pregnancy*. Bala Cynwyd, PA: Center for Assessment and Policy Development; d) Saewyc, E. M., et al (2004) Teenage Pregnancy and Associated Risk Behaviors among Sexually Abused Adolescents. *Perspectives on Sexual and Reproductive Health* 36 (3): 98–105.

53. a) Dube, S.R., et al (2005) Consequences of Childhood Sexual Abuse by Gender *American Journal of Preventive Medicine*. 28: 430–438; b) Teicher, M. (2002) Scars that Won't Heal. *Scientific American* March: 68–75.

54. a) Caspi, A., et al. (2002) Role of Genotype in the Cycle of Violence in Maltreated Children. *Science* 297: 851–854; b) Dube, S.R., et al (2005) Long-term Consequences of Childhood Sexual Abuse by Gender of Victim *American Journal of Preventive Medicine*. 28 (5): 430–438.

55. Rogers, A.G. (2006) *The Unsayable*. New York: Random House.

56. Cline, F. (1995) *Conscienceless Acts Societal Mayhem*. Golden, CO: The Love and Logic Press, pp. 2–3.

57. Silveri, M.M. & Spear, L.P. (1998) Decreased Sensitivity to the Hypnotic Effects of Ethanol Early in Ontogeny. *Alcohol Clinical Experimental Research* 22: 670–676.

58. a) World Health Organization (2004) *Neuroscience of Psychoactive Substance Use and Dependence*. Geneva: World Health Organization, p.247; b) Nestler, E.J. & Malenka, R.C. (2004) The Addicted Brain. *Scientific American* 290 (3): 78–85; c) Office of Applied Studies (2007) *Depression and the Initiation of Alcohol and Other Drug Use among Youths Aged 12 to 17*. Rockville, MD: Substance Abuse and Mental Health Services Administration; d) Nestler, E.J. (2006) The Neurobiology of Cocaine Addiction. *Science and Practice Perspectives* 3 (1): 4–10.

59. The National Center on Addiction and Substance Abuse at Columbia University (2006) *Women under the Influence*. Baltimore, MD: The Johns Hopkins University Press.

60. Greene, J.P. & Forster, G. (2004) Sex, Drugs, and Delinquency in Urban and Suburban Public Schools. *Education Working Paper No. 4*. New York: The Manhattan Institute.

61. The National Center on Addiction and Substance Abuse (2006) *National Survey of American Attitudes on Substance Abuse XI: Teens and Parents*. New York: Columbia University, p. 8.

62. Miller, T.R., et al (2006) Societal Costs of Underage Drinking. *Journal of Studies on Alcohol* 67 (4): 519–528.

63. National Center for Injury Prevention and Control (2007) *Teen Drivers*. Atlanta, GA: Centers for Disease Control and Prevention.

64. a) National Institute on Alcohol Abuse and Alcoholism (2006) *Why Do Adolescents Drink, What Are the Risks, and How Can Underage Drinking Be Prevented? Alcohol Alert No.67*. Washington, DC: National Institutes of Health; b) Foster, S.E., et al (2006) Estimate of the Commercial Value of Underage Drinking and Adult Abusive and Dependent Drinking to the Alcohol Industry. *Archives of Pediatric Adolescent Medicine* 160: 473–478; c) Faden, V.B. (2006) Trends in Initiation of Alcohol Use in the United States, 1975 to 2003. *Alcoholism*. 30 (6): 1011–1022; d) Center on Alcohol Marketing and Youth (2006) *Underage Drinking in the United States*. Washington, DC: Georgetown University; e) Federal Interagency Forum on Child and Family Statistics (2006) *America's Children in Brief*. Washington, DC: Office of Management and Budget.

65. a) Hingson, R.W., et al (2006) Age at Drinking Onset and Alcohol Dependence. *Archives of Pediatric and Adolescent Medicine* 160: 739–746; b) Alati, R., et al. (2006) In Utero Alcohol Exposure and Prediction of Alcohol Disorders in Early Adulthood. *Archives of General Psychiatry* 63: 1009–1016.

66. a) News from Child Trends (2008) *New Data on Teen Substance Abuse, Math Proficiency, and School Activities*. Washington, DC: Child Trends, April 8; b) Johnston, L.D., et al (2007) Overall, Illicit Drug Use by American Teens Continues Gradual Decline in 2007. Ann Arbor, MI: University of Michigan News Service [Online]; c) Federal Interagency Forum on Child and Family Statistics (2006) *America's Children in Brief*. Washington, DC: Author; d) PATS Teens Report (2006) *Generation Rx*. New York: Partnership for a Drug-Free America; e) Lynskey M.T., et al (2003) A Longitudinal Study of the Effects of Adolescent Cannabis Use on High School Completion. *Addiction* 98 (5): 685–692.

67. CASA Teen Survey (2005) *National Survey of American Attitudes on Substance Abuse X*. New York: The National Center on Addiction and Substance Abuse.

68. Woodall, M. (2006) Drug Woes Growing in City's Grade Schools. *Philadelphia Inquirer* March 29.

69. Crime in the United States (2004) *Arrests of Juveniles for Drug Abuse Violations from 1994 to 2003*. Washington, DC: Department of Justice, Federal Bureau of Investigation.

70. a) Aria A.M., et al (2006) Methamphetamine and other Substance Use During Pregnancy. *Maternal and Child Health Journal Online* January 6, 2006. b) Tronick, E. Z., et al (2005) Cocaine Exposure Is Associated With Subtle Compromises of Infants' and Mothers' Social-Emotional Behavior. *Developmental Psychology* 41: 711–722

71. a) Friedman, R.A. (2006) The Changing Face of Teenage Drug Abuse. *New England Journal of Medicine* 354 (14): 1448–1450; b) PATS Teens Report 2004 Report (2006) *Generation Rx*. New York: Partnership for a Drug-Free America; c) Johnston, L. D., et al (2007) *Illicit Drug Use By American Teens Continues Gradual Decline*. Ann Arbor, MI: University of Michigan News Service; d) Office of Applied Studies (2008) *The NSDUH Report: Misuse of Over-the-Counter Cough and Cold Medications among Persons Aged 12 to 25*. Rockville, MD: Substance Abuse and Mental Health Services Administration; e) Critzer, G. (2005) *Generation Rx*. New York: Houghton Mifflin.

72. a) American Lung Association. (2003) *Adolescent Smoking Statistics*. New York, NY: Author; b) Federal Interagency Forum on Child and Family Statistics (2006) *America's Children in Brief*. Washington, DC: Author.

73. a) Belluzzi, J.D., et al (2005) Acetaldehyde Enhances Acquisition of Nicotine Self-Administration in Adolescent Rats. *Neuropsychopharmacology* 30 (4): 705–712; b) Audrian-McGovern, J., et al (2004) Interacting Effects of Genetic Predisposition and Depression on Adolescent Smoking Progression. *American Journal of Psychiatry* 161 (7): 1224–1230; c) National Center for HIV/AIDS, Viral Hepatitis, STD and TB Prevention (2008) *1 in 4 Teenage Girls Has a Sexually Transmitted Disease*. Atlanta, GA: Centers for Disease Control and Prevention.

74. a) *Protecting America's Youth*. Lexington, KY: Council of State Governments; b) Weinstock, H., et al. (2004) Sexually Transmitted Diseases among American Youth. *Perspectives on Sexual & Reproductive Health* 36: 6–10.

75. a) HIV/AIDS Fact Policy Sheet. (2006) *Women and HIV/AIDS in the United States*. Menlo Park, CA: The Henry J. Kaiser Family Foundation. February; b) National Center for HIV, STD and TB Prevention (2005) AIDS Public Information Data Set. U.S. Surveillance Data for 1981–2002, CDC WONDER On-line Database, December.

76. a) Darroch, J.E., et al (2001) Differences in Teenage Pregnancy Rates Among Five Developed Countries. *Family Planning Perspectives* 33: 244–250, 281; b) Darroch, J.E., et al (2001) Teenage Sexual and Reproductive Behavior in Developed Countries. New York, NY: Alan Guttmacher Institute; c) Ryan, S., et al (2008) Older Sexual Partners during Adolescence. *Perspectives on Sexual and Reproductive Health* 40: 17–26; d) Sandfort, T.G.M., et al (2008) Long-Term Health Correlates of Timing of Sexual Debut. *American Journal of Public Health* 98: 155–161.

77. a) American Academy of Pediatrics (1999) *Handbook of Pediatric Environmental Health*. Evanston, IL: Author; b) Needleman H.L. & Gatsonis, C.A. (1990) Low-Level Lead Exposure and the IQ of Children. *Journal of the American Medical Association* 263 (5): 673–678; c) Thacker, S.B., et al (1992) Effect of Low-level Body Burdens of Lead on the Mental Development of Children. *Archives of Environmental Health* 47 (5): 336–346; d) Colborn, T., et al (1996) *Our Stolen Future*. New York, N.Y.: Dutton.

78. a) Garbarino, J. (1995) *Raising Children in a Socially Toxic Environment*. San Francisco: Jossey-Bass Publishers; b) Garbarino, J. (2001) Supporting Parents in a Socially Toxic Envi-

ronment. In Westman, J.C. (Ed.) *Parenthood in America*. Madison, WI: University of Wisconsin Press, pp. 224–228; c) Garbarino, J. (2008) *Children and the Dark Side of Human Experience*. New York: Springer.

79. Rexford, E.N. (1969) Children and Our Brave New World. *Archives of General Psychiatry* 20: 25–37.

80. *USA Today* November 28, p. 9D.

81. Moynihan, D.P. (1993) Defining Deviancy Down. *The American Scholar* Winter: 17–30.

82. Westman, J.C. (1994) *Licensing Parents*. New York: Perseus Publishing, pp. 123–148.

CHAPTER 2. ADOLESCENT PREGNANCY AND CHILDBIRTH TRENDS

1. Mill, J.S. (1859) *On Liberty*. In Hutchins, R.M. (Ed.) *Great Books of the Western World, Volume 43*. Chicago, IL: University of Chicago Press, p. 318.

2. a) *U.S. Teenage Pregnancy Statistics National and State Trends and Trends by Race and Ethnicity*. New York: Guttmacher Insitute, September 2006; b) Ventura, S.J., et al (2006) *Recent Trends in Teenage Pregnancy in the United States, 1990–2002. Health E-stats*. Hyattsville, MD: National Center for Health Statistics. September 200

3. a) Brown, B.B., et al (2002) *The World's Youth*. New York: Cambridge University Press, p. 330; b) Santelli, J.S., et al (2007) Explaining Recent Declines in Adolescent Pregnancy in the United States. *American Journal of Public Health* 97 (1): 150–156.

4. The National Campaign To Prevent Teen Pregnancy (2006) Pregnancy Among Sexually Experienced Teens. *Science Says* 23, April. Washington, DC.

5. East, P.L. & Felice, M.E. (1996) *Adolescent Pregnancy and Parenting*. Mahwah, NJ: Lawrence Erlbaum.

6. Putting Together What Works (2006) *It's a Guy Thing*. Washington, DC: National Campaign to Prevent Teen Pregnancy, February.

7. U.S. Department of Health and Human Services (1995) *Report to Congress on Out-of-wedlock Childbearing*. Hyattsville, MD: U.S. Department of Health and Human Services.

8. National Center for Health Statistics (2007) *Births: Preliminary Data for 2006*. Volume 56, No. 7.

9. a) Ibid; b) Schelar, E., et al (2007) *Repeat Teen Childbearing*. Publication #2007–23. Washington, DC: Child Trends; b) National Center for Health Statistics (2007) *Teen Birth Rate Rises for First Time in 15 Years*. Washington, DC: Centers for Disease Control and Prevention.

10. Child Stats (2006) *America's Children in Brief* Washington, DC: Federal Interagency Forum on Child and Family Statistics.

11. a) Hamilton, B.E., et al (2006) Births. *Health E-Stats* November 21; b) Martin, J.A., et al (2006) *Births. National Vital Statistics Report* 55 (1). Washington, DC: Centers for Disease Control, Division of Vital Statistics.

12. National Campaign to Prevent Teen Pregnancy (2002) *Not Just Another Single Issue*. Washington, DC: Author.

13. a) Franzetta, K., et al (2006) *Trends and Recent Estimates*. Washington, DC: Child Trends Research Brief #2006–04; b) Finer, L.B. & Henshaw, S.K. (2006) Disparities in Rates of Unintended Pregnancy in the United States, 1994 and 2001. *Perspectives on Sexual and Reproductive Health* 38 (2): 90–96.

14. East, P.L. & Felice, M.E. (1996) *Adolescent Pregnancy and Parenting*. Mahwah, NJ: Lawrence Erlbaum.

15. a) Moore, K. (2005) *What's Behind the Decline in the Teen Birth Rate?* Washington, DC: Brookings Institution Presentation, March 30; b) National Survey of Family Growth (1997) *Vital and Health Statistics* Series 23: No. 19. Hyattsville, MD: Department of Health and Human Services.

16. Westman, J.C. (2005) *Maternal Status of Girls Ages 15–17 in Madison and Milwaukee, Wisconsin.* Madison, WI: Wisconsin Cares, Inc.

17. Federal Interagency Forum on Child and Family Statistics (2007) *America's Children.* Washington, DC: U.S. Government Printing Office.

18. National Center for Health Statistics (1994) *Advance Report of Final Natality Statistics 43, no. 5, 1992, Supplement* October 25.

19. a) Martin, J.A., et al (2003) *Births: Vol 52, No. 10.* Hyattsville, MD: National Center for Health Statistics; b) National Campaign to Prevent Teen Pregnancy (2002) *Not Just another Single Issue.* Washington, DC: Author; c) Gallagher, M. (1999) *The Age of Unwed Mothers.* New York: Institute for American Values.

20. a) Coley, R. & Chase-Lansdale, P.L.(1998) Adolescent Pregnancy and Parenthood. *American Psychologist* 53 (2): 152–166; b) Martin J.A., et al. (2005) Births. *National Vital Statistics Reports* 54 (2) Hyattsville, MD: National Center for Health Statistics. Tables 13, 14 & 17.

21. Putting What Works to Work (2003) The Sexual Attitudes and Behavior of Male Teens. *Science Says* 6 October. Washington, DC: National Teen Pregnancy Prevention Campaign.

22. George, A. (2005) Going All the Way. *New Scientist*, March 15: 44–48.

23. Mabin, C. (2005) Teen Pregnancies Test Experts, Parents, Students. *Wisconsin State Journal* Sept. 2, p. A3.

24. Bureau of Health Information and Policy (2006) *Wisconsin Youth Sexual Behavior and Outcomes 1993–2005.* Madison, WI: Division of Public Health, Department of Health and Family Service, February.

25. Santow, G. & Bracher, M. (1999) Explaining Trends in Teenage Childbearing in Sweden. *Studies in Family Planning* 30 (3): 169–182.

26. Kaufman, C., et al (2001) Adolescent Pregnancy and Parenthood in South Africa. *Studies in Family Planning* 32 (2): 147–160.

27. Demographic and Health Surveys. Calverton, MD: Measure DHS, Macro International Inc. August 24, 2005.

CHAPTER 3. THE DENIGRATION OF PARENTHOOD

1. Hutchins, R.M. (Ed.) *Great Books of the Western World, Volume 7.* Plato, The Republic V. Chicago, IL: University of Chicago Press, p. 362.

2. a) Richards, D.A.J. (1980) The Individual, the Family, and the Constitution. *New York University Law Review* 55: 1, 28; b) West, C. & Hewlett, S.A. (1998) *The War Against Parents.* New York: Houghton Mifflin.

3. Rosenblum, K.L. & Olshansky, E. (2007) Building Families. *Zero to Three* 17 (5): 16–21.

4. a) Terman, L.M. & Oden, M.H. (1959). *The Gifted Group at Mid-Life.* Stanford, CA: Stanford University Press; b) Sears, P.S. & Barbee, A.H. (1975) Career and Life Satisfactions of Terman's Gifted Women. Louis M. Terman Memorial Symposium, Johns Hopkins University, November 6; c) Sears, R.R. (1977) Sources of Life Satisfactions of the Terman Gifted Men. *American Psychologist* 32: 119–128.

5. Brazelton, T.B. & Greenspan, S.I. (2000) *The Irreducible Needs of Children*. New York: Da Capo Press, pp. xviii-xix.

6. Mason, M., et al (Eds.) *All Our Families, Second Edition*. New York: Oxford University Press, p. 2.

7. Steiner, L.M. (2006) *Mommy Wars*. New York: Random House.

8. a) Hirshman, L.R. (2005) Homeward Bound. *The American Prospect. December*. Washington, DC: The American Prospect. b) Hirshman, L.R. (2006) *Get to Work*. New York: Viking.

9. Bennetts, L. (2007) *Feminine Mistake*. New York: Hyperion Books.

10. Lareau, A. (2003) *Unequal Childhoods*. Berkeley, CA: University of California Press, p. 13.

11. Westman, J.C. (1989) The Risks of Day Care for Children, Parents, and Society. In Christiansen, Bryce J. (Ed.) *Day Care*. Rockford, IL: The Rockford Institute, pp. 18–20.

12. Westman, J.C. (1979) *Child Advocacy*. New York: Free Press, pp. 107–108.

13. a) Breiner, S. J. (1990) *Slaughter of the Innocents*. New York: Plenum; b) Berger, B. (1988) Multiproblem Families and the Community. In Wilson, J.Q. & Loury, G.C. (Eds.) *From Children to Citizens, Volume III*. New York: Springer-Verlag, p. 277; c) Westman, J.C. & Kaye, D. (1990) The Termination of Parental Rights as a Therapeutic Option. In Westman, J.C. (Ed.) *Who Speaks for the Children?* Sarasota, FL: Professional Resources Exchange, Inc., pp. 257–259; d) Keltner, B. (1990) Family Characteristics of Preschool Social Competence among Black Children in a Head Start Program. *Child Psychiatry and Human Development* 21: 95–108.

14. Westman, J.C. (1994) *Licensing Parents*. New York: Insight Books, p. 33.

15. Sarah A. (2002) The Price of Motherhood. *Social Science in the Public Interest* 2 (1). Ann Arbor, MI: Institute of Social Research.

16. Hewlett, S.A. (2007) *Off Ramps and On Ramps*. Cambridge, MA: Harvard Business School Publishing.

17. Cabrera, N.J., et al (2000) Fatherhood in the Twenty-First Century. *Child Development* 71 (1): 127–136.

18. Lamb, M.E., et al (1987) A Biosocial Perspective on Paternal Behavior and Involvement. In Lancaster, J. B., et al (Eds.) *Parenting across the Lifespan*. New York: Aldine de Gruyter, pp. 111–142.

19. a) World Trends & Forecasts. *The Futurist*. 39 (5): 12; b) Gupta, S., et al (2005) *Panel Study of Income Dynamics between 1968 and 1997*. Ann Arbor, MI: Institute of Social Research.

20. Tucker, P. (2005) Stay-at-home Dads: At-home Dads Can Benefit Children and Mothers. *Futurist* Sept. 1.

21. Roberts, P. (2004) No Minor Matter. *Childbearing and Reproductive Health Series, Brief No. 2*. Washington, DC: Center for Law and Social Policy.

22. Anderson, K.G. (2006) How Well Does Paternity Confidence Match Actual Paternity? *Current Anthropology* 48 (3): 511–518.

23. Baker, K.K. (2006) Asymmetric Parenthood. In Wilson, R. Fretwell (Ed.) *Reconceiving the Family*. New York: Cambridge University Press, p. 141.

24. Roberts, P. (2004) No Minor Matter. *Childbearing and Reproductive Health Series, Brief No. 2*. Washington, DC: Center for Law and Social Policy.

25. a) Center of Law and Social Policy (2005) *Update on Uniform Parentage Act*. Washington, DC: Author; b) Child Support Enforcement and Fragile Families (2003) *Fragile Families Research Brief Number 15* April. Princeton, NJ: Princeton University.

26. Corrigan, M.D. (2006) A Formula for Fool's Gold. In Wilson, Robin Fretwell (Ed.) *Reconceiving the Family*. New York: Cambridge University Press, p. 419.

27. David, H.P., et al (l988) *Born Unwanted.* New York: Springer.
28. Levitt, S.D. & Dubner, S J. (2005) *Freakonomics.* New York: William Morrow.

CHAPTER 4. DIVERGENT PARENTHOOD STYLES

1. More, T. (1949) *Utopia* 1551—Ogden, H.V.S. Arlington Heights, IL: AHM Publishing Corporation, p. 58.
2. Coontz, S. (2005) *Marriage, a History.* New York: Viking, p. 309.
3. Ibid, p. 32–33.
4. Ibid, p. 7, 40.
5. Ibid, p. 9.
6. Ibid, p.11.
7. Ibid, p. 307.
8. Wu, L.L. & Li, J. (2005) "Modern" Family Paths Not So New After All. In Settersten Jr., et al (Ed.) *On the Frontier of Adulthood.* Chicago: University of Chicago Press.
9. a) Coontz, S. (2005) *Marriage, a History.* New York: Viking, p. 313; b) Fisher, Helen (2004) *Why We Love.* New York: Henry Holt, p. xix; c) Schneider, C.E. (2006) Afterword: Elite Principles. In Wilson, R.F. (Ed.) *Reconceiving the Family.* New York: Cambridge University Press, p. 505; d) Wilson, J.Q. (2002) *The Marriage Problem.* New York: HarperCollins Publishers, p.103.
10. Zinsmeister, K. (1990) Growing Up Scared. *Atlantic Monthly* June: 49–66.
11. Ettelbrick, P. (1997) Since When Is Marriage a Path to Liberation? In Sullivan, A. (Ed.) *Same-Sex Marriage.* New York: Vintage Books, p. 118.
12. Opinion of the Justices, no. SJC-08860, in Goodridge v. Department of Public Health. Massachusetts Supreme Judicial Court (Boston: November 18, 2003), p. 10.
13. Coontz, S. (2005) *Marriage, a History.* New York: Viking, p. 49.
14. Whitehead, B.D. (2006) *The State of Our Unions.* New Brunswick, NJ: Rutgers University.
15. Hymowitz, K.S. (2006) *Marriage and Caste in America.* Chicago, IL: Ivan R. Dee Publisher.
16. Fields, J. (2004) America's Families and Living Arrangements: 2003. *Current Population Reports, P20–553.* Washington, DC: U.S. Census Bureau.
17. Population Division, Fertility & Family Statistics Branch (2006) *America's Families and Living Arrangements: 2005, Table H1.* Washington, DC: U.S. Bureau of the Census.
18. a) Johnson, T. & Dye, J.(2005) *Indicators of Marriage and Fertility in the United States from the American Community Survey.* Washington, DC: U.S. Bureau of the Census; b) DHHS Pub No. (PHS) 95–127 (2005) *Report to Congress on Out-of-Wedlock Childbearing.* Washington, DC: Department of Health and Human Services; c) Stevenson, B. & Wolfers, J. (2007) Divorced From Reality. *New York Times* September 29, p. A-27.
19. Dobson, R. (2007) Five-Year Itch. *The Independent* 07:39.
20. Center for Research on Child Wellbeing (2006) The Prevalence and Correlates of Multipartnered Fertility Among Urban U.S. Parents. *Fragile Families Research Brief* Number 35. Princeton, NJ: Princeton University.
21. Division of Labor Force Statistics (2006) Table 5. Employment Status of the Population by Sex, Marital Status, and Presence and Age of Own Children Under 18. Washington, DC: U.S. Bureau of Labor Statistics.
22. Mincieli, L. (2007) *The Relationship Context of Births Outside of Marriage.* Washington, DC: Child Trends.

23. Blankenhorn, D. (2007) *The Future of Marriage*. New York: Encounter Books, p. 218.

24. Pew Research Center (2007) As Marriage and Parenthood Drift Apart. Washington, DC: Author.

25. Attitudes toward Marriage. *Social Science in the Public Interest* 2 (1) 2002.

26. a) Twenge, J.M. (2006) *Generation Me*. New York: Free Press, p. 215; b) Thornton, A. & Young-DeMarco, L. (2001) Four Decades of Trends in Attitudes toward Family Issues in the United States. *Journal of Marriage and the Family* 63 (4): 1009–1037.

27. Science Says (2002) *Teens' Attitudes Toward Marriage, Cohabitation and Divorce 16*, July. Washington, DC: The National Campaign To Prevent Teen Pregnancy.

28. Whitehead, B. & Popenoe, D. (2002) *Why Men Won't Commit*. Piscataway, NJ: The National Marriage Project.

29. Bumpass, L. (2001) The Changing Contexts of Parenting in the United States. In Westman, J.C. (Ed.) *Parenthood in America*. Madison, WI: University of Wisconsin Press, p. 212.

30. Whitehead, B.D. & Pearson, M. (2006) *Making a Love Connection*. Washington, DC: The National Campaign To Prevent Teen Pregnancy.

31. Garfinkel, I. (2004) Policy and the Family. In Moynihan, Daniel P., et al (Eds.) *The Future of the Family*. New York: Russell Sage Foundation, p. 279.

32. Sigle-Rushton, W. & McLanahan, S. (2002) For Richer or Poorer? *Population* 57 (3): 509–526.

33. Folbre, N. (2004) Disincentives to Care. In Moynihan, D.P., et al (Eds.) *The Future of the Family*. New York: Russell Sage, p. 249.

34. Sigle-Rushton, W. & McLanahan, S. (2002) For Richer or Poorer? *Population* 57 (3): 509–526.

35. a) Leiderman, Sally (2001) *Interpersonal Violence and Adolescent Pregnancy*. Bala Cynwyd, PA: Healthy Teen Network; b) Moore, K.A., et al (2004) *What is a Healthy Marriage?* Washington, DC: Child Trends.

36. a) Furstenberg, Jr. F.F., et al (1999) *Managing to Make It*. Chicago, IL: University of Chicago Press, p. 217; b) Loprest, P. (2003) *Fewer Welfare Leavers Employed in Weak Economy*. Washington, DC: Urban Institute Press.

37. a) Haskins, R., et al (2005) The Decline in Marriage: What to Do. *Policy Brief: Fall*. Princeton, NJ: The Future of Children; b) The Retreat from Marriage among Low-Income Families (2003) *Fragile Families Research Brief 17*. Princeton, NJ: Princeton University.

38. a) Gallagher, M. (1999) *The Age of Unwed Mothers*. New York, NY: Institute for American Values; b) National Campaign to Prevent Teen Pregnancy (2002) *Not Just Another Single Issue*. Washington, DC: Author.

39. Furstenberg, Jr., F.F., et al (2004) Values, Policy, and the Family. In Moynihan, D.P., Smeeding, T.M. & Rainwater, L. (Eds.) *The Future of the Family*. New York: Russell Sage Foundation, p. 275.

40. Roberts, P. (2007) Out of Order? *Couples and Marriage Series Policy Brief No. 9*. Washington, DC: Center for Law and Social Policy.

41. Rainwater, L. & Yancey, W. (1967) *The Moynihan Report and the Politics of Controversy*. Cambridge: Massachusetts Institute of Technology.

42. Gottlieb, L. (2005) The XY Files. *The Atlantic* 296 (2): 141–150.

43. Fields, J. (2004) America's Families and Living Arrangements: 2003. *Current Population Reports, P20–553*. Washington, DC: U.S. Census Bureau.

44. Coontz, S. (2005) *Marriage, a History*. New York: Viking.

45. Holoway, S.D., et al (1997) *Through My Own Eyes*. Cambridge, MA: Harvard University Press, p. 226.

46. Rainwater, L. & Smeeding, T.M. (2004) Single Parent Poverty, Inequality, and the Welfare State. In Moynihan, D.P., et al (Eds.) *The Future of the Family*. New York: Russell Sage Foundation, pp. 112–113.

47. Chivers, C.J. (2006) Russians Are Asked to Make Babies. *New York Times* May 14, p. 4 WK.

48. Glenn, N. & Sylvester, T. (2008) *The Shift and the Denial. Research Brief No 8*. New York: Center for Marriage and Families.

49. a) McLanahan, S. & Sandefur, G. (1994) *Growing Up with a Single Parent*. Cambridge, MA: Harvard University Press, p. 154; b) Wilcox, W.B. & Dew, J. (2008) *Protectors or Perpetrators?* New York: Institute for American Values.

50. Lang, K. & Zagorsky, J.L. (2001) Does Growing Up with a Parent Absent Really Hurt? *Journal of Human Resources* 36 (2): 253–273.

51. a) Morrison, D.R. & Cherlin, A.J. (1995) The Divorce Process and Young Children's Well-Being. *Journal of Marriage and the Family* 57: 800–812; b) Entwisle, D.R. & Alexander, K.L. (1995) A Parent's Economic Shadow. *Journal of Marriage and the Family* 57:399–40; c) Lang, K. & Zagorsky, J.L. (2001) Does Growing Up with a Parent Absent Really Hurt? *Journal of Human Resources* 36: 253–273; d) Aughinbaugh, A., et al (2001) *The Impact of Family Structure and School Quality on Youth Achievement in Mathematics*. Mimeo. Washington, DC: United States Bureau of Labor Statistics; e) Pong, S., et al (2002) *Family Policies and Academic Achievement by Young Children in Single-Parent Families*. Population Research Institute, Pennsylvania State University; f) Thompson, E., et al (1994) Family Structure and Child Well-Being. *Social Forces* 73: 221–242.

52. a) DeLeire, T. & Kalil, A. (2002) Good Things Come in Threes. *Demography* 39: 393–413; b) Astone, N.M. & McLanahan, S.S. (1991) Family Structure, Parental Practices and High School Completion. *American Sociological Review* 6:309–320; c) Painter, G. & Levine, D.I. (2000) Family Structure and Youths' Outcomes. *Journal of Human Resources* 35:524–549; d) McLanahan, S.S. & Sandefur, G. (1994) *Growing Up with a Single Parent*. Cambridge, MA: Harvard University Press; e) McLanahan, S.S. (1997) Parent Absence or Poverty? In Duncan, G. & Brooks-Gunn, J. (Eds.) *Consequences of Growing Up Poor*. New York: Russell Sage Foundation; f) Bjorklund, A., et al (2002) *Family Structure and Children's Educational Attainment*. Presented at the ESPE meetings in Bilbao, June.

53. a) DeLeire, T. & Kalil, A. (2002) Good Things Come in Threes. *Demography* 39: 393–413; b) Antecol, H., Bellard, K. & Helland, E. (2002) *Does Single Parenthood Increase the Probability of Teenage Promiscuity, Drug Use, and Crime?* Claremont, CA: Claremont McKenna College; c) Wu, L.L. (1996) Effects of Family Structure and Income on the Risks of a Premarital Birth. *American Sociological Review* 58: 210–232; d) Painter, G. & Levine, D.I. (1999) *Daddies, Dedication, and Dollars*. Berkeley, CA: University of California Institute for Industrial Relations.

54. a) Painter, G. & David I.L. (2000) Family Structure and Youths' Outcome. *Journal of Human Resources* 35: 524–549; b) Goldscheider, FK. & Goldscheider, C. (1998) The Effects of Childhood Family Structure on Leaving & Returning Home. *Journal of Marriage and the Family* 60: 745.

55. a) Lang, K. & Zagorsky, J.L. (2001) Does Growing Up with a Parent Absent Really Hurt? *Journal of Human Resources* 36: 253–273; b) Biblarz, T.J. & Raftery, A. (1999) Family Structure, Educational Attainment, and Socioeconomic Success. *American Journal of Sociology* 105: 321–365; c) McLanahan, S.S. & Sandefur, G. (1994) *Growing Up with a Single Parent*. Cambridge, MA: Harvard University Press.

56. a) Powell, M.A. & Parcel, T.L. (1997) Effects of Family Structure on the Earnings Attainment Process. *Journal of Marriage and the Family* 59: 419–433; b) Lang, K. & Zagorsky,

J.L. (2001) Does Growing Up with a Parent Absent Really Hurt? *Journal of Human Resources* 36: 253–273.

57. a) Royse, D. & Wiehe, V.R. (1988) Impulsivity in Felons and Unwed Mothers *Psychological Reports* 62: 335–336; b) Boxill, N.A. (l987) "How Would You Feel...?" In Battle, S.F. (Ed.) *The Black Adolescent Parent*. New York: Haworth, pp. 48–49; c) Search Institute (1993) *Youth in Single-parent Families*. Minneapolis, MN: Search Institute; d) Musick, J.S. (1990) Adolescents as Mothers. *Zero to Three* 11 (2) 21–28.

58. Entwisle, D.R. & Alexander, K.L. (1996) Family Type and Children's Growth in Reading and Math over the Primary Grades. *Journal of Marriage and the Family* 58: 341–355.

59. Institute for Marriage and Public Policy (2005) Can Married Parents Prevent Crime? Recent Research on Family Structure and Delinquency 2000–2005. *Policy Brief September 21*.

60. a) Amato, P.R. & Keith, B. (1991) Parental Divorce and Adult Well-being. *Journal of Marriage and the Family* 53: 43–58; b) Cherlin, A.J., et al (1998) Effects of Parental Divorce on Mental Health throughout the Life Course. *American Sociological Review* 63: 239–249.

61. a) Corral, J. & Miya-Jervis, L. (2001) *Young Wives Tales*. Seattle: Seal Press, p. xiii; b) Hertz, R. (2006) *Single by Chance, Mothers by Choice*. New York: Oxford University Press, pp. xviii, 191, 192.

62. <http://singlemothers.org/>.

63. a) Glendon, M.A. (2006) Foreword. In Wilson, R.F. (Ed.) *Reconceiving the Family*. New York: Cambridge Press, pp. xiii-xv; b) Blankenhorn, D. (1995) *Fatherless America*. New York: Basic Books; c) Preston, S.H. (2004) The Value of Children. In Moynihan, D.P., et al (Eds.) *The Future of the Family*. New York: Russell Sage, p. 265.

64. a) Shulman, S. & Seiffgre-Krenke, I. (1997) *Fathers and Adolescents*. London: Routledge, p. 219; b) Sigle-Rushton, W. & McLanahan, S. (2004) Father Absence and Child Well-being: A Review. In Moynihan, D.P., et al (Eds.) *The Future of the Family*. New York: Russell Sage, p. 142.

65. a) Carlson, M.J. (2006) Family Structure, Father Involvement, and Adolescent Behavioral Outcomes. *Journal of Marriage and Family* 68 (1): 137–154; b) Marsiglio, W. (1995) Fatherhood Scholarship. In Marsiglio, W. (Ed.) *Fatherhood*. Thousand Oaks, CA: Sage Publications.

66. Erikson, J. (1964) Nothing to Fear: Notes on the Life of Eleanor Roosevelt. *Daedalus* 93: 781–801.

67. a) Comanor, W.S. & Philllips, L. (1998) *The Impact of Family Structure on Delinquency*. Santa Barbara, CA: University of California; b) Carlson, M. (1999) Do Fathers Really Matter? *Center for Research on Child Wellbeing*. Princeton, NJ: Princeton University; c) Harper, C. & McLanahan, S.S. (1999) Father Absence and Youth Incarceration. *Center for Research on Child Well-being Working Paper #99–03*. Princeton, NJ: Princeton University; d) Simons, R.L., et al (1999) Explaining the Higher Incidence of Adjustment Problems Among Children of Divorce Compared with Those in Two-Parent Families. *Journal of Marriage and the Family* 61:1020–1033; e) Antecol, H., et al (2002) *Does Single Parenthood Increase the Probability of Teenage Promiscuity, Drug Use, and Crime?* Princeton, NJ: Princeton University Center for Research on Child Wellbeing.

68. a) Simons, R.L., et al (1994) The Impact of Mothers' Parenting, Involvement by Non-residential Fathers, and Parental Conflict on the Adjustment of Adolescent Children. *Journal of Marriage and the Family* 56: 356–374; b) McLeod, J.D., et al (1994) Does Parenting Explain the Structural Conditions on Children's Antisocial Behavior? *Social Forces* 73 (2): 575–604; c) Barnes, G.M., et al (1990) Parent-Adolescent Interactions in the Development of Alcohol Abuse and Other Deviant Behaviors. In Barber, B.K. & Rollins, B.C. (Eds.) *Parent-Adolescent Relationships*. Lanham, MD: University Press of America.

69. a) Kelly, J.B. (2000) Children's Adjustment in Conflicted Marriage and Divorce. *Journal of the American Academy of Child & Adolescent Psychiatry* 39 (8): 963–973; b) Westman, J.C. (1971) Divorce is a Family Affair. *Family Law Quarterly* 5:110.

70. U.S. House of Representatives, Committee on Ways and Means, Subcommittee on Human Resources (2005) *Hearing on Welfare Reform Reauthorization Proposals.* Washington, D.C.: Government Printing Office.

71. Secunda, V. (1992) *Women and Their Fathers.* New York: Delacorte Press.

72. a) Shulman, S. & Seiffgre-Krenke, I. (1997) *Fathers and Adolescents.* London: Routledge, pp. 29, 86; b) Bohan, Ca., et al (2007) Predicting School Dropout and Adolescent Sexual Behavior in Offspring of Depressed and Nondepressed Mothers. *Journal of the American Academy of Child and Adolescent Psychiatry* 46 (1): 15–14.

73. Pruett, K.D. (2000) *Fatherneed.* New York: The Free Press, p. 213.

74. Shulman, S. & Seiffgre-Krenke, I. (1997) *Fathers and Adolescents.* London: Routledge, pp. 217, 204.

75. Corneau, G. (1991) *Absent Fathers, Lost Sons.* Boston: Shambala, pp. 168–169.

76. Balcom, D.A. (1998) Absent Fathers: Effects on Abandoned Sons. *Journal of Men's Studies* 6 (3): 283–296.

77. Pruett, K.D. (2000) *Fatherneed.* New York: The Free Press, p. 210.

78. a) Corneau, G. (1991) *Absent Fathers, Lost Sons.* Boston: Shambala, p.14; b) Gee, H. (1991) The Oedipal Complex in Adolescence. *Journal of Analytical Psychology* 36: 193–210.

79. Drexler, P. (2005) *Raising Boys without Men.* New York: Rodale.

80. Kraemer, S. (2005) Narratives of Fathers and Sons. In Vetere, A. & Dowling, E. (Eds.) *Narrative Therapies with Children and their Families.* London, Brunner/Routledge.

81. Erikson, J. (1964) Nothing to Fear. *Daedalus* 93: 781–801.

82. Heath, D. (1994) The Impact of Delayed Fatherhood on the Father-Child Relationship. *Journal of Genetic Psychology* 155 (4): 511–530.

83. Bradshaw, J., et al (1999) *Absent Fathers?* New York: Routledge, p p. 232, 227.

84. Mandell, D. (2002) *"Deadbeat Dads".* Toronto, Canada: University of Toronto Press, pp. 215–216.

85. a) Wilson, J.Q. (2002) *The Marriage Problem.* New York: HarperCollins; b) Bumpass, L. (2001) The Changing Contexts of Parenting in the United States. In Westman, J.C. (Ed.) *Parenthood in America.* Madison, WI: University of Wisconsin Press, p. 215; c) Garrison, M. (2006) Marriage Matters. In Wilson, R.F. (Ed.) *Reconceiving the Family.* New York: Cambridge University Press, p.141.

86. Bumpass, L. (1998) The Changing Significance of Marriage in the United States. In Mason, K.O., et al (Eds.) *The Changing Family in Comparative Perspective.* Honolulu: University of Hawaii Press.

87. a) Thornton, A. & Young-DeMarco, L. (2001) Four Decades of Trends in Attitudes toward Family Issues in the United States. *Journal of Marriage and the Family* 63 (4): 1009–1037; b) *The State of Our Unions 2005.* Piscataway, NJ: The National Marriage Project, Rutgers.

88. Center for Research on Child Wellbeing (2005) Young Children's Behavioral Problems in Married and Cohabiting Families. *Fragile Families Research Brief 33*, June. Princeton, NJ: Princeton University.

89. *The State of Our Unions 2005.* Piscataway, NJ: The National Marriage Project, Rutgers.

90. Popenoe, D. (2005) *Marriage and Family.* Piscataway, NJ: The National Marriage Project.

91. Kiernan, K. (2002) Cohabitation in Western Europe. In Booth, A. & Crouter, A. (Eds.) *Just Living Together.* New Jersey: Lawrence Erlbaum Associates.

CHAPTER 5. DYSFUNCTIONAL SOCIAL POLICIES AND SERVICES

1. Reinhold N. (1932) *Moral Man, Immoral Society*. New York: Charles Scribner's Sons.

2. Edgerton, R.B. (2000) Traditional Beliefs and Practices Are Some Better than Others? In Harrison, L.E. & Huntington, Samuel P. (Eds.) *Culture Matters*. New York: Basic Books, p. 138.

3. Epstein, W.M. (2002) *American Policy Making*. Lanham: Rowman and Littlefield Publishers, p. 214.

4. Donovan, D.M. & McIntyre, D.(1990) *Healing the Hurt Child*. New York: W.W. Norton.

5. Epstein, W.M. (1993) *The Dilemma of American Social Welfare*. New Brunswick, NJ: Transaction, p. 204.

6. Ibid, p. 189.

7. Thayer, L. (1976) The Functions of Incompetence. In Laszlo, E. & Sellon, E.B. (Eds.) *Vistas in Physical Reality*. New York: Plenum Press.

8. a) Davis, D .(2007) *The Secret History of the War on Cancer*. New York: Basic Books, p. 15; b) Brandt, A.M. (2007) *The Cigarette Century*. New York: Basic Books.

9. Rhodes, W.C. (1972) *Behavior Threat and Community Response*. New York: Behavioral Publications.

10. Elizur, J. & Minuchin, S. (l989) *Institutionalizing Madness*. New York: Basic Books.

11. Kaufman, L. (2006) New Procedure Takes Children from Parents. *New York Times* Jan.27, p. A17.

12. a) Gordon, D.R. (1990) *The Justice Juggernaut*. New Brunswick, NJ: Rutgers University Press; b) Pew Center on the States (2008) *One in 100*. Washington, DC: Pew Charitable Trusts; (c) Bureau of Justice Statistics (2007) *Correctional Surveys*. Washington, DC: U.S. Department of Justice.

13. a) Travis, J. & Waul, M. (2004) (Eds.) *Prisoners Once Removed*. Washington, DC: The Urban Institute, p. 59; b) Bureau of Justice Statistics (2007) *Prison Statistics*. NCJ 219416. Washington, DC: U.S. Department of Justice.

14. Gibbons, J. J. & Katzenback, N. (2006) *Confronting Confinement*. New York: Vera Institutes of Justice.

15. Langan, P.A. & Levin, D.J. (2002) *Recidivism of Prisoners Released in 1994*. Washington, DC: Bureau of Justice Statistics.

16. Lovell, D. & Johnson, C. (2004) *Felony and Violent Recidivism among Supermax Prison Inmates in Washington State*. Seattle, WA: University of Washington, April 2004.

17. Toch, H. (2001) The Future of Supermax Confinement. *Prison Journal* 81: 376–388.

18. Jones, V. (2006) Con Game. *Forbes* April 24, p. 34.

19. Gottfried, M. (2006) Stuck in the Slammer. *Forbes* May 22, p. 195.

20. Mobley, A. & Geis, G. (2001) The Corrections Corporation of America aka The Prison Realty Trust, Inc. In Shichor, D. & Gilbert, M.J. (Eds.) *Privatization in Criminal Justice*. Cincinnati, OH: Anderson Publishing, p. 226.

21. Bogenschneider, K. & Normadin, H. (2007) *Cost-Effective Approaches in Juvenile and Adult Corrections*. Madison, WI: University of Wisconsin-Extension Family Impact Seminars.

22. Hanson, R. (Ed.) (l982) *Institutional Abuse of Children and Youth*. New York: Haworth, p. 3.

23. McKnight, J. (1995) *The Careless Society*. New York: Basic Books, p. ix.

24. Thomas, B.R. (l982) Protecting Abused Children. In Hanson, Ranae (Ed.) *Institutional Abuse of Children & Youth*. New York: Haworth.

25. a) Polier, J.W. (1989) *Juvenile Justice in Double Jeopardy.* Hillsdale, NJ: Erlbaum, p. 159; b) Forer, L.G. (1991) *Unequal Protection.* New York: Norton; c) Jacobs, M.D. (1990) *Screwing the System and Making It Work.* Chicago, IL: University of Chicago Press.

26. Groner, J. (1991) *Hilary's Trial:* New York: Simon & Schuster.

27. a) *In Re Application of Gault,* 387 U. S. 1, 87s. Ct. 1428, 1967; b) Snyder, H.N. & Sickmund, M. (2006) *Juvenile Offenders and Victims.* Washington, DC: National Center for Juvenile Justice.

28. Iceland, J. (2003) *Poverty in America.* Berkeley, CA: University of California Press, pp. 2, 8.

29. Fromm, S. (2001) *Total Estimated Cost of Child Abuse and Neglect in the United States.* Chicago, IL: Prevent Child Abuse America.

30. a) Roberts, D.(2002) *Shattered Bonds.* New York: Basic Civitas Books, p. 74; b) Children's Bureau (2005) *General Findings from the Federal Child and Family Services Review.* Washington, DC: Administration for Children and Families.

31. Mason, M., et al (Eds.) *All Our Families, Second Edition.* New York: Oxford University Press, p. 11.

32. Hofferth, S.L. & Hayes, C.D. (Eds.) (1987) *Risking the Future, Volume I.* Washington, DC: National Academy Press, pp. 2, 7, 138.

33. a) Miller, S.H. (1983) *Children as Parents.* New York: Child Welfare League, p. 112; b) Musick, J.S. (1993) *Young, Poor, and Pregnant.* New Haven, CT: Yale University Press, p. 203.

PART 2. THEORETICAL FOUNDATION

1. Hock, D. (1999) *Birth of the Chaordic Age.* San Francisco: Berret-Koehler Publishers, p. 120.

CHAPTER 6. CHAOS/COMPLEXITY THEORY

1. White House. Moynihan, D.P. (1973) *The Politics of a Guaranteed Income.* New York: Random House.

2. Feist, G. (2006) *The Psychology of Science and the Origins of the Scientific Mind.* New Haven, CT: Yale Press.

3. Gazzaniga, M.S. (2005) *The Ethical Brain.* New York: Harper Perennial, pp. 161, 168, 177, 172.

4. a) Tavris, C. & Aronson, E. (2007) *Mistakes Were Made (But Not by Me).* Orlando, FL: Harcourt; b) Hamilton Papers, Volume II, December 1979–March 1980 (New York, 1961–1978), p. 242.

5. Forrester, J.W. (1971) *World Dynamics.* Cambridge, MA: Wright-Allen Press.

6. Kelly, E.F. (2007) *Irreducible Mind.* Lanham, MD: Rowman & Littlefield.

7. a) Lerner, R. (1998) Theories of Human Development: Contemporary Perspectives. In Damon, W. & Lerner, R. (Eds.) *Handbook of Child Psychology.* New York: John Wiley & Sons, p. 19; b) Watts, D.J. (2003) *Six Degrees.* New York: W.W. Norton; c) Weiner, N. (1948) *Cybernetics.* Cambridge, MA: MIT Press.

8. a) Von Bertalanffy, L. (1968) *General Systems Theory.* New York: Braziller; b) Miller, J.G. (1978) *Living Systems.* New York: McGraw-Hill.

9. a) Devall, B. & Sessions, G. (1985) *Deep Ecology*. Salt Lake City: Peregrine Smith; b) Capra, F. (1996) *The Web of Life*. New York: Anchor Books; c) Bateson, G. (1979) *Mind and Nature*. New York: Dutton; d) Bronfenbrenner, U. (Ed.) (2005) *Making Human Beings Human*. Thousand Oaks, CA: Sage Publications.

10. Halfon, N. & Hochstein, M. (2002) Life Course Health Development. *The Milbank Quarterly* 80 (3).

11. Scannapieco, M. & Connell-Carrick, K. (2005) *Understanding Child Treatment*. New York: Oxford University Press, pp. 6–31.

12. a) Gleick, J. (1987) *Chaos*. New York: Penguin Books, pp. 3, 5; b) Capra, F., et al (Eds.) (2007) *Reframing Complexity*. Mansfield, MA: ISCE Publishing.

13. a) Kossman, M.R. & Bullrich, S.(1997) Systematic Chaos. In Masterpasqua, F. & Perna, P.A. (Eds.) *The Psychological Meaning of Chaos*. Washington, DC: American Psychological Association; b) Lipton, B.H. (2005) Embracing the Immaterial Universe. *Shift* 9: 8–12.

14. Csikszentmihalyi, M. & Rathunde, K. (1998) The Development of the Person. In Damon, W. & Lerner, R.(Eds.) *Handbook of Child Psychology, Fifth Edition*. New York: John Wiley & Sons, p. 652.

15. Henry, J. (1964) *Culture against Man*. New York: Random House, p. 477.

16. Waldrop, M. M. (1992) *Complexity*. New York: Simon and Schuster, p. 329.

17. Watts Miller, W. (1996) *Durkheim, Morals and Modernity*. Montreal, Buffalo: McGill-Queens University Press.

18. Strauss, W. & Howe, N.(1997) *The Fourth Turning*. New York: Broadway Books, pp. 3, 318.

19. Cooley, C.H. (1966) *Social Process*. Carbondale, IL: Southern Illinois University Press, p. xiv.

20. Caplan, G. (1964) *Principles of Preventive Psychiatry*. New York: Basic Books, pp. 31–34.

21. a) Shonkoff, J.P. & Phillips, D.A. (Eds.) (2000) *From Neurons to Neighborhoods*. Washington, DC: National Academies Press; b) Center on the Developing Child (2007) *A Science-Based Framework for Early Childhood Policy*. Cambridge, MA: Harvard University.

22. Harrison, L.E. & Huntington, S.P. (2000) *Culture Matters*. New York: Basic Books, p. xv.

23. a) Florida, R. (2005) *The Flight of the Creative Class*. New York: HarperBusiness, pp. 72–73; b) Inglehart, R. (2000) Modernization, Cultural Change and Traditional Values. *American Sociological Review* 65: 19–51.

24. Berreby, D. (2005) *Us and Them*. New York: Little, Brown & Company.

25. Sarwer-Foner, G. J. (1972) On Human Territoriality. *Canadian Psychiatric Association Journal* 17: SS-169–183.

26. Milne, E. & Grafman, J. (2001) Ventromedial Prefrontal Cortex Lesions in Humans Eliminate Implicit Gender Stereotyping. *Journal of Neuroscience* 21, RC150: 1–6.

27. Jones, M. & Fabian, A. (Eds.) (2006) *Conflict*. New York: Cambridge University Press.

28. Dugatkin, L.A. (2006) *The Altruism Equation*. Princeton, NJ: Princeton University Press.

29. Rohmer, R.P. (1975) *They Love Me, They Love Me Not*. New Haven, CT: Human Relations Area Files Press.

30. a) Anderson, S.W., et al (1999) Impairment of Social and Moral Behavior Related to Early Damage in Human Prefrontal Cortex. *Nature Neuroscience* 2: 1032–1037; b) Hinde, R.A. (2007) *Bending the Rules*. Oxford, UK: Oxford University Press.

31. Linden, D.J. (2007) *The Accidental Mind*. Cambridge, MA: Harvard University Press.

32. Institute of Noetic Sciences (2007) *The 2007 Shift Report*. Petaluma, CA, p.74.

33. Henry, J. (1964) *Culture against Man*. New York: Random House, p. 12.

34. a) United Nations (1991) *Convention on the Rights of the Child*. New York: United Nations, No. DPI/1101—December—10M; b) Gazzaniga, M.S. (2005) *The Ethical Brain*. New York: Harper Perennial, p. 174.

35. a) Hauser, M.D. (2006) *Moral Minds*. New York: HarperCollins, pp. xviii, 420, 417; b) Wilson, D.S. (2007) *Evolution for Everyone*. New York: Delacorte Press.

36. Haidt, J. (2007) The New Synthesis of Moral Psychology. *Science* 316: 998–1002.

37. a) Fitzgibbon, S. (2006) a City without Duty, Fault, or Shame. In Wilson, R.F. (Ed.) *Reconceiving the Family*. New York: Cambridge University Press, p. 45; b) Schneider, C.E. (2006) Afterword: Elite Principles. In Wilson, R.F. (Ed.) *Reconceiving the Family*. New York: Cambridge University Press, p. 504.

38. Ibid b), p. 503.

39. Gilbert, M. (2006) *The Disposable Male*. Atlanta, GA: The Hunter Press, pp. ix, x, xii, 282–283.

40. Kuhn, T. (1962) *The Structure of Scientific Revolution*. Chicago: University of Chicago Press.

41. Capra, F. (1996) *The Web of Life*. New York: Anchor Books, p.10.

42. Bernstein, J. (2006) *All Together Now*. San Francisco, CA: Berrett-Koehler Publishers, pp. 3–7.

43. a) Lewis, H.R. (2006) *Excellence without a Soul*. New York: PublicAffairs; b) Stiles, Paul (2005) *Is the American Dream Killing You?* New York: HarperCollins.

44. Hacker, J.S. (2006) *The Great Risk Shift*. New York: Oxford University Press.

45. a) McKnight, J. (1995) *The Careless Society*. New York: Basic Books, p. 117; b) de Tocqueville, A., trans. by Reeve, H. (1901) *Democracy in America, Volume 2*. New York: D. Appleton & Company, pp. 825, 786.

46. Kagan, S.L. & Lowenstein, A.E. (2006) Cultural Values and Parenting Education. In Harrison, L.E. & Kagan, J. (Eds.) *Developing Cultures*. New York: Routledge, p. 52.

47. a) Ormerod, P. (2006) *Why Most things Fail*. New York: Pantheon; b) Hart, S.D., et al (2007) Precision of Actuarial Risk Assessment Instruments. *British Journal of Psychiatry* 190: s60—s65.

CHAPTER 7. THE RIGHTS OF ADOLESCENTS

1. Children's Defense Fund (1991) *A Vision for America's Future*. Washington, DC: Author, p. xii.

2. Cunningham, H. (1995) *Children and Childhood in Western Society since 1500*. Harlow, Essex: Pearson.

3. Tanenhaus, D.S. (2002) Creating the Child, Constructing the State. In Alaimo, K. & Klug, B. (Eds.) *Children as Equals*. Lanham, MD: University Press of America, pp. 127, 138.

4. a) Key, E. (1909) *The Century of the Child. Ninth Edition*. New York: G.P. Putnam's Sons; b) Smuts, A. (2006) *Science in the Service of Children, 1893–1935*. New Haven: Yale University Press.

5. Cunningham, H. (1995) *Children and Childhood in Western Society since 1500*. Harlow, UK: Pearson, p.163.

6. Bellon, C. (2002) The Promise of Rights for Children. In Alaimo, K. & Klug, B. (Eds.) *Children as Equals*. Lanham, MD: University Press of America, p.119.

7. a) Brown, D.E. (1991) *Human Universals.* New York: McGraw-Hill; b) Andre, C. & Velasquez, M. (1990) Rights Stuff. *Issues in Ethics* 3 (1). Santa Clara, CA: Santa Clara University, Markkula Center for Applied Ethics.

8. Ibid b).

9. Levin, L. (1988) The Rights of the Child. In Davies, Peter (Ed.) *Human Rights.* London: Routledge, p. 40.

10. a) Westman, J.C. (1979) *Child Advocacy* New York: Free Press, pp. 257–262; b) United Nations General Assembly Resolution 1386 (XIV). *Fourteenth Session, Supplement No.16. 1960*, p.19; c) Child Rights Information Network (1990) *Convention on the Rights of the Child.* London, UK: Author.

11. a) Freeman, M.D.A. (1983) *The Rights and Wrongs of Children.* London: Frances Printer, p. 150; b) Archard, D. (1993) *Children.* London: Routledge; c) Wolfson, S.A. (1992) Children's Rights. In Freeman, M. & Veerman, P. (Eds.) *The Ideologies of Childrens' Rights.* Boston: Martinus Nijhhoff, p. 23; d) Dwyer, J.G. (2006) *The Relationship Rights of Children.* New York: Cambridge University Press, p.131.

12. a) Hunt, L. (2007) *Inventing Human Rights.* New York: W.W. Norton; b) Andre, C. & Velasquez, M. (1990) Rights Stuff. *Issues in Ethics* 3 (1): Winter. Santa Clara, CA: Santa Clara University.

13. Dwyer, J.G. (2006) *The Relationship Rights of Children.* New York: Cambridge University Press, p.124.

14. a) Raphael, D.D. (1967) *Political Theory and the Rights of Man.* London: Macmillan, p. 54; b) Houlgate, Laurence D. (1980) *The Child and the State.* Baltimore, MD: Johns Hopkins Press, pp. 99–100.

15. U.S. Supreme Court. *Roper v. Simmons, Case No. 03–63.*

16. a) Vito, G. & Wilson, D.G. (1985) *The American Juvenile Justice System.* Beverly Hills, CA: Sage Publications, p. 47, 56; b) Polier, J. Wise (1989) *Juvenile Justice in Double Jeopardy.* Hillsdale, NJ: Lawrence Erlbaum.

17. *Ginsberg v. New York* (1969) 390 U. S. 629, 88 S. Ct. 1274, 20 L. Ed. 2d 195. *Prince v. Massachusetts* (1944) 321 U. S. 158, 170.

18. Davis, S.M. & Schwartz, M.D. (1987) *Children's Rights and the Law.* Lexington, MA: Lexington, pp. 207–208.

19. Meyer, D.D. (2003) The Modest Promise of Children's Relationship Rights. *William & Mary Bill of Rights Journal* 11 (3): 1117.

20. Dwyer, J.G. (2006) *The Relationship Rights of Children.* New York: Cambridge University Press, p. 2.

21. Andre, C. & Velasquez, M. (1990) Rights Stuff. *Issues in Ethics* 3 (1): Winter. Santa Clara, CA: Santa Clara University, Markkula Center for Applied Ethics.

22. a) Guggenheim, M. (2005) *What's Wrong With Children's Rights.* Cambridge, MA: Harvard University Press; b) Rodman, H., et al (1984) *The Sexual Rights of Adolescents.* New York: Columbia University Press, p. 50.

23. Zimring, F.E. (1982) *The Changing World of Adolescence.* New York: Free Press, p. 100.

24. Westman, J.C. & Kaye, D. (1990) The Termination of Parental Rights as a Therapeutic Option. In Westman, J.C. (Ed.) *Who Speaks for the Children?* Sarasota, FL: Professional Resources Exchange, pp. 257–259.

25. Shepard, R.E. (Ed.) (1996) *Juvenile Justice Standards.* Chicago, IL: American Bar Association.

26. a) Sigman G.S. & O'Connor C. (1991) Exploration for Physicians of the Mature Minor Doctrine. *Journal of Pediatrics* 119 (4): 520–525; b) Michigan Mental Health Code 330.1707.

27. a) Guggenheim, M. (2005) *What's Wrong with Children's Rights*. Cambridge, MA: Harvard University Press, p. 41; b) Goldstein, R., et al (1979) *Before the Best Interests of the Child*. New York: Free Press.

28. Wright, A.M. (2004) What Voluntary Acts of Child, Other than Marriage or Entry into Military Service, Terminate Parent's Obligation to Support. *55 American Law Reports ALR5th 557*.

29. 67 C. J. S., *Parent and Child*, p. 815, sec. 89; Annot. (1946) *What Amounts to Implied Emancipation of Minor Child* 165 A. L. R. 723.

30. a) Legal Information Institute. *State Marriage Statutes*. Ithaca, NY: Cornell University Law School; b) *39 American Jurisprudence*, Parent and Child, p. 704, sec. 64.

31. a) Cohen, S.& Taub, N. (1988) *Reproductive Laws for the 1990s*. Clifton, NJ: Humana. pp. 381–384; b) Rodman, H., et al. (1984) *The Sexual Rights of Adolescents*. New York: Columbia University Press.

32. Dailard, C. & Richardson, C.T. (2005) Teenagers' Access to Confidential Reproductive Health Services. *The Guttmacher Report on Public Policy*. November.

33. a) *Poe v. Gerstein* (1975) 517 F. 2D 787; b) *Planned Parenthood v. Danforth* (1976) 428 US 52, 72–75; c) 5th Cir. *Hodgson et al v. Minnesota et al* (1990) U.S. Supreme Court 88–1125, June 25; d) *Ohio v. Akron Center for Reproductive Health et al* (1990) U.S. Supreme Court 88–805, June 25; e) Council on Ethical and Judicial Affairs (1993) Mandatory Parental Consent to Abortion *Journal of the American Medical Association* 269: 82–86.

34. 546 U.S. 04–1144 (2006)

35. Guttmacher Institute (2005) Parental Involvement in Minors' Abortions. *State Policies in Brief* November 1. Washington, DC.

36. a) *Planned Parenthood v. Danforth*, 428 U.S. 52 (1976). *Bellotti v. Baird II*, 443 U.S. 662 (1979); b) Guggenheim, M. (2002) Minor Rights. *Hofstra Law Review* 30: Spring; c) Redding, R.E. (2005) Where the Action Is. *The Gavel Gazette*. February 14. Villanova, PA: Villanova University School of Law.

37. Goodnough, A. (2005) Florida Halts Fight to Bar Girl's Abortion. *New York Times* May 4, 2005, p. A15.

38. a) Liptak, A. (2005) On Moral Grounds, Some Judges Are Opting Out of Abortion Cases. *New York Times*, September 4, p. A11; b) Center for Health Statistics (2007) *Final Resident Data for Selected Induced Termination of Pregnancy Data 2006*. Montgomery, AL: Alabama Department of Public Health.

39. Roberts, P. (2005) No Minor Matter. *Childbearing and Reproductive Health Series* March 2004, Brief No. 2. Washington, DC: Center for Law and Social Policy.

40. Troup-Leasure, K., et al (2005) Statutory Rape Known to Law Enforcement. *Juvenile Justice Bulletin*. Washington, DC: U.S. Department of Justice, Office of Justice Programs, Office of Juvenile Justice and Delinquency Prevention.

41. a) Oliveri, R. (2000) Statutory Rape Law and Enforcement In The Wake Of Welfare Reform. *Stanford Law Review* 52: 463–508; b) Child Trends (2005) *A Demographic Portrait of Statutory Rape*. The Office of Population Affairs, a Division of the United States Department of Health & Human Services. March.

42. Troup-Leasure, K. & Snyder, H.N. (2005) Statutory Rape Known to Law Enforcement. *Juvenile Justice Bulletin*. Washington, DC: U.S. Office of Juvenile Justice and Delinquency Prevention. August.

43. Oliveri, R. (2000) Statutory Rape Law and Enforcement in the Wake of Welfare Reform. *Stanford Law Review* 52: 463–508.

44. Wisconsin Statutes 940.225 (3m), 948.09, 48.981.

45. a) Wisconsin Statutes 948.02 (1), (2); b) Wisconsin Statutes 48.981(2), (2m), (3), 253.07 (1) (c), 940.225 (3m), 948.02 (1), (2), (3), 948.025; 948.09; b) DHFS Office of Legal Counsel letter 3/15/94; c) Opinions of the Attorney General, 1983; DOJ Memorandum 4/14/05. d) Burmaster, E. (2005) *Reporting Requirements for Sexually Active Adolescents*. Madison, WI: Student Services/Prevention & Wellness Team, Department of Public Instruction.

46. Wilgoren, J. (2005) Rape Charge Follows Marriage to a 14–Year-Old. *New York Times* August 19, p 1A.

47. Roberts, P. (2005) No Minor Matter. *Childbearing and Reproductive Health Series* March 2004 Brief No. 2. Washington, DC: Center for Law and Social Policy.

48. Oliveri, R. (2000) Statutory Rape Law and Enforcement in the Wake of Welfare Reform. *Stanford Law Review* 52: 463–508.

49. Cunningham, H. (2006) *The Invention of Childhood*. London: BBC Books, p. 245.

50. Bartholet, E. (2004) The Challenge of Children's Rights Advocacy. *Whittier Journal of Child and Family Advocacy* 3: 215–230.

51. State of New York (2007) Title 8–A, Article 6 of the Social Services Law, Section 447. *Safe Harbour for Exploited Children Act*.

52. Smith, J.M. (2002) A Child-Centered Jurisprudence. In Alaimo, K. & Klug, B. (Eds.) *Children As Equals*. Lanham, MD: University Press of America, p. 160.

CHAPTER 8. THE RIGHTS OF PARENTS

1. Abrahamsen, D. (1952) *Who Are the Guilty?* New York: Grove Press, p. 309.

2. a) Hollinger, J.H. (1993) Adoption Law. *The Future of Children* 3: 43–61; b) Hollinger, J.H. (2004) Note on the Revised Uniform Parentage Act. In Cahn, N.R. & Hollinger, J.H. (Eds.) *Families by Law*. New York: New York U. Press, pp. 294–296; c) Markens, S. (2007) *Surrogate Motherhood*. Berkeley, CA: U. of California Press, p. 180.

3. Glendon, M.A. (1991) *Rights Talk*. New York: Free Press.

4. Bartlett, K.T. (2004) Re-expressing Parenthood. In Cahn, Naomi R. & Hollinger, J. Heifetz (Eds.) *Families by Law*. New York: New York University Press, pp. 259–264.

5. Guggenheim, M., et al (1996) *The Rights of Families*. Carbondale IL: Southern Illinois University Press. p. 87.

6. Garbarino, J. (2001) Supporting Parents in a Socially Toxic Environment. In Westman, J.C. (Ed.) *Parenthood in America*. Madison, WI: University of Wisconsin Press, pp. 224–228.

7. a) Guggenheim, M. (2005) *What's Wrong with Children's Rights*. Cambridge, MA: Harvard University Press, p. 21, 23; b) Parham v. J.R., 442 U.S. 548, 602 (1979); c) Troxel v. Granville. 530 U.S. 558, 562 (2003).

8. a) House and Senate as H.R. 1946 and S. 984. (1995/1996) Parental Rights Drama Unfolds. *Home School Court Report* 11 (6): 16; b) Erken, G.D. & Westman, J.C. (1995) Does the U.S. Need a Parental-Rights Amendment? *Insight on the News* May 15; c) McCarthy, M.H. (2005) *Parental Rights Legislation*. Camano Island, WA: Washington Natural Learning Association.

9. Mason, M.A. (1994) *From Father's Property to Children's Rights*. New York: Columbia University Press.

10. Shanley, M.L. (2001) *Making Babies, Making Families*. Boston: Beacon Press, p. 7.

11. Dwyer, J.G. (2003) Children's Rights. In Curren, R. (Ed.) *A Companion to the Philosophy of Education*. Oxford, UK: Blackwell Publishing, pp. 444–447.

12. Cahn, N.R. & Hollinger, J. (2004) *Families by Law*. New York: New York University Press, p. 39.

13. a) Dwyer, J.G. (1996) Setting Standards for Parenting. *Child Psychiatry and Human Development* 27 (3): 165–176; b) *Winkelman v. Parma City School District* (2007) U.S. Supreme Court No. 05–983.

14. Scott, E.S. (2003) Parental Autonomy and Children's Welfare. *William & Mary Bill of Rights Journal* 11: 1072; b) Dwyer, J.G. (1996) Setting Standards for Parenting. *Child Psychiatry and Human Development* 27: 165–176.

15. Ibid.

16. Westman, J.C. (1998) Children's Rights, Parental Prerogatives, and Society's Obligations. *Child Psychiatry and Human Development* 29 (4): 315–328.

17. Shanley, M.L. (2001) *Making Babies, Making Families*. Boston: Beacon Press, pp. 156, 10.

18. Dwyer, J.G. (2003) A Taxonomy of Children's Existing Rights in State Decision Making about their Relationships. *William & Mary Bill of Rights Journal* 11 (3): 859–865.

19. State of New York Department of Corrections Services (1993) *Profile of Participants: The Bedford Hills and Taconic Nursery Program in 1992*.

20. Galietta, M. (2005) When Families Cannot Be Healed. In Mason, M.A. (1994) *From Father's Property to Children's Rights*. New York: Columbia University Press, pp. 161–174.

21. Dwyer, J.G. (2003) A Taxonomy of Children's Existing Rights in State Decision Making about their Relationships. *William & Mary Bill of Rights Journal* 11 (3): 866–881.

22. Lewin, T. (2006) Unwed Fathers Fight for Babies Placed for Adoption. *New York Times* March 19, A-1.

23. *Michael H.,* 491 U.S. at 131.

24. a) *Wilson by Wilson v. Wilson* (1984) C. A. Tenn. 742 F.2d 1004; b) Horowitz, R. (1992) Families, Infants and the Justice System. *Zero to Three* 13: 1–7; c) Russ, G.H. (1993) Through the Eyes of a Child. *Family Law Quarterly* 27: 365–394.

25. *Zepeda v. Zepeda* (1963) 41 Ill App 2d 240, 190 NE 2d 849, 379 U.S. 945.

26. a) *Illinois National Bank & Trust v. Turner* (1981) 38 Ill. Dec. 653, 403 N.E. 2d 1256, 83 Ill. App. 3d 234; b) Russ, G.H. (1993) Through the Eyes of a Child. *Family Law Quarterly* 27: 365–394.

27. Ladd, R. Ekman (2002) Rights of the Child. In Alaimo, K. & Klug, B. (Eds.) *Children as Equals*. Lanham, MD: University Press of America, pp. 97–98.

28. a) Vito, G. & Wilson, D.G. (1985) *The American Juvenile Justice System*. Beverly Hills, CA: Sage Publications, p. 16; b) Zimring, F. E. (1982) *The Changing World of Adolescence*. New York: Free Press, pp. 31–32.

29. a) King v. Low 1 S.C.R. 87 (1985); b) Wynne, E.E. (1996) Children's Rights and the Biological Bias. *Connecticut Journal of International Law* 11:367.

30. *DeShaney v. Winnebago County Department of Social Services* (1989) U.S. Supreme Court No. 87–154.

31. *Smith v. Alameda County Social Services Agency* (1979) 90 Cal. App. 3d 929; 153 Cal. Rptr. 712; March.

32. Gorner, P. (1981) How Illinois Turned Its back on Billy. *Chicago Tribune* December 14.

33. a) Ave, M. (2008) Foster Care Laws Attacked. *St. Petersburg Times* January 26, 1B; b) Grimm, W. (1992) Recent Federal Lawsuits Prompt Child Welfare Reform. *Protecting Children* 8: 3–5.

34. Bureau of Milwaukee Child Welfare (2005) *Vision, Commitment and History*. Madison, WI: Wisconsin Department of Health and Family Services.

PART 3. THE HUMAN DEVELOPMENTAL PROCESS

1. Johnson, Paul (2006) Let's Have More Babies. *Forbes* April 17, p. 31.

CHAPTER 9. DEVELOPING HUMAN RELATIONSHIPS: ATTACHMENT BONDING

1. Bronfenbrenner, U. (1976) *The Ecology of Human Development.* Cambridge, Massachusetts: Harvard Press.
2. Chamberlain, D. (1998) *The Mind of Your Newborn Baby.* Berkeley, CA: North Atlantic Books, p. xviii.
3. a) Hauser, M.D. (2006) *Moral Minds.* New York: Ecco; b) Dugatkin, L.A. (2006) *The Altruism Equation.* Princeton, NJ: Princeton University Press.
4. Fletcher, G. (2002) *The New Science of Intimate Relationships.* Malden, MA: Blackwell, p. 168.
5. Ibid, p. 168.
6. Shermer, M. (2007) *The Mind of the Market.* New York: Times Books.
7. a) Miller, W.B. & Rodgers, J.Lee (2001) *The Ontogeny of Human Bonding Systems.* Boston, MA: Kluver Academic Publishers, p. 2; b) Zak, P.J. (2008) The Neurobiology of Trust. *Scientific American* 298 (6):88–95
8. Nathanielsz, P.W. (1999) *Life in the Womb.* Ithaca, New York, pp. 33–55.
9. a) Chamberlain, D. (1998) *The Mind of Your Newborn Baby.* Berkeley, CA: North Atlantic Books, p. xiv; b) Hepper, P.G., et al (1993) Newborn and Fetal Responses to Maternal Voice. *Journal of Reproductive Infant Psychology* 11 (3): 147–153; c) Chamberlain, D. (1998) *The Mind of Your Newborn Baby.* Berkeley, CA: North Atlantic Books, p. xx.
10. Haidt, J. (2005) *The Happiness Hypothesis.* New York: Basic Books, p. 113.
11. Miller, W.B. & Rodgers, J.L. (2001) *The Ontogeny of Human Bonding Systems.* Boston, MA: Kluver, p.16.
12. Goleman, D. (2006) *Social Intelligence.* New York: Bantam.
13. Hrdy, S.B. (2001) *The Past, Present, and Future of the Human Family.* Tanner Lectures. Salt Lake City, UT: University of Utah, February 27 and 28.
14. Hrdy, S.B. (1999) *Mother Nature.* New York: Ballantine, p. 536.
15. a) Hepper, P.G., et al (1993) Newborn and Fetal Response to Maternal Voice. *Journal of Reproductive and Infant Psychology* 11: 147–153; b) Kisilevsky, B. S., et al (2003) Effects of Experience on Fetal Voice Recognition. *Psychological Science* 14 (3): 220–224; c) Ward, C.D. & Cooper, R.P. (1999) A Lack of Evidence in 4–Month-Old Human Infants for Paternal Voice Preference. *Developmental Psychobiology* 35 (1): 49–59; d) Kaitz, M., et al (1994) Fathers Can Also Recognize their Newborns by Touch. *Infant Behavior and Development* 17 (2): 205–207.
16. Haidt, J. (2005) *The Happiness Hypothesis.* New York: Basic Books, p. 120.
17. a) Storey, A.E., et al (2000) Hormonal Correlates of Paternal Responsiveness in New and Expectant Fathers. *Evolution and Human Behavior* 21 (2): 79–95; b) Wynne-Edwards, K. & Reburn, C.J. (2000) Behavioral Endocrinology of Mammalian Fatherhood. *Trends in Ecology and Evolution* 15 (11): 464–68.
18. a) Arredondo, D. & Edwards, L.P. (2000) *Journal of the Center for Families, Children, and the Court* 2: 109–127; b) Gallese, V. (2006) Intentional Attunement. *Brain Research* 1079 (1): 15–24; c) Rizzolatti, G., et al (2006) Mirrors in the Mind. *Scientific American* 295 (5): 54–61;

d) Greenspan, S.I. (1999) *Building Healthy Minds*. New York: Perseus, pp. 85–129; e) Perry, B.D. (2000) *Maltreated Children*. New York: Norton.

19. Ramachandran, V. S. & Oberman, L. M. (2006) Broken Mirrors. *Scientific American* 295 (5): 62–69.

20. a) Nelson, K. (2007) *Young Minds in Social Worlds*. Cambridge, MA: Harvard University Press; b) Siegel, D.J. (1999) *The Developing Mind*. New York: The Guilford Press, pp. 336, 337, 217.

21. Ibid, pp. 218, 221.

22. Ibid, pp. 275, 278, 280.

23. a) Ibid, pp. 280–281; b) Alvy, K.(2007) *The Positive Parent*. New York: Teachers College Press, pp. 66–67.

24. Parker, K.J., et al (2005) Mild Early Life Stress Enhances Prefrontal-Dependent Response Inhibition in Monkeys. *Biological Psychiatry* 57:848–855.

25. Hobson, P. (2004) *The Cradle of Thought*. New York: Oxford University Press, p. 274.

26. a) Singer, D. & Singer, J.L. (2005) *Imagination and Play in the Electronic Age*. Cambridge, MA: Harvard University Press, pp. 5, 6; b) Schmidt, M. & Vandewater, E.A. (2008) Media and Attention, Cognition, and School Achievement. *The Future of Children* 18 (1).

27. Solomon, J. & George, C. (1999) The Measurement of Attachment Security in Infancy and Childhood. In Cassidy, J. & Shaver, P.R. (Eds.) *Handbook of Attachment*. New York: Guilford Publications, pp. 287–316.

28. a) Zeanah, C.H. & Emde, R.N (1994) Attachment Disorders in Infancy and Childhood. In Rutter, M., et al. (Eds.) *Child and Adolescent Psychiatry: Modern Approaches, 3d Edition*. London: Blackwell, pp. 490–504; b) Berlin, L.J, et al (2005) *Enhancing Attachment*. New York: The Guilford Press, p. 331.

29. Haidt, J.(2005) *The Happiness Hypothesis*. New York: Basic Books, p. 117.

30. Siegel, D.J. (1999) *The Developing Mind*. New York: The Guilford Press, p. 224.

31. Zahn-Waxler, C. (2006) Becoming Compassionate. *Shift* (13): 21–23.

32. Holtzman, D. & Kulish, N. (2000) The Femininization of the Female Oedipal Complex. *Journal of American Psychoanalytic Association* 48: 1413–1437.

33. Fisher, H. (2004) *Why We Love*. New York: Henry Holt & Company. p. 151.

34. Ibid, p. 76

35. Haidt, J. (2005) *The Happiness Hypothesis*. New York: Basic Books, p.125.

36. Fisher, H. (2004) *Why We Love*. New York: Henry Holt & Company, p. xii.

37. Entwisle, D.R. & Doering, S.G. (1981) *The First Birth*. Baltimore, MD: Johns Hopkins University Press.

38. a) Pruett, K.D. (2000) *Fatherneed*. New York: Free Press, p. 70; b) Parke, R.D. & Tinsley, B.J. (1987) Parent-Infant Interaction. In Osofsky, J. (Ed.) *Handbook of Infancy*. New York: Wiley. c) Parke, R.D. (1996) *Fatherhood*. Cambridge, MA: Harvard University Press.

39. Berreby, D. (2005) *Us and Them*. New York: Little, Brown & Company.

40. Harmon, A. (2006) Love You, K2a2a, Whoever You Are. *New York Times* January 22, p. 4–1.

41. a) Caspi, A., et al (2003) Influence of Life Stress on Depression: Moderation by a Polymorphism in the 5–HTT Gene. *Science* 301: 386–389; b) Kaufman, J., et al (2006) Brain-Derived Neurotrophic Factor-5–HTTLPR Gene Interactions and Environmental Modifiers of Depression in Children. *Biological Psychiatry* 59 (8): 673–80.

42. Kim-Cohen, J., et al. (2006) *MAOA*, Maltreatment, and Gene–Environment Interaction Predicting Children's Mental Health. *Molecular Psychiatry* 11: 903–913.

43. a) Siegel, D.J. (1999) *The Developing Mind*. New York: Guilford Press; b) Karr-Morse, R. & Wiley, M.S. (1997) *Ghosts from the Nursery*. New York: Atlantic Monthly Press; c) Lo-

gan, C., et al (2007) Conceptualizing a "Strong Start". *Research Brief, Publication #2007–10.* Washington, DC: Child Trends; d) Mendizza, M. & Pearce, J.C. (2001) *Magical Parent, Magical Child.* Nevada City, CA: Touch the Future.

CHAPTER 10. ADOLESCENT DEVELOPMENT

1. Shakespeare, W. *The Winter's Tale,* Act III, Scene III. In Rowse, A.L (1984) *The Annotated Shakespeare.* New York: Greenwich House, p. 2364.

2. Hall, G.S. (1904) *Adolescence.* 2 vols. New York, Appleton.

3. a) Richter, L.M. (2006) Studying Adolescence. *Science* 312: 1902–1905; b) Schlegel, A. & Barry. H. (1991) *Adolescence.* The Free Press. New York.

4. a) Graham, P. (2004) *The End of Adolescence.* New York: Oxford University Press; b) Epstein, R. (2007) *The Case against Adolescence.* Sanger, CA: Quill Driver.

5. a) Masten, A.S. (2007) Competence, Resilience, and Development in Adolescence. In Romer, D. & Walker, E.F. (Eds.) *Adolescent Psychopathology and the Developing Brain.* New York: Oxford University Press, p. 46; b) Bjorklund, DF. (2007) *Why Youth is Not Wasted on the Young.* Oxford, UK: Blackwell.

6. Hong, K. L. (2005) *Life Freaks Me Out.* Minneapolis, MN: Search Institute.

7. a) Arnett, J.J. (1999) Adolescent Storm and Stress, Reconsidered. *American Psychologist* 54: 317–326; b) Steinberg, Lawrence (2004) The Study of Developmental Psychopathology. In Cicchetti, D. (Ed.) *Handbook of Developmental Psychopathology.* New York: John Wiley; c) Osgood, D., et al (2004) Six Paths to Adulthood. In Settersten, Jr., Richard A., et al (Eds.) *On the Frontier of Adulthood.* Chicago, IL: University of Chicago Press.

8. Steinberg, L. (1991) Developmental Considerations in Youth Advocacy. In Westman, Jack C. (Ed.) *Who Speaks for the Children?* Sarasota, FL: Professional Resource Exchange, pp. 26–27.

9. a) Bakan, D. (1971) Adolescence in America. *Daedalus* 100: 979–995; b) Kroger, Jane (1990) *Identity in Adolescence.* London: Routledge; c) Csikzentmihalyi, M. (1993) Contexts of Optimal Growth in Childhood. *Daedalus* 122: 31–56.

10. Herman-Giddens, M.E., et al (1997) Secondary Sexual Characteristics and Menses in Young Girls Seen in Office Practice. *Pediatrics* 99 (4): 505–512.

11. a) Hrdy, S.B. (2001) *The Past, Present, and Future of the Human Family.* Tanner Lectures. Salt Lake City, UT: University of Utah, February 27 & 28; b) Eveleth, P.B. & Tanner, J.M. (1976) *Worldwide Variation in Human Growth.* London: Cambridge University Press, p. 229; c) Eveleth, P. B. & Tanner, J. M. (1990) *Worldwide Variation in Human Growth.* New York: Cambridge University Press, p. 217; d) Eveleth, P. B. & Tanner, J. M. (1990) *Worldwide Variation in Human Growth, 2nd Edition.* New York: Cambridge University Press, pp. 145–175.

12. a) Chumlea, W.C., et al (2003) Age at Menarche and Racial Comparisons in Girls. *Pediatrics* 111 (1): 110–113; b) Prior to 1800 the average menarche probably was 16.7 in Serbia: Laslett, P. (1971/2) Age of Menarche in Europe since the Eighteenth Century. *Journal of Interdisciplinary History* 2: 221–236; c) In 1830, the mean menarche probably was 17.5 in England: Tanner, J.M. (1962) *Growth at Adolescence.* Oxford, UK: Oxford Press, pp. 152–153; d) Dewhurst, J. (1984) *Female Puberty and Its Abnormalities.* Edinburgh: Churchill Livingstone, p. 27.

13. a) Schonfeld, W.A. (1971) Adolescent Development. In Feinstein, S., et al (Eds.) *Adolescent Psychiatry, Vol. 1.* New York: Basic Books; b) Falkner, F. & Tanner, J.M. (1986) *Human Growth, 2nd Edition, Vol. 2.* New York: Plenum, pp. 389–390; c) Anastasiow, N.J. (Ed.) (1982) *The Adolescent Parent.* Baltimore, MD: Brookes, pp. 2–31.

14. a) Koutras, D.A. (1997) Disturbances of Menstruation in Thyroid Disease. *Annals of the New York Academy of Sciences* 816: 280–4; b) Herman-Giddens, M.E., et al (1997) Secondary Sexual Characteristics and Menses in Young Girls Seen in Office Practice. *Pediatrics* 99 (4): 505–512.

15. a) Houppert, K. (1999) *The Curse*. New York: Farrar, Strauss and Giroux, pp. 242–243; b) Lee, J. & Sasser-Cohen, J. (1996) *Blood Stories*. New York: Routledge, p.181.

16. a) Phinney, V.G., et al (1990) The Relationship Between Early Development and Psychosexual Behaviors in Adolescent Females. *Adolescence* 25: 321–332; b) Ge, X., et al (1996) Coming of Age Too Early. *Child Development* 67: 3386–3400; c) Sonis, W.A., et al. (1985) Behavior Problems and Social Competence in Girls with True Precocious Puberty. *Journal of Pediatrics* 106: 156–160; d) Wierson, M. & Long, P.J. (1993) Toward a New Understanding of Early Menarche. *Adolescence* 28 (112): 913–24.

17. a) Herman-Giddens, M., et al (2001) Secondary Sexual Characteristics in Boys. *Archives of Pediatrics & Adolescent Medicine* 155: 1022–1028; b) Marty, M.S., et al (2003) Development and Maturation of the Male Reproductive System. *Birth Defects Research on Behavioral and Developmental Reproductive Toxicology* 68 (2): 125–36; c) Ramsey, G. V. (1943) The Sexual Development of Boys. *American Journal of Psychology* 56: 217–233.

18. Graber, J., et al (1997) Is Psychopathology Associated with the Timing of Pubertal Development? *Journal of the American Academy of Child & Adolescent Psychiatry* 36: 1768–1776.

19. a) Kaplowitz, P.B., et al (2001) Earlier Onset of Puberty in Girls. *Pediatrics* 108: 347–353; b) Sjöberg, R.L., et al (2005) Obesity, Shame, and Depression in School-Aged Children. *Pediatrics* 116 (3): e389—e392; c) Setchel, K.D., et al (1997) Exposure in Infants to Phyto-oestrogens from Soy-Based Infant Formula. *Lancet* 350 (9070): 23–27; d) Guillette, E. (2005) Pesticide Linked to Breast Growth. *New Scientist* 2528 (3–9): 21; e) Ellis B.J. & Garber J. (2000) Psychosocial Antecedents of Variation in Girls' Pubertal Timing. *Child Development* 71 (2): 485–501; f) Zabin, L., et al (2005) Childhood Sexual Abuse and Early Menarche. *Journal of Adolescent Health* 36: 393–400; g) Herman-Giddens, M.E., et al (1998) Sexual Precocity in Girls. *American Journal of Diseases of Children* 142: 431–433; h) Tremblay, L. & Frigon, J. (2005) Precocious Puberty in Adolescent Girls. *Child Psychiatry and Human Development* 36 (1): 73–94; i) Wei-Chu Chie, L., et al (1997) Predictive Factors for Early Menarche in Taiwan. *Journal of the Formosan Medical Association* 96: 446–450; i) Pescovitz, O.H. & Walvoord, E.C. (Eds.) (2007) *When Puberty is Precocious*. Totowa, NJ: Humana Press.

20. a) Draper, P. & Harpending, H. (1982) Father Absence and Reproductive Strategy. *Journal of Anthropological Research* 38: 255; b) Belsky, J., et al (1991) Childhood Experience, Interpersonal Development, and Reproductive Strategy. *Child Development* 62: 647–670; c) Belsky, J., et al (1991) Further Reflections on an Evolutionary Theory of Socialization. *Child Development* 62: 682–685; d) Moffitt, T.E., et al (1992) Childhood Experience and the Onset of Menarche. *Child Development* 63 (1): 47–58; e) Maestripieri, D. (2004) Developmental and Evolutionary Aspects of Female Attraction to Babies. *APA OnLine Psychological Science Agenda* 18: (1).

21. a) Diamond, M. & Hopson, J. (1998) *Magic Trees of the Mind*. New York: Dutton, pp. 238–239; b) fMRI (functional magnetic resonance imaging), PET scans (positron emission tomography), and SPECT (single photon emission computerized tomography); c) Gogtay, N., et al (2004) Mapping of Human Cortical Development during Childhood through Adulthood. *Proceedings of the National Academy of Science* 101: 8174–8179.

22. Walker, D., et al (1994) Prediction of School Outcomes Based on Early Language Production and Socioeconomic Factors. *Child Development* 65: 606–621.

23. Giedd, J.N. (2004) Structural Magnetic Resonance Imaging of the Adolescent Brain. *Annals of the New York Academy of Sciences* 1021: 77–85.

24. a) Walsh, D. (2004) *Why Do They Act That Way?* New York: Free Press, pp. 3, 65; b) Giedd, J.N. (2004) Structural Magnetic Resonance Imaging of the Adolescent Brain *Annals of the New York Academy of Sciences* 1021: 77–85; c) Yurgelun-Todd, D. (2004) *Inside the Teenage Brain.* Mc Clean Hospital, Boston. January 26.

25. Dahl, R. (2003) Beyond Raging Hormones. *The Dana Forum on Brain Science* 5 (3) Summer. Dana Press.

26. a) Dahl, R.E. (2001) Affect Regulation, Brain Development, and Behavioral/Emotional Health in Adolescence. *CNS Spectrums* 6 (1): 60–61; b) Carskadon, M.A. (2002) (Ed.) *Adolescent Sleep Patterns.* New York. Cambridge University Press, p. xvii.

27. a) Gurian, M. (2002) *The Wonder of Girls.* New York: Pocket Books, pp. 78–82; b) Niehoff, Debra (2002) *The Biology of Violence.* New York: Simon & Schuster, pp. 158–161.

28. a) Gurian, M. (2002) *The Wonder of Girls.* New York: Pocket Books, p. 6; b) New York Academy of Science (2003) Adolescent Brain Development. *Update.* November/December: 2–5.

29. a) Marcus, G. (2004) *The Birth of the Mind.* New York: Basic Books, p. 61; b) Powers, S. (2006) What Can We Learn from Studying Twins? *Zero To Three* 26 (5): 9–14.

30. Hyde, J.S. (2005) The Gender Similarities Hypothesis. *American Psychologist* 60 (6): 581–592.

31. Brizendine, L. (2006) *The Female Brain.* New York: Random House.

32. a) Cahill, L. (2005) His Brain, Her Brain. *Scientific American* 293 (5): 40–47; b) Becker, J.S., et al (Eds.) (2008) *Sex Differences in the Brain.* Oxford, UK: Oxford University Press.

33. Tyre, P. (2006) The Trouble With Boys. *Newsweek* January 30, pp. 44–52.

34. Pollack, W. (2005) *Real Boys.* New York: Henry Holt & Company.

35. Corneau, G. (1991) *Absent Fathers, Lost Sons.* Boston: Shambala, pp.1–2.

36. a) Hudspeth, W. & Pribram, K. (1992) Psychophysiological Indices of Brain Maturation. *International Journal of Psychophysiology* 12: 19–29; b) Fischer, K. & Rose, S. (1994) Dynamic Development of Coordination of Components in Brain and Behavior. In Dawson, G. & Fischer, K.W. (Eds.) *Human Behavior and the Developing Brain.* New York: Guilford Press. Chapter 1.

37. Erikson, E.H. (1968) *Identity Youth and Crisis.* New York: W.W. Norton, p. 156.

38. a) Dahl, R.E. & Spear, L.P. (Eds.) (2004) Adolescent Brain Development. *Annals of the New York Academy of Sciences* 1021: xi-469; b) Knoch, D. & Fehr, E. (2007) The Right Prefrontal Cortex and Self-Control. *Annals of the New York Academy of Science* 1104: 123–134.

39. a) Wilbrecht, L. (2007) Conference on Linking Affect to Action. March 11–14. New York: New York Academy of Sciences; b) Strauch, B. (2004) *The Primal Teen.* Westminster, MD: Knopf; c) Eshel, N., et al (2007) Neural Substrates of Choice Selection in Adults and Adolescents. *Neuropsychologia* 45 (6): *1270–1279.*

40. a) Steinberg, L. (1991) Developmental Considerations in Youth Advocacy. In Westman, J.C. (Ed.) *Who Speaks for the Children?* Sarasota. FL: Professional Resource Exchange, pp. 32–33. b) Gordon, D.E. (1990) Formal Operational Thinking. *American Journal of Orthopsychiatry* 60: 346–356; c) Jacobs, J.E. & Klaczynski, P.A. (2002) The Development of Judgment and Decision Making during Childhood and Adolescence. *Current Directions in Psychological Science* 11: 145–149.

41. a) Engel, S. (2005) *Real Kids.* Cambridge, MA: Harvard University Press; b) Johnson, S. (2005) *Everything Bad Is Good for You.* New York: Riverhead Books; c) Singer, D. & Singer, J.L. (2005) *Imagination and Play in the Electronic Age.* Cambridge, MA: Harvard University Press, p. 167.

42. Cherniss, C. (2000) *Emotional Intelligence*. Annual Meeting of the Society for Industrial and Organizational Psychology, New Orleans, LA. April 15. Consortium for Research on Emotional Intelligence in Organizations.

43. a) Salovey, P., et al (2002). Emotional Intelligence. In Fletcher, G. & Clark, M.S. (Eds.) *The Blackwell Handbook of Social Psychology. Vol. 2: Interpersonal Processes*. Oxford, England: Blackwell Publishers; b) Goleman, D. (1998) *Working with Emotional Intelligence*. New York: Bantam Books.

44. Goleman, D. (2006) *Social Intelligence*. New York: Bantam Books.

45. Snarey, J. R. & Vaillant, G. E. (1985) How Lower- and Working-Class Youth Become Middle-Class Adults. *Child Development* 56 (4): 899–910.

46. Feist, G. J. & Barron, F. (1996) *Emotional Intelligence and Academic Intelligence in Career and Life Success*. Presented at the Annual Convention of the American Psychological Society, San Francisco, CA. June.

47. Rogers, A.G. (2006) *The Unsayable*. New York: Random House.

48. Tangney, J.P. & Mashek, D.J. (2004). In Search of the Moral Person. In Greenberg, J., et al (Eds.), *Handbook of Experimental Existential Psychology*. New York: Guilford Press, pp. 156–166.

49. Lynd, H.M. (1961) *On Shame and the Search for Identity*. New York: Science Editions, pp. 22, 257.

50. McClintock, M. (1996) Rethinking Puberty. *Current Directions in Psychological Science* 5: 178–183.

51. Christiani, M. (2003) *A Life History Perspective on Dating and Courtship among Albuquerque Adolescents*. Ph.D. Dissertation, Department of Anthropology. Albquerque, NM: University of New Mexico.

52. LeDoux, J. (1996) *The Emotional Brain*. New York: Simon & Schuster.

53. Fisher, H. (2004) *Why We Love*. New York: Henry Holt & Company.

54. a) Peele, S. (1981) *Love and Addiction*. New York: Signet; b) Fisher, H. (2004) *Why We Love*. NY: Henry Holt.

55. Ibid, b).

56. Mitchell, J. (1998) *The Natural Limitations of Youth*. London: Ablex Publishing Company, pp. 32–34, 89–91.

57. a) Lucente, R. L. (1986) Self-transcending and the Adolescent Ego Ideal. *Child and Adolescent Social Work Journal* 3 (3): 161–176; b) Rodrigues, E. & Mendes, P. (2002) Contemporary Adolescence and the Crisis of Ideals. *International Forum of Psychoanalysis* 11 (2): 125–134.

58. Smetana, J. G. (1999) The Role of Parents in Moral Development. *Journal of Moral Education* 28: 311–321.

59. a) Kohlberg, L. (1984) *Essays on Moral Development*. San Francisco: Harper & Row. b) Gilligan, Carol (1993) *In a Different Voice*. Cambridge, MA: Harvard University Press.

60. Zimring, F.E. (2005) *American Juvenile Justice*. New York: Oxford University Press, p. 17.

61. a) Llewellyn, D.J. & Sanchez, X. (2007) Individual Differences and Risk Taking in Rock Climbing. *Psychology of Sport and Exercise*. Online 26 July; b) Galvan, A., et al (2006) Earlier Development of the Nucleus Accumbens Relative to the Orbitofrontal Cortex. *The Journal of Neuroscience* 26 (25): 6885–6892.

62. a) Eaton, D.K., et al (2006) Youth Risk Behavior Surveillance US 2005. *MMWR: Morbidity & Mortality Weekly Report* June 9. 55 (SS05): 1–108. Atlanta, GA: Centers for Disease Control and Prevention; b) National Highway Traffic Safety Administration. *Traffic Safety*

Facts 2005. Washington, DC: U.S. Department of Transportation; c) Davis, R. & O'Donnel, J. (2005) Black Boxes for Cars Slow to Catch On. *USA Today*, June 3, p. B1.

63. a) Dahl, R. E. (2004) Adolescent Brain Development. *Annals of the New York Academy of Sciences* 1021: 1–22; b) Reyna, V. F. & Farley, F. (2006) Is the Teen Brain Too Rational? *Scientific American Mind* November 29.

64. Hallowell, E. M. (2002) *The Childhood Roots of Adult Happiness.* New York: Ballantine Books.

65. a) Small, S. (1992) *The Teen Assessment Project* Madison, WI: Department of Child & Family Studies, University of Wisconsin-Madison; b) Institute for Social Research (2006) *Men, Women and Children after 9–11.* Ann Arbor, MI: University of Michigan.

66. Petersen, W. (1990) Malthus: The Reactionary Reformer. *The American Scholar* Spring: 275–282.

67. Rose, S. (2005) *The Future of the Brain.* New York: Oxford University Press, pp. 6, 186.

68. Sherraden, M. (1990) *Individual Developmental Accounts.* Washington, DC: Corp. for Enterprise Development.

CHAPTER 11. EMERGING ADULTHOOD

1. de Tocqueville, A.(1969) *Democracy in America, 1840.* Mayer, J. P. (Ed.) *Democracy in America.* Garden City, NY: Doubleday.

2. Robbins, A. & Wilner, A. (2001) *Quarterlife Crisis.* New York: Tarcher/Putnam.

3. Arnett, J.J. (2004) *Emerging Adulthood.* New York: Oxford University Press, p. 15.

4. Wuthnow, R. (2007) *After the Baby Boomers.* Princeton, NJ: Princeton University Press.

5. a) Sax, L. (2006) What's Happening to Boys? *Washington Post* March 31, p. A19; b) Shaffer, S.M. (2004) *Mom, Can I Move Back in with You?* New York: Penguin; c) Furman, E. (2005) *Boomerang Nation.* New York: Fireside.

6. 60 Minutes (2005) *The Echo Boomers.* New York: CBS. Sept. 4.

7. a) Quindlan, A. (2006) The Face in the Crowd. *Newsweek* March 20, p. 80; b) Howe, N., et al (2006) *Millennials and the Pop Culture.* Great Falls, VA: LifeCourse Associates; c) Dodes, R. (2006) The 'Me' Mother's Day. *Wall Street Journal* May 13, p.1; d) Howe, N., et al (2000) *Millennials Rising.* New York: Random House, p. 76; e) Twenge, J.M. (2006) *Generation Me.* New York: Free Press, p. 6.

8. a) Howe, N., et al (2000) *Millennials Rising.* New York: Random House; b) Toppe, C. (2006) *The National Volunteer Index.* Washington, DC: Points of Light. c) Winograd, M. & Hais, M. (2008) *Millennial Makeover.* Piscataway, NJ: Rutgers University Press; d) Twenge, J.M. (2006) *Generation Me.* New York: Free Press, pp. 5, 21.

9. a) Reynolds, John, et al (2006) Have Adolescents Become Too Ambitious? *Social Problems* 53 (2): 186–206; b) Kadison, R. (2004) The Mental Health Crisis. *Chronicle of Higher Education* December 10; c) American College Health Association (2007) *Healthy Campus 2010.* Baltimore, MD: Author.

10. Fitzsimmons, W., et al (2000) Time Out or Burn Out for the Next Generation. *New York Times* December 6.

11. Levine, M. (2005) *Ready or Not, Here Life Comes.* New York: Simon & Schuster.

12. Schlegel, A. & Barry, III, H. (1991) *Adolescence.* New York: Free Press.

13. Zimring, F.E. (1982) *The Changing Legal World of Adolescence.* New York: Free Press.

14. a) Sandefur, G., et al (2005) Higher Education Versus Single Motherhood. In Settersten Jr., R.A., et al (Ed.) *On the Frontier of Adulthood.* Chicago: University of Chicago Press; b) Arnett, J.J. (2004) *Emerging Adulthood.* New York: Oxford University Press.

15. Settersten Jr., R.A., et al (Eds.) (2005) *On the Frontier of Adulthood.* Chicago: University of Chicago Press.

16. Schoeni, R. & Ross, K. (2005) Family Support during the Transition to Adulthood. In Settersten Jr., R.A., et al (Eds.) (2005) *On the Frontier of Adulthood.* Chicago: University of Chicago Press.

17. a) Thornton, A., et al (2002) *Determinants of Marriage and Childbearing Attitudes.* Ann Arbor, MI: Institute for Social Research, University of Michigan; b) Fussell, E. & Gauthier, A. (2005) Women Moving into Adulthood. In Settersten Jr., R.A., et al (Ed.) *On the Frontier of Adulthood.* Chicago: University of Chicago Press.

18. a) Thornton, A. & Young-DeMarco, L. (2001) Four Decades of Trends in Attitudes Toward Family Issues in the United States. *Journal of Marriage and the Family* 63 (4): 1009–1037; b) Schulenberg, J.E., et al (2004) Taking Hold of Some Kind of Life. *Development and Psychopathology* 16: 1119–1140.

19. Csikszentmihalyi, M. & Schneider, B. (2000) *Becoming Adult.* New York: Basic Books, pp. 213, 228.

20. Ibid, pp. 218, 221–222.

21. a) James, W. (1890) *Principles of Psychology.* New York: Holt; b) Csikszentmihalyi, M. & Schneider, B. (2000) *Becoming Adult.* New York: Basic Books, p. 236.

22. Levine, M. (2005) *Ready or Not, Here Life Comes.* New York: Simon & Schuster.

23. Csikszentmihalyi, M. & Schneider, B. (2000) *Becoming Adult.* New York: Basic Books, p. 224.

24. Arnett, J.J. (2004) *Emerging Adulthood.* New York: Oxford University Press, pp. 94–95, 116.

25. Schulenberg, J. (2004). Taking Hold of Some Kind of Life. *Development and Psychopathology* 16: 1119–1140.

26. Schulenberg, J., et al (2005) Early Adult Transitions and Their Relation to Well-Being and Substance Use. In Settersten Jr., R.A., et al (Eds.) *On the Frontier of Adulthood.* Chicago, IL: University of Chicago Press.

27. Barber, B.L., et al (2001) Whatever Happened to the Jock, the Brain, and the Princess? *Journal of Adolescent Research* 16: 429–455.

28. Kerckhoff, A.C. (2002) The Transition from School to Work. In Mortimor, J.T. & Larson, R.W. (Eds.) *The Changing Adolescent Experience.* New York: Cambridge University Press, p. 70.

29. Kids Count 2004 Data Book Online. Annie E. Casey Foundation Analysis of the U.S. Census Bureau's 2002 American Community Survey.

30. James, W. (1910) The Moral Equivalent of War. *McClure's Magazine,* August, pp. 463–468.

31. Erikson, E. (1968) *Identity: Youth and Crisis.* New York: W.W. Norton, pp. 156–158.

32. a) The Council for Excellence in Government (2002) *Young Americans' Call to Public Service.* Washington, DC: Author; b) The USA Freedom Corps. 1600 Pennsylvania Avenue NW, Washington, DC 20500.

33. Youth Service America. 1101 15th Street, Suite 200, Washington, DC 20005.

34. International Association for National Youth Service. Innovations in Civic Participation, 1776 Massachusetts Avenue, NW, Suite 201, Washington, DC 20036.

CHAPTER 12. PARENTHOOD AS A DEVELOPMENTAL STAGE IN LIFE

1. St. Petersburg Times, May 2, 2005, p. 9A.

2. Lino, M. (2005) *Expenditures on Children by Families, 2004*. Miscellaneous Publication. No. 1528–2004. Washington, DC: U.S. Department of Agriculture, Center for Nutrition Policy and Promotion.

3. Thomas, R., et al (2005) Strengthening Parent-Child Relationships: The Reflective Dialogue Parent Education Design. *Zero to Three* 26 (1): 27–34.

4. a) Benedek, T. (1959) Parenthood as a Developmental Phase *Journal of the American Psychoanalytic Association* 7: 389–417; b) Anthony, E.J. & Benedek, T. (Eds.) (1970) *Parenthood*. Boston, MA: Little, Brown; c) Ruddick, W. (1979) Parents and Life Prospects. In O'Neill, O. & Ruddick, W. (Eds.) *Having Children*. New York: Oxford University Press, pp. 124–137.

5. a) Newberger, C.M. (1977) Parental Conceptions of Children and Childrearing. Doctoral Dissertation. Cambridge, MA: Harvard University; b) Newberger, C.M. (1980) The Cognitive Structure of Parenthood. In Selman R. & Yando, R., (Eds.) *New Directions For Child Development, Number 7, Clinical-developmental Psychology*. San Francisco: Jossey-Bass, pp. 45–67; c) Newberger, C.M. & Cook, S.J. (1983) Parental Awareness and Child Abuse and Neglect. *American Journal of Orthopsychiatry* 53: 512–524; d) Newberger, C.M. & White, K.M. (1989) Cognitive Foundations for Parental Care. In: Cicchetti, D. & Carlson, V. (Eds.) *Child Maltreatment*. Cambridge University Press, pp. 302–316.

6. Mitchell, J.J. (1998) *The Natural Limitations of Youth*. London: Ablex Publishing Company, pp. xii-xiv.

7. Cohen, S. & Taub, N. (1988) *Reproductive Laws for the 1990s*. Clifton, NJ: Humana, p. 5.

8. Skinner v. Oklahoma *exrel*. Williamson, 316 U.S. 535 (1942).

9. Luker, K. (1996) *Dubious Conceptions*. Cambridge, MA: Harvard University Press, pp. 15–16, 131.

10. Ruddick, S. (1993) Procreative Choice for Adolescent Women. In Lawson, A. & Rhode, D.L. (Eds.) *The Politics of Pregnancy*. New Haven, CT: Yale University Press, p.138.

11. a) Legal Information Institute. *Mariage Laws of the Fifty States, District of Columbia and Puerto Rico*. Ithaca, NY: Cornell Law School; b) *39 American Jurisprudence*, Parent and Child, p. 704, sec. 64.

12. Rude-Antoine, E. (2005) *Forced Marriages in Council of Europe Member States*. Strasbourg, France: Directorate General of Human Rights.

13. Zimring, F.E. (2005) *American Juvenile Justice*. New York: Oxford University Press, p. 127.

14. Ibid, p. 130.

15. Title XX of the Public Health Service Act: Adolescent Family Life Demonstration Projects. *Federal Register* June 1, 2006, 71 (105): 31897–31906.

PART 4. THE DYNAMICS OF ADOLESCENT PARENTHOOD

1. Mill, J.S. (1859) On Liberty. In Hutchins, R.M. (Ed.) (1952) *Great Books of the Western World, Volume 43*. Chicago, IL: University of Chicago Press, p. 318.

CHAPTER 13. CHOOSING TO BE AN ADOLESCENT PARENT

1. Lerman, E. (1997) *Teen Moms*. Buena Park, CA: Morning Glory Press, pp. 142, 147.

2. Upchurch, D.M. & McCarthy, J. (1990) The Timing of a First Birth and High School Completion. *American Sociological Review* 55:224–234.

3. a) Becker, G. (1992) *The Economic Way Of Looking At Life*. Department of Economics. Chicago, IL: University of Chicago, pp. 46, 42; b) Simon, H. (1996) *Models of My Life*. Cambridge, MA: MIT Press.

4. Gladwell, M. (2005) *Blink*. Boston: Little Brown.

5. Mauldon, J. (2003) Families Started by Teenagers. In Mason, M., et al (Eds.) *All Our Families, Second Edition*. New York: Oxford University Press, p. 43.

6. a) Ibid, p. 48; b) Montgomery, K.S. (2001) Planned Adolescent Pregnancy. *Issues in Comprehensive Pediatric Nursing* 24: 19–29.

7. Rosengard, C., et al (2006) Concepts of the Advantages and Disadvantages of Teenage Childbearing among Pregnant Adolescents: A Qualitative Analysis. *Pediatrics* 118 (2): 503–510.

8. Males, M. (2006) The Ugly Eugenics of "Teen Pregnancy Prevention". *Youth Today* November, p. 18.

9. Edin, K. & Kefalas, M. (2005) *Promises I Can Keep*. Berkeley, CA: University of California Press.

10. De Parle, J. (2004) Raising Kevion. *New York Times Magazine* August 22, pp. 26–53.

11. Moynihan, D. P. (1993) Defining Deviancy Down. *The American Scholar* Winter: 17–30.

12. Horowitz, R. (1995) *Teen Mothers*. Chicago: University of Chicago Press, p. 259.

13. Abrahamse, A. (1988) Teenagers Consider Single Parenthood. *Family Planning Perspectives* 20: 13–18.

14. Williams, L.B. & Pratt, W.F. (1990) *Wanted and Unwanted Childbearing in the United States, 1973–1988*. Hyattsville, MD: National Center for health Statistics, p. 5, Table 4.

15. Horowitz, R. (1995) *Teen Mothers*. Chicago: University of Chicago Press, p. 183.

16. Bingenheimer, J.B., et al (2005) Firearm Violence Exposure and Serious Violent Behavior. *Science* 308 (27): 1323–1326.

17. Edin, K. & Kefalas, M. (2005) *Promises I Can Keep*. Berkeley, CA: University of California Press.

18. Ibid, pp. 10, 7–8.

19. Rosengard, C., et al (2005) Psychosocial Correlates of Adolescent Males' Pregnancy Intention. *Pediatrics* 116 (3): e414–e419.

20. Lindsay, J.W. (1989) *Parents, Pregnant Teens and the Adoption Option*. Buena Park, CA: Morning Glory Press.

21. Stout, M. (2000) *The Feel Good Curriculum*. Cambridge, MA: Perseus Books, p. 119.

22. De Parle, J. (2004) Raising Kevion. *New York Times Magazine* August 22, pp. 26–53.

23. Irvine, W.B. (2005) *On Desire*. New York: Oxford University Press.

24. a) Eigsti, I., et al (2006). Predictive Cognitive Control from Preschool to Late Adolescence and Young Adulthood; b) Seligman, M.E.P. & Duckworth, A.L. (2005) Self-Discipline Outdoes IQ in Predicting Procrastination. *Psychological Science* 17 (6): 478–484; c) Tice, D.M. & Baumeister, R.F. (1997) Longitudinal Study of Procrastination, Performance, Stress, and Health. *Psychological Science* 8 (6): 454–458.

25. *Interfaith Hospitality Network Newsletter*. Madison, WI: Interfaith Hospitality Network, Spring, 2006

26. a) de Bruin, W.B., et al (2007) Can Adolescents Predict Significant Life Events? *Journal of Adolescent Health* 41 (2): 208–210; b) Joiner, W. (2006) I Hid My Pregnancy. *Seventeen* December, pp. 104–106.

27. a) Flach, F. (2002) *The Secret Strength of Depression*. Long Island City, NY: Hatherleigh Press, p.; b) Tavris, C. & Aronson, E. (2007) *Mistakes Were Made (But Not by Me)*. New York: Harcourt.

28. a) Waller, M.W., et al (2006) Gender Differences in Associations Between Depressive Symptoms and Patterns of Substance Use and Risky Sexual Behavior. *Archives of Women's Mental Health* 9 (3): 139–150; b) Lehrer, J.A., et al (2006) Depressive Symptomatology as a Longitudinal Predictor of Sexual Risk Behavior. *Journal of Adolescent Health* 38 (2): 109; c) Furstenberg, Jr., F.F., et al (1990) The Children of Teenage Mothers. *Family Planning Perspectives* 22:54–61; d) Barnet, B. et al (2008) Double Jeopardy. *Archives of Pediatrics and Adolescent Medicine* 162 (3): 246–252.

29. a) Siegel, D.J. (1999) *The Developing Mind*. New York: The Guilford Press, pp. 119–120; b) McCart, M., et al (2007) Do Urban Adolescents Become Desensitized to Community Violence? *American Journal of Orthopsychiatry* 77: (3): 434–442; c) Kenney, J.W., et al (1997) Ethnic Differences in Childhood and Adolescent Sexual Abuse and Teenage Pregnancy. *Journal of Adolescent Health* 21: 3–4; d) Leiderman, S. (2007) *Adolescent Pregnancy*. Bala Cynwyd, PA: Center for Assessment and Policy Development.

30. Ross, G.R. (1994) *Treating Adolescent Substance Abuse*. Boston: Allyn & Bacon, p. 26.

31. Ibid, p. xii.

32. Blos, P. (1962) *On Adolescence*. Glencoe, IL: Free Press.

33. a) Herzog, J.M. (1984) Boys Who Make Babies. In Sugar, Max (Ed.) *Adolescent Parenthood*. New York: SP Medical & Scientific Books, p. 71; b) Substance Use during Pregnancy. (2005) *The NSDUH Report*, June.

34. Ross, G.R. (1994) *Treating Adolescent Substance Abuse*. Boston: Allyn & Bacon, p. 188.

35. a) Wallerstein, G. (2003) *Mind, Stress, & Emotions*. Boston: Commonwealth Press, p. 172; b) Peele, S. (1985) *The Meaning of Addiction*. San Francisco: Jossey-Bass Publishers, p. 156.

36. Ross, G.R. (1994) *Treating Adolescent Substance Abuse*. Boston: Allyn & Bacon, p. 90.

CHAPTER 14. PROFILES OF ADOLESCENT PARENTS

1. Bernstein, L. & Sondheim, S. (1956, 1957) *Somewhere*. © Amberson Holdings LLC and Stephen Sondheim. New York: Leonard Bernstein Music Publishing Company LLC, Publisher.

2. a) Quay, H.C. (1981) Psychological Factors in Teenage Pregnancy. In Scott, K.G., et al (Eds.) *Teenage Parents and Their Offspring*. New York: Grune & Stratton, pp. 88–89; b) Fineman, J.A.B. & Smith, M.A. (1984) Object Ties and Interaction of the Infant and Adolescent Mother. In Sugar, M. (Ed.) *Adolescent Parenthood*. New York: SP Medical & Scientific Books; c) Merrick, E. (2001) *Reconceiving Black Adolescent Development*. Boulder, CO: Westview Press; d) Williams, C.W. (1991) *Black Teenage Mothers*. Lexington, MA: Lexington Books.

3. Sander, J. (1991) *Before Their Time*. New York: Harcourt Brace Jonvanovich.

4. Ibid.

5. Resnick, M.D., et al (1990) Characteristics of Unmarried Adolescent Mothers. *American Journal of Orthopsychiatry* 60: 577–584.

6. a) McLaughlin, S.D., et al (1986) The Effects of Sequencing of Marriage and First Birth during Adolescence. *Family Planning Perspectives* 18: 12–18; b) Weeks, J.R. (1976) *Teenage Marriages*. Westpoint, CT: Greenwood; c) Glick, P. & Norton, A. (1977) *Marrying, Divorcing and Living Together in the U.S. Today*. Washington, DC: Population Reference Bureau, October.

7. Julia S. (2005) Next Generation. *Boulder Weekly* August 18.

8. Underwood, M.K., et al (1996) Childhood Peer Sociometric Status and Aggression as Predictors of Adolescent Childbearing. *Journal of Research on Adolescence* 6: 201–223.

9. LeBlanc, A.N. (2003) *Random Family*. New York: Scribner.

10. Merkin, D. (2005) Passion and the Prisoner. *New York Times Magazine*, August 28, pp. 9–10.

11. DeParle, J. (2004) *American Dream*. New York: Viking, pp. 5–6, 338.

12. a) Marsiglio, W. (1994) Young Nonresident Biological Fathers. *Marriage & Family Review* 20 (3/4): 325–348; b) Weinman, M.L., et al (2002) Young Fathers. *Child and Adolescent Social Work Journal* 19 (6): 437–453.

13. a) Rosengard, C., et al (2005) Psychosocial Correlates of Adolescent Males' Pregnancy Intention. *Pediatrics* 116: e414–e419; b) Simons, R.L., et al (1991) Parenting Factors, Social Skills, and Value Commitments as Precursors to School Failure. *Journal of Youth and Adolescence* 20 (6): 645–664; c) Whitbeck, L.B. (1987) Modeling Efficacy. *Journal of Early Adolescence* 7 (2): 165–177.

14. a) Sonenstein, F.L., et al (1993) Paternity Risk among Adolescent Males. In Lerman & T.J. Ooms, R.I. (Eds.) *Young Unwed Fathers*. Philadelphia, PA: Temple University Press, pp. 99–116; b) Parikh, S.S. (2005) The Other Parent. *Praxis* 5: 1–21; c) Landry, D.J. & Forest, J.D. (1995) How Old Are U.S. fathers? *Family Planning Perspectives* 27: 159–165; d) Lerman, R.I. (1993) A National Profile of Unwed Fathers. In Lerman, R.I. & Ooms, T.J. (Eds.) *Young Unwed Fathers*. Philadelphia: Temple University Press, pp. 27–51.

15. Allen, W.D. & Doherty, W.J. (2004) "Being There." *The Prevention Researcher* 11 (4): 6–9.

16. Nilsson, K.W., et al (2006) Role of Monoamine Oxidase in Male Adolescent Criminal Activity. *Biological Psychiatry* 59 (2): 121–7.

17. a) Mazza, C. (2002) Young Dads. *Adolescence* 37: 681–693; b) Carlson, Marcia J. (2004) Involvement by Young, Unmarried Fathers Before and After Their Baby's Birth. *The Prevention Researcher* 11 (4): 14–17.

18. Teenadvice.about.com.

CHAPTER 15. THE IMPACT OF PARENTHOOD ON ADOLESCENTS

1. Roberts, D. (1997) *Killing the Black Body*. New York: Vintage Books, p. 3.

2. Hofferth, S.L. (Ed.) (1987) *Risking the Future*. Washington, DC: National Academy Press, pp. 2, 7, 138.

3. Chisholm, J.S. (1999) *Death, Hope and Sex*. Cambridge, UK: Cambridge University Press, p. 237.

4. Healthy Teen Network. 1501 St. Paul Street, Suite 124, Baltimore, MD.

5. Kandel, D.B. & Raveis, V.H. (1989) Cessation of Illicit Drug Use in Young Adulthood. *Archives of General Psychiatry* 46: 109–121.

6. Kinsley, C.H. & Lambert, K.G. (2005) The Maternal Brain. *Scientific American* 294 (1): 72–79.

7. Bowen, R. (2007) Oxytocin. The Hypothalamus and Pituitary Gland. Fort Collins: Colorado State University.

8. Science Says (2006) Teens' Attitudes toward Pregnancy and Childbearing, 1988–2002. *Putting What Works To Work. Number 21, March*. Washington, DC: National Campaign To Prevent Teen Pregnancy.

9. a) SmithBattle, L. (2005) Viewpoint: Examining Assumptions About Teen Mothers. *American Journal of Nursing* 105 (4): 13; b) Lerman, E. (1997) *Teen Moms*. Buena Park, CA: Morning Glory Press, p. 133.

10. 24. Catherine Z. (2006) *Resilience in Children Conference*. New York: New York Academy of Sciences.

11. a) Werner, E.E. & Smith, R.S. (1992) *Vulnerable but Invincible*. New York: McGraw-Hill; b) 25. Hauser, S. & Allen, J. (2007) Overcoming Adversity in Adolescence. *Psychoanalytic Inquiry* January. Mahwah, NJ: Analytic Press. Milne, D. (2007) Some Troubled Teens Tap Well of Resilience. *Psychiatric News* May 18, p. 33.

12. Maton, K.I., et al (2004) *Investing in Children, Youth, Families, and Communities*. Washington, DC: American Psychological Association, p. 120.

13. Whitman, T.L., et al (2001) *Interwoven Lives*. Mahwah, NJ: Lawrence Erlbaum, p. 191.

14. Thomas, R.A. (2001) *Academic Success*. Alameda, CA: Aliant University. Presented to The African-American Success Foundation, November 3.

15. Singer, B., et al (1998) Linking Life Histories and Mental Health. In Raftery, A. (Ed.) *Sociological Methodology*. Washington, DC: American Sociological Association.

16. Coley, R.L. & Chase-Lansdale, P.L. (1998) Adolescent Pregnancy. *American Psychologist* 53 (2): 152–166.

17. Whitman, T.L., et al (2001) *Interwoven Lives*. Mahwah, NJ: Lawrence Erlbaum, pp. 46, 94.

18. a) Gunnar, M.R. (2007) Stress Effects on the Developing Brain. In Romer, D. & Walker, E.F. (Eds.) *Adolescent Psychopathology and the Developing Brain*. New York: Oxford University Press, pp. 127–143; b) Yehuda, R. & McEwen, B. (Eds.) (2005) *Behavioral Stress Response, Volume 784*. New York: New York Academy of Sciences.

19. a) Lynch, J.W., et al (1997) Cumulative Impact of Sustained Economic Hardship. *New England Journal of Medicine* 337: 1889–1895; b) Felitti, V.B., et al (1998) Relationship of Child Abuse and Household Dysfunction to Leading Causes of Death in Adults. *American Journal of Preventive Medicine* 14: 245–258; c) Wallerstein, G. (2003) *Mind, Stress, & Emotions*. Boston: Commonwealth Press, p. 70. d) Gunnar, M.R. & Donzella, B. (2002) Social Regulation and the Cortisol Levels in Early Human Development. *Psychoneuroendocrinology* 27: 199–220.

20. a) McEwen, B. (2002) *The End of Stress As We Know It*. Washington, DC: Joseph Henry Press, pp. 85, 95, 116, 119; b) Vines, A.I., et al (2007) Associations of Abdominal Fat with Perceived Racism and Passive Emotional Responses to Racism in African American Women. *American Journal of Public Health* 997 (3): 526–530.

21. Williams, L.A. (2005) *Broken China*. New York: Simon & Schuster.

22. Matsuhashi, Y. & Felice, M.E. (1991) Adolescent Body Image during Pregnancy. *Journal of Adolescent Health* 12: 313–315.

23. Borkowski, J.G., et al (2002) The Adolescent as Parent. In Borkowski, J.G., et al (Eds.) *Parenting and the Child's World*. Mahwah, NJ: Lawrence Erlbaum.

24. Kimball, C. (2004) Teen Fathers. *The Prevention Researcher* 11 (4): 3–5.

25. Schlegel, A. & Barry, III, H. (1991) *Adolescence*. New York: Free Press.

26. a) Kaplan, A. (1997) Teen Parents and Welfare Reform Policy. *Welfare Information Network* 1 (3); b) Furstenberg, Jr., F.F., et al (1997) Adolescent Mothers in Later Life. New York: Cambridge University Press; c) Maynard, R.A. (Ed.) *Kids having Kids*. Washington, DC: The Urban Institute Press.

27. Shapiro, D.L. & Marcy, H.M. (2002) *Knocking on the Door*. Chicago, IL: Center for Impact Research.

28. a) Miller, B.C. & Moore, K.A. (1990) Adolescent Sexual Behavior, Pregnancy, and Parenting. *Journal of Marriage and the Family* 52 (4): 1025–1044. b) Testa, M.F. (1992) Racial and Ethnic Variation in the Early Life Course of Adolescent Welfare Mothers. In Rosenheim, MK. & Testa, MF. (Eds.) *Early Parenthood and Coming of Age in the 1990s*. New Brunswick, NJ: Rutgers University Press.

29. Maynard, R.A. (1997) *Kids Having Kids*. New York: Robin Hood Foundation, p. 20.

30. a) Whitman, T.L., et al (2001) *Interwoven Lives*. Mahwah, NJ: Lawrence Erlbaum, pp. 83–86, 216, 178; b) Coley, R.C. & Chase-Lansdale, P.L. (2004) Adolescent Pregnancy and Parenthood. *American Psychologist* 53: 152.

31. a) Landry, D.J. & Forest, J.D. (1995) How Old Are U.S. Fathers? *Family Planning Perspectives* 27: 159–165; b) Lerman, R.I. (1993) A National Profile of Unwed Fathers. In Lerman, R.I. & Ooms, T.J. (Eds.) *Young Unwed Fathers*. Philadelphia: Temple University Press, pp. 27–51; b) Bronte-Tinkew, J., et al (2007) *Men's Pregnancy Intentions and Prenatal Behaviors*. Research Brief; Publication #2007–18. Washington, DC: Child Trends.

32. Thornberry, T.P., et al (2004) Teenage Fatherhood and Involvement in Delinquent Behavior. *The Prevention Researcher* 11 (4): 10–13.

33. Maynard, R.A. (1997) *Kids Having Kids*. New York: Robin Hood Foundation.

34. a) Kiselica, M.S. (1995) *Multicultural Counseling with Teenage Fathers*. Thousand Oaks, CA: Sage Publications; b) Lowenthal, B. & Lowenthal R. (1997) Teenage Parenting. *Childhood Education* 74: 29–32.

CHAPTER 16. THE IMPACT OF ADOLESCENT PARENTHOOD ON CHILDREN

1. Schorr, L.B. & Schorr, D. (1988) *Within Our Reach*.New York: Anchor Press, Doubleday, p. 15.

2. a) Furstenberg, Jr., F.F., et al (1999) *Managing to Make It*. Chicago, IL: University of Chicago Press, p. 216; b) Furstenberg, Jr., F.F., et al (1990) The Children of Adolescent Mothers. *Family Planning Perspectives* 22:54–61; c) Maynard, R. (1996) *Kids Having Kids*. New York: The Robin Hood Foundation; d) Jaffee, S., et al (2001) Why Are Children Born to Teen Mothers at Risk for Adverse Outcomes in Young Adulthood? *Development and Psychopathology* 13: 377–97; e) Levine, J.A., et al (2001) Academic and Behavioral Outcomes among Children of Young Mothers. *Journal of Marriage and the Family* 63: 355–69.

3. a) Turley, R.N.L. (2003) Are Children of Young Mothers Disadvantaged Because of their Mother's Age or Family Background? *Child Development* 74: 465–74; b) Geronimus, A., et al (1994) Does Young Maternal Age Adversely Affect Child Development? *Population and Development Review* 20 (3): 585–602.

4. a) Jaffee, S., et al (2001) Why Are Children Born to Teen Mothers at Risk for Adverse Outcomes in Young Adulthood? *Development and Psychopathology* 13: *377–97, Table 3*; b) Terry-Humen, E., et al (2005) *Playing Catch-Up*. Washington, DC: National Campaign to Prevent Teen Pregnancy; c) Levine, J.A., et al (2001) Academic and Behavioral Outcomes among Children of Young Mothers. *Journal of Marriage and the Family* 63: 355–69.

5. a) Chamberlain, D. (1998) *The Mind of Your Newborn Baby*. Berkeley, CA: North Atlantic Books; b) Nathanielsz, P.W. (1999) *Life in the Womb*. Ithaca, NY: Promethean Press.

6. a) East, P.L. & Felice, M.E. (1996) *Adolescent Pregnancy and Parenting*. Mahway, NJ: Lawrence Erlbaum; b) Maynard, R.A. (1997) *Kids Having Kids*. New York: Robin Hood Foundation; c) Bergvall, N., et al (2006) Birth Characteristics and Risk of Low Intellectual Perfor-

mance in Early Adulthood. *Pediatrics* 117: 714–721; c) Scholl, T.O., et al (1989) Association between Low Gynaecological Age and Preterm Birth. *Paediatric and Perinatal Epidemiology* 3: 357–366; d) Perry, R.L, et al (1996) Pregnancy in Early Adolescence. *The Journal of Maternal-Fetal Medicine* 5: 333–339; e) Overpeck, M.D., et al (1998) Risk factors for Infant Homicide in the United States. *New England Journal of Medicine* 339 (17): 1211–17.

7. a) Volkow, N.D. (2005) Drug-Related Damage that Begins Before Birth. *NIDA Notes* 19 (4): 3; b) Huizink, A.C. & Mulder, E.J.H (2006) Maternal Smoking, Drinking or Cannabis Use during Pregnancy and Neurobehavioral and Cognitive Functioning in Human Offspring. *Neuroscience and Biobehavioral Reviews* 30: 24–41; c) Office of Justice Programs (1997) *New Survey Documents Dramatic Rise in Drug Courts*. Washington, DC: U.S. Department of Justice; d) Janovsky, E. & Kalotra, C. (2003) *Information Relevant to Female Participants in Drug Courts*. Washington, DC: Bureau of Justice Assistance Drug Court Clearinghouse.

8. Journal Watch (2008) Prevention of Perinatal HIV Infection. *New England Journal of Medicine* February 27.

9. a) Whitman, T. L., et al (2001) *Interwoven Lives*. Mahwah, NJ: Lawrence Erlbaum; b) Lounds, J.J., et al (2005) Adolescent Parenting and Attachment. *Parenting: Science and Practice* 5 (1): 91–118.

10. a) Whitman, T.L., et al (2001) *Interwoven Lives*. Mahwah, NJ: Lawrence Erlbaum Associates, Inc., p. 168; b) Fries, Alison B., et al (2005) Early Experience in Humans Is Associated with Changes in Neuropeptides Critical for Regulating Social Behavior. *Proceedings of the National Academy of Sciences* 102 (47): 17237–17240.

11. a) George, R.M. & Lee, B.G. (1999) Poverty, Early Child Bearing, and Child Maltreatment. *Children and Youth Services Review* 21 (9/10): 755–780; b) Drake, B. & Pandley, S. (1996) Understanding the Relationship between Neighborhood Poverty and Specific Types of Child Maltreatment. *Child Abuse and Neglect* 20 (11): 1003–1018.

12. a) Lenthal, J. (1989) *Are Children of Teenage Mothers at Increased Risk of Child Maltreatment?* New Haven, CT: Yale University Department of Pediatrics; b) Goerge, R.M. & Lee, B.G. (1999) Poverty, Early Child Bearing, and Child Maltreatment. *Children and Youth Services Review* 21 (9/10): 755–780; c) Bolton, F.G. (1990) The Risk of Child Maltreatment in Adolescent Parenting. *Advances in Adolescent Mental Health* 4: 223–237.

13. Goerge, R.M, et al (2007) Effects of Early Childbearing on Child Maltreatment and Placement into Foster Care. In Maynard, R. & Hoffman, S. (Eds.) *Kids Having Kids: Revised Edition*. Washington, DC: Urban Institute Press.

14. Ellis, B.J. & Bjorklund, D.F. (Eds.) (2005) *Origins of the Social Mind*. New York: Guilford Press.

15. Whitman, Thomas L., et al (2001) *Interwoven Lives*. Mahwah, NJ: Lawrence Erlbaum, pp. 128, 147.

16. Terry-Humen, E., et al (2005) *Playing Catch-Up*. Washington, DC: Campaign to Prevent Teen Pregnancy.

17. Lenthal, J. (1989) *Are Children of Teenage Mothers at Increased Risk of Child Maltreatment?* Research Grant Status Report (NCCAN Grant No. 90–CA-1374). New Haven, CT: Yale University Department of Pediatrics.

18. Ryan, S., et al (2004). *Science Says: The Relationship between Teenage Motherhood and Marriage*. Washington, DC: National Campaign to Prevent Teen Pregnancy.

19. Schnitzer, P.G. & Ewigman, B.G. (2005) Child Deaths from Inflicted Injuries. *Pediatrics* 116 (5): e687–e693.

20. a) Horowitz, S. McCue, et al (1991) Intergenerational Transmission of School-Age Parenthood. *Family Planning Perspectives* 23: 168–172. b) Bolton, F.G., Jr. (1983) *When Bonding Fails*. Beverly Hills, CA: Sage, pp. 150–155.

21. Hoffman, S.D. & Scher, L.S. (2007) Children of Early Childbearers as Young Adults-Updated Estimates. In Maynard, R.A. & Hoffman, S. (Eds.) *Kids Having Kids: Revised Edition*, Washington, DC: Urban Institute Press.

22. a) Porgosky, G., et al (2003) The Delinquency of Children Born to Young Mothers. *Criminology* 41 (4): 1249–1286; b) Scher, L.S. & Hoffman, S.D. (2007) Incarceration-Related Costs of Early Childbearing. In Maynard, R.A. & Hoffman, S.D. (Eds) *Kids Having Kids: Revised Edition.* Washington, DC: The Urban Institute Press.

23. Carothers, S.S., et al (2005) Religiosity and the Socioemotional Adjustment of Adolescent Mothers and their Children. *Journal of Family Psychology* 19 (2): 263–275.

24. a) Gelles, R.J. (1989) Child Abuse and Violence in Single-Parent Families. *American Journal of Orthopsychiatry* 59: 492–501; b) Hare, N. & Hare, J. (1984) *The Endangered Black Family.* San Francisco, CA: Black Think Tank; c) Davidson, N. (1990) Life without Fathers. *Policy Review* 51: 40–41. d) Rose, H. & Mc Clain, P.D. (1990) *Race, Place, and Risk.* Albany, NY: State University of New York Press, p. 198.

25. a) Carlson, M.J. (2006) Family Structure, Father Involvement, and Adolescent Behavioral Outcomes. *Journal of Marriage and Family* 68 (1): 137–154; b) Marsiglio, W. (1995) Fatherhood Scholarship. In Marsiglio, W. (Ed.) *Fatherhood.* Thousand Oaks, CA: Sage Publications.

PART 5. FAMILIES

1. Moynihan, D.P. (1987) *Family and Nation.* New York: Harcourt Brace Jovanovich, pp. 188–189.

CHAPTER 17. THE FAMILIES OF ADOLESCENT PARENTS

1. Gibran, K. (1923) *The Prophet.* New York: Alfred A. Knopf.

2. a) Maccoby, E.E. (2002) Parenting Effects. In Borkowski, J.G., et al (Eds.) *Parenting and the Child's World.* Mahwah, NJ: Lawrence Erlbaum; b) Allis, C. David, et al (Eds.) *Epigenetics.* Cold Spring Harbor, NY: Cold Spring Harbor Laboratory Press; c) Aufseeser, D., et al (2006). *The Family Environment and Adolescent Well-Being.* Washington, D.C.: Child Trends; d) Hair, E., et al (2005). The Parent-Adolescent Relationship Scale. In Moore, K. & Lippman, L. (Eds.) *What Do Children Need to Flourish.* New York: Springer Science, pp. 183–202.

3. Schneider, C.E. (2006) Afterword: Elite Principles. In Wilson, R.F. (Ed.) *Reconceiving the Family.* New York: Cambridge University Press, p. 501.

4. Simons, R. L., et al (1991) Parenting Factors, Social Skills, and Value Commitments as Precursors to School Failure. *Journal of Youth and Adolescence* 20 (6): 645–664.

5. Resnick, Michael D., et al (1990) Characteristics of Unmarried Adolescent Mothers. *American Journal of Orthopsychiatry* 60: 577–584.

6. Larson, R. W. & Richards, M. H. (1994) Family Emotions. *Journal of Research on Adolescence* 4 (4): 567–583.

7. Hair, E., et al (2005) The Parent-adolescent Relationship Scale. In Moore, K. & Lippman, L. (Eds.) *What Do Children Need to Flourish.* New York: Springer Science, pp. 183–202.

8. Bronson, P. (2005) *Why Do I Love These People?* New York: Random House.

9. Ge, X., et al (1996a) Parenting Behaviors and the Occurrence and Co-Occurence of Adolescent Depressive Symptoms and Conduct Problems. *Developmental Psychology* 32 (4): 717–731.

10. a) Dodge, K.A. (2002) Mediation, Moderation, and Mechanism in How Parenting Affects Children's Aggressive Behavior. In Borkowski, J.G., et al (Eds.) *Parenting and the Child's World*. Mahwah, NJ: Lawrence Erlbaum; b) Guttman-Steinmetz, S. & Crowell, J.A. (2006) Attachment and Externalizing Disorders. *Journal of the American Academy of Child and Adolescent Psychiatry* 45 (4): 440–451.

11. Benedek, T. (1970) The Family as a Psychological Field. In Anthony, E.J. & Benedek, T. (Eds.) *Parenthood*. Boston: Little Brown, pp. 134–135.

12. Cummings, E.M., et al (2002) Interparental Relations as a Dimension of Parenting. In Borkowski, J.G., et al (Eds.) *Parenting and the Child's World*. Mahwah, NJ: Lawrence Erlbaum.

13. Rexford, E.N. (1966) *A Developmental Approach to Problems of Acting Out*. Monograph No.1 of the American Academy of Child Psychiatry. New York: International Universities Press, pp. 200–201

14. Bogan, Z. & Krohn, F. (2001) The Effects Absent Fathers Have on Female Development and College Attendance. *College Student Journal* 35 (4): 598.

15. Ellis, B.J., et al (2003) Does Father Absence Place Daughters at Special Risk for Early Sexual Activity and Teenage Pregnancy? *Child Development* 74 (3): 801–821.

16. a) Herrenkohl, E., et al (1998) The Relationship Between Early Maltreatment and Teenage Parenthood. *Journal of Adolescence* 21: 291–303; b) Kelley, B., et al (1997) *In the Wake of Child Maltreatment*. Washington, DC: Department of Justice, Office of Juvenile Justice and Delinquency Prevention; c) McFarlane, Judith (1991) Violence during Teen Pregnancy. In Levy, Barrie (Ed.) *Dating Violence*. Toronto, Canada: Publishers Group West, p. 141.

17. a) Moore, K.A., et al (1995) Welfare and Adolescent Sex. *Journal of Family and Economic Issues* 16: 207; b) Coley, R.L. & Chase-Lansdale, P.L. (1998) Adolescent Pregnancy and Parenthood. *American Psychologist* 53: 152; c) Leiderman, S. (2007) *Adolescent Pregnancy*. Bala Cynwyd, PA: Center for Assessment and Policy Development.

18. Kahn, Abby & Paluzzi, Pat (2007) *Understanding the Impact of Child Maltreatment and Family Violence on the Sexual, Reproductive, and Parenting Behaviors of Young Men*. Washington, DC: Healthy Teen Network.

19. Repetti, R.L., et al (2002) Risky Families. *Psychological Bulletin* 128 (2): 330–66.

20. Mincy, R.B. & Wiener, S.J. (1990) *A Mentor, Peer Group, Incentive Model for Helping Underclass Youth*. Washington. DC: Urban Institute; b)

21. a) Furstenberg, Jr., F.F., et al (1999) *Managing to Make It*. Chicago, IL: University of Chicago Press, p. 606; b) Amato, P.R. & Booth, A. (1997) *A Generation at Risk*. Cambridge, MA: Harvard Press, pp. 215–221.

22. Duncan, G.J. & Brooks-Gunn J. (Eds.) (1997) *Consequences of Growing Up Poor*. New York: Russell Sage Foundation, pp. 597, 601.

CHAPTER 18. THE IMPACT OF ADOLESCENT PARENTHOOD ON FAMILIES

1. Moynihan, D.P. (1987) *Family and Nation*. New York: Harcourt Brace Jovanovich, p. 173.

2. Lindsay, J.W. (1989) *Parents, Pregnant Teens and the Adoption Option*. Buena Park, CA: Morning Glory Press.

3. a) Analysis of data from Cycle 5 of the National Survey of Family Growth and the 1995 National Survey of Adolescent Males-New Cohort. Washington, DC: National Campaign to Prevent Teen Pregnancy; b) Putting What Works to Work (2003) Younger Siblings of Teen Parents. *Science Says 13*, November. Washington, DC: The National Campaign To Prevent Teen Pregnancy.

4. a) East, P.L., et al (1993) Sisters' and Girlfriends' Sexual and Childbearing Behavior. *Journal of Marriage and the Family* 55: 953–963; b) East, P. & Jacobson, L. (2001) The Younger Siblings of Teenage Mothers. *Developmental Psychology* 37 (2): 254–264.

5. East, P. (1996) The Younger Sisters of Childbearing Adolescents. *Child Development* 67: 267–282.

6. East, P. (1999) The First Teenage Pregnancy in the Family. *Journal of Marriage and the Family* 61: 306–319.

7. Goyer, A. (2007) *State Fact Sheets for Grandparents and Other Relatives Raising Children*. Washington, DC: American Association of Retired Persons.

8. Apfel, N.H. & Seitz, V. (1996) African-American Adolescent Mothers, their Mothers, and their Daughters. In Leadbeater, B.J.R. & Way, N. (Eds.) *Urban Girls*. New York: Cambridge University Press, pp. 486–506.

9. a) R1001. *Percent of Grandparents Responsible for their Grandchildren*. Data Set: 2004. Washington, DC: The United States Census Bureau, American Community Survey; b) Minkler, M. & Fuller-Thomson, E. (2000) Second Time around Parenting. *International Journal of Aging and Human Development* 50 (3): 185–200.

10. East, P. (1999) The First Teen Pregnancy In The Family. *Journal of Marriage and the Family* 61: 306–319.

11. a) Duncan, G.J. & Hoffman, S.D. (1990) Teenage Welfare Receipt and Subsequent Dependence Among Black Adolescent Mothers. *Family Planning Perspectives* 22: 16–20; b) Dunston, P.J., et al (1987) Black Adolescent Mothers. In Battle, S.F. (Ed.) *The Black Adolescent Parent*. New York: Haworth, p. 99; c) Wilson, M.N. & Tolson, T.F.J. (1988) Single Parenting in the Context of Three-generational Black Families. In Hetherington, E.M. & Arasteh, J. (Eds.) *The Impact of Divorce, Single Parenting, and Stepparenting on Children*. Hillsdale, NJ: Erlbaum; d) Franklin, D.L. (1992) Early Childbearing Patterns among African Americans. In Rosenheim, M.K. & Testa, M.F. (Eds.) *Early Parenthood and Coming of Age in the 1990s*. New Brunswick, NJ: Rutgers Press.

12. Children's Bureau (2000) Secretary's Report to Congress on Kinship Foster Care. Washington, DC: U.S. Department of Health and Human Services.

13. Smithgal, C., et al (2006) *Caring for their Children's Children*. Chicago, Illinois: Chapin Hall.

14. Chase-Lansdale, P.L., et al (1994) Young African-American Multigenerational Families in Poverty. *Child Development* 65: 374–393.

15. a) Emick, M.A. & Hayslip, B. Jr. (1996) Custodial Grandparenting. *International Journal of Aging and Human Development* 43: 135–154; b) Hayslip, B. Jr., et al (1998) Custodial Grandparenting and the Impact of Grandchildren with Problems. *Journal of Gerontology: Psychological Sciences* 53: S164–173; c) Whitley, D.M., et al (2001) Grandmothers Raising Grandchildren. *Health and Social Work* 26: 105–114; d) Minkler, M. & Fuller-Thomson, E. (1999) The Health of Grandparents Raising Grandchildren. *American Journal of Public Health* 89: 1384–1389.

16. a) Emick, M. & Hayslip, B.J.(1999) Custodial Gradparenting. *Journal of Aging and Human Development* 48 (1): 35–61; b) Minkler, M., et al (1997) *Archives of Family Medicine* 6

(5): 445–452; c) Fuller-Thomson, E. & Minkler, M. (2000) African-American Grandparents Raising Grandchildren. *Health and Social Work* 25 (2): 109–118.

17. a) Musil, C.M. (1998) Health, Stress, Coping, and Social Support in Grandmother Care-givers. *Health Care Women International* 19 (5): 441–455; b) Kelley, S.J., et al (1997) To Grandmother's House We Go . . . and Stay. *Journal of Gerontological Nursing* 23 (9): 12–20; c) Minkler, M., et al (1994) Raising Grandchildren from Crack-Cocaine Households. *American Journal of Orthopsychiatry* 64 (1): 20–29.

18. a) Minkler, M., et al (1992) The Physical and Emotional Health of Grandparents Rais-ing Grandchildren. *Gerontologist* 32 (6): 752–761; b) Warner, V., et al (1999) Grandparents, Parents, and Grandchildren at High Risk for Depression. *Journal of the American Academy of Child and Adolescent Psychiatry* 38 (3): 289–296.

19. Burnette, D. (1999) Physical and Emotional Well-Being of Custodial Grandparents in Latino Families. *American Journal of Orthopsychiatry* 69 (3): 305–318.

20. LeBlanc, A.N. (2003) *Random Family*. New York: Scribner, p. 388.

21. Johnson, N. (2006) Adults-Only Park Stands Firm against Soldier's Kids. *St. Petersburg Times* Feb. 25, p. 3B.

22. *Moore v. City of East Cleveland* 431 U.S. 494, 1977; *Troxel V. Granville* 530 U.S. 57 (2000) 137 Wash. 2d 1, 969 P.2d 21, 1976.

23. Stanton, A.M. (1998) Grandparents' Visitation Rights and Custody. *Child and Adoles-cent Psychiatric Clinics of North America* 7 (2): 409–422.

24. Wallace, G. (2004) *Relatives Caring For Children*. 35 John Street, West Hurley, NY. 845.496.0355.

25. Ibid, Title 15 of the General Obligations Law.

26. Washington S.H.B. 1281 & SHB 3139.

27. a) Miner, M. & Wallace, G. (1998) *The Dilemma of Kinship Care*. Albany, NY: Albany Law School, The Government Law Center; b) Mullen, F. & Einhorn, M. (2000) *The Effect of State TANF Choices on Grandparent-Headed Households*. Washington, DC: Public Policy Institute.

28. a) Green, R., et al (2001) *On their Own Terms*. Washington, DC: The Urban Institute; b) Sawisza, C. (2001) *Relative Caregiving*. Fort Lauderdale, Florida: Nova Southeastern Uni-versity, Children First Project.

29. a) Maine Statutes: *Me Rev Stat. Ann, tit. 18–A, p. 5. Parts One and Two*; b) SECTION 2. Subarticle 1, Article 11, Chapter 7, Title 20 of the 1976 South Carolina Code amended by adding: Section 2071540. 4.

30. Wilhelmus, M. (1998) Mediating Kinship Care. *Social Work* 43: 117–118.

31. Main, R., et al (2006) Trends in Service Receipt. *New Federalism, National Survey of America's Families. Series B, No. B-68*. Washington, DC: The Urban Institute.

32. Malm, K., et al (2001, October). *Running to Keep in Place*. Washington, DC: The Ur-ban Institute.

33. a) Conway, T. & Hutson, R.Q. (2007) *Is Kinship Care Good for Kids?* Washington, DC: Center for Law and Social Policy; b) Heger, R. & Scannapieco, M. (1995) From Family Duty to Family Policy. *Child Welfare* 74: 200.

34. Adoption and Safe Families Act of 1997; Public Law 105–89; Amendments to Title IV-B Subparts 1 and 2 and Title IV-E of the Social Security Act; State Automated Child Welfare Information System (SACWIS)

35. Hegar, R.L. (1999) Kinship Foster Care. In Hegar, R.L. & Scannapieco, M. (Eds.) *Kin-ship Foster Care*. New York: Oxford University Press, pp. 234–235.

36. a) Brooks, S. L. (2001). The Case for Adoption Alternatives. *Family Court Review* 39 (1): 43–57; b) Fact Sheet (2006) *Grandfamilies: Subsidized Guardianship Programs*. Wash-ington, DC: Generations United.

37. Hegar, R.L. & Scannapieco, M.(1995) From Family Duty to Family Policy. *Child Welfare* 74 (1): 200–216.

38. Mullen, F. & Einhorn, M. (2000). *The Effect of State TANF Choices on Grandparent-headed Households*. Washington, DC: Public Policy Institute.

39. Takas, M. & Hegar, R.L. (1999) The Case for Kinship Adoption Laws. In Hegar, R.L. & Scannapieco, M. (Eds.) *Kinship Foster Care*. New York: Oxford University Press, pp. 54–67.

40. Morgan, L.W. (1999) Fork It Over, Granny. *Divorce Litigation* July p. 129.

41. Wisconsin Statute 49.90 Liability of relatives; enforcement.

42. a) Champagne v. Passons, 95 Cal. App. 15, 272 P. 353 (3d Dist. 1928; Anonymous (1983–6), 39 Conn. Supp. 35, 467 A.2d 687 (Super. Ct. 1983); b) 718 So. 2d 1091 (Miss. 1998) Code 1972, § 93–5–23.

43. In re Marriage of Clay, 670 P.2d 31 (Colo. Ct. App. 1983).

44. Wulff v. Wulff, 243 Neb. 616, 500 N.W.2d 845 (1993).

45. Thompson v. Thompson, 94 Misc. 2d 911, 405 N.Y.S.2d 974 (Fam. Ct. 1978); (Purdy v. Purdy, 578 S.E.2d 30 (S.C. Ct. App. 2003).

46. a) The National Committee of Grandparents for Children's Rights. Stony Brook, NY: Stony Brook University School of Social Welfare; b) GrandFamilies of America. 6525 Fish Hatchery Road, Thurmont, MD 21788; c) Grandfamilies State Law and Policy Resource Center. <http://www.grandfamilies.org/>.

47. Personal communication.

PART 6. NEIGHBORHOODS AND COMMUNITIES

1. Benson, P.L. (2006) *All Kids Are Our Kids, Second Edition*. San Francisco, CA: Jossey-Bass, p.1.

CHAPTER 19. SOCIAL CLASS AND ADOLESCENT PARENTHOOD

1. Moynihan, D.P. (1986) *Family and Nation*. New York: Harcourt Brace, chapter 3.

2. a) Lareau, A. (2003) *Unequal Childhoods*. Berkeley: University of California Press, p. 256; b) Scott, J. & Leonhardt, D.L. (2005) Class in America. *New York Times* May 15, p. A1.

3. a) Kagan, J. (2006) *An Argument for Mind*. New Haven, CT: Yale University Press; b) Tilly, C. (1998) *Durable Inequality*. Berkeley, CA: University of California Press, p. 24; c) Barrett, M. & McIntosh, M.(1991) *The Anti-social Family*. London: Verso, pp. 43, 80.

4. Heckman, J.J. (2006) Catch 'em Young. *Wall Street Journal* January 10.

5. Weissbourd, R. (1996) *The Vulnerable Child*. Reading, MA: Addison-Wesley Publishing Company, p. 221.

6. a) Rouse, C., et al (2005) Introducing the Issue. *Future of Children* 15 (1): 5–13; b) Lareau, A. (2003) *Unequal Childhoods*. Berkeley, CA: University of California Press, p. 13.

7. a) Crosby, R.A. & Holtgrave, D.R. (2006) The Protective Value of Social Capital against Teen Pregnancy. *Journal of Adolescent Health* 38: 556–559; b) Lareau, A. (2003) *Unequal Childhoods*. Berkeley, CA: University of California Press, p. 256.

8. Scott, J. & Leonhardt, D.L. (2005) Class in America. *New York Times* May 15. A1.

9. Economic Mobility Project (2007) *Key Findings for the Economic Mobility of Families across Generations, Men and Women, Black and White Families*. Washington, DC: Pew Charitable Trusts.

10. Murray, C. (1988) The Coming of Custodial Democracy. *Commentary* 86: 19–24.

11. a) Epstein, W.M. (1993) *The Dilemma of American Social Welfare*. New Brunswick, NJ: Transaction, pp. 142–142, 146–147; b) Rank, M.R. (2004) *One Nation, Underprivileged*. New York: Oxford Press, pp. 179, 252; c) Newman, K.S. (2007) *The Missing Class*. Boston, MA: Beacon Press.

12. Dew-Becker, I. & Gordon, R.J. (2005) *Where Did the Productivity Growth Go?* London, UK: Centre for Economic Policy Research.

13. a) Glenn, J.C. & Gordon, T.J. (2006) Update on the State of the Future. *The Futurist* Jan-Feb; b) Piketty, T. & Saez, E. (2006) *The Evolution of Top Incomes, Paper 11955*. Cambridge, MA: Nat'l Bureau of Economic Research.

14. Housing and Household Economic Statistics Division (2006) *The Effects of Government Taxes and Transfers on Income and Poverty: 2004*. Washington, DC: U.S. Census Bureau.

15. Ibid.

16. a) Children's Defense Fund *(2006) The State of America's Children 2005*. Washington, DC: Children's Defense Fund; b) Rank, M.R. (2004) *One Nation, Underprivileged*. New York: Oxford University Press, pp. 25, 32; c) Woolf, S.H., et al (2006) The Rising Prevalence of Severe Poverty in America. *American Journal of Preventive Medicine* 31 (4): 332; d) Newman, K. & Chen, V.T. (2007) *The Missing Class*. Boston, MA: Beacon Press.

7. a) U.S. Census Bureau (2006) Current Population Survey, Housing and Household Economic Statistics. Washington, DC; b) Iceland, J. (2003) *Poverty in America*. Berkeley, CA: University of California Press, pp. 2, 144, 3; c) U.S. Census Bureau, Current Population Survey, 1981–2005. Annual Social and Economic Supplements.

18. Children's Defense Fund (2006) *The State of America's Children 2005*. Washington, DC: Author.

19. Federal Interagency Forum on Child and Family Statistics (2006) *America's Children in Brief*. Washington, DC: Office of Management and Budget.

20. a) Rank, M.R. (2004) *One Nation, Underprivileged*. New York: Oxford University Press, p. 5; b) Danziger, S.H. & Haveman, R.H. (Eds.) (2001) *Understanding Poverty*. New York: Russell Sage Foundation, pp. 6–8, 29; c) Ibid, p. 53; d) Iceland, J. (2003) *Poverty in America*. Berkeley, CA: University of California Press, p. 145.

21. Payne, R.K. (2005) *A Framework for Understanding Poverty*. Highlands, TX: aha' Process, Inc.

22. Corcoran, Mary (2001) Mobility, Persistence, and the Consequences of Poverty for Children. In Danziger, S.H. & Haveman, R.H. (Eds.) *Understanding Poverty*. New York: Russell Sage Foundation, pp. 160–161.

23. a) Ibid, p. 163; b) Iceland, J. (2003) *Poverty in America*. Berkeley, CA: University of California Press, p. 2.

24. a) Eberstadt, N. (2006) The Mismeasure of Poverty. *Policy Review* August and September. Stanford, CA: Hoover Institution. b) Iceland, J. (2003) *Poverty in America*. Berkeley, CA: University of California Press, p. 3.

25. a) Mendel, D. (2006) *Double Jeopardy*. New York: Annie E. Casey Foundation; b) Newman, K. S. (2007) *The Missing Class*. Boston: Beacon Press.

26. a) Scott, J. & Leonhardt, D.L. (2005) Class in America. *New York Times* May 15, A1; b) Sapolsky, R. (2005) Sick of Poverty. *Scientific American* 203 (6): 93–99; c) Kruger, P.M. & Chang, V.W. (2008) Being Poor and Coping with Stress. *American Journal of Public Health* 98: 889–896.

27. a) Miech, R.A., et al (2006) Trends in the Association of Poverty with Overweight among U.S. Adolescents, 1971–2004. *Journal of the American Medical Association* 295: 2385–2393; b) Ratey, J.J. (2002) *Users Guide to the Brain*. New York: Vintage Books.

28. Sattler, B. (2005) The Risky Business of Reproduction. *Zero to Three* 26 (2): 20–25.

29. a) Faris, R.E. & Dunham, W. (1939, 1965) *Mental Disorders in Urban Areas.* Chicago, IL: University of Chicago Press; b) Silver, E., et al (2002). Neighborhood Structural Characteristics and Mental Disorder. *Social Science and Medicine* 55: 1457–1470.

30. Lykken, D. (2000) *Happiness.* New York: Golden Guides from St. Martin's Press.

31. a) McMahon, D. (2006) *Happiness.* New York: Atlantic Monthly Press; b) Layard, R. 2005) *Happiness.* New York: Penguin Press; c) Economics Discovers Its Feelings (2006) *The Economist* December 23, pp. 33–35; d) Montgomery, R. (2006) Rich vs. Super Rich. *Wisconsin State Journal* December 26, p. A7; e) Kahneman, D., et al (2006) Would You Be Happier If You Were Richer? *Science* 312: 1908–1910; f) Layard, R. (2005) *Happiness.* New York: Penguin; g) Wilson, E.G. (2008) *Against Happiness.* New York: Farrar, Straus & Giroux.

32. a) Csikszentmihalyi, M. (2003) *Good Business.* New York: Viking; b) Flescher, A.A. & Worthen, D.L. (2007) *The Altruistic Species.* West Conshohocken, PA: Templeton Foundation; c) Klein S. (2006) *The Science of Happiness.* New York: Marlow, p. 252; d) Seligman, M.E.P. (2002) *Authentic Happiness.* New York: Free Press.

33. a) Cox, W.M. & Alm, R. (1999) *Myths of Rich and Poor.* New York: Basic Books; b) Cassidy, J. (2006) Relatively Deprived. *The New Yorker* April 3, p. 44.

34. Stiles, P. (2005) *Is the American Dream Killing You?* New York: Harper Collins.

35. Marmot, M. (2004) *The Status Syndrome.* New York: Times Books.

36. Chisholm, J.S. (1999) *Death, Hope and Sex.* Cambridge, UK: Cambridge University Press, p. 186.

37. Luker, K. (1996) *Dubious Conceptions.* Cambridge, MA: Harvard University Press, p. 39.

38. Ibid, pp. 82–83.

39. Whitman, T.L., et al (2001) *Interwoven Lives.* Mahwah, NJ: Lawrence Erlbaum.

40. a) Turley, R.N.L. (2003) Are Children of Young Mothers Disadvantaged Because of the Mother's Age or Family Background? *Child Development* 74: 465–474; b) SmithBattle, L. (2005) Viewpoint: Examining Assumptions about Teen Mothers. *American Journal of Nursing* 105 (4):13.

41. Kelly, D.M. (1996) Stigma Stories. *Youth and Society* 27 (4): 421–49.

42. Males, M. (2006) "Teen Pregnancy" Prevention's Ugly Eugenics. *Youth Today* October 1.

43. Furstenburg, Jr., F.F., et al (1987) *Adolescent Mothers in Later Life.* Cambridge, UK: Cambridge Press, p. 99.

44. a) Maynard R.A. (Ed.) (1997) *Kids Having Kids.* Washington, DC: The Urban Institute; b) Moore, K.A., et al (1993) Age at First Childbirth and Later Poverty. *Journal of Research on Adolescence* 3: 393–422.

45. Steep Decline in Teen Birth Rate Significantly Responsible for Reducing Child Poverty and Single-Parent Families. *Committee on Ways and Means. Issue Brief* April 23, 2004.

46. Williams, Linda B. & Pratt, William F. (1990) *Wanted and Unwanted Childbearing in the United States, 1973–1988.* Hyattsville, MD: National Center for Health Statistics, p. 5, Table 4.

47. Westman, J.C. (2003) *A Comparison of Adolescent Pregnancy and Childbirth in Madison and Milwaukee, Wisconsin.* Madison, WI: Wisconsin Cares, Inc.

48. Hoffman, S.D. (1998) Teenage Childbearing Is Not so Bad After All . . . or Is It? *Family Planning Perspectives* 30: 236–239.

49. Roehlkepartain, E.C., et al (2004) *Building Strong Families.* Minneapolis, MN: Search Institute in Collaboration with YMCA of the USA.

50. Moore, K.A. & Kahn, J. (2008) Family and Neighborhood Risks. *Research to Results Fact Sheet, Publication #2008–06*. Washington, DC: Child Trends.

51. Douglas, S. & Michaels, M. (2004) *The Mommy Myth*. New York: The Free Press.

52. a) Maynard, R. (Ed.) (1993) *Building Self-Sufficiency among Welfare-Dependent Teenage Parents*. Princeton, N.J.: Mathematica Policy Research, Inc.; b) Wertheimer, R. & Moore, K. (1998) *Childbearing by Teens*. Washington, DC: Urban Institute.

53. a) Harris, K.M., et al (2002) Evaluating the Role of "Nothing to Lose" Attitudes on Risky Behavior in Adolescence. *Social Forces*, 80 (3): 1005–1039; b) Parker, S. & Sasaki, T.T. (1965) Society and Sentiments in Two Contrasting Socially Disturbed Areas. In Murphy J.M. & Leighton, A. (Eds.) *Approaches to Cross-Cultural Psychiatry*. Ithaca, NY: Cornell University Press, pp. 329–359.

54. Kozol, J. (2005) *The Shame of the Nation*. New York: Crown Publishers.

55. Harris, K.M., et al (2002) Evaluating the Role of "Nothing to Lose" Attitudes on Risky Behavior in Adolescence. *Social Forces* 80 (3): 1005–1039.

56. Carlson, M.: Unpublished figures from the *Fragile Families and Child Well-Being Study*. Princeton, NJ: Princeton University.

57. a) Douthat, R. (2005) Does Meritocracy Work? *The Atlantic Monthly* 296 (4): 125; b) Commission on Substance Abuse at Colleges and Universities II (2007) *Wasting the Best and the Brightest*. New York: National Center on Addiction and Substance Abuse at Columbia University.

58. Payne, R.K. (1995) *A Framework for Understanding and Working with Students and Adults from Poverty*. Baytown, TX: RFT Publishing.

59. Dao, J. (2005) Instant Millions Can't Halt Winners' Grim Slide. *New York Times* December 5, A-1.

60. Courtney, M.E. & Dworsky, A. (2006) Those Left Behind. *Chapin Hall Issue Brief: May*. Chicago, IL: University of Chicago.

61. a) Mead, L.M. (2004) *Government Matters*. Princeton, NJ: Princeton Press, p. 276; b) Rank, M.R. (2004) *One Nation, Underprivileged*. New York: Oxford Press, pp.15, 10; c) Ibid, p.170; b) Holoway, S.D., et al (1997) *Through My Own Eyes*. Cambridge, MA: Harvard Press, p. 207; d) Stern, A. (2006) A Country that Works. New York: Free Press; e) 36. Blank, R.M. (1997) *It Takes a Nation*. Princeton, NJ: Princeton Press, p. 293; e) Schorr, L. (1998) *Common Purpose*. New York: Random House.

62. a) Lipset, S.M. (1996) *American Exceptionalism*. New York: W. W. Norton; b) Lipset, S.M. & Marks, G. (2001) *It Didn't Happen Here*. New York: W. W. Norton.

63. a) Haskins, R. & Sawhill, I.V. (2003) *Work and Marriage. Policy Brief #28–2003*. Washington, DC: The Brookings Institution; b) Mead, L.M. (2004) *Government Matters*. Princeton, NJ: Princeton University Press, p. 277.

64. a) Murray, C. (1995) *Losing Ground*. New York: Basic Books. b) Murray, C. (2006) *In Our Hands*. Washington, DC: AEI Press.

65. a) Furstenberg, Jr., F. F., et al (1999) *Managing to Make It*. Chicago, IL: University of Chicago Press, p. 608; b) Wessel, D. (2006) In Poverty Tactics, an Old Debate. *Wall Street Journal* June 15, p. A1.

66. Rank, M.R. (2004) *One Nation, Underprivileged*. New York: Oxford University Press, p. 230.

67. Florida, R. (2005) *The Flight of the Creative Class*. New York: HarperBusiness, pp. 77–78.

68. a) Amabile, T. (1996) *Creativity in Context*. Boulder, CO: Westview Press, pp. 77, 89; b) Advisory Council (2004) Smart Advice. *Information Week* February 2.

69. a) Appiah, K.A. (2007) *Experiments in Ethics*. Cambridge, MA: Harvard University Press; b) Wilson, W.J. (2006) *There Goes the Neighborhood*. New York: Vintage Books, p. 184, 186.

70. Hoem, B. (1992) Early Phases of Family Formation in Contemporary Sweden. In Rosenheim, M. K. & Testa, M.F. (Eds.) *Early Parenthood and Coming of Age in the 1990s*. New Brunswick, NJ: Rutgers University Press.

71. Sung, K. 1992) Teenage Pregnancy and Premarital Childbirth in Korea. In Rosenheim, M.K. & Testa, M.F. (Eds.) *Early Parenthood and Coming of Age in the 1990s*. New Brunswick, NJ: Rutgers University Press.

72. Thorner, J. (2007) Furniture Giant Ikea Has Big Tampa Plan. *St. Petersburg Times* March 27, pp. D1–2.

CHAPTER 20. PEER INFLUENCES ON ADOLESCENT PARENTHOOD

1. De Becker, G. (2002) *Fear Less*. Boston: Little, Brown & Company, p. 180.

2. Harris, J.R. (1998) *The Nurture Assumption*. New York: Free Press.

3. a) Vigdor, J. (2006) Peer Effects in Neighborhoods and Housing. In Dodge, K.A., et al (Eds.) Deviant Peer Influences in Programs for Youth. New York: Guilford Press, p.198; b) Borkowsky, J., et al (Eds.) (2002). *Parenting and the Child's World*. Mahwah, NJ: Lawrence Erlbaum.

4. Harris, J.R. (1995) Where Is the Child's Environment? *Psychological Review* 102 (3): 458–489.

5. a) Rayo, L. & Becker, G.S. (2005) *Evolutionary Efficiency and Happiness*. Chicago, IL: University of Chicago Department of Economics working paper; b) Brown, D.E. (1999) Human Universals. In Wilson, R.A. & Keil, F.C. (Eds.) *The MIT Encyclopedia of the Cognitive Sciences*. Cambridge, MA: MIT Press.

6. Cohen-Sandler, R. (2005) *Stressed-out Girls*. New York: Viking.

7. Lieberman, M.D. & Eisenberger, N.I. (2006) A Pain by any other Name Still Hurts the Same. In Capioppo, J.T., et al (Eds.) *Social Neuroscience*. Cambridge, MA: MIT Press, pp. 167–188.

8. Shrier, L.A., et al (2005) Improved Affect Following Coitus. *Journal of Adolescent Health* 36 (2): 108.

9. a) Wyshak, G. & Frisch, R.E. (1982) Evidence for a Secular Trend in Age of Menarche. *New England Journal of Medicine* 306: 245–306; b) Hindu, M.A. & Smith, D.S. (1975) Premarital Pregnancy in America 1640–1971. *Journal of Interdisciplinary History* 5: 537–570; c) Vinovskis, M.A. (1988) *An "Epidemic" of Adolescent Pregnancy?* New York: Oxford University Press, pp. 11–15; d) Juster, S.M. (1988) *Disorderly Women*. Presented at the Social Science History Association Meeting. Chicago, October; e) Alcott, W.A. (1856) *Physiology of Marriage*. Boston, MA: John P. Jewett; f) Massachusetts (1887) *Census of Massachusetts, 1885. 4 vols*. Boston, MA: Wright & Potter.

10. Laumann, E.O., et al (1994) *The Social Organization of Sexuality*.Chicago: University Press.

11. Pike, L.B. (1999) Why Abstinent Adolescents Report They Have Not Had Sex. *Youth Family Relations* 48: 295.

12. a) Putting Together What Works (2006) *It's a Guy Thing*. Washington, DC: National Campaign to Prevent Teen Pregnancy; b) Leitenberg H. & Saltzman H. (2000) A Statewide Survey of Age at First Intercourse for Adolescent Females and Age of Their Male Partners.

Archives of Sexual Behavior 29 (3): 203–215; c) Ryan, S, et al (2003) *The First Time*. Washington, DC: Child Trends Research Brief #2003–16.

13. Panchaud, C., et al (2000) Sexually Transmitted Diseases among Adolescents in Developed Countries. *Family Planning Perspectives* 32 (1): 24–32, 45.

14. a) National YRBS (2008) Trends in the Prevalence of Sexual Behaviors: 1991—2007. Washington, DC: National Center for Chronic Disease Prevention and Health Promotion; b) Science Says (2006) Teens' Sexual Experience, 1995–2002. *Putting What Works To Work. Number 22, March*. Washington, DC: National Campaign to Prevent Teen Pregnancy.

15. a) Healthy Youth (2007) *YRBSS*. Washington, DC: National Center for Chronic Disease Prevention and Health Promotion; b) Science Says (2006) *Parent-Child Communication About Sex and Related Topics. Number 25*. Washington, DC: The National Campaign To Prevent Teen Pregnancy; c) Putting Together What Works (2006) *It's a Guy Thing*.Washington, DC: National Campaign to Prevent Teen Pregnancy, February.

16. Terry-Humen, E., et al (2006) *Trends and Recent Estimates*. Washington, DC: Child Trends Research Brief, Publication #2006–08.

17. a) Putting What Works to Work (2006) Teen Contraceptive Use. *Science Says Number 29 September*. Washington, DC: National Campaign to Prevent Teen Pregnancy; b) Putting Together What Works (2006) *It's a Guy Thing*. Washington, DC: National Campaign to Prevent Teen Pregnancy, February; c) Franzetta, K., et al (2006) *Trends and Recent Estimates*. Washington, DC: Child Trends Research Brief #2006–04; d) Manlove, J., et al (2005) Sex Between Young Teens and Older Individuals. *Child Trends Research Brief 2005–07*.

18. a) Weinberger, D.R., et al (2005) *The Adolescent Brain*. Washington, DC: The National Campaign to Prevent Teen Pregnancy; b) Sonnerstein, F.L., et al (1989) *At Risk of Aids*. Presented at the Population Association of America, March 31, Baltimore, MD; c) Ager, J.W., et al (1982) Method Discontinuance in Teenage Women. In Stuart, I.R. & Wells, C.F. (Eds.) *Pregnancy in Adolescence*. New York: Van Nostrand Reinhold, p. 237.

19. Greene, J.P. & Forster, G. (2004) Sex, Drugs, and Delinquency in Urban and Suburban Public Schools. *Education Working Paper No. 4*. New York: The Manhattan Institute.

20. Division of Public Health, Bureau of Health Information and Policy (2008) *Wisconsin Youth Sexual Behavior and Outcomes, 1993–2007* (PPH 5706–07). Madison, WI: Wisconsin Department of Health and Family Services.

21. a) Collins, R.L. (2005) Sex on Television. *Child and Adolescent Psychiatric Clinics of North America* 143: 371; b) Centers for Disease Control and Prevention (2005) Sexual Behavior and Selected Health Measures. *Advance Data from Vital and Health Statistics* 362: 1-S6; c) Putting Together What Works (2006) *It's a Guy Thing*. Washington, DC: National Campaign to Prevent Teen Pregnancy, February; d) Mosher, W.D., et al (2005) Sexual Behavior and Selected Health Measures. *Advance Data* 362: 1–55; e) Brady, S. & Halpern-Felsher, B.L. (2007) Adolescents' Reported Consequences of Having Oral Sex. *Pediatrics* 119 (2): 229–236; f) Gates, G. & Sonenstein, F. (2000) Heterosexual Genital Sexual Activity among Adolescent Males. *Family Planning Perspectives* 34: 6.

22. Science Says (2006) *Parent-Child Communication About Sex and Related Topics. Number 25*. Washington, DC: The National Campaign to Prevent Teen Pregnancy.

23. Science Says (2006) Teens' Attitudes toward Pregnancy and Childbearing, 1988–2002. *Putting What Works To Work. Number 21, March*. Washington, DC: National Campaign to Prevent Teen Pregnancy.

24. Seventeen/Candie's Foundation Survey. *Seventeen* February 2008.

25. Robertson, M. (2005) *Motherhood*. New York: Karibu Books.

26. Dahl, J.E. (2006) Pregnancy High. *Seventeen*, May, pp. 148–151.

27. Mabin, C. (2005) Ohio School Struggling with Teen Pregnancy. *Northwest Herald* September 2.

28. a) Gloucester WBZ Newsroom/AP. Monday, June, 23, 2008 1:31PM. b) Anderson, P. (2008) Gloucester High School's Day-care Center Overflowing in September. *Gloucester Daily Tribune*, June 19.

29. Robinson, P. (1976) *The Modernization of Sex*. New York: Harper Colophon.

30. Putting What Works to Work (2006) *Religiosity and Teenagers' Sexual Behavior*. Washington, DC: National Campaign to Prevent Teen Pregnancy.

31. APA Task Force on the Sexualization of Girls (2007) *Report of the APA Task Force on the Sexualization of Girls*. Washington, DC: American Psychological Association.

32. a) Shopper, M. (1984) From Discovery to Ownership of the Vagina. In Sugar, M. (Ed.) *Adolescent Parenthood*. New York: SP Medical & Scientific Books, p. 53; b) Scharff, D.E. (1982) *The Sexual Relationship*. London: Routledge, pp. 211–212.

33. Centers for Disease Control (2004) Surveillance Summaries. MMWR 2004: 53 (No. SS-2): Table 10.

34. Levy, B. (Ed.) (1991) *Dating Violence*. Toronto, Canada: Publishers Group West, p. 5.

35. a) Levy, B.(1993) *In Love and In Danger*. Seattle, WA: Seal Press; b) Murray, J. (2005) *But I Love Him*. New York: Regan Books.

36. Levy, B. (1993) *In Love & In Danger*. Seattle, WA: Seal Press, pp. 29, 73.

37. Graham, L.R. & Rawlings, E.I. (1991) Bonding with Abusive Dating Partners. In Levy, B. (Ed.) *Dating Violence*. Seattle, WA: Seal Press, p. 121–122.

38. NiCarthy, G. (1991) Addictive Love and Abuse. In Levy, B. (Ed.) *Dating Violence*. Toronto, Seattle, WA: Seal Press, pp. 214–142.

39. Levy, B. (1993) *In Love & In Danger*. Seattle, WAL Seal Press, p. 81.

40. a) Choose Respect. Atlanta. GA: Centers for Disease Control and Prevention. <www.chooserespect.org>; b) Jaycox, L., et al (2006) Impact of a School-Based Dating Violence Prevention Program among Latino Teens. *Journal of Adolescent Health* 39 (5): 694–704.

41. a) Hill, C. & Silva, E. (2005) *Drawing The Line*. Washington, DC: American Association of University Women; b) Tjaden, P. & Thoennes, N. (1998) *Prevalence, Incidence, and Consequences of Violence Against Women*. Washington, DC: National Institute of Justice Centers for Disease Control and Prevention; c) Blythe, M.J., et al (2006) Incidence and Correlates of Unwanted Sex in Relationships of Middle and Late Adolescent Women. *Archives of Pediatric and Adolescent Medicine* 160: 591–595.

42. a) Harris Interactive, Inc. (2006) *Drawing the Line*. Washington, DC: American Association of University Women Educational Foundation; b) Warshaw, R. (1988) *I Never Called it Rape*. New York: Harper & Row.

CHAPTER 21. GANG INFLUENCES ON ADOLESCENT PARENTHOOD

1. Eysenck, S.B.G. (1989) Foreword, in Eysenck, H.J. & Gudjonsson, G.H. *The Causes and Cures of Criminality*. New York: Plenum.

2. Knox, G.W. (2000) *An Introduction to Gangs*. Peotone, IL: New Chicago School Press.

3. Egley, A., et al (2006) National Youth Gang Survey: 1999–2001. (NCJ 209392) Washington, DC: Office of Juvenile Justice and Delinquency Prevention.

4. Moffitt, T.E. & Caspi, A. (2001) Childhood Predictors Differentiate Life-Course Persistent and Adolescence-Limited Antisocial Pathways among Males and Females. *Development and Psychopathology* 13: 355–375.

5. OJJDP Summary (2000) *Youth Gang Programs and Strategies,* August. Washington, DC: Office of Juvenile Justice and Delinquency Prevention.

6. National Alliance of Gang Investigators Associations. *2005 National Gang Threat Assessment.* Grant Number 2003–DD-BX-031. Washington, DC: Bureau of Justice Assistance, U.S. Department of Justice.

7. Regional Organized Crime Information Center (2006) *ROICIC Gang Report 2006.* Nashville, TN: Regional Organized Crime Information Center.

8. Editorial (2006) Capital Gangs. *The News and Observer.* Raleigh, North Carolina, June 10, p. 20A.

9. Knox, G.W. (2000) *An Introduction to Gangs.* Peotone, IL: New Chicago School Press, p. 298.

10. a) Nunnally, D.(2007) Fatal Intersection/The Arc of a Crime Crew. *Milwaukee Journal Sentinel* April, p.1; b) Venkatesh, S. (2008) *Gang Leader for a Day.* New York: Penguin.

11. Seabright, P. (2004) *The Company of Strangers.* Princeton, NJ: Princeton University Press.

12. Gang and Security Threat Group Awareness (2007) *Los Angeles-based Gangs.* Talahassee, FL: Florida Department of Corrections.

13. Levitt, S.D. & Venkatesh, S.A. (2000) An Economic Analysis of a Drug-Selling Gang's Finances. *The Quarterly Journal of Economics,* August 115: 755–789.

14. a) Whyte, W.F. (1943) *Street Corner Society.* Chicago: University of Chicago Press; b) Gang and Security Threat Group Awareness (2007) *Los Angeles-based Gangs.* Talahassee, FL: Florida Department of Corrections.

15. Lawton Police Gang Unit (2007) *Street Gangs.* Lawton, Oklahoma: Lawton Police Department.

16. National Gang Crime Research Center (1997) *A National Study of over 4,000 Gang Members.* Peotone, IL: National Gang Crime Research Center.

17. a) Thrasher, F.M. (1927) *The Gang.* Chicago, IL: University of Chicago Press; b) Thornberry, T.P., et al (2003) *Gangs and Delinquency in Developmental Perspective.* Cambridge, UK: Cambridge University Press, pp. 1–2.

18. Sherman, A. (2006) Teaching Empathy. *Miami Herald* March 4, p. 1E.

19. Brooks, D. (2205) Gangsta, in French. *New York Times* November 10, A 31.

20. Smith, E. & Sanders, P. (2006) Leaving Las Vegas? *Wall Street Journal* March 28, p. 1.

21. Knox, G.W. (2000) *An Introduction to Gangs.* Peotone, IL: New Chicago School Press, pp. 292, 294.

22. a) Moore, J. & Hagedorn, J.M. (2001) Female Gangs. *Juvenile Justice Bulletin.* Washington, DC: Office of Juvenile Justice and Delinquency Prevention; b) Moore, J. & Hagedorn, J. (1995) *Milwaukee Drug Posse and Homegirl Studies.* Washington. DC: The National Criminal Justice Reference Service Abstracts Database; c) Treleven, Ed (2006) Mother Gets Jail for Drive-by Shooting Role. *Wisconsin State Journal* October 13, p. B3.

23. Knox, G.W. (2000) *An Introduction to Gangs.* Peotone, IL: New Chicago School Press, pp. 316–318, 320.

24. Thornberry, T.P., et al (2003) *Gangs and Delinquency in Developmental Perspective.* Cambridge, UK: Cambridge University Press, p. 31, 169–171.

25. OJJDP Summary (2000) *Youth Gang Programs and Strategies.* Washington, DC: Office of Juvenile Justice and Delinquency Prevention; b) Youth Service of America. 1101 15th Street, Suite 200; Washington, DC 20005; c) Philadelphia Millions More Movement. P.O. Box 42853, Philadelphia, PA 19101.

26. CeaseFire (2007) *Report to the State of Illinois.* Chicago, IL: University of Illinois, School of Public Health.

PART 7. CULTURE

1. http://www.columbia.edu/itc/music/NYCO/butterfly/luther.html

CHAPTER 22. CULTURAL INFLUENCES ON
ADOLESCENT PARENTHOOD

1. Harrison, L. & Huntington, S.P. (Eds.) (2000) *Culture Matters*. Cambridge, MA: Harvard University Press.

2. Weisfeld, G.E. & Woodward, L. (2003) Current Evolutionary Perspectives on Adolescent Romantic Relations and Sexuality. *Journal of the American Academy of Child and Adolescent Psychiatry* 43: 11–18.

3. Hirschman, C., et al (Eds.) *The Handbook of International Migration*. New York: Russell Sage Foundation, p. 13.

4. Matthews, H. & Ewen, D. (2006) *Reaching All Children?* Washington, DC: Center for Law and Social Policy.

5. a) Hansen, M.L. (1942) *The Immigrant in American History*. Cambridge, MA: Harvard University Press, p. 188; b) U.S. Census Bureau Statistical Abstract of the United States 2006.

6. a) Table 15. Resident Population by Race, Hispanic Origin Status, and Age—Projections: 2005 and 2010. Washington, DC: U. S. Census Bureau; b) Table 37. Selected Characteristics of Racial Groups and Hispanic/Latino Population: 2003. Washington, DC: U. S. Census Bureau.

7. a) Gans, H. (1999) Toward a Reconciliation of "Assimilation" and "Pluralism". In Hirschman, C., et al (Eds.) *The Handbook of International Migration*. New York: Russell Sage Foundation, p. 162; b) Vermeulen, H. & Perlman, J. (Eds.) (2001) *Immigrants, Schooling and Social Mobility*. New York: St. Martin's Press, p.15.

8. a) Fisher, C.B., et al (1998) The Study of African American and Latin American Children and Youth. In Damon, W. & Lerner, R. (Eds.) *Handbook of Child Psychology, Fifth Edition*. New York: John Wiley & Sons, p. 1186; b) Harrison, L.E. (2006) *The Central Liberal Truth*. New York: Oxford University Press. c) Horton, J.O. & Horton, L.E. (1997) *In Hope of Liberty*. New York: Oxford University Press, p. ix; d) Takaki, R. (1993) *A Different Mirror*. Boston, MA: Little, Brown.

9. a) Florida, R. (2005) *The Flight of the Creative Class*. New York: HarperBusiness, p. 86; b) Gates, G.J. (2003) *Racial Integration, Diversity, and Social Capital*. Washington, DC: Urban Institute; c) Lara, M., et al (2005) Acculturation and Latino Health in the United States. *Annual Review of Public Health* 26: 367–397.

10. a) Zhou, M. (1999) Segmented Assimilation. In Hirschman, C., et al (Eds.) *The Handbook of International Migration*. New York: Russell Sage Foundation, p. 210. b) Portes, A. & Rumbaut, R.G. (2001) *Legacies*. Berkeley, CA: University of California Press.

11. Gerstle, G. (1999) Liberty, Coercion, and the Making of Americans. In Hirschman, C., et al (Eds.) *The Handbook of International Migration*. New York: Russell Sage Foundation, p. 291.

12. a) Vermeulen, H. & Perlman, J. (Eds.) (2001) *Immigrants, Schooling and Social Mobility*. New York: St. Martin's Press, p. 10. b) Cohen, D.K. (1970) Immigrants and the Schools. *Review of Educational Research* 40: 13–27; c) Hirschman, C., et al (Eds.) (1999) *The Handbook of International Migration*. New York: Russell Sage, p. 9.

13. Olneck, M.R. & Lazerson, M. (1974) The School Achievement of Immigrant Children, 1900–1930. *History of Education Quarterly* 14: 453–482.

14. Takeuchi, D.T., et al (2007) Immigration and Mental Health. *American Journal of Public Health* 97 (1): 11–12.

15. Jacoby, T. (Ed.) (2004) *Reinventing the Melting Pot.* New York: Basic Books, pp. 15–16, 314.

16. Borjas, G.J. (2006) Making It in America. *Future of Children* 16 (2): 55–71.

17. Child Trends News Release (2007) *Children in Immigrant Families Firmly Rooted in America.* Washington, DC: Child Trends, April 12.

18. a) Appiah, K.A. (2006) *Cosmopolitanism.* New York: W.W. Norton. b) Mollenkopf, M.C., et al (2005) The Dynamics of Assimilation. In Settersten Jr., R.A., et al (Ed.) (2005) *On the Frontier of Adulthood.* Chicago: University of Chicago Press; b) Kristof, N. D. (2006) The Model Students. *New York Times* May 14, 13WK.

19. Diplomas Count. *Education Week* 25 (41S): 3, June 22, 2006.

20. Greene, J.P. & Winters, M.A. (2006) *Leaving Boys Behind.* New York: Manhattan Institute.

21. Mishel, L. & Roy, J. (2006) *Rethinking High School Graduation Rates and Trends.* Washington, DC: Economic Policy Institute.

22. Erickson, P.I. (1998) *Latina Adolescent Childbearing in East Los Angeles.* Austin, Texas: University of Texas Press, p. 22.

23. Chong, E. & Haberland, N. (2005) Child Marriage. *Promoting Healthy, Safe, and Productive Transitions to Adulthood. Brief No. 14.* New York: Population Council.

24. a) Forum on Marriage and the Rights of Women and Girls 2000; UNICEF 2005; b) 26. Paige, K. & Paige, J.M. (1981) *The Politics of Reproductive Ritual.* Berkeley, CA: University of California Press, pp. 49–50.

25. Universal Declaration of Human Rights (1948), the United Nations Convention on the Elimination of All Forms of Discrimination Against Women (1979), the United Nations Convention on the Rights of the Child (1989) and the African Charter on the Rights and Welfare of the Child (1990).

26. a) Chung, P.J., et al (2007) Acculturation and Parent-Adolescent Communication About Sex in Filipino-American Families. *The Journal of Adolescent Health* 40 (6): 543–550; b) Brown, B.B., et al (2002) *The World's Youth.* New York: Cambridge University Press, pp. 183, 164.

27. Kumar, A. (2002) Adolescence and Sexuality in the Rajasthani Context. In Manderson, L. & Liamputtong, P. (Eds.) *Coming of Age in South and Southeast Asia.* Richmond, British Columbia, Canada: Curzon, p. 63.

28. Ibid, pp. 92–93.

29. Ibid, p. 14.

30. Lancaster, J.B. & Hamburg, B. A. (Eds.) (1986) *School-Age Pregnancy and Parenthood.* New York: Aldine.

31. Cohen, J.E. (2005) Human Population Grows Up. *Scientific American* 293 (3): 54.

32. Gleich, J. (1999) *Faster.* New York: Pantheon Books, p.11.

33. Ablow, K. (2005) Speaking in the Third Person. *New York Times* November 1, p. D-5.

34. Rader, D. (2006) "I Can Create Who I Am." *Parade* April 9, pp. 6–8.

35. a) Kitwana, B. (2002) *The Hip Hop Generation.* New York: BasicCivitas Books; b) Reeves, Marcus (2007) *Somebody Scream.* London, UK: Faber & Faber.

36. Change, J. (2005) *Can't Stop Won't Stop.* New York: St. Martin's Press.

37. a) Martino, S.C., et al (2006) Exposure to Degrading Versus Nondegrading Music Lyrics and Sexual Behavior Among Youth. *Pediatrics* 118 (2): e430–e441; b) Herd D. (1993) Contesting Culture. *Contemporary Drug Problems* 20: 739–758.

38. Hilary Magazine (2008) *Rap Culture.* February 11.

39. Deggans, E. (2007) Words Can Hurt. *St. Petersburg Times* February 20, p. E1.

40. CBS (2007) Stop Snitchin'. *60 Minutes* April 19.

41. God Bless the Child Productions, Inc., Plainfield, NJ.

42. Jones, E.F., et al (1986) *Teenage Pregnancy in Industrialized Countries.* New Haven, CT: Yale Press.

43. Huesmann, L.R. & Taylor, L.D. (2006) The Role of Media Violence In Violent Behavior. *Annual Review of Public Health* 27: 393–415.

44. a) Escobar-Chaves, S.L., et al (2005) Impact of the Media on Adolescent Sexual Attitudes and Behaviors. *Pediatrics* 116 (1): 303–326. b) Brown, J.D., et al (2006) Sexy Media Matters. *Pediatrics* 117: 1018–1027; c) Collins, R.L. (2005) Sex on Television and Its Impact on American Youth. *Child and Adolescent Psychiatric Clinics of North America* 14 (3): 371–385.

45. Associated Press (2005) In America, Good Manners Disappearing. *St. Petersburg Times* October 16, p. 12A.

46. a) International Communications Research (2001) *Generation Rx.com.* New York: Kaiser Family Foundation; b) Paul, Pamela (2005) *Pornified.* New York: Times Books, pp. 188, 274.

47. Thrash, R. (2005) Baby Mamas. *St. Petersburg Times* May 8, E 1.

48. CD *Free Yourself* by Fantasia Barrino.

49. National Center for Health Statistics (1993) *Advance Report of Final Natality Statistics 41, No. 9, Supplement.* February 25, Table 16.

50. La Barre, M. (l968) Pregnancy Experiences among Married Adolescents *American Journal of Orthopsychiatry* 38: 47–55.

51. a) Associated Press (2005) Judge Faces Discipline for Remarks to Women. *St. Petersburg Times*, May 21, p. 1A; b) Herbert, B. (2006) Why Aren't We Shocked? *New York Times* October 16, p. A23.

52. Males, M. (2006) "Teen Pregnancy" Prevention's Ugly Eugenics. *Youth Today* October 1.

CHAPTER 23. BLACK ADOLESCENT PARENTHOOD

1. Edelman, M.W. (1995) *Guide My Feet.* Boston: Beacon Press, p. xxviii.

2. Hawkins-Leon, C.G. (1998) The Indian Child Welfare Act and the African American Tribe. *Brandeis Journal of Family Law* 36: 201–218.

3. Coontz, S. (2005) *Marriage, a History.* New York: Viking.

4. Roberts, D. (1997) *Killing the Black Body.* New York: Vintage, pp. 30, 34–36.

5. Patterson, O. (1998) *Rituals of Blood.* Washington, DC: Civitas/Counterpoint, pp. 32–35.

6. Roberts, D. (1997) *Killing the Black Body.* New York: Vintage, p. 21.

7. a) Burton, L.M. (1990) Teenage Childbearing as an Alternative Life Course Strategy in Multigenerational Black Families. *Human Nature* 1: 123; b) Janis, F. (2004) *Cotton Field of Dreams.* Chicago: Writing Our World Press.

8. a) Frazier, E.F. (1939) *The Negro Family in the United States.* Notre Dame, IN: University of Notre Dame Press; b) Morgan, S.P., et al (1993) Racial Differences in Household and Family Structure at the Turn of the Century *American Journal of Sociology* 98: 799–828: c) Edelman, M.W. (1992) *The Measure of Our Success.* Boston, MA: Beacon Press, pp. 50–52; d) Mandara, J. & Murray, C. B. (2000) Effects of Parental Marital Status, Income and Family Functioning on African American Adolescent Self-Esteem. *Journal of Family Psychology* 14: 475–490; e) Tolnay, S. E. (1997) The Great Migration and Changes in the Northern Black Fam-

ily. *Social Forces* 75: 1213–1238; f) DeParle, J. (2004) *American Dream*. New York: Viking, p. 34.

9. a) Testimony of Ron Haskins, Senior Fellow, Brookings Institution, Before the Social Security and Family Policy Subcommittee of the Committee on Finance, U.S. Senate, May 5, 2004; b) Billingsley, A. (1992) *Climbing Jacob's Ladder*. New York: Simon & Schuster; c) South, S. (1993) Racial and Ethnic Differences in the Desire to Marry. *Journal of Marriage and the Family* 55 (2):357–370.

10. Jones, J. (2006) Marriage Is for White People. *Washington Post*, March 26.

11. a) Frazier, E.F. (1938) Some Effects of the Depression on the Negro in Northern Cities. *Science and Society* 2: 495–496; b) Graham, L.O. (2000) *Our Kind of People*. New York: HarperCollins.

12. a) Edelman, M.W. (1995) We Must Not Lose What We Knew Was Right Then. *Ebony 50th Anniversary Issue*, November; b) News and Views (2005) The Progress of Black Student Enrollments at the Nation's Highest-Ranked Colleges and Universities. *The Journal of Blacks in Higher Education* 49, Autumn.

13. Williams, B.F. & Woodson, D.G. (1993) *After Freedom*. Madison, WI: University of Wisconsin Press.

14. a) Patterson, O. (2000) Taking Culture Seriously. In Harrison, L.E. & Huntington, S.P. (Eds.) *Culture Matters*. New York: Basic Books, p. 218; b) Holzer, H.J., et al (2006) *Reconnecting Disadvantaged Young Men*. Washington, DC: Urban Institute Press.

15. *National Urban League's State of Black America 2006*. Washington, DC: Urban League.

16. Lindsay, J.W. (1989) *Parents, Pregnant Teens and the Adoption Option*. Buena Park, CA: Morning Glory Press.

17. a) Rhode, D.L. (1993) Adolescent Pregnancy and Public Policy. In Lawson, A. & Rhode, D.L. (Eds.) *The Politics of Pregnancy*. New Haven, CT: Yale University Press, p. 314; b) Gordon, L. (1992) Teenage Pregnancy: Morals, Moralism, Experts. *MacArthur Foundation Conference on Morality and Health*. Santa Fe, NM, June 22–23.

18. The State of the American Dream 2004. *United for a Fair Economy*, January, p. 20.

19. a) Nisbett, R.E. (1998) Race, Genetics, and IQ. In Jencks, C. & Phillips, M. (Eds.) *The Black-White Test Score Gap*. Washington, DC: Brookings Institution Press, p. 101; b) op cit, p. 509.

20. a) Dyson, M.E .(2005) *Is Bill Cosby Right?* New York: Basic Civitas Books, p. 65; b) Vital Signs (2005) Statistics That Measure the State of Racial Inequality. *The Journal of Blacks in Higher Education* 47, Summer.

21. Crawford, A. (2006) What Have Your Experiences Been Like in Advanced Placement Courses? *Simpson Street Free Press*. Madison, Wisconsin, p. 11.

22. a) Edin, K. & Kefalas, M. (2005) *Promises I Can Keep*. Berkeley, CA: University of California Press, pp. 211–213; b) Graefe, D.R. & Lichter, D.T. (2002) Marriage among Unwed Mothers. *Perspectives on Sexual and Reproductive Health* 34: 286–293; c) Bramlett, M.D. & Mosher, W.T. (2001) First Marriage Dissolution, Divorce, and Remarriage. *Advance Data from Vital and Health Statistics. No 323*. Hyattsville, MD: National Center for Health Statistics; d) Malone-Colon, L., et al (2006) *Consequences of Marriage for African Americans*. New York: Institute for American Values.

23. a) Mincy, R. & Pouncy, H. (2003) The Marriage Mystery. In Clayton, O., et al (Eds.) *Black Fathers in Contemporary American Society*. New York: Russell Sage, pp. 45–70; b) Williams, J., et al (2000) African American Family Structure. *Journal of Family Issues* 21: 838–857; c) Broman, C. (1988) Satisfaction among Blacks. *Journal of Marriage and the Family* 50: 45–51; d) Chatters, L. & Jackson, J. (1989) Quality of Life and Subjective Well-Being among Black Adults. In Jones, R. (Ed.) *Adult Development and Aging*. Berkeley, CA: Cobb and

Henry, pp. 191–214; d) Swaidan, Z., et al (2003) Consumer Ethics. *Journal of Business Ethics* 46: 175–186; e) Sampson, R. (1995) Unemployment and Imbalanced Sex Ratios. In Tucker, M. & Kernan, C. (Eds.) *The Decline in Marriage Among African Americans*. New York: Russell Sage.

24. a) Teachman, J., et al (1998) Sibling Resemblance in Behavioral and Cognitive Outcomes. *Journal of Marriage and the Family* 60: 835–848; b) Dunifon, R. & Kowaleski-Jones, L. (2002) Who's in the House? *Child Development* 73: 1249–1264; c) Malone-Colon, L. & Roberts, A. (2006) Marriage and the Well-Being of African American Boys, *Research Brief 2*. New York: Center for Marriage and Families at Institute for American Values, November.

25. Malone-Colon, L. (2007) *Responding to the Black Marriage Crisis.* Research Brief No. 6, June. New York: Institute for American Values, Center for Marriage and Families.

26. Roberts, D. (1997) *Killing the Black Body*. New York: Vintage Books, p. 3.

27. Ibid, pp. 6, 4, 2, 152,

28. Ibid, p.72.

29. Ibid, pp. 191, 167.

30. Du Bois, W.E.B. (1996) *The Philadelphia Negro*. Philadelphia: University of Pennsylvania Press, pp. 392–393.

31. Pew Report (2007) *Blacks See Growing Values Gap between Poor and Middle Class*. Washington, DC: Pew Research Center, November 13.

32. a) Personal communication; b) Dyson, M.E. (2005) *Is Bill Cosby Right?* New York: Basic Civitas Books, p. xv; c) Raspberry, William (2005) Will Black Middle Class Show Others the Way Up? *St. Petersburg Times* April 11, p.7A; d) Pattillo-McCoy, M. (1999) *Black Picket Fences*. Chicago, IL: University of Chicago Press.

33. Williams, J. (2006) *Enough*. New York: Crown.

34. Dyson, M.E. (2005) *Is Bill Cosby Right?* New York: Basic Civitas Books, pp. xii–xiv, 30, 180.

35. a) Smiley, T. (2006) *What I Know for Sure*. New York: Doubleday; b) Smiley, T. (2006) *The Covenant with Black America*. Chicago: Third World Press, pp. 89,138.

36. Williams, J. (2006) *Enough*. New York: Random House.

37. Daniels, C. (2004) *Black Power, Inc*. New York: John Wiley & Sons, p. xv.

38. National Center for Black Philanthropy. 1313 L Street NW, Suite 110, Washington, DC 20005–4110.

39. a) Daniels, C. (2004) *Black Power, Inc*. New York: John Wiley & Sons, pp. 69–70; b) Cose, E. (2003) The Black Gender Gap. *Newsweek* March 3, p. 46.

40. Clingman, J. (2005) *Black-O-Knowledge*. Milligan Books.

41. Jones, D. (2005) Seeing Ourselves through Our Own Black Eyes. *The Black Commentator* 156—October 27.

42. Michael, A. & Eccles, J.S. (2003) When Coming of Age Means Coming Undone. In Hayward, C. (Ed.) *Gender Differences at Puberty*. New York: Cambridge University Press.

43. a) Geronimus, A., et al (1996) Excess Mortality Among Blacks and Whites in the United States. *New England Journal of Medicine* 335:1552–1558; b) Racial and Ethnic Differences in Marriage among New, Unwed Parents (2004) *Fragile Families Research Brief 25*. Princeton, NJ: Princeton University.

44. a) Ardelt, M. & Eccles, J.S. (2001) Effects of Mothers' Parental Efficacy Beliefs on Inner-City Youth. *Journal of Family Issues* 22: 944–972; b) Gutman, L.M., et al (2002) The Academic Achievement of African American Students during Early Adolescence. *American Journal of Community Psychology* 30: 367–400.

45. Hughes, D. (2003) Correlates of Black and Latino Parents' Messages to Children about Ethnicity and Race. *American Journal of Community Psychology* 31 (1/2) March.

46. a) Martin, K.A. (1996) *Puberty, Sexuality and the Self.* New York: Routledge; b) Michael, A. (1997) Family Relations during Puberty. Poster at the Society for Research in Child Development. Washington, DC.

47. Cook, P.J. & Ludwig, J. (1997) Weighing the Burden of "Acting White." *Journal of Policy Analysis and Management* Spring: 256–278.

48. Staples, B. (2005) Making a Killing in Hip-hop. *St. Petersburg Times* May 13, p.15A.

49. Sennett, R. (2003) *Respect in a World of Inequality.* New York: W.W. Norton & Company, p. 34.

50. Ogbu, J.H. (1990) Minority Status and Literacy in Comparative Perspective. *Daedalus* 119 (2): 141–165.

51. Herbert, B. (2003) Breaking Away. *New York Times* July 10, p. A23.

52. Fordham, S. & Ogbu, J. (1986) Black Students and School Success. *Urban Review* 18: 176–206.

53. Austen-Smith, D. & Fryer, R.G. (2003) The Economics of "Acting White." *National Bureau of Economic Research, Inc. Working Paper 9904.*

54. Tyson, K., et al (2004) Breeding Animosity. *Sanford Institute Working Paper Series: SAN04–03.* Durham, NC: Duke University. Terry Sanford Institute of Public Policy.

55. Fryer, R.G. (2006) "Acting White." *Education Next, Winter.* Stanford, California: Hoover Institution.

56. King, R. (2003) Problem: Teens Shun Academic Achievement. *Wisconsin State Journal* December 8.

57. Majors, R. & Billson, J.M. (1992) *Cool Pose.* New York: Lexington Books.

58. a) Patterson, O. (2006) A Poverty of the Mind. *New York Times* March 26, p. WK 13; b) McShepard, R., et al (2007) *The Rap on Culture.* Cleveland, OH: PolicyBridge.

59. Sansone, L. (2001) The Internationalization of Black Culture. In Vermeulen, H. & Perlman, J. (Eds.) *Immigrants, Schooling and Social Mobility.* New York: St. Martin's Press, pp. 176–177.

60. Stevenson, H.C. (2004) Boys in Men's Clothing. In Way, N. & Chu, J.Y. (Eds.) *Adolescent Boys.* New York: New York University Press, p. 60–61.

61. Comer, J.P. & Poussaint, A.F. (1992) *Raising Black Children.* New York: Plume.

62. Sharpley-Whiting, T.D. (2007) *Pimps Up, Ho's Down.* New York: New York University Press, p. 147.

63. Ibid, p. 84.

64. Ikard, D. (2007) *Breaking the Silence.* Baton Rouge, LA: Louisiana State University Press, p. 27.

65. Morgan, J. (1999) *When Chickenheads Come Home to Roost.* New York: Simon and Schuster, pp. 161, 231.

66. Steele, S. (2006) *White Guilt.* New York: HarperCollins.

67. a) McWhorter, J.(2000) *Losing the Race.* New York: Free Press; b) McWhorter, J. (2006) *Winning the Race.* New York: Gotham Books; c) Ford, R.T. (2007) *The Race Card.* New York: Farrar, Straus & Giroux; c) Blackman, M.B. (2005) *Urban Suicide.* Phoenix, AZ: Amber Books.

68. Cosby, B. & Poussaint, A.F. (2007) *Come on People.* Nashville, TN: Thomas Nelson.

69. Unmarried African-American Fathers' Involvement with their Infants. *Fragile Families Research Brief* January 2004, Number 21. Princeton, NJ: Princeton University.

70. a) Orfield, G. (Ed.) (2004) *Dropouts in America.* Cambridge, MA: Harvard Education Press; b) Mincy, R.B. (Ed.) (2006) *Black Males Left Behind.* Washington, DC: Urban Institute Press.

71. Western, B. (2006) *Punishment and Inequality in America.* New York: Russell Sage Press.

72. Holzer, H.J., et al (2006) *Reconnecting Disadvantaged Young Men*. Washington, DC: Urban Institute Press.

73. Eckholm, E. (2006) Plight Deepens For Black Men, Studies Warn. *New York Times* March 20, p 1–A.

74. a) Geronimus, A., et al (1996) Excess Mortality Among Blacks and Whites in the United States. *New England Journal of Medicine* 335:1552–1558; b) Minkler, M., et al (2006) Gradient of Disability across the Socioeconomic Spectrum in the United States. *New England Journal of Medicine* 355 (7): 695–703.

75. Lowe, W. (2000) Detriangulation of Absent Fathers in Single-Parent Black Families. *The American Journal of Family Therapy* 28:29–40.

76. Miller, O.A. (2007) A Celebration of African American Fathers! *Perspectives on Our Work*. 7, June 22. Upper Marlboro, MD: Institute for Family and Child Well-Being.

77. a) Neal, M.A. (2005) *New Black Man*. New York: Routledge, p.159; b) Coates, T.N. (2008) *The Beautiful Struggle*. New York: Spiegel & Grau.

78. Hilfiker, D. (2002) *Urban Injustice*. New York: Seven Stories Press.

79. Wilson, William Julius (1987) *The Truly Disadvantaged*. Chicago: University of Chicago.

80. Dash, L. (1989) *When Children Want Children*. New York: Morrow, pp. 9–10.

81. Comer, J.P. (1972) *Beyond Black and White*. New York: Quadrangle Books.

82. Motivational Educational Entertainment Productions, Inc. (2004) *This Is My Reality*. Philadelphia, PA.

83. Hagedorn, J. M. (2002). Gangs and the Informal Economy. In Huff, R. (Ed.) *Gangs in America III*. Beverly Hills, CA: Sage, pp. 101–120.

84. Jacobs, J.B. (1977) *Stateville*. Chicago: University of Chicago Press.

85. a) Marsh, C. (1996) *From Black Muslims to Muslims*. Maryland: Scarecrow Press, Inc.; b) White, V.L. (2001) *Inside the Nation of Islam*. Gainesville: University Press of Florida.

86. a) Young, M. (2001) *What's in a Name?* Islam for Today; b) Baldwin, J. (1963) *The Fire Next Time*. New York: Vintage International Press.

CHAPTER 24. LATINO ADOLESCENT PARENTHOOD

1. Suro, Roberto (1994) *Strangers among Us*. New York: Alfred A. Knopf.

2. Horwitz, Tony (2006) Immigration – and the Curse of the Black Legend. *New York Times* July 9, p. WK 13.

3. De Genova, N. & Ramos-Zayas, A.Y. (2003) *Latino Crossings*. New York: Routledge, p. 214.

4. Gallardo-Cooper, M. (1999) *Latino Perspectives*. In Kromash, S. Cultural/Spiritual Diversity. Symposium at the National Association of Social Workers. Melbourne, Florida.

5. a) Camp-Flore, A. & Fineman, H. (2005) A Latin Power Surge. *Newsweek*, May 30, pp. 25–31; b) U.S. Census Bureau (2008) *2007 American Community Survey Data Profile Highlights*.

6. Camp-Flore, A. & Fineman, H. (2005) A Latin Power Surge. *Newsweek* May 30, pp. 25–31.

7. Suro, R. (1998) *Strangers among Us*. New York: Knopf.

8. Smith J.P. (2003) Assimilation across the Latino Generations. *American Economic Review* 93 (2): 315–319.

9. Vexler, E.J. & Suellentrop, K. (2006) *Bridging Two Worlds*. Washington, DC: The National Campaign to Prevent Teen Pregnancy.

10. Rodriguez, G. (2005) Why We're the New Irish. *Newsweek*, May 30, p. 35.

11. a) Smith J.P. (2003) Assimilation Across the Latino Generations. *American Economic Review* 93 (2): 315–319; b) Quirk, M. (2007) The Mexican Connection. *The Atlantic* 299 (3): 26–27.

12. Mindiola, Jr., T., et al (2002) *Black-Brown Relations and Stereotypes*. Austin, TX: University of Texas Press, pp. 100–101, 120.

13. Sosa, L. (1998) *The Americano Dream*. New York: Penguin.

14. Badillo, H. (2007) *One Nation, One Standard*. New York: Sentinel.

15. Tobar, H. (2005) *Translation Nation*. New York: Riverhead Books.

16. a) Thernstrom, A. & Thernstrom, S. (2003) *No Excuses*. New York: Simon & Schuster, p. 105; b) Besharov, D. J. (2007) The Rio Grande Rises. *New York Times* October 1, p. A27.

17. a) Vexler, E.J. & Suellentrop, K. (2006) *Bridging Two Worlds*. Washington, DC: The National Campaign to Prevent Teen Pregnancy; b) Tienda, M. & Mitchell, F. (Eds.) (2006) *Hispanics and the Future of America*. Washington, DC: Committee on Transforming Our Common Destiny, National Research Council.

18. a) Pew Hispanic Center and Kaiser Family Foundation (2002) *2002 National Survey of Latinos*. Washington, DC & Menlo Park, CA; b) Jacoby, T. (Ed.) (2003) *Reinventing the Melting Pot*. New York: Basic Books, p. 28, 137.

19. Smith J.P. (2003) Assimilation across the Latino Generations. *American Economic Review* 93 (2): 315–319.

20. a) Lara, M., et al (2005) Acculturation and Latino Health in the United States. *Annual Review of Public Health* 26: 367–397; b) Grieco, E.M. (2004) *The Hispanic Challenge?* Washington, DC: Woodrow Wilson International Center for Scholars, pp. 10–12; c) Renoso, T.C., et al (1993) Does American Acculturation Affect Outcome of Mexican-American Teenage Pregnancy? *Journal of Adolescent Health* 14: 257–261.

21. De Genova, N. & Ramos-Zayas, A.Y. (2003) *Latino Crossings*. New York: Routledge, pp. 4, 157.

22. Horowitz, R. (1983) *Honor and the American Dream*. New Brunswick, NJ: Rutgers Press, pp. 219, 235, 230.

23. Pavich, E.G. (1986) A Chicana Perspective on Mexican Culture and Sexuality. *Journal of Social Work and Human Sexuality* 4 (3): 47–65.

24. Erickson, P.I. (1998) *Latina Adolescent Childbearing in East Los Angeles*. Austin, TX: University of Texas Press, pp. 66–71.

25. a) Alvarez, J. (2007) *Once Upon a Quinceañera*. New York: Viking Press; b) Suro, R. (1994) *Strangers Among Us*. New York: Alfred A. Knopf.

26. Erickson, P.I. (1998) *Latina Adolescent Childbearing in East Los Angeles*. Austin, TX: University of Texas Press, p. 29.

27. Vexler, E. (2007) *Voices Heard*. Washington, DC: The National Campaign to Prevent Teen Pregnancy.

28. a) Aufseeser, D., et al (2006). *The Family Environment and Adolescent Well-Being*. Washington, D.C.: Child Trends and San Francisco, CA: National Adolescent Health Information Center, University of California; b) Vexler, E.J., & Suellentrop, K. (2006) *Bridging Two Worlds*. Washington, DC: Campaign to Prevent Teen Pregnancy.

29. Suro, R. (1994) *Strangers among Us*. New York: Alfred A. Knopf.

30. Vexler, E.J. & Suellentrop, K. (2006) *Bridging Two Worlds*. Washington, DC: National Campaign to Prevent Teen Pregnancy.

31. a) Wilson, W.J. (1991) Poverty, Joblessness, and Family Structure in the Inner City. *Chicago Urban Poverty and Family Life Conference*, October; b) For Puerto Ricans see: Lemann, Nicholas (1991) The Other Underclass *The Atlantic Monthly* December: 96–110.

32. a) Williams, N. (1990) *The Mexican-American Family*. Dix Hills, NY: General Hall, p. 27; b) Erickson, P.I. (1998) *Latina Adolescent Childbearing in East Los Angeles*. Austin, TX: University of Texas Press, p. 28.

33. Sylvia C. (1994) Women, Work and Household Survival Strategies in Mexico 1982–1992. *Bulletin of Latin American Research* 13 (2): 203–233.

34. a) Smith, P.B., et al (2002) Targeting Males for Teenage Pregnancy Prevention in a School Setting. *School Social Work Journal* 27 (1): 23–36; b) Ryan, S., et al (2005) Hispanic Teen Pregnancy and Birth Rates. *Child Trends* No. 2005–01, February 2005.

35. a) Vexler, E.J. & Suellentrop, K. (2006) *Bridging Two Worlds*. Washington, DC: National Campaign to Prevent Teen Pregnancy; b) Erickson, P.I. (1998) *Latina Adolescent Childbearing in East Los Angeles*. Austin, TX: University of Texas Press, p. 27.

36. a) Martinez, A.L. (1981) The Impact of Adolescent Pregnancy on Hispanic Adolescents and their Families. In Ooms, T. (Ed.) *Teenage Pregnancy in a Family Context* Philadelphia, PA: Temple Press, pp. 335–336; b) Erickson, P.I. (1998) *Latina Adolescent Childbearing in East Los Angeles*. Austin, TX: University of Texas Press, p. 34.

37. Vexler, E.J. & Suellentrop, K. (2006) *Bridging Two Worlds*. Washington, DC: The National Campaign to Prevent Teen Pregnancy.

38. a) Way, S., et al (2006) Hispanic Concentration and the Conditional Influence of Collective Efficacy on Adolescent Childbearing. *Archives of Pediatrics & Adolescent Medicine* 160 (9): 925–930; b) Vexler, E.J. & Suellentrop, K. (2006) *Bridging Two Worlds*. Washington, DC: The National Campaign to Prevent Teen Pregnancy.

39. a) Hallcom, F. (2000) *An Urban Ethnography of Latino Street*. Northridge, CA: California State University; b) Mydans, S. (1995) For Hispanic Gang Members, Family Ties Are Strong. *New York Times* September 11: p. A12

40. Moore, J.W. (1991) *Going Down to the Barrio*. Philadelphia: Temple University Press, p. 114.

41. Moore, J.W. (1994) The Chola Life Course. *The International Journal of the Addictions* 29 (9): 1115–1126.

42. Domash, S.F. (2005) *America's Most Dangerous Gangs*. Washington, D.C: Terror Alert Response Center.

43. Mindiola, Jr., T., et al (2002) *Black-Brown Relations and Stereotypes*. Austin, TX: University of Texas Press, pp. 117–118, 120.

CHAPTER 25. AMERICAN INDIAN ADOLESCENT PARENTHOOD

1. Hilger, S.M. (1992) *Chippewa Child Life and Its Cultural Background*. St. Paul, MN: Minnesota Historical Society Press, p. 53.

2. *Invisible Tribes*. Seattle: Urban Indian Health Commission, 2007.

3. 417 U.S. 535 (1974).

4. National Indian Education Association (2003) *Education Facts & History*. Washington, DC: National Indian Education Association.

5. Niethammer, C. (1977) *Daughters of the Earth*. New York: MacMillan Publishing Co., p. 207.

6. Schwarz, M.T. (1997) *Molded in the Image of Changing Women*. Tucson, AZ: University of Arizona Press, pp. 229, 387, 384, 348.

7. Frisbie, C. J. (1967) *Kinaaldá*. Middletown, CT: Wesleyan University Press, p. 7.

8. Begay, C. (2006) Navajo Blessing Way Ceremony. *Native Youth Magazine* March 3.

9. Johnston, B. (1990) *Ojibway Ceremonies*. Lincoln, NB: University of Nebraska Press, pp. 1–4.

10. Buckley, T. (1988) Menstruation and the Power of Yurok Women. In Buckley, T. & Gottlieb, A. (Eds.) *Blood Magic*. Berkeley, CA: University of California Press, p. 207.

11. Underhill, R. (1979) *Papago Woman*. Prospect Heights, IL: Waveland Press, Inc.

12. Niethammer, C. (1977) *Daughters of the Earth*. New York: MacMillan Publishing Co., pp. 57, 64, 67, 68.

13. a) Willeto, A.A. & Goodluck, C. (2003) *Indian Children's Well-Being Indicators Data Book for 14 States*. New York: Annie E. Casey Foundation; b) Geronimus, A.T. (1987) On Teenage Childbearing and Neonatal Mortality in the United States. *Population and Development Review* 13 (2): 245–279; c) Kimminau, K.S. & Satzler, C.J. (2005) *Racial and Minority Health Disparities in Kansas*. Topeka, Kansas: Kansas Health Institute.

14. Cross, Te. (2006) Personal communication. Washington, DC: National Congress of American Indians.

15. a) Kimminau, K.S. & Satzler, C.J. (2005) *Racial and Minority Health Disparities in Kansas*. Topeka, KS: Kansas Health Institute; b) Kaufman, C.E. et al (2007) Within the Hidden Epidemic. *Sexually Transmitted Diseases* 34 (10): 767–777; c) Dixon, M. & Iron, P.E. (2006) *Strategies for Cultural Competency in Indian Health Care*. Washington, DC: American Public Health Association; d) Jones, D.S. (2006) The Persistence of American Indian Health Disparities. *American Journal of Public Health* 96 (12): 2122–2134.

16. The NHSDA Report (2003) *Substance Use among American Indians or Alaska Natives*. Washington, DC: Office of Applied Studies, Substance Abuse and Mental Health Services Administration.

17. Associated Press (2005) Numbers Paint Bleak Picture of Teen Life. *St. Petersburg Times* March 27, p. 4A.

18. May, P. (2007) Cited in Nieves, E.: Indian Reservation Reeling in Wave of Youth Suicides and Attempts. *New York Times* June 9, A9.

19. a) Webster Jr., B.H. & Bishaw, A. (2006) *Income, Earnings, and Poverty Data from the 2005 American Community Survey*. Washington, DC: U.S. Census Bureau.

20. a) Greene, J.P. & Winters, M.A. (2006) *Leaving Boys Behind*. New York: Manhattan Institute; b) National Center on Education Statistics (2005) *Status and Trends in Education of American Indians and Alaska Natives*. Washington, DC: U. S. Department of Education.

21. Kimminau, K.S. & Satzler, C.J. (2005) *Racial and Minority Health Disparities in Kansas*. Topeka, KS: Kansas Health Institute.

22. a) Tribal Law & Policy Institute (2003) *Tribal Healing to Wellness Courts*.Washington, DC: Bureau of Justice Assistance, U.S. Department of Justice; b) Lovell, A. (2005) Personal communication with C.W. Huddleston. In Huddleston C.W., et al (2005) *Painting the Current Picture.1, No. 2*. Alexandria, VA: National Drug Court Institute.

23. a) Major, A.K. & Egley, Jr., A. (2002) *2000 Survey of Youth Gangs in Indian Country*. Washington, DC: Office of Juvenile Justice and Delinquency Prevention, OJJDP Fact Sheet, June #01; b) Shay, B. (2006) Expert: Crack Down on Indian Gangs. Casper, WY: *Jackson Hole Star Tribune* May 20.

24. Bureau of Indian Affairs, U.S. Department of Interior.1849 C Street, NW, Washington, DC.

25. National Congress of American Indians. 1301 Connecticut Avenue, NW, Washington, DC.

26. National Indian Child Welfare Association, 5100 S.W Macadam Avenue, Suit, Portland, OR 97239.

27. National Indian Education Association. 110 Maryland Avenue, NE, Suite 104, Washington, D.C. 20002.

28. National Indian Gaming Association. 224 Second Street, SE, Washington, DC.

29. a) Reynolds, J. (2005) NIGA Tribal Gaming Impact Analysis. *Indian Country Today* March 1; b) Stiffman, A.R., et al (2007) From Early to Late Adolescence. *Journal of the Academy of Child and Adolescent Psychiatry* 46: 849.

30. Willeto, A.A. & Goodluck, C. (2003) *Indian Children's Well-Being Indicators Data Book for 14 States*. New York: Annie E. Casey Foundation.

CHAPTER 26. MUSLIM ADOLESCENT PARENTHOOD

1. Muslim Women's League (1995) *Sex and Sexuality in Islam*. Los Angeles, CA.

2. Al-Munajjid, Sheikh Muhammed Salih (2007) Al-Siyaam: 70 Rules for Fasting. <http://islamqa.com/>.

3. Booth, M. (2002) Arab Adolescents Facing the Future. In Brown, B. Bradford, et al (Eds.) *The World's Youth*. New York: Cambridge University Press, pp. 207–208.

4. Muslim Women's League (1995) *Sex and Sexuality in Islam*. Los Angeles, CA.

5. Ahmed, Leila (1992) *Women and Gender in Islam*. New Haven, CT: Yale University Press, p. 35.

6. Muslim Women's League USA (1998) Our Religion Teaches Equality and Peace. *Feminism and Nonviolence Studies*. Special Issue on Spiritual Diversity.

7. a) Kecia, A. (2003) *Muslim Sexual Ethics*. Waltham, MA: Brandeis University. The Feminist Ethics Sexuality Project; b) *Ahmad khan vs. Shah Bano Begum, A.I.R 1985. S.C.945.*

8. Ali, K. (2002) Rethinking Women's Issues in Muslim Communities. In Wolfe, M. (Ed.) *Taking Back Islam*. Emmaus, PA: Rodale Press.

9. a) Kelek, N. (2005) *Die Fremde Braut*. Berlin: Kiepenheuer & Witsch; b) Welch Report (2002) *New Law Raises Legal Muslim Marriage Age For Females From 9 To 13*. June 24.

10. Tibi, B. (2006) Cultural Change in Islamic Civilization. In Harrison, L.E. & Kagan, J. (Eds.) *Developing Cultures*. New York: Routledge, pp. 245, 258–259.

11. Pew Report (2007) *Muslim Americans*.Washington, DC: Pew Research Center, May 22.

12. Ali, K. (2002) Rethinking Women's Issues in Muslim Communities. In Wolfe, M. (Ed.) *Taking Back Islam*. Emmaus, PA: Rodale Press.

13. Dar al Islam. < http://www.daralislam.org/>.

CHAPTER 27. HMONG ADOLESCENT PARENTHOOD

1. Pfaff, T. (1995) *Hmong in America*. Eau Claire, WI: Chippewa Valley Museum Press.

2. Julian, R. (2005) Hmong Transnational Identity. *Hmong Studies Journal* 5: 1–23.

3. Ranard, D.A. (Ed.) (2004) *The Hmong*. Washington, DC: The Cultural Orientation Resource Center, p. 2.

4. a) Pfeifer, M. Minneapolis, MN: Hmong Resource Center; b) Xiong, Z.B. & Tuicomepee, A. (2004) Hmong Families in America. In *Hmong Census Publication*. Saint Paul, MN: Hmong Resource Center, pp. 12–20.

5. Ranard, D.A. (Ed.) (2004) *The Hmong*. Washington, DC: The Cultural Orientation Resource Center, p.1.

6. Keown-Bomar, J. (2004) *Kinship Networks among Hmong-American Refugees*. New York: LFB Publ., p. 167.

7. a) Keown-Bomar, J.A. (2003) *Relative Abilities*. Ph.D. Dissertation. Minneapolis, MN. University of Minnesota; b) Xiong, Z.B, et al (2005). Southeast Asian Perceptions of Good Adolescents and Good Parents. *Journal of Psychology* 139 (2): 159–175; c) Kaiser, T.L. (2005) Caught Between Cultures. *Hmong Studies Journal* 5: 1–14.

8. Xiong, Z.B. & Detzner, D.F. (2005) Southeast Asian Fathers' Experiences. *Hmong Studies Journal* 6: 1–23.

9. Chan, S. (2003) Scarred, Yet Undefeated Hmong and Cambodian Women and Girls in the United States. In Hune, S. & Nomura, G.M. (Eds.) *Asian/Pacific Islander American Women*. New York: New York University Press, p. 265.

10. Uno, K. (2003) Unlearning Orientalism. In Hune, S. & Nomura, G. M. (Eds.) *Asian/Pacific Islander American Women*. New York: New York University Press, p. 54.

11. Lo, K. (2002) *Across the Ocean*. Paper M.S. Menomonie, WI: University of Wisconsin-Stout.

12. Corlett, J.L. (1999). *Landscapes and Lifescapes*. Ph.D. dissertation. University of California–Davis.

13. Rice, P.L. (2002). Gender, Sexuality, and Marriage among Hmong Youth in Australia. In Manderson, L. & Liamputtong, P. (Eds.) *Coming of Age in South and Southeast Asia*. Richmond, BC, Canada: Curzon, p. 261.

14. Hutchinson, R. & McNall, M. (1994) Early Marriage in a Hmong Cohort. *Journal of Marriage and the Family* 65 (3): 579–590.

15. Vue, M. (2000) *Perception of Early Marriage and Future Educational Goals Attainment for Hmong Female Adolescents*. Paper for M.S. Menomonie, WI: University of Wisconsin-Stout.

16. Ngo, B. (2002) Contesting "Culture." *Anthropology & Education Quarterly* 33 (2): 163–188.

17. a) Foo, L.J. (2002) Hmong Women in the U.S. In Foo, L.J. (Ed.) *Asian American Women*. New York: Ford Foundation, pp. 145–161; b) Lo, K. (2002) *Across the Ocean*. Paper for M.S. Menomonie, WI: University of Wisconsin-Stout.

18. Julian, R. (2005) Hmong Transnational Identity. *Hmong Studies Journal* 5: 1–23.

19. Moua, T. (2003) *The Hmong Culture*. Paper for M.S. Eau Claire, WI: University of Wisconsin-Eau Claire.

20. Higgins, M.B. & Vang, K. (1999) *An Examination of Gangs in Eau Claire, Wisconsin and the Community's Racial Perception of Gangs*. Paper for M.S. Menomonie, WI: University of WI- Stout.

21. Xiong, S. (2002) *Hmong Family Processes and Their Impact on Hmong Adolescents' Delinquent Behaviors*. Paper for M.S. Menomonie, WI: University of Wisconsin-Stout.

22. Memmo, M., Park, J. & Small, S. (2000) *Dane County Youth Survey 2000*. Madison, WI: Dane County Youth Commission & University of Wisconsin-Madison, Dept. of Human Development & Family Studies.

PART 8. SOCIETY

1. Cadyand, E.H. & Budd, L.J. (1987) *On Whitman*. Durham, NC: Duke University Press.

CHAPTER 28. IMPACT OF ADOLESCENT PARENTHOOD ON SOCIETY

1. Thayer, L. (1976) The Functions of Incompetence. In Laszlo, E. & Sellon, E.B. (Eds.) *Vistas in Physical Reality*. New York: Plenum Press, p. 186.

2. Lerner, R.M., et al (2001) Parenting Adolescents and Adolescents as Parents. In Westman, J.C. (Ed.) *Parenthood in America*. Madison, WI: University of Wisconsin Press, pp. 106–108.

3. a) Vinovskis, M.A. (1988) *An "Epidemic" of Adolescent Pregnancy?* New York: Oxford University Press; b) Vinovskis, M.A. (2003) Historical Perspectives on Adolescent Pregnancy. *History of the Family* 8: 399–421.

4. a) Jackson, J. & Vinovskis, M.A. (1983) Public Opinion, Elections, and the "Single-Issue". In Steiner, G.Y. (Ed.) *The Abortion Dispute and the American System*. Washington, DC: The Brookings Institution; b) Vinovskis, M. A. (1988) *An "Epidemic" of Adolescent Pregnancy?* New York: Oxford University Press, pp. 211, 217.

5. Vinovskis, M.A. (2003) Historical Perspectives on Adolescent Pregnancy. *History of the Family* 8: 399–421.

6. a) Rowe, J. (2004) *W-2 Participants Who Had Their First Child as Minors*. Madison, Wisconsin: Department of Workforce Development; b) Furstenberg, F.F., et al (1987) Adolescent Mothers in Later Life. New York: Cambridge University Press. c) Maynard, R.A. (Ed.) (1997) *Kids having Kids*. Washington, DC: Urban Institute.

7. Harris, K.M. (1997) *Teen Mothers and the Revolving Welfare Door*. Philadelphia, PA: Temple University Press, pp. 127, 65, 74, 128, 131–132.

8. Gottschalk, P. (1992) The Intergenerational Transmission of Welfare Participation. *Journal of Policy Analysis and Management* 11: 254–272.

9. Maynard, R.A. (1997) *Kids Having Kids*. New York: Robin Hood Foundation, p. 20.

10. a) Whitman, T.L., et al (2001) *Interwoven Lives*. Mahwah, NJ: Lawrence Erlbaum. pp. 216, 83–86; b) Ibid, p. 178; c) Coley, R.C. & Chase-Lansdale, W. (1998) Adolescent Pregnancy and Parenthood. *American Psychologist* 53 (2): 152–66.

11. Hotz, V.J., et al (1996) The Cost and Consequences of Teenage Childbearing for Mothers and the Government. *Social Policy Review* Volume 1.1. Chicago, IL: University of Chicago.

12. Hoffman, S.D. (2006) *By the Numbers*. Washington, DC: National Campaign to Prevent Teen Pregnancy. When the costs of educating adolescent mothers are taken into account the estimate is increased to $20 billion.

13. a) Moretti, E. (2005) Social Returns to Human Capital. *NBER Reporter*, Spring, p. 13–15; b) College Degree Nearly Doubles Annual Earnings. *U.S. Census Bureau News* CB05–38. Washington, DC: Department of Commerce.

14. a) Zeckhauser, R.J. & Viscusi, W.K. (1990) Risk Within Reason. *Science* 248: 559–564; b) Brandt, AM. (1990) The Cigarette, Risk, and American Culture. *Daedalus* 119: 155–176, p. 161; c) Steenland, K. (1992) Passive Smoking and the Risk of Heart Disease. *Journal of the American Medical Association* 267: 94–99.

15. Hume, D. (1964) *David Hume, The Philosophical Works*. Darmstadt: Scientia Verlag Aalen, pp. 117–118.

16. Bowles, S. (2007) *Social Preferences and Public Economics*. Santa Fe, NM: Santa Fe Institute, January 14.

CHAPTER 29. PROGRAMS FOR ADOLESCENT PARENTS

1. *Hamilton Papers, Volume 2* (1961–1978) Burlington, Ontario: Canada: TannerRitchie Publishing, p. 242.

2. Kaplan, A. (1997) Teen Parents and Welfare Reform Policy. *Welfare Information Network, Issue Notices.* 1 (3).

3. Ibid.

4. Rothenberg, A. (2005) Bryan's First Two Years. *Zero to Three* 25 (4): 22–29.

5. Horowitz, R. (1995) *Teen Mothers.* Chicago: University of Chicago Press, pp. 195, 256–257, 260.

6. Musick, J. (1991) *Young, Poor, and Pregnant.* New Haven, CT: Yale University Press, p. 234.

7. Maton, K.I., et al (2004) *Investing in Children, Youth, Families, and Communities.* Washington, DC: American Psychological Association, p. 344.

8. Harvard Family Research Project. Cambridge, MA: Harvard Graduate School of Education.

9. National Youth Development Information Center. Washington, DC: National Collaboration for Youth.

10. a) Campbell, S. (2005) Caretaking in a Nurturing Way. *Zero to Three* 25 (5): 17–28; b) Harding, K., et al (2004). *Initial Results of the HFA Implementation Study.* Chicago, IL: Prevent Child Abuse America.

11. Duggan, A.K., et al (1999) Evaluation of Hawaii's Healthy Start Program. *Future of Children* 9 (1): 66–90.

12. Visiting Programs Help Reduce Child Maltreatment (2003) *Children's Bureau Express* 4 (3).

13. Nurse Family Partnership. Denver, CO: Nurse-Family Partnership National ServiceOffice.

14. Boo, K. (2006) Swamp Nurse. *The New Yorker* February 6, pp. 54–65.

15. a) Olds, D.L. (2002) Prenatal and Infancy Home Visiting by Nurses. *Preventive Science* 3 (3): 153–72; b) Olds, D.L., et al. (2007) Effects of Nurse Home Visiting on Maternal and Child Functioning. *Pediatrics* 120 (4): 832–45.

16. Korfmacher, J., et al (1999) Differences in Program Implementation between Nurses and Paraprofessionals Providing Home Visits during Pregnancy and Infancy. *American Journal of Public Health* 89 (12): 1847–1851.

17. Parents as Teachers National Center, Inc. St. Louis, M0. <www.patnc.org>.

18. O'Brien, T., et al (2002) *Impact of the Parents as Teachers Program.* Canon City, CO: Center for Human Investment Policy, Graduate School of Public Affairs, University of Colorado-Denver.

19. Colorado Bright Beginnings 2006 Program Evaluation. 730 Colorado Boulevard, Suite 202, Denver, CO 80206.

20. Sergio, A. (2006) *5 Year Comprehensive Performance Report October 1, 2000–September 15, 2005.* Milwaukee, WI: Rosalie Manor Community & Family Services.

21. Daro, D., et al (2005*) Welcome Home and Early Start.* Chicago, IL: Chapin Hall Working Paper.

22. Meredith K., et al (2001) *The Potential of Home Visitor Services to Strengthen Welfare-to-Work Programs for Teenage Parents on Cash Assistance.* Philadelphia, PA: University of Pennsylvania, Mathematica Policy Research, Inc. & the Health Federation of Philadelphia.

23. McCormick, M.C., et al (2006) Early Intervention in Low Birth Weight Infants. *Pediatrics* 117: 771–780.

24. McGonigel, M. (2005) Replication in Practice. *Zero to Three* 25 (5): 9–16.

25. Levenstein, P., et al (1998) Long-term Impact of a Verbal Interaction Program for an Exploratory Study of High School Outcomes. *Journal of Applied Developmental Psychology* 19 (2): 267–285.

26. a) McGonigel, M. (2005) Replication in Practice. *Zero to Three* 25 (5): 9–16; b) Center for Health Services (2004) *The Effectiveness of Mental Infant Health Outreach Worker Program.* Nashville, TN: Vanderbilt University.

27. a) The Ounce of Prevention Fund (2005) Adding Doulas to Early Childhood Programs, *Zero to Three* 25 (5): 43–45; b) Wilgoren, J. (2005) "Mothering the Mother." *New York Times* September 25, p. YT 11.

28. Wisconsin Center for Education Research. *Families and Schools Together (FAST) Project.* Madison, WI: University of Wisconsin School of Education.

29. Cardone, I., et al (2007) Know Yourself. *Zero to Three* 28 (2): 39–44).

30. National Center for Family Literacy. Louisville, KY. <http://www.famlit.org.>.

31. McGonigel, M. (2005) Replication in Practice: Lessons from Five lead Agencies. *Zero to Three* 25 (5): 9–16.

32. Black, M.M., et al (2006) Delaying Second Births among Adolescent Mothers. *Pediatrics* 118: e1087–e1099.

33. a) Rouse, C., et al (2005) Introducing the Issue. *Future of Children* 15 (1): 5–13; b) Korfmacher, J. (2005) Teen Parents in Early Childhood Interventions. *Zero to Three* 25 (4): 7– 13; c) Maynard, R. (1995) Teenage Childbearing and Welfare Reform. *Children and Youth Services Review* 17: 309–332.

34. Trupin, C. & Levin-Epstein, J. (2007) *Early Head Start and Teen Parent Families.* Washington, DC: Center for Law and Social Policy.

35. Policy Brief (2007) *2006 Head Start Program Information.* Washington, DC: Center for Law and Social Policy.

36. a) Love, J.M., et al (2005) Effectiveness of Early Head Start. *Developmental Psychology* 41: 885; b) Administration for Children and Families (2007) Preliminary Findings from the Early Head Start Follow-up. Washington, D.C.: Department of Health and Human Services; c) Center for Law and Social Policy (2007) *Early Head Start and Teen Parent Families.* Washington, DC: Author; d) Administration for Children and Families (2002) *Making a Difference in the Lives of Infants and Toddlers.* Washington, DC: Department of Health and Human Services.

37. Muir, M. (2004) School-Based Child Care. *The Principals' Partnership.* Principals' Partnership and Union Pacific Foundation. Maine Center for Meaningful Engaged Learning.

38. Williams, E.G. & Sadler, L.S. (2001) Effects of an Urban High School-Based Child Care Center on Self-Selected Adolescent Parents and Their Children. *Journal of School Health* 71 (2): 47–52.

39. Wisconsin Statutes: Chapter PI 19 *Education for School Age Parents.*

40. a) Batten, S. & T. Stowell, B.G. (1996) *School-Based Programs for Adolescent Parents and their Young Children.* Trenton, NJ: Center for Assessment and Policy Development; b) Adolescent Parent Network. St. Paul, MN: Minnesota Organization on Adolescent Pregnancy, Prevention and Parenting.

41. Potter, Tim (2006) Personal communication. Madison, WI: Madison Metropolitan School District.

42. Bosman, J. (2007) New York's Schools for Pregnant Girls Will Close. *New York Times* May 24, p. 1A.

43. San Francisco, CA: Administrative Offices for Florence Crittenton Services.

44. The Gladney Center for Adoption. Fort Worth, TX.

45. Interfaith Hospitality Network. 1121 University Avenue, Madison, WI 53715

46. a) Office for Planning and Evaluation (2000) *Second Chance Homes*. Washington, DC: Department of Health and Human Services; b) Reich, K. & Kelly, L. (2000) *A Place to Call Home*. Washington, DC: Social Policy Action.

47. Hulsey, L.K., et al (2005) *The Implementation of Maternity Group Home Programs*. Washington, DC: Assistant Secretary for Planning and Evaluation, U.S. Department of Health and Human Services.

48. a) Massachusetts Alliance on Teen Pegnancy (2002) *Teens and Sex in Massachusetts,* Boston, MA: Massachusetts Alliance on Teen Pegnancy; b) Probert, M.S. (2005) *Teen Living Program Network Monitoring Report*. Boston, MA: Department of Social Services & Department of Transitional Assistance.

49. Marsh, J.C. & Wirick, M.A. (1991) Evaluation of Hull House. *Evaluation and Program Planning* 14: 49–61.

50. Bureau of Child and Adolescent Health. *Teen Parent Services*. Springfield, IL: Department of Human Services.

51. a) Wechsler, N. (2005) Passing It On. *Zero to Three* 25 (4): 14–21; b) Lynn, L. (1990) The Rhetoric of Welfare Reform. *Social Science Review* 64 (2): 175–188.

52. Mayers, H. & Siegler, A.L. (2004) Finding Each Other. *Journal of Infant, Child, and Adolescent Psychotherapy* 3 (4): 444–465.

53. a) Quint, J.C., et al (1994) *New Chance*. New York: Manpower Demonstration Research Corporation; b) Quint, J.C., Bos, J.M., & Polit, D.F. (1997) *New Chance*. New York, NY: Manpower Demonstration Research Corporation.

54. Office of Family Planning (2008) *Adolescent Family Life Budget*. Washington, DC: Department of Health and Human Services.

55. Zaslow, M., et al (1998) Implications of the 1996 Welfare Legislation for Children. *Social Policy Report* 12 (3). Society for Research in Child Development.

56. Leiderman, S. (2001) *Interpersonal Violence and Adolescent Pregnancy*. Bala Cynwyd, PA: Center for Assessment and Policy Development & National Organization on Adolescent Pregnancy, Parenting and Prevention.

57. Turetsky, V. (2006) *Child Support Assignment and Distribution Provisions in the Deficit Reduction Act*. Washington, DC: Center for Law and Social Policy.

58. a) Wisconsin Works Fact Sheet (2007) *Wisconsin Works (W-2): Minor Parents*. Madison, WI: Department of Workforce Development; b) Teens and TANF. *The Henry J. Kaiser Family Foundation*. December 2003.

59. Shapiro, D.L. & Marcy, H.M. (2002) *Knocking on the Door*. Chicago, IL: Center for Impact Research.

60. Doran, M.B.W. & Roberts, D. (2001) Welfare Reform and Families in the Child Welfare System. *Institute for Policy Research Working Paper WP-02–08*. Evanston, IL: Institute for Policy Research, Northwestern University.

61. Bos, J.M. & Fellerath, V. (1997) *Final Report on Ohio's Welfare Initiative to Improve School Attendance among Teenage Parents*. New York, NY: Manpower Demonstration Research Corporation.

62. Cal-Works (2008) *Cal-Learn*. Sacramento, CA: Department of Social Services.

63. Mauldon, J., et al (2000) *Impact of California's Cal-Learn Demonstration Project*. Berkeley, CA: University of California Archive & Technical Assistance & California Department of Social Services.

64. a) Duffy, J. & Levin-Epstein, J. (2002) *Add It Up*. Washington, DC: Center for Law and Social Policy; b) Pawasarat, J., et al (1992) *Experiment on the School Attendance of Teenagers*

Receiving Aid to Families with Dependent Children. Milwaukee, WI: Employment and Training Institute, University of Wisconsin-Milwaukee.

65. Saleh, M., et al (2005) The Nature of Connections. *Adolescence* 40 (159): 513–523.

66. Sander, J.H. & Rosen, J.L. (1987) Teenage Fathers. *Family Planning Perspectives* 19 (3): 107–110.

67. Buzi, R.S., et al (2004) Young Fathers in a Fatherhood Program. *The Prevention Researcher* 11 (4): 18–20.

68. Center for Urban Families. Baltimore, MD. <http://www.cfwd.org/>.

69. Klerman, L.V. (2004) *Another Chance*. Washington, DC: National Campaign to Prevent Teen Pregnancy.

70. a) Looney, S. (2004) *Supporting Responsible Fatherhood in Austin, TX*. For the M.P.A., University of Texas; b) Smith, P.B., et al (2002) Programs for Young Fathers. *North American Journal of Psychology* 4 (1): 81–92.

71. a) Besharov, D.J. (1996) Work, Not Job Training. *AEI Online*. Washington, DC: February 28. b) Warrick, L., et al (1993). Educational Outcomes in Teenage Pregnancy and Parenting Programs. *Family Planning Perspectives* 25: 148–155.

72. a) Coley, R.L. & Chase-Lansdale, P.L. (1998) Adolescent Pregnancy and Parenthood. *American Psychologist* 53 (2): 152–166; b) Bruns, E.J. (2008) State Implementation of Evidence-Based Practice for Youths, Part I. *Journal of the Academy of Child and Adolescent Psychiatry* 47 (4): 369–373.

73. Lesesne, C.A., et al (2008) Promoting Science-Based Approaches to Teen Pregnancy Prevention. *American Journal of Community Psychology* Feb 27, DOI 10.1007/s10464–008–9175–y.

74. *What Do Children Need to Flourish?* Washington, DC: Child Trends.

75. Moore, K.A. (2008) Quasi Experimental Evaluations. *Research Brief #2008–04*. Washington, DC: Child Trends.

76. Summerville, G. (2006) *Copy That*. Washington, DC: Campaign to Prevent Teen Pregnancy.

77. Lohr, S. (2006) Academia Dissects the Service Sector, but Is It a Science? *New York Times* April 18, p. C-1.

CHAPTER 30. DAMPENING AND AMPLIFYING TRENDS

1. Coleman, J.S. (1982) *The Asymmetric Society*. Syracuse, NY: Syracuse University Press.

2. Hatcher, R.A., et al (1989) *Contraceptive Technology 1988–1989, 14th Ed*. New York: Irvington Publishers.

3. Facts at a Glance (2006) *Teen Birth Rate*. Washington, DC: Child Trends April, Publication # 2006–03.

4. Bianchi, S.M., et al (2006) *Changing Rhythms in American Family Life*. New York: Russell Sage.

5. Annie E. Casey Foundation. *Making Connections* in Denver, CO; Des Moines, IA; Hartford, CT; Indianapolis, IN; Louisville, KY; Oakland, CA; Providence, RI; San Antonio, TX; and Seattle, WA.

6. News from Child Trends (2008) *New Data on Teen Substance Abuse, Math Proficiency, and School Activities*. Washington, DC: Child Trends.

7. Kirby, D., et al (2006) *The Impact of Sex and HIV Education Programs in Schools and Communities on Sexual Behaviors Among Young Adults*. Research Triangle Park, NC: Family Health International, ETR Associates.

8. *FBI Annual Uniform Crime Report 2005*. Washington, DC: Federal Bureau of Investigation.

9. Donohue III, J.J. & Levitt, S.D. (2000) The Impact of Legalized Abortion on Crime. *The Quarterly Journal of Economics* 116 (2): 379–420.

10. a) Teen Drug Abuse Continues its Three-Year Decline. *NIDA Notes*. 19 (6): 10, 15; b) Becker, Gary S., et al (2004) *The Economic Theory of Illegal Goods*. NBER Working Paper No. 10976.

11. a) Moffitt, R. (1988) The Effect of Welfare on Marriage and Fertility. In *Welfare, the Family, and Reproductive Behavior*. Washington, D.C.: National Academy Press; b) Garfinkel, I., et al (Eds.) (1998) *Fathers Under Fire*, New York: Russell Sage; c) Aizer, A. & McLanahan, S. (2005) The Impact of Child Support on Fertility, Parental Investments and Child Health. *Journal of Human Resources*. 41: 28–45; d) McLanahan, S. (2007) Single Mothers. In Edwards, J., et al (Eds.) *Ending Poverty*. Chapel Hill, NC: University of North Carolina Center on Poverty.

12. a) Gennetian, L. & Knox, V. (2003) *Staying Single*. New York: Manpower Demonstration Research Corp.; b) Harknett, K. & Gennetian, L.A. (2003) How Earnings Supplement Affects Union Formation Among Low-Income Single Mothers. *Demography* 40: 451–478; c) Duncan, G., et al (2007) *Higher Ground*. New York: Russell Sage.

13. Cowan, P., et al (1998) Parenting Interventions. In Damon, W. (Ed.) *Handbook of Child Psychology, Volume 5*. New York: Wiley, 1998.

14. Basic Facts about Child Support (2007) *OCSE Annual Reports to Congress and 2005 and 2006 Preliminary Data Reports*. Washington, DC: Center for Law and Social Policy.

15. Jones, E.F., et al (1986) *Teenage Pregnancy in Industrialized Countries*. New Haven, CT: Yale Press, p. 7.

16. Sourander, A., et al (2006) Childhood Predictors of Male Criminality. *Journal of the American Academy of Child and Adolescent Psychiatry* 45 (5): 578–586.)

17. Bird, H.R. (1980) Stranger Reaction versus Stranger Anxiety. *Journal of the American Academy of Psychoanalysis* 8 (4): 555–63.

18. a) *National Center for Cultural Competence*. Washington, DC: Georgetown Center for Child and Human Development; b) Kennedy, E., et al (2007) Enhancing Cultural Competence in Out-Of-School Time Programs: What Is It, and Why Is It Important? *Research to Results #2007–03*. Washington, DC: Child Trends.

19. a) Gans, H.J. (1988) *Middle American Individualism*. New York: Free Press; b) Mitchell, L. (1998) *Stacked Deck*. Philadelphia: Temple Press, p. 11.

20. a) Epstein, W. M. (2002) *American Policy Making*. Lanham: Rowman & Littlefield Publishers, pp. 97, 103, 112; b) Rothkopf, D. (2008) *Superclass*. New York: Farrar, Straus and Giroux.

21. Henderson, W. (2006) Rethinking the "Juvenile" in Juvenile Justice. *WisKids Journal*, April.

22. National Center for Juvenile Justice (2006) *Models for Change*. Washington, DC: National Council of Juvenile and Family Court Judges.

23. Lakoff, George (2002) *Moral Politics. Second Edition*. Chicago: University of Chicago Press.

24. Childers, M. (2005) *Welfare Brat*. New York: Bloomsbury, pp. 1–3.

25. Wolff, V.E. (1993) *Make Lemonade*. New York: Scholastic Inc.

26. Robertson, M. (2005) *Motherhood, What You Don't Know*. Melinda Robertson.

27. Jones, E.F., et al (1986) *Teenage Pregnancy in Industrialized Countries*. New Haven, CT: Yale Press, p. 7.

PART 9. SOLUTIONS

1. Ellis, J.J. (2007) *American Creation*. New York: Alfred A. Knopf.

CHAPTER 31. PREVENTING ADOLESCENT PREGNANCY AND PARENTHOOD

1. Comer, J.P. (1972) *Beyond Black and White.* New York: Quadrangle Books, p. xv.

2. a) Heckman, J. J. (2006) Skill Formation and the Economics of Investing in Disadvantaged Children. *Science* 312: 1900–1902; b) Heckman, J. J. (2006) Catch 'em Young. *Wall Street Journal* January 10; c) Carneiro, P. & Heckman, J.J. (2003) Chapter 2. In Heckman, J.J., et al (Eds.) (2003) *Inequality in America*. Cambridge, MA: MIT Press, pp. 77–237; d) Rolnick, A. & Grunewald, R. (2003) Early Childhood Development. *FedGazette*. Sept. 9.

3. Galbraith, J.K. (1996) *The Good Society*. Boston: Houghton Mifflin.

4. a) Karoly, L.A., et al (2005) *Early Childhood Interventions*. Santa Monica, CA: RAND Corporation; b) Kilburn, M.R. & Karoly, L.A. (2008) *The Economics of Early Childhood Policy*. Santa Monica, CA: RAND Corporation.

5. Allen, J P., et al (2004). The Sexually Mature Teen as a Whole Person. In Phillips, D., et al (Eds.) *Child Development and Social Policy across Four Decades*. New York: Pergamon.

6. Maton, K.I., et al (2004) *Investing in Children, Youth, Families, and Communities*. Washington, DC: American Psychological Association, p. 200.

7. Fukuyama, F. (2000) Social Capital. In Harrison, Lawrence E. & Huntington, Samuel P. (Eds.) *Culture Matters*. New York: Basic Books, p. 98.

8. a) Miranne, K. & Young, A. (2002) Teen Mothers and Welfare Reform. *Occasional Paper 2002–1*. Detroit, MI: Wayne State University College of Urban and Metropolitan Affairs; b) Hoffman, S. (1998). Teenage Childbearing Is Not So Bad After All. . . Or Is It? *Family Planning Perspectives* 30: 236–241.

9. Bachrach, C.A. (l986) Adoption Plans, Adopted Children, and Adoptive Mothers. *Journal of Marriage and the Family* 48: 243–25.

10. The National Campaign to Prevent Teen Pregnancy (2005) *What's It Going to Take?* Washington, DC: Author.

11. a) Rothschild, M.L. (2004) *Overcoming the Tyranny of Small Decisions*. Madison, WI: University of Wisconsin School of Business Working Paper; b) Evans, W.D. (2008) Social Marketing Campaigns and Children's Media Use. *The Future of Children* 18 (1).

12. Burnham, T. (2005) *Mean Markets and Lizard Brains*. New York: Wiley.

13. Select Media (2007) *Tanisha's Choice*. New York: Select Media.

14. Putting What Works to Work (2006) *Curriculum-Based Programs That Prevent Teen Pregnancy*. Washington, DC: The National Campaign to Prevent Teen Pregnancy.

15. Brady, M. (1998) Laying the Foundation for Girls' Healthy Futures. *Studies in Family Planning* 29 (1): 79–82.

16. Adolescent Pregnancy Prevention Committee (2007) *Youth Confirmation Sessions*. Madison, Wisconsin: Division of Public Health; Impact Strategies, Inc.

17. Luker, K. (2006) *When Sex Goes to School*. New York: W.W. Norton & Company.

18. Maternal and Child Health Section (2002) *Minnesota Education Now and Babies Later*. St. Paul, MN: Minnesota Department of Health.

19. a) Kirby, D., et al (2006) *Sex and HIV Education Programs*.Scotts Valley, CA: ETR Associates; b) Kirby, D. (2007) *Emerging Answers*. Washington, DC: National Campaign to Pre-

vent Teen Pregnancy; c) Mueller, T.E., et al (2008) The Association Between Sex Education and Youth's Engagement in Sexual Intercourse. *Journal of Adolescent Health* 42: 89–96.

20. Get Real Indiana (2007) *Working for Comprehensive Sex Education in Your Community.* Indianapolis, IN: Indiana Department of Education.

21. a) Bleakley, A., et al (2006) Public Opinion on Sex Education. *Archives of Pediatric and Adolescent Medicine* 160: 1151–1156; b) Santelli, J., et al (2006) Abstinence and Abstinence Only Education. *Journal of Adolescent Health* 38: 72–81; c) Trenholm, C., et al (2007) *Impacts of Four Abstinence Education Programs.* Princeton, NJ: Mathematica Policy Research; d) Kohler, P. K., et al (2008) Abstinence-Only and Comprehensive Sex Education. *Journal of Adolescent Health* 42: 344–351; e) Weed, S.E., et al (2008) An Abstinence Program's Impact on Cognitive Mediators and Sexual Initiation. *American Journal of Health Behavior* 32: 60–73.

22. Zezima, K. (2007) Not All Are Pleased at Plan to Offer Birth Control at Maine Middle School. *New York Times* October 21, p. 14.

23. Duberstein, L., et al (2006) Changes in Formal Sex Education: 1995–2002. *Perspectives on Sexual and Reproductive Health* 38 (4): 182–189.

24. a) Infant Simulators. Eau Claire, WI: Realityworks, Inc.; b) Chavaudra, N. (2007) The Impact of Virtual Infant Simulators. *Journal of Family Planning and Reproductive Health Care* 33 (1):35.

25. Coyle, K.K., et al (2004) Draw the Line/Respect the Line. *American Journal of Public Health* 94 (5): 843–851.

26. Wise Guys. Greensboro, NC: Family Life Council of Greater Greensboro, Inc.

27. Ngwe, J.E., et al (2003) Evaluation of the Effects of the Aban Aya Youth Project in Reducing Violence among African American Adolescent Males. *Evaluation Review* 20 (10): 1–21.

28. a) Shaffer D., et al (1996) The NIMH Diagnostic Interview Schedule for Children Version 2.3. *Journal of the American Academy of Child and Adolescent Psychiatry* 35: 865–877; b) Kessler, R.C., et al (2005) Lifetime Prevalence and Age-Of-Onset Distributions of DSM-IV Disorders. *Archives of General Psychiatry* 62: 593–602.

29. a) Friedman, R.A. (2006) Uncovering an Epidemic. *New England Journal of Medicine* 355: 2717–2719; b) Velez, C.N. & Cohen. P. (1988) Suicidal Behavior and Ideation in a Community Sample of Children. *Journal of the American Academy of Child and Adolescent Psychiatry* 27: 349–356.

30. a) MENTOR/National Mentoring Partnership. Alexandria, VA. <www.mentoring.org>; b) Students Against Destructive Decisions. Marlborough, MA: SADD National.

31. a) Big Brothers Big Sisters of America. 230 North 13th Street, Philadelphia, PA. 19107; b) Tierney, J.P., Grossman, J.B. & Resch, N.L. (1995) *Making a Difference.* Philadelphia, PA: Public/Private Ventures.

32. Beating the Odds Foundation. *Beating the Odds Mentoring Program.* Hollidaysburg, PA: Author.

33. Alpha Phi Alpha Fraternity, Inc. 2313 Saint Paul Street, Baltimore, MD 21218.

34. a) Billig, S., et al (2005) The Impact of Participation in Service-Learning on High School Students' Civic Engagement. *Circle Working Paper 33.* Denver, CO: RMC Research Corporation, Denver, CO; b) Harris Interactive (2006) *Growing to Greatness.* St. Paul, MN: National Youth Leadership Council.

35. O'Donnell, L., et al (2002) Long-Term Reductions in Sexual Initiation and Sexual Activity among Urban Middle Schoolers in The Reach For Health Service Learning Program. *Journal of Adolescent Health* 31: 93–100.

36. a) Wyman Teen Outreach Program. Wyman Center. Eureka, Missouri < www.wymanteens .org>; b) Allen, J.P. & Philliber, S. (2001) Who Benefits Most from a Broadly Targeted Prevention Program? *Journal of Community Psychology* 29 (6): 637–655.

37. National 4–H Headquarters. Washington, DC: Cooperative State Research, Education, and Extension Service, United States Department of Agriculture.

38. Carrera Adolescent Pregnancy Prevention Program. 219 Sullivan St # 1. New York, NY 10012.

39. a) The Children's Aid Society. *Carrera High Graduation and College Admission Results*. Philliber Research Associates, 16 Main Street, Accord, NY12404; b) Beckett, M.K. (2008) *Current-GenerationYouth Programs*. Santa Monica, CA: RAND Corporation.

40. Boys and Girls Clubs. 1275 Peachtree Street NE, Atlanta, GA 30309–3506.

41. Wisconsin National Guard Challenge Academy. Fort McCoy, WI.

42. Tsoi-A-Fatt, R. (2008) *A Collective Responsibility, A Collective Work*. Washington, DC: Center for Law and Social Policy.

43. a) Brooks-Gunn, J. & Furstenberg, Jr., F.F. (l987) Continuity and Change in the Context of Poverty. In Gallagher, J. & Ramey, C. (Eds.) *The Malleability of Children* Baltimore, MD: Paul H. Brookes; b) Mincy, R.B. & Wiener, S.J. (1990) *A Mentor, Peer Group, Incentive Model for Helping Underclass Youth*. Washington. DC: Urban Institute; c) Barth, R.P. (2008) Outcomes for Youth Receiving Intensive Home Therapy or Residential Care. *American Journal of Orthopsychiatry* 77 (4) 497–505.

44. Schemo, D. J. (2006) More than Schools to Close the Achievement Gap. *New York Times* August 9, p. A15.

45. Rothstein, R. (2004) *Class and Schools*. Washington, DC: Economic Policy Institute, 2004.

46. Goldstein, S.E., et al (2005) Parents, Peers, and Problem Behavior. *Developmental Psychology* 41 (2): 401–413.

47. Albert, B. (2007) *With One Voice 2007*. Washington, DC: National Campaign to Prevent Teen Pregnancy.

48. a) Rothschild, M. L. (1999) Carrots, Sticks and Promises. *Journal of Marketing* 63: 24–37; b) Rolleri, L., et al (2006) *A Logic Model of Parent-Child Connectedness*. Santa Cruz, CA: ETR Associates; c) Fasula, A.M. (2006) African-American and Hispanic Adolescents' Intentions to Delay First Intercourse. *Journal of Adolescent Health* 38 (3): 193–200; d) *Terms of Engagement*. Washington, DC: The National Campaign to Prevent Teen Pregnancy.

49. Altoosa (2006) Sometimes What You Need the Most is the Last Thing You Want. *Seventeen* March, p, 131.

50. a) Brody, G. H., et al (2006). The Strong African-American Families Program. *Journal of Family Psychology* 20 (1): 1–11.; b) Spoth, R., et al (2005). Randomized Study of Combined Universal Family and School Preventive Interventions. *Psychology of Addictive Behaviors* 19 (4): 372–381.

51. Wisconsin Center for Education Research. *Families and Schools Together (FAST) Project*. Madison, WI: School of Education, University of Wisconsin-Madison.

52. Motivational Educational Entertainment Productions, Inc. (2004) *This Is My Reality*. Philadelphia, PA: Author.

53. a) Coontz, S. & Folbre, N. (2002) Marriage, Poverty, and Public Policy. *Fifth Annual CCF Conference*, April 26–28; b) Institute for Family-Centered Care. 7900 Wisconsin Avenue, Suite 405. Bethesda, Maryland 20814.

54. a) Commission on Children at Risk (2007) Hardwired to Connect. *The New Scientific Case for Authoritative Communities*. New York, NY: Institute for American Values; b) Pittman, K., et al (2007) *Core Principles for Engaging Young People in Community Change*. Washington, DC: The Forum for Youth Investment.

55. Jean-Louis, B. (2006) *Harlem Children's Zone Evaluation*. New York, NY: Harlem Children's Zone.

56. a) Time Dollar Newsletter (2004) *Time to Unite*. Washington, DC: Time Dollar Institute; b) Henderson, Henderson (2006) 21st Century Strategies for Sustainability. *Foresight*, February. Cambridge, U.K.; c) Cahn, E.S. (2000) *No More Throw-Away People*. Washington, DC: Essential Books; d) TimeBanks USA, 5500 39th St. NW.Washington, DC 20015.

57. a) Finn, Jr., C.E. (2005) Things Are Falling Apart. *Education Next*. Stanford, CA: Hoover Foundation; b) Wise, B. (2008) *Raising the Grade*. San Francisco: Jossey-Bass.

58. a) The Teaching Commission (2004) *Teaching at Risk*. New York: The CUNY Graduate Center; b) Cetron, M. & Davies, O. (2008) *Trends: Looking at the Future of Education*. Alexandria, VA: Educational Research Service.

59. a) Henderson, A.T. & Mapp, K.L. (2002) *A New Wave of Evidence*. Austin, Texas: Southwest Educational Development Laboratory; b) Center on School, Family, and Community Partnerships. Baltimore, MD: National Network of Partnership Schools, Johns Hopkins University; c) Martin, N. & Halperin, S. (2006). *Whatever It Takes*. Washington, DC: American Youth Policy Forum.

60. a) Mirel, J. (2006) The Traditional High School. *Education Next* 6 (1). Stanford, CA: Hoover Foundation; b) Powell, A., et al (1985) *The Shopping Mall High School*. Boston, MA: Houghton Mifflin.

61. a) Finn, Jr., C.E. (2005) Things Are Falling Apart. *Education Next* 6 (1). Stanford, CA: Hoover Foundation; b) Finn, S.E., Jr. (2008) *Troublemaker*. Princeton, NJ: Princeton University Press.

62. a) Maton, K.I., et al (2004) *Investing in Children, Youth, Families, and Communities*. Washington, DC: American Psychological Association, p. 245; b) Angus, D.J. & Mirel, J. (1999) *The Failed Promise of the American High School, 1890–1995*. New York: Teachers College Press.

63. Mirel, J. (2006) The Traditional High School. *Education Next* 6 (1). Stanford, CA: Hoover Foundation.

64. Saulny, S. (2006) Tutor Program Offered By Law Is Going Unused. *New York Times* February 12.

65. a) Philp, R. (2007) *Engaging Tweens and Teens*. Thousand Oaks, CA: Corwin Press; b) Roberts, R.E., et al (2008) Chronic Insomnia and Its Negative Consequences. *Journal of Adolescent Health* 42: 294–302.

66. Thernstrom, A. & Thernstrom, S. (2003) *No Excuses*. New York: Simon & Schuster, p. 274.

67. Knowledge Is Power Program. San Francisco, CA: KIPP Foundation. <http://www.kipp.org/>.

68. Eaton, S. E. (2001) *The Other Boston Busing Story*. New Haven, CT: Yale University Press, pp. 220–221, 225.

69. Comer, J. (2004) *Leave No Child Behind*. New Haven, CT: Yale University Press.

70. Martin, N. & Halperin, S. (2006) *Whatever It Takes*. Washington, DC: American Youth Policy Forum, p. 7.

71. Eagle Academy for Young Men. 244 E. 163rd Street. Bronx, NY.

72. a) The Technical Assistance & Leadership Center. 2620 W. North Ave. Milwaukee WI 53205: b) Martin, N. & Halperin, S. (2006). *Whatever It Takes*. Washington, DC: American Youth Policy Forum, p. 112.

73. a) Birmingham, J., et al (2005) *Shared Features of High-Performing After-School Programs*. Washington, DC: Policy Studies Associates; b) Durlak, J.A. & Weissberg, R.P. (2007). *The Impact of After-School Programs that Promote Personal and Social Skills.* Chicago, IL: Collaborative for Academic, Social, and Emotional Learning.

74. Beckett, M.K. (2008) *Current-GenerationYouth Programs.* Santa Monica, CA: RAND Corporation.

75. Community Building Resource Exchange. < http://www.commbuild.org>.

76. a) Chambers, E.T. (2003) *Roots for Radicals.* New York: Continuum; b) Industrial Areas Foundation. 220 West Kinzie Street, Chicago, IL 60610.

77. Communities Organized for Public Service. 2300 West Commerce. San Antonio, Texas 78283.

78. a) YouthBuild USA. 58 Day Street Somerville, MA 02144; b) Ferguson, R.F., et al (1996) *YouthBuild in Developmental Perspective.* Cambridge, MA: Harvard University Department of Urban Studies and Planning; c) Hahn, Andrew, et al (2004) *Life after YouthBuild.* Somerville, MA: YouthBuild USA.

79. a) New York City Department of Homeless Services. 33 Beaver Street. New York 10004; b) Rew, Lynn (2001) Sexual Health Practices of Homeless Youth. *Issues in Comprehensive Pediatric Nursing* 24: 1–18.

80. a) Goering J. & Kraft, J. (1999) *Moving to Opportunity for Fair Housing Demonstation Program.* Washington, DC: Office of Policy Development and Research, U.S. Department of Housing and Urban Development; b) Orr, L., et al (2003) *Moving to Opportunity Interim Impacts Evaluation.* Washington, DC: Office of Policy Development & Research, Department of Housing and Urban Development; c) Sanbonmatsu, L., et al (2006) *Neighborhoods and Academic Achievement.* Cambridge, MA: National Bureau of Economic Research.

81. Cassell, C., et al (2005) Mobilizing Communities. *Journal of Adolescent Health* 37: S3–S10.

82. Rao, V. & Walton, M. (2004) Culture and Public Action. In Rao, V. & Walton, M. (Eds.) *Culture and Public Action.* Stanford, CA: Stanford University Press, pp. 29, 361–362.

83. Think MTV: It's Your Sex Life. <http://www.mtv.com/thinkmtv/sexual_health>.

84. a) Motivational Educational Productions. Philadelphia, PA. <http://www.meeproductions.com>; b) Be on the Safe Side. MEE Productions Inc. 1608 20th Street, NW, 2nd Floor, Washington, DC 20009.

85. a) Wilson, W.J. (1996) *When Work Disappears.* New York: Knopf, pp. 43, 238; b) Holzer, Harry J., et al (2006) *Reconnecting Disadvantaged Young Men.* Washington, DC: Urban Institute Press.

86. *National Urban League's State of Black America 2006.* Washington, DC: Urban League.

87. Haskins, R. (2006) *Work over Welfare.* Washington, DC: Brookings Institution Press.

88. Courtney, M.E. (2006) Welfare Reform's Shortcoming. *Washington Post* July 24, p. A19.

89. The Commission on Adult Basic Education. Syracuse, NY.

90. Western, B. (2006) *Punishment and Inequality in America.* New York: Russell Sage Foundation.

91. a) Mumola, C.J. & Karberg, J.C. (2007) *Drug Use and Dependence, State and Federal Prisoners, 2004.* Washington, DC: Bureau of Justice Statistics Special Report; b) Number of Women in Prisons Is on Rise. *New York Times* October 27, 2005, p. A-18; c) Center for Research on Child Wellbeing (2008) Parental Incarceration and Child Wellbeing in Fragile Families. *Fragile Families Research Brief* #42. Princeton, NJ: Princeton University.

92. a) National Helping Individuals with Criminal Records Re-enter through Employment Network. New York, NY: Legal Action Center; b) Johnson, E. I. (2006) Youth with Incarcerated Parents. *The Prevention Researcher* 13: 3–6.

93. a) Travis, J. & Waul, M. (Eds.) *Prisoners Once Removed*. Washington, DC: The Urban Institute Press, pp. ix-x; b) Currie, E. (1998) *Crime and Punishment in the United States*. New York: Henry Holt, p. 191.

94. a) Ehrensaft, M. et al (2003) *Patterns of Criminal Conviction and Incarceration.* New York: Vera Institute of Justice; b) Ross, T., et al (2004) *Hard Data on Hard Times*. New York: Vera Institute of Justice.

95. National Collaboration for Youth (2001) *Making a Difference in the Lives of Youth*. Washington, DC: Author.

96. a) The National Association of Drug Court Professionals. *Talking Points/Statistics on Drug Courts*. Alexandria, VA: National Drug Court Institute; b) *Drug Use Forecasting Study* (1996) Washington, DC: Department of Justice; c) Mumola, C.J. & Karberg, J.C. (2007) *Drug Use and Dependence, State and Federal Prisoners, 2004*. Washington, DC: Bureau of Justice Statistics Special Report.

97. a) Huddleston III, C., et al (2005) *Painting the Current Picture, Volume 1, No. 2*. Alexandria, VA: National Drug Court Institute; b) Greene, J. & Pranis, K. (2006) *Treatment Instead of Prison*. Brooklyn, NY: Justice Strategies; c) Skipp, C. & Campo-Flores, A. (2006) A 'Meth Prison' Movement. *Newsweek* April 24, p. 9.

98. a) Office of Justice Programs Drug Court Clearinghouse and Technical Assistance Project (1998) *Juvenile and Family Drug Courts*. Washington, DC: American University; b) Kelly, J.F., et al (2005) Substance Use Disorder Patients Who Are Mandated to Treatment. *Journal of Substance Abuse Treatment* 28 (3): 213–223.

99. Office of Justice Programs Drug Court Clearinghouse and Technical Assistance Project (2001) *Drug Court Activity Update*. Washington, DC: American University.

100. a) National Association of Youth Courts, Inc., 345 N. Charles Street, Baltimore, MD 21201; b) Vickers, M.M. (2004) *An Overview of School-Based Youth Court Program Design Options*. Washington DC: National Youth Court Center, Department of Justice.

101. Turner, S. & Fain, T. (2005) *Accomplishments in Juvenile Probation in California over the Last Decade*. Santa Monica, CA: RAND Corporation.

102. a) Levitt, S.D. (2004) Understanding Why Crime Fell in the 1990s. *Journal of Economic Perspectives* 18: 163–190; b) Zehr, H. (Ed.) (2004) *Critical Issues in Restorative Justice*. Monsey, NY: Criminal Justice Press.

103. a) McCold, P. & Wachtel, T. (2003) *In Pursuit of Paradigm*. Bethlehem, PA: International Institute for Restorative Practices; b) Langan, P.A. & Durose, M.R. (2004) *The Remarkable Drop in Crime in New York City*. Washington, DC: Bureau of Justice Statistics, U. S. Department of Justice.

104. a) Henggeler, S.W. Multisystemic Therapy. *Consortium on Children, Families and the Law*. Charleston, SC: Family Services Research Center, Medical University of South Carolina; b) Patchin, J.W. (2006) *The Family Context of Childhood Delinquency*. New York: LFB Scholarly Publishing, p. 117.

105. Marshall, W. & Sawhill, I.V. (2004) Progressive Family Policy in the Twenty-first Century. In Moynihan, D.P., et al (Eds.) *The Future of the Family*. New York: Russell Sage Foundation, p. 207.

106. a) Devantier, P. (2005) *Adoption Awareness Training*. Washington, DC: National Council for Adoption; b) Infant Adoption Training Initiative. Spaulding for Children, 16250 Northland Drive, Southfield, MI 48075.

107. Resnick, M.D., et al (1990) Characteristics of Unmarried Adolescent Mothers. *American Journal of Orthopsychiatry* 60: 577–584.

CHAPTER 32. VALUING PARENTHOOD

1. Crittenden, A. (2001) *The Price of Motherhood*. New York: Henry Holt & Company, p. 258.

2. Charlton, B.G. (2006) The Rise of the Boy-genius. *Medical Hypotheses* 67 (4): 679–681.

3. Fineman, M. (2000) Cracking the Foundational Myths. *Journal of Gender, Social Policy and the Law* 8: 13–29.

4. a) Westman, J.C. (1994) *Licensing Parents*. New York: Perseus Books, p. 85; b) Cohen, M. (1998) The Monetary Value of Saving a High Risk Youth. *Journal of Quantitative Criminology* 14: 5–33.

5. a) Knudsen, E.I., et al (2006) Economic, Neurobiological, and Behavioral Perspectives on Building America's Workforce. *Perspectives of the National Academy of Sciences* 103 (27): 10155–10162; b) Committee on Science, Engineering & Public Policy (2005) *Rising above the Gathering Storm*. Washington DC: National Academies Press.

6. Ibid, p. 162.

7. Ibid, p. 172.

8. de Tocqueville, A. (1969) *Democracy in America, 1840*. In Mayer, J.P. (Ed.) *Democracy in America*. Garden City, NY: Doubleday.

9. Florida, R. (2005) *The Flight of the Creative Class*. New York: HarperBusiness, pp. 16, 269.

10. Ibid, p. 144.

11. Epstein, W.M. (1993) *The Dilemma of American Social Welfare*. New Brunswick, NJ: Transaction, p. 2.

12. Ozment, S. (2001) *Ancestors*. Cambridge, MA: Harvard University Press.

13. a) Chambers, E.T. (2003) *Roots for Radicals*. New York: Continuum, p. 31; b) Lakoff, G. (2006) *Thinking Points*. New York: Farrar, Straus and Giroux.

14. Ibid, p. 22.

15. Johann Wolfgang von Goethe's last letter, 17 March 1832, to Wilhelm von Humboldt.

16. Chambers, E.T. (2003) *Roots for Radicals*. New York: Continuum, p. 42.

17. Ibid, p. 125.

18. Marglin, S.A. (2008) *The Dismal Science*. Cambridge, MA: Harvard University Press.

19. Chambers, E.T. (2003) *Roots for Radicals*. New York: Continuum, p. 61.

20. Ibid, pp. 134–140.

21. a) Hewlett, S.A. & West, C. (2001) Parent Power. In Westman, J.C. (Ed.) *Parenthood in America*. Madison, WI: Univ. of Wisconsin Press, pp. 270–271; b) Longman, P. (2004) Raising Hell. *Washington Monthly* March, p. 256.

22. Aviezer, O., et al (1994) "Children of the Dream" Revisited. *Psychological Bulletin* 116: 99–116.

23. National Child Abuse and Neglect Data System (2005) *Summary Child Maltreatment 2004*. Ithaca, NY: Cornell University Family Life Development Center.

24. Haidt, J. (2005) *The Happiness Hypothesis*. New York: Perseus, p.117.

25. Hrdy, S.B. (2001) *The Past, Present, and Future of the Human Family*. The Tanner Lectures on Human Values. Salt Lake City, UT: University of Utah, February 27 and 28.

26. Marquardt, E. (2007) *The Revolution in Parenthood*. New York: Institute for American Values.

27. Nightingale, C.H. (1993) *On the Edge*. New York: Basic Books.

28. Schelling, T.C. (2006) *Strategies of Commitment and Other Essays*. Cambridge, MA: Harvard University Press.

29. Winn, Marie (1983) *Children without Childhood*. New York: Pantheon, p. 210.

30. a) Brooks-Gunn, J. & Furstenberg, F.F. (1987) Continuity and Change in the Context of Poverty. In Gallagher, J. & Ramey, C. (Eds.) *The Malleability of Children*. Baltimore, MD: Paul H. Brookes; b) Mincy, R.B. & Wiener, S. J. (1990) *A Mentor, Peer Group, Incentive Model for Helping Underclass Youth*. Washington. DC: Urban Institute.

31. a) Warner, J. (2006) *Perfect Madness*. New York: Riverhead Books; b) Skocpol, T. (1997) *Lessons from History*. Washington, DC: The Children's Partnership.

32. Lally, J. (2005) The Human Rights of Infants and Toddlers. *Zero to Three* 25 (3): 43–46.

33. a) Presser, H.B. (2003) *Working in a 24/7 Economy*. New York: Russell Sage Foundation; b) National Association of Child Care Resource & Referral Agencies (2007) *We Can Do Better*. Arlington, VA: Author.

34. Weissbourd, R. (1999) Distancing Dad. *The American Prospect* 11 (2): December 6.

35. The Black Star Project, 3509 S. King Drive, Suite 2B, Chicago, IL. 60653.

36. Erickson, P. (1998) *Latina Adolescent Childbearing in East Los Angeles*. Austin, TX: U. of Texas Press, p. 162.

37. Marquardt, E. (2006) *The Emerging Global Clash between Adult Rights and Children's Needs*. New York: Commission on Parenthood's Future, Institute for American Values.

CHAPTER 33. PARENTHOOD PLANNING TEAMS AND CERTIFICATION OF PARENTHOOD

1. Greider, W. (1992) *Who Will Tell the People*. New York: Simon & Schuster, pp. 13–14.

2. Hine, T. (2000) *The Rise and Fall of the American Teenager*. New York: Bard/Avon.

3. Trad, P.V. (1995) Mental Health of Adolescent Mothers. *Journal of the American Academy of Child and Adolescent Psychiatry* 34: 130–142.

4. Grad, F.P. (1990) *Public Health Law Manual*. Washington, DC: American Public Health Association, p. 4.

5. National Clearinghouse on Child Abuse and Neglect Information (2006) Child Abuse Prevention and Treatment Act (CAPTA) of 1974, P.L. 93–247; Amended 1978, 1984, 1988, 1992, 1996, 2003.

6. a) New Jersey Public Law 2006 c12; b) Bayer, R. & Fairchild A.L. (2006) Changing the Paradigm for HIV Testing. *New England Journal of Medicine* 355: 674.

7. a) Broder, D. (2006) Do We Really Have to Add This to our Worry List? *St. Petersburg Times* April 15; b) Maynard, R. (1997) The Role for Paternalism in Teen Pregnancy Prevention and Teen Parent Services. In Mead, L. (Ed.) *The New Paternalism*. Washington, DC: The Brookings Institution Press.

8. a) Frankfurt, H. (1971) Freedom of the Will and the Concept of a Person. *The Journal of Philosophy* 68 (1): 5–20; b) Frankfurt, H. (2006) *On Truth*. New York: Random House.

9. a) Title XX: Adolescent Family Life Demonstration Projects. *Federal Register June 1, 2006*, 71 (105): 31897–31906; b) Zabin, L.S., et al (1996) Adolescents with Negative Pregnancy Test Results. *Journal of the American Medical Association* 275: 113–117; c) Wisconsin Medicaid (2001) Wisconsin Medicaid and BadgerCare Prenatal Care Coordination Services Handbook. Madison, WI: Department of Health and Family Services; d) Olds, D., et al (1998) Long-term Effects of Nurse Home Visitation. *Journal of the American Medical Association* 280:1238–1244.

10. a) Alvy, K.T. i) *Effective Black Parenting Program Parent Handbook*; ii) *Los Niños Bien Educados Parent Handbook*; iii) *South East Asian Parent Handbook*. Studio City, CA: Center for the Improvement of Child Caring; b) Alvy, K.T. (2007) *The Positive Parent*. New York: Teachers College Press; c) Santiago-Rivera, A.L., et al (2002) *Counseling Latinos and la familia*. Thousand

Oaks, CA: Sage Publications; d) National Indian Child Welfare Association. *Positive Indian Parenting*. Portland, OR: Author.

11. Nadelson, C.C. (1975) The Pregnant Teenager. *Psychiatric Opinion* 12 (2): 6–12.

12. Fessler, A. (2006) *The Girls Who Went Away*. New York: The Penguin Press, p. 189.

13. Leary, M. (2004) *The Curse of the Self*. New York: Oxford University Press, pp. vi, 163.

14. Wall, T. (2000) Transcending Ideals about Trans-Racial Adoptions. *New Visions Commentary*. Washington, DC: The National Center for Public Policy Research.

15. *1 Kings* 3:16–28

16. Wilson, T.D. (2006) The Power of Social Psychological Interventions. *Science* 313: 1251–1252.

17. Wisconsin Chapter 48.415 Grounds for involuntary termination of parental rights: (10) Prior involuntary termination of parental rights to another child.

18. *Carey v. Population Services International* (1977) 431 U.S. 678, p. 694.

19. Baker, S.P., et al (2006) Graduated Driver Licensing Programs and Fatal Crashes. *Pediatrics* 118: 56–62.

20. Maine Statutes: Title 18–A: Probate Code, Article V: Protection of Persons under Disability and their Property, Part 2: Guardians of Minors, §5–204. Court appointment of guardian of minor; conditions for appointment.

21. Children Come First Advisory Committee (2005) *Annual Report On Integrated Services Projects and Coordinated Services Teams*. Madison, WI: Bureau of Mental Health and Substance Abuse Services.

22. Ray, B. (2003) Mothers in Prison. *Harris View*. Chicago, IL: School of Public Policy, University of Chicago.

23. Vital Statistics of the U.S. (2008) *Table 5. Trends in Total Births and Out-of-Wedlock Births among Women under 30 Years of Age*. Washington, DC: National Center for Health Statistics.

24. Dwyer, J. (2006) *Children's Relationship Rights*. New York: Cambridge University Press, pp. 254–258.

25. My estimates of annual births to dependent mothers are: minors—145,000; adjudicated child abuse and neglect—40,500; mentally retarded—32,000; incarceration—8,400; termination of parental rights—6,600.

26. a) Appelbaum, P.S. (2007) Assessment of Patients' Competence to Consent to Treatment. *New England Journal of Medicine* 357: 1834–1840; b) Grisso, T. & Appelbaum, P.S. (1998) Assessing Competence to Consent to Treatment. New York: Oxford University Press; c) Grisso, T. & Appelbaum, P.S. (1998) *MacArthur Competence Assessment Tool for Treatment (MacCAT-T)*. Sarasota, FL: Professional Resource Press; d) Ostler, T. (2007) *Assessment of Parenting Competency in Mothers with Mental Illness*. Baltimore, MD: Brookes.

27. National Center for Health Statistics (2008) *2003 Revisions of the U.S. Standard Certificates of Live Birth and Death and the Fetal Death Report*. Hyattsville, MD: U.S. Department Of Health And Human Services, Centers for Disease Control and Prevention.

28. Medical Professionalism in the New Millenium. *Annals of Internal Medicine* 136: 243–246, 2002.

CHAPTER 34. ADOPTION

1. Schooler, J.E. & Norris, B.L. (2002) *Journeys after Adoption*. Westport, CT: Bergin & Garvey, pp. xix – xx.

2. Pertman, A. (2000) *Adoption Nation*. New York: Basic Books.

3. a) Donovan, D.M. (2000) Rethinking Adoption. *Adoption/Medical News* 6: 1–11. Reprinted in Atwood, T.C. (Ed.) *Adoption Factbook IV*. Alexandria, VA: National Council for Adoption; b) Donovan, D.M. (2007) *The Adoption Assumption*. Unpublished manuscript. St. Petersburg, FL: EOCT Institute.

4. Pruett, K.D. (2000) *Fatherneed*. New York: The Free Press, p. 26.

5. Ridely, M. (2003) *Nature Via Nurture*. New York: HarperCollins Publisher, p. 4.

6. a) Donor Sibling Registry, PO Box 1571, Nederland CO 80466; b) Harmon, A. (2005) Sperm Bank Half Siblings Can Connect. *Wisconsin State Journal* November 20, p. A-5.

7. a) Pruett, K.D. (2001) *Fatherneed*. New York: Broadway; b) Wilcox, W.B. (2005) Who's Your Daddy? *The Weekly Standard* December 12.

8. Egan, J. (2006) Wanted: A Few Good Sperm. *New York Times Magazine* March 19, p. 44.

9. a) Nickman, Steven, et al (2005) Children in Adoptive Families. *Journal of the American Academy of Child & Adolescent Psychiatry* 44 (10): 987–995; b) *The Adoption History Project*. <www.adoptionopen.com>; c) Carp, E.W. (Ed.) (2002) *Adoption in America*. Ann Arbor, MI: University of Michigan Press.

10. Fessler, A. (2006) The *Girls Who Went Away*. New York: Penguin Press.

11. a) Shanley, M.L. (2001) *Making Babies, Making Families*. Boston: Beacon Press, p. 41; b) National Adoption Information Clearinghouse (2004) *Access to Family Information by Adopted Persons*. Washington, DC.

12. Bachrach, C.A., et al (1992). Relinquishment of Premarital Births. *Family Planning Perspectives* 24: 27–32, 48.

13. Pecora, P.J., et al (2005) *Improving Family Foster Care*. Seattle, WA: Casey Family Programs.

14. Summary of The Adoption and Safe Families Act of 1997. <http://library.adoption.com>.

15. a) Nickman, S.L., et al (2005) Children in Adoptive Families. *Journal of the American Academy of Child & Adolescent Psychiatry* 44 (10): 987–995; b) Section 1808 of the Personal Responsibility and Work Opportunity Reconciliation Act of 1996; c) Smith, S., et al (2008) *Finding Families for African American Children*. New York: Evan B. Donaldson Adoption Institute.

16. Davenport, D. (2004) African-American Babies Are Going to Parents Overseas. *Christian Science Monitor* October 27.

17. Cahn, N.R. & Hollinger, J. (2004) *Families by Law*. New York: New York University Press, p. 2.

18. a) American Academy of Adoption Attorneys. P.O. Box 33053, Washington, DC 20033; b) Marshner, C. & Pierce, W.L. (Eds.) (1999) *Adoption Fact Book III*. Alexandria, VA: National Council for Adoption; c) Hollinger, J.H.(1993) Adoption Law. *The Future of Children* 3 (1): 43–61.

19. a) National Adoption Information Clearinghouse (2000) *Placing Children for Adoption*. Washington, DC: Departmetn of Health and Human Services; b) Bachrach, C.A., et al (1992) Relinquishment of Premarital Births. *Family Planning Perspectives* 24: 26; c) Mosher, W.D. & Bachrach, C.A. (1996) Understanding U.S. Fertility. *Family Planning Perspectives* 28 (1); d) Moore, K.A., et al (1995) *Adolescent Sex, Contraception, and Childbearing*. Washington, DC: Child Trends, June; e) Stolley, K.S. (1993) Statistics on Adoption in the United States. *The Future of Children* 3 (1): 26–42.

20. Webber, L. (2004) Bush Administration Pushes Grabbing Babies From Poor Women So Wealthy Can Adopt. <http://www.opednews.com>.

21. Solinger, R. (1992) *Wake Up Little Susie*. New York: Routledge.

22. a) Kunzel, R. (1993) *Fallen Women, Problem Girls*. New Haven: Yale University Press; b) Fessler, A. (2006) *The Girls Who Went Away*. New York: The Penguin Press, pp. 142–143, 208.

23. a) Dwyer, J.G. (2003) A Taxonomy of Children's Existing Rights in State Decision Making about Their Relationships. *William & Mary Bill of Rights Journal* 11 (3): 882; b) Hollinger, J.H. (2004) *Families by Law*. New York: New York University Press.

24. Pierce, W.L. (1999) Open Adoption. In Marshner, C. & Pierce, W.L. (Eds.) *Adoption Fact Book III*. Alexandria, VA: National Council for Adoption.

25. Powers, A. (2007) Sharing Rebecca. *Parenting* December/January: 126–130.

26. AAA Partners in Adoption, Inc. 5665 Hwy 9, Suite 103–351 Alpharetta, GA 30004.

27. Berry, M. & Dylla, D.J.C. (1998) The Role of Open Adoption in the Adjustment of Adopted Children and Their Families. *Children and Youth Services Review* 20: 151–171.

28. a) Pertman, A. (2000) *Adoption Nation*. New York: Basic Books, p. 211; b) Schooler, J.E. & Norris, B.L. (2002) *Journeys After Adoption*.Westport, CT: Bergin & Garve, p. 29.

29. Ibid, p.14.

30. a) Winkler, R. & van Keppel, M. (1984) *Relinquishing Mothers in Adoption. (Monograph No. 3)*. Melbourne, Australia: Institute of Family Studies; b) Askren, H.A. & Bloom, K.C. (1999) Postadoptive Reactions of the Relinquishing Mother. *Journal of Obstetric, Gynecological, and Neonatal Nursing* 28 (4): 395–400; c) Winkler, R.C., et al (1988) *Clinical Practice in Adoption*. New York: Pergamon; d) Winkler, R. & van Keppel, M. (1984) *Relinquishing Mothers in Adoption (Monograph No. 3)*. Melbourne, Australia: Institute of Family Studies.

31. Luker, K. (1996) *Dubious Conceptions*. Cambridge, MA: Harvard University Press, p. 164.

32. a) Blum, R.W. & Resnick, M.D. (1982) Adolescent Sexual Decision Making. *Pediatric Annals* 11: 797–805; b) Robinson, E.B. *(2000) Adoption and Loss*. Christies Beach, South Australia: Clova Books.

33. David, H.P., et al (1988) *Born Unwanted*. New York: Springer.

34. Clapton, G. (2001) Birth Fathers' Lives after Adoption. *Adoption & Fostering Abstracts* 25 (4): 50–59.

35. *Stanley v. Illinois*, 405 U.S. 645 (1972); *Quilloin v. Walcott*, 434 U.S. 246 (1978); *Caban v. Mohammed*, 441 U.S. 380 (1979); *Lehr v. Robertson*, 463 U.S. 248 (1983).

36. a) Freundlich, M. (1998) Supply and Demand. *Adoption Quarterly* 2 (1): 13–42; b) Shanley, M.L. (2001) *Making Babies, Making Families*. Boston: Beacon Press, p. 74.

37. National Adoption Information Clearinghouse (2004) *State Statutes Series 2004: The Rights of Presumed (Putative) Fathers*. Washington, DC: Children's Bureau.

38. Brinich, P.M. (1994) Adoption from the Inside Out. In Brodzinsky, D.M. & Schechter, M.D. (Eds) *The Psychology of Adoption*. New York: Oxford University Press, pp. 43–61.

39. Ibid, pp. 43–61.

40. a) Gateways to Information (2004) *Searching for Birth Relatives*. Washington, DC: National Adoption Information Clearinghouse; b) Muller, U. & Perry, B. (2001) Adopted Persons' Search for and Contact with their Birth Parents I. *Adoption Quarterly* 4: 5–37, 39–62; c) Bastard Nation, P.O. Box 1469, Edmond, OK 73083–1469; d) Clapton, Gary (2001) Birth Fathers' Lives After Adoption. *Adoption & Fostering Abstracts* 25: 50–59; e) OmniTrace Corporation, 23123 State Rd. #7, Boca Raton, FL 33428.

41. a) Schooler, J.E. & Norris, B.L. (2002) *Journeys After Adoption*. Westport, CT: Bergin & Garvey, p. 172; b) Boisvert, B., et al (2002) Who Am I? *Focal Point* Spring 16 (1): 25–27.

42. Brinich, P.M. (1994) Adoption from the Inside Out. In Brodzinsky, D.M. & Schechter, M.D. (Eds) *The Psychology of Adoption*. New York: Oxford University Press, pp. 43–61.

43. a) Kaye, K. (1994) Acknowledgement or Rejection of Differences? In Brodzinsky, D.M. & Schechter, M.D. (Eds.) *The Psychology of Adoption*. New York: Oxford Press, pp. 121–143; b) Donovan, Denis. In preparation.

44. a) Hawkins-Leon, C.G. (1998) The Indian Child Welfare Act and the African American Tribe. *Brandeis Journal of Family Law* 36: 201–218; b) McKelvey, C. & Stevens, J. (1994) *Adoption Crisis*. Golden, CO: Fulcrum, p. 147.

45. Simon, R.J., et al (1994) *The Case for Transracial Adoption*. Washington, DC: The American University Press.

46. a) Ibid, p. 1; b) Mabry, C.R. (1996) Love Alone Is Not Enough! *Wayne Law Review* 42: 1347–1394.

47. a) Inter-Ethnic Adoption Act: IEAA. P.L. 103–382 [42 USC 622]; b) Hawkins-Leon, C. & Bradley, C. (2002) Race and Transracial Adoption. *Catholic University Law Review 51*: 1227–1286.

48. Fogg-Davis, H. (2002) *The Ethics of Transracial Adoption*. Ithaca, New York, p. 12.

49. a) Hawkins-Leon, C. & Bradley, C. (2002) Race and Transracial Adoption. *Catholic University Law Review* 51: 1227–1286; b) Hollinger, J.H. (1998) A Guide to the Multiethnic Placement Act of 1994 as Amended in 1996. Washington, DC: National Resource Center on Legal and Court Issues; c) Maple, J. (2002) Adoption of Adolescents. New York, NY: National Resource Center for Foster Care & Permanency Planning, Hunter College School of Social Work; d) Campbell, S.B. (2000) Taking Race Out of the Equation. *Southern Methodist University Law Review* 53: 1599; e) Shanley, M.L. (2001) *Making Babies, Making Families*. Boston: Beacon Press, p. 4.

50. Simon, R.J., et al (1994) *The Case for Transracial Adoption*. Washington, DC: The American University Press.

51. Mabry, C. R. (1996) Love Alone Is Not Enough! *Wayne Law Review* 42: 1347–1394.

52. Simon, R.J. (1994) *The Case for Transracial Adoption*. Washington, DC: American University Press, p. 248.

53. Ibid, pp. 39–40.

54. a) Roberts, D. (2002) *Shattered Bonds*. New York: Basic Civitas Books, p. 253; b) Simon, R.J., et al (1994) *The Case for Transracial Adoption*. Washington, DC: American University Press, p. 171; c) Bartholet, E. (1991) Where Do Black Children Belong? *University of Pennsylvania Law Review* 139: 1163.

55. a) Herzog, E., et al (1971) Some Opinions on Finding Homes for Black Children. *Children* 18: 143–48. b) Howard, A., et al (1977) Transracial Adoption. *Social Work* 22: 184–89; b) Whatley, M., et al (2003) College Student Attitudes toward Transracial Adoption. *College Student Journal* 37: September.

56. a) Steinberg, G. & Hall, B. (2000) *Inside Transracial Adoption*. Indianapolis, IN: Perspectives Press; b) Silverman, A.R. (1993) Outcomes of Transracial Adoption. *The Future of Children* 3 (1): 104–118; c) Sharma, A.R., et al (1996). The Emotional and Behavioral Adjustment of United States Adopted Adolescents: Part 1. *Children & Youth Services Review* 18: 83–100.

57. a) Payne, R.J. (1998) *Getting Beyond Race*. Boulder, CO: Westview Press; b) Bagley, C., et al (1993) *International and Transracial Adoptions*. Brookfield, VT: Ashgate Publishing Company.

58. Fogg-Davis, H. (2002) *The Ethics of Transracial Adoption*. Ithaca, New York, p. 15.

59. Steinberg, G. & Hall, B. (2000) *Inside Transracial Adoption*. Indianapolis, IN: Perspectives Press, p. 31.

60. Patton, S. (2000) *Birthmarks*. New York: New York University Press, p. 98.

61. Wall, T. (2000) *Transcending Ideals about Trans-Racial Adoptions*. Washington, DC: The National Center for Public Policy Research.

62. Crumbley, J. (1999) *Transracial Adoption and Foster Care*. Washington, DC: CWLA Press, p. 15, 7–8.

63. a) Patton, S. (2000) *Birthmarks*. New York: New York University Press, p. 189; b) Vonk, M.E. (2001) Cultural Competence for Transracial Adoptive Parents. *Social Work* 46 (3): 246–255; c) Crumbley, J. (1999) *Transracial Adoption and Foster Care*. Washington, DC: CWLA Press, p. 9; d) Kirton, D., et al (2000) Searching, Reunion, and Transracial Adoption. *Adoption & Fostering Abstracts* 24 (3): 6–18.

64. Steinberg, G. & Hall, B. (2000) *Inside Transracial Adoption*. Indianapolis, IN: Perspectives Pres, p. 382.

65. a) Crumbley, J. (1999) *Transracial Adoption and Foster Care*. Washington, DC: CWLA Press, pp. 94–95; b) McKelvey, C. & Stevens, J. (1994) *Adoption Crisis*. Golden, CO: Fulcrum Publishers, p. 147.

66. NABSW Task Force on Foster Care and Adoption, Toni Oliver, Co-Chair. *Preserving Families of African Ancestry*. Washington, DC: National Association of Black Social Workers, Inc.

67. a) Gilles, T. & Kroll, J. (1991) *Barriers to Same Race Placement*. St. Paul, MN: North American Council on Adoptable Children; b) Crumbley, J. (1999) *Transracial Adoption and Foster Care*. Washington, DC: CWLA Press, p. 96; c) Davenport, Dawn (2004) African-American Babies Are Going to Parents Overseas. *Christian Science Monitor* October 27; d) One Church, One Child of Florida, Tallahassee, FL 32399, <http://www.ococfl.org>; e) Homes for Black Children, 511 E. Larned Street, Detroit, Michigan 48226, (313) 961–4777; f) Another Choice for Black Children, Charlotte, NC 28216; g) Rejoice, Inc., Harrisburg, Pennsylvania 17103; h) Roots Adoption Agency, Atlanta, GA 30349; i) North American Council on Adoptable Children, St. Paul, MN 55114.

68. Adoption-Link, 1113 South Boulevard, Oak Park, IL 60302.

69. 417 U.S. 535 (1974).

70. Metteer, C. (1996) Pigs in Heaven. *Arizona State Law Journal* 28: 589, 596.

71. a) Hawkins-Leon, C.G. (1998) The Indian Child Welfare Act and the African American Tribe. *Brandeis Journal of Family Law* 36: 201–218; b) Title 25: Chapter 21 § 1901, § 1915. Congressional Fndings 2005–08–18.

72. a) *In re* Adoption of D.M.J., 741 P.2d 1386, 1389 (Okla. 1985); b) *In re* Adoption of a Child of Indian Heritage, 543 A. 2d 925, 933–38 (N.J. 1988).

73. Bohman, M. & Sigvardsson, S. (1994) Outcome in Adoption Lessons from Longitudinal Studies. In Brodzinsky, D.M. & Schechter, M.D. (Eds) *The Psychology of Adoption*. New York: Oxford University Press, pp. 93–106.

74. a) Hamilton, Laura, et al (2007) Adoptive Parents, Adaptive Parents. *American Sociological Review* 72:95–116; b) Brodzinsky, D.M. (1993) Long-Term Outcomes in Adoption. *The Future of Children* 3 (1): 153–166.

75. a) Brooks, D. & Barth, R. (1999) Adult Transracial and Inracial Adoptees. *American Journal of Orthopsychiatry* 69: 87–99; b) Ingersoll, B.D. (1997) Psychiatric Disorders among Adopted Children. *Adoption Quarterly* 1: 57–73.

76. Duyme, M, (1999) How Can We Boost IQs of "Dull Children"? *Proceedings of the National Academy of Science* 96: 8790–8794.

77. a) Rushton, A. & Dance, C. (2006) The Adoption of Children from Public Care. *Journal of the Academy of Child and Adolescent Psychiatry* 45 (7): 877–883; b) Rosenthal, J.A. (1993) Outcomes of Adoption of Children with Special Needs. *The Future of Children* 3 (1).

78. Wilson, S.L. (2004) A Current Review of Adoption Research. *Children & Youth Services Review* 26: 687–696.

79. Rosenthal, J.A. (1993) Outcomes of Adoption of Children with Special Needs. *The Future of Children* 3 (1).

80. Bohman, M. & Sigvardsson, S. (1994) Outcomes in Adoption. In Brodzinsky, D.M. & Schechter, M.D. (Eds.) *The Psychology of Adoption.* New York: Oxford University Press, pp. 93–106.

81. Juffer, F. & van Ijzendoorn, M.H. (2005) Behavior Problems and Mental Health Referrals of International Adoptees. *Journal of the American Medical Association* 293: 2501–2515.

82. Reilly, T. & Platz, L. (2004) Post-Adoption Service Needs of Families with Special Needs Children. *Journal of Social Service Research* 30 (4): 51–67.

83. a) Silverman, A.R. (1993) The Outcomes of Transracial Adoption. *Future of Children* 3 (1); b) Patel, Tina, et al (2004) Identity, Race, Religion, and Adoption. *Adoption and Fostering Abstracts* 28: 6–15.

84. Shireman, J.F. & Johnson, P.R. (1986) A Longitudinal Study of Black Adoptions. *Social Work* 62: 172.

85. Simon, R. & Altstein, H. (2002) *Adoption, Race, and Identity, Second Edition.* Somerset, NJ: Transaction Pub.

86. a) Sharma, A.R., et al (1996) The Emotional And Behavioral Adjustment of United States Adopted Adolescents: Part 1. *Children and Youth Services Review* 18: 83–100; b) Barth, R.P. & Brooks, D. (1997) A Longitudinal Study of Family Structure, Family Size, and Adoption Outcomes. *Adoption Quarterly* 1: 29–56.

87. Silverman, A.R. (1993) The Outcomes of Transracial Adoption. *Future of Children* 3 (1).

88. Hrdy, S.B. (2001) *The Past, Present, and Future of the Human Family.* Tanner Lectures on Human Values. Salt Lake City, UT: University of Utah, February 27 and 28.

89. The Gloria M. Silverio Foundation. A Safe Haven for Newborns. 6801 N.W. 77th. Ave., Miami, FL 33166.

90. Shanley, M.L. (2001) *Making Babies, Making Families.* Boston: Beacon Press.

91. Hsu, M., et al (2005) Neural Systems Responding to Degrees of Uncertainty in Human Decision-Making. *Science* 310: 1680–1683.

92. Brown, B.B., et al (2002) *The World's Youth.* New York: Cambridge University Press, p. 43.

93. Donovan, D.M. (1998–2002) *The Choice Model.* St. Petersburg, FL: Center for Developmental Psychiatry.

94. AAA Partners in Adoption, Inc. 5665 Hwy 9, Suite 103–351 Alpharetta, GA 30004.

95. Baran, A. & Pannor, R. (2000) Perspectives on Open Adoption. In Cahn, N.R. & Hollinger, J.H. (Eds.) *Families by Law.* New York: New York University Press, p. 166.

96. Hollinger, J.H. (2004) State and Federal Adoption Laws. In Cahn, N. R. & Hollinger, J.H. (Eds.), op cit, p. 39.

PART 10. CONCLUSION

1. Grubb, W.N. & Lazerson, M. (1982) *Broken Promises.* New York: Basic Books, pp. 5, 269.

2. Maynard, R.A. (1997) The Role for Paternalism in Teen Pregnancy Prevention and Teen Parent Services. *In the New Paternalism.* Washington. DC: The Brookings Institute, pp. 89–129.

3. Christensen, C.M. (1997) *The Innovators Dilemma.* Boston: Harvard Business School Press.

Index